Clinical Biomarkers of Neurological Disorders

Clinical Biomarkers of Neurological Disorders

Editor: Abbie Bardsley

FOSTER ACADEMICS
www.fosteracademics.com

www.fosteracademics.com

FOSTER ACADEMICS

Cataloging-in-Publication Data

Clinical biomarkers of neurological disorders / edited by Abbie Bardsley.
p. cm.
Includes bibliographical references and index.
ISBN 978-1-64646-612-2
1. Nervous system--Diseases. 2. Brain--Diseases. 3. Biochemical markers.
4. Neurology. I. Bardsley, Abbie.
RC346 .C55 2023
616.8--dc23

Foster Academics,
118-35 Queens Blvd., Suite 400,
Forest Hills, NY 11375, USA

ISBN 978-1-64646-612-2 (Hardback)

Contents

Preface

This book has been a concerted effort by a group of academicians, researchers and scientists, who have contributed their research works for the realization of the book. This book has materialized in the wake of emerging advancements and innovations in this field. Therefore, the need of the hour was to compile all the required researches and disseminate the knowledge to a broad spectrum of people comprising of students, researchers and specialists of the field.

A neurological disorder refers to any disorder of the nervous system. A variety of symptoms can occur during these disorders due to biochemical, structural or electrical abnormalities in the spinal cord, brain or other nerves. Biomarkers offer a dynamic and powerful approach for gaining a better knowledge of a range of neurological disorders. They are also used in prognosis, screening, observational and analytic epidemiology, diagnosis, and randomized clinical trials. These markers are defined as changes in the constituents of body fluids or tissues, which provide a way to classify diseases and risk factors uniformly. They can help in learning more about the underlying pathogenesis of a disease. Biomarkers can also reflect the entire disease spectrum from the earliest manifestations to the final stages. The validity of biomarkers must be carefully evaluated in relation to the stage of disease. This book aims to shed light on the clinical biomarkers of neurological disorders. Those in search of information to further their knowledge will be greatly assisted by this book.

At the end of the preface, I would like to thank the authors for their brilliant chapters and the publisher for guiding us all-through the making of the book till its final stage. Also, I would like to thank my family for providing the support and encouragement throughout my academic career and research projects.

Editor

1

Understanding the Physiopathology Behind Axial and Radial Diffusivity Changes—What do we Know?

Pawel J. Winklewski[1,2,3], Agnieszka Sabisz[3], Patrycja Naumczyk[4], Krzysztof Jodzio[4], Edyta Szurowska[3] and Arkadiusz Szarmach[3]*

[1] Department of Human Physiology, Medical University of Gdan´sk, Gdan´sk, Poland, [2] Department of Clinical Anatomy and Physiology, Pomeranian University in Słupsk, Słupsk, Poland, [3] 2-nd Department of Radiology, Medical University of Gdan´sk, Gdan´sk, Poland, [4] Institute of Psychology, University of Gdan´sk, Gdan´sk, Poland

***Correspondence:**
Pawel J. Winklewski
pawelwinklewski@wp.pl

The use of the diffusion tensor imaging (DTI) is rapidly growing in the neuroimaging field. Nevertheless, rigorously performed quantitative validation of DTI pathologic metrics remains very limited owing to the difficulty in co-registering quantitative histology findings with magnetic resonance imaging. The aim of this review is to summarize the existing state-of-the-art knowledge with respect to axial ($\lambda_{\parallel}$) and radial ($\lambda_{\perp}$) diffusivity as DTI markers of axonal and myelin damage, respectively. First, we provide technical background for DTI and briefly discuss the specific organization of white matter in bundles of axonal fibers running in parallel; this is the natural target for imaging based on diffusion anisotropy. Second, we discuss the four seminal studies that paved the way for considering axial ($\lambda_{\parallel}$) and radial ($\lambda_{\perp}$) diffusivity as potential *in vivo* surrogate markers of axonal and myelin damage, respectively. Then, we present difficulties in interpreting axial ($\lambda_{\parallel}$) and radial ($\lambda_{\perp}$) diffusivity in clinical conditions associated with inflammation, edema, and white matter fiber crossing. Finally, future directions are highlighted. In summary, DTI can reveal strategic information with respect to white matter tracts, disconnection mechanisms, and related symptoms. Axial ($\lambda_{\parallel}$) and radial ($\lambda_{\perp}$) diffusivity seem to provide quite consistent information in healthy subjects, and in pathological conditions with limited edema and inflammatory changes. DTI remains one of the most promising non-invasive diagnostic tools in medicine.

Keywords: diffusion tensor imaging, axial diffusivity, radial diffusivity, myelin dysfunction, axonal injury

INTRODUCTION

The number of studies using diffusion tensor imaging (DTI) has grown exponentially. A search for the term "diffusion tensor imaging" yields 13,841 records in PubMed. This is not surprising as DTI represent a highly promising method for characterizing microstructural evolution in neuropathology and treatment (1).

For instance, DTI allows developmental changes in the prefrontal cortex to be tracked. It is believed that brain maturation is associated with augmented myelination, organization, and integrity of frontal white matter; this is confirmed by DTI indices, such as fractional anisotropy, mean diffusivity, radial diffusivity ($\lambda_{\perp}$), and axial diffusivity ($\lambda_{\parallel}$). Therefore, DTI provides a tool to highlight patterns associated with the developmental time course of the frontal structural integrity, which correlates with the improvements in higher level cognitive functions taking place between adolescence and early adulthood (2). Interestingly, DTI studies reveal some consistent patterns in subjects exhibiting antisocial behavior. In particular, adult antisocial behavior was shown to be associated with greater diffusivity within several white matter tracts, including the inferior fronto-occipital fasciculus, uncinate fasciculus, cingulum, thalamic radiations, corticospinal tract, and corpus callosum (3).

At the same time, a clinical meta-analysis in subjects with mild-traumatic brain injury produced conflicting results. This large review, consisting of 86 studies, concluded that "DTI is sensitive to a wide range of group differences in diffusion metrics, but currently lacks the specificity necessary for meaningful clinical application" (4). There is a clear lack of consensus among the experts about the use of DTI indices in a specific region of the brain as biomarkers for post-concussion syndrome, because no consistent trends for DTI variables in these subjects have been defined (5). On the contrary, in subjects suffering from cerebral small vessel disease, associations between DTI parameters and cognition have been confirmed in a multicenter study (6).

When reviewing the DTI studies it is quite striking that rigorous quantitative validation of DTI pathologic metrics remains very limited, most likely due to the difficulty in co-registering quantitative histopathology data with magnetic resonance imaging (MRI). It seems obvious that heterogenic pathologies within the brain white matter, including changes, such as brain edema and the inflammatory response, can potentially affect the consistency of DTI metrics. The aim of this review is to summarize the existing state-of-the-art knowledge with respect to axial ($\lambda_{\parallel}$) and radial ($\lambda_{\perp}$) diffusivity as DTI markers of axonal and myelin damage, respectively.

TECHNICAL CONSIDERATIONS

The principles of diffusion-weighted MRI were first described in the mid-1980s (7–9); they were based on the concept of MRI imaging combined with bipolar magnetic field gradient pulses that were introduced earlier to encode molecular diffusion effects on the spin-echo experiment (10). In ideal conditions, diffusion can be considered a truly three-dimensional process. However, in biological materials like tissues, molecular mobility may be constrained or facilitated in particular directions. Such anisotropy results from the presence of obstacles that influence molecular movement. The MRI signal is generated from water molecules by combining radiofrequency pulses with magnetic field gradients. Importantly, only molecular movements occurring within the direction of the gradient pulses are encoded in MRI generated signal. Consequently, the effect of diffusion anisotropy is easily measured by alternating the direction of the gradient pulses and observing variations in diffusivity parameters in the three planes. This feature makes diffusion-weighted MRI unique and distinguishes it from routine T1 or T2 weighted images (11).

Optimization of MRI sequences and fine tuning of the processing and display of recorded MRI signals allows for the full extraction of diffusion anisotropy effects, and thus, provides details on tissue microstructure. This more rigorous and elaborated diffusion-weighted MRI technique is named DTI (12, 13). The DTI matrix is obtained from a series of diffusion-weighted images in various gradient directions. The three diffusivity parameters (λ_1, λ_2, and λ_3), are generated by matrix diagonalization. Diffusivities are scalar indices describing water diffusion in a specific voxels (the smallest volumetric elements in the image) associated with the geometry of white matter tracts (14, 15). The diffusivities (λ_1, λ_2, and λ_3) obtained by DTI matrix diagonalization can be delimitated into parallel (λ_1) and perpendicular (λ_2 and λ_3) components to the axonal tract (16–18). Axial diffusivity, $\lambda_{\parallel} \equiv \lambda_1 > \lambda_2, \lambda_3$, describes the mean diffusion coefficient of water molecules diffusing parallel to the tract within the voxel of interest. Similarly, radial diffusivity, $\lambda_{\perp} \equiv (\lambda_2 + \lambda_3)/2$, can be defined as the magnitude of water diffusion perpendicular to the tract (19, 20). Fractional anisotropy in brain measures the total magnitude of water directional movement along the axonal fibers (16), while mean diffusivity is a measure of mean diffusion of each direction. Therefore, fractional anisotropy may be enhanced in situations of facilitated parallel diffusivity, restricted perpendicular diffusivity, or as a result of combination of both factors (21).

White matter in the brain, organized in bundles of axonal fibers running in parallel, is the natural target for imaging based on diffusion anisotropy. In principle, diffusion along the fibers should be faster than in the perpendicular direction. Based on the assumption that the direction of the fastest diffusion indicates the overall orientation of the fibers, color-coded maps of white matter tracts in the brain are created [**Figure 1** (22)]. A non-invasive method to objectively quantify white matter abnormalities greatly support studies aiming at clarification of mechanisms of damage, matching pathology with neurologic function, and assessing therapeutic interventions.

EARLY EXPERIMENTAL STUDIES

White matter impairment leading to neurological disorders can be categorized according to myelin abnormality (demyelination), axonal injury, or a combination of both (23, 24). There are several animal experimental models that allow for at least partial differentiation of these processes. One such model, congenitally dysmyelinated Shiverer mutant mice, was used by Song et al. (19) in his first study on radial ($\lambda_{\perp}$) and axial ($\lambda_{\parallel}$) diffusivity. Radial diffusivity ($\lambda_{\perp}$) was significantly increased, while axial diffusivity ($\lambda_{\parallel}$) was not altered in congenitally dysmyelinated shiverer

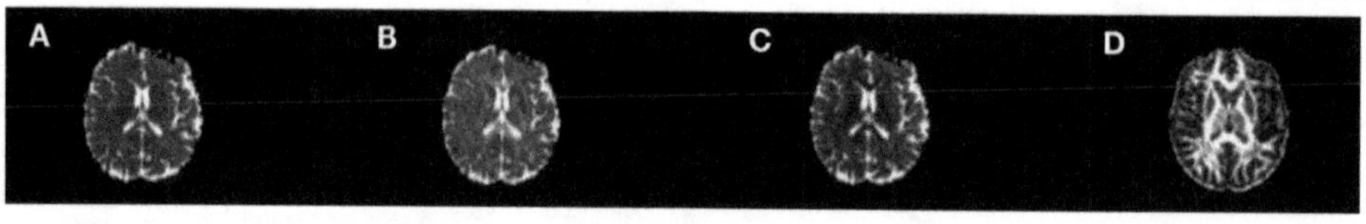

FIGURE 1 | Example of maps computed from diffusion tensor imaging of the brain: **(A)** mean diffusivity, **(B)** axial diffusivity ($\lambda_{\parallel}$), **(C)** radial diffusivity ($\lambda_{\perp}$), and **(D)** fractional anisotropy.

mutant mice, as compared to wild-type mice (19), suggesting that radial diffusivity ($\lambda_\perp$) may represent a potential non-invasive marker of myelin disintegration.

In a second study, Song et al. (20) used a mouse model of retinal ischemia. This model is characterized by acute inner retinal degeneration (25, 26) with initial axonal degeneration in the optic nerve, and secondary myelin fragmentation following retinal degeneration (27). Song et al. (20) observed distinct evolution patterns of axial ($\lambda_\parallel$) and radial ($\lambda_\perp$) diffusivity during the progression of optic nerve degeneration. Axial diffusivity ($\lambda_\parallel$) diminished in the injured optic nerve by day 3 following ischemia, while change in radial diffusivity ($\lambda_\perp$) between the injured optic nerves and control nerves was not detected until day 5. Radial diffusivity ($\lambda_\perp$) reached its minimal value on day 5, and remained on this level on day 7 after ischemia. Importantly, this longitudinal DTI examination of the optic nerve was positively linked with neurofilament and myelin basic protein immunostaining (28) results at day 3 (axonal degeneration) and 7 (myelin fragmentation) after the injury.

The notion that demyelination might be associated with a marked increase in radial diffusivity ($\lambda_\perp$), and modest often insignificant changes in axial diffusivity ($\lambda_\parallel$), was further reinforced by the third seminal study of Song et al. (29). In this study, the cuprizone model, which is characterized by consistent demyelination of the corpus callosum in mouse brains, was used. Demyelination after several weeks of diet, including cuprizone (neurotoxicant that chelates copper) is extensive, yet can be reversed if the mice are back to normal chow (30–32). The axonal's damage time course was clearly different from the radial diffusivity time course, demonstrating that radial diffusivity ($\lambda_\perp$) recognizes demyelination as distinct from axonal damage. However, although changes in axial diffusivity measured at the initial stage of cuprizone administration suggested acute axonal damage in white matter, the diminished axial diffusivity ($\lambda_\parallel$) did not reach statistical significance (29). The uncertainty about the potential of axial diffusivity ($\lambda_\parallel$) as a marker of axon damage was further clarified in the study by Sun et al. (33), from the same group using the same cuprizone mouse model. Biweekly *in vivo* DTI examinations showed a transient decrease in axial diffusivity ($\lambda_\parallel$) in the corpus callosum after 2–6 weeks of cuprizone administration, while immunostaining for non-phosphorylated neurofilaments demonstrated corresponding axonal damage after 4 weeks of treatment.

In summary, in four seminal studies, Song and colleagues demonstrated that axial ($\lambda_\parallel$) and radial ($\lambda_\perp$) diffusivity may be useful *in vivo* surrogate markers of axonal and myelin damage, respectively, in selected mouse experimental models of white matter abnormalities.

CRITIQUE OF THE METHOD

Interestingly, when a synthetic model of crossing fibers is used, the three diffusivities (λ_1, λ_2, and λ_3) may not detect the same underlying structural characteristics in particular datasets, because orientation of the related principal eigenvector (a characteristic vector whose direction does not change in the linear transformation and has got the largest magnitude) may differ (34). According to these authors, axial ($\lambda_\parallel$) and radial ($\lambda_\perp$) diffusivities, i.e., the water diffusion coefficient parallel and perpendicular to the axons, may provide an acceptable approximation if the voxel includes a healthy fiber bundle determining the diffusion characteristic of the voxel. However, if the signal-to-noise ratio is low, if crossing fibers are present, or if pathology causes a decrease in anisotropy, such an approach can lead to misinterpretation of the results (35). This is an important statement as the latter situation occurs within brain lesions, characteristic, for instance, of multiple sclerosis (36).

Inflammation, often present in diseases associated with white matter impairment, poses another difficulty for the interpretation of DTI signals (37). In a cuprizone experimental mouse model, it has been shown that axial diffusivity ($\lambda_\parallel$) values were diminished in the beginning of demyelination process in corpus callosum regions characterized by nonuniform axonal edema, beads, varicosities parallel to the axon segments, and microglia/macrophage activation. In the same animals, axial diffusivity ($\lambda_\parallel$) was not decreased during prolonged demyelination, in which axonal atrophy was evident. The radial diffusivity ($\lambda_\perp$) values generally were enhanced in chronically demyelinated corpus callosum voxels, but in regions with extensive axonal edema and prominent inflammatory cell presence, radial diffusivity ($\lambda_\perp$) did not change, likely because of reduced intra-axonal water diffusivity following injury and/or the enhanced restriction related to the presence of infiltrating cells (38).

A combination of oligodendrocyte apoptosis and the development of vasogenic edema could also result in enhanced diffusivity across the axons, leading to discrepancies between radial diffusivity ($\lambda_\perp$) and the histological picture (39). Thus, DTI-derived radial diffusivity ($\lambda_\perp$) may not be specific to myelin integrity and may actually reflect both myelin integrity and extra-axonal water content (40–42). Finally, cerebrospinal fluid contamination represents another challenge. Cheng et al. (43) proposed a combination of the DTI technique and a FLAIR $b = 0$ image to suppress cerebrospinal fluid partial volume effects and improve white matter fiber tractography.

Summing up, experimental studies from different pathogenic events: acute injury (ischemia, trauma), short term/progressive injury (cuprizone model), and congenial and long-term chronic injury (Shivered mice) are part of different cellular responses which can result in different DTI scalars anomalies (**Table 1**). In addition, some of the acute processes (trauma), include complex acute multicellular processes (inflammation) and chronic processes (scarring) which could radically change the white matter matrix structure and temporal course of the DTI parameters. Moreover, trophic iteration between neuronal and glial cell populations in the nervous tissue should be taken into consideration. The pathological changes occurring in one population may defectively alter another cell group and affect axial ($\lambda_\parallel$) and radial ($\lambda_\perp$) diffusivity.

CLINICAL ASPECTS OF AXIAL AND RADIAL DIFFUSIVITY

Pathophysiological changes in multiple sclerosis encompass the dynamic evolution of inflammation, axonal injury, and myelin

TABLE 1 | Summary of findings from specific experimental reports cited in the review.

Experimental model/disease	Axial diffusivity ($\lambda_{\|}$)	Radial diffusivity ($\lambda_{\perp}$)	Histopathological correlation	Reference
Congenitally demyelinated Shiverer mutant mice	Not changed	Increased	Yes, for axial (no axon damage—no $\lambda_{\|}$ change) and radial (demyelination) diffusivity	(19)
Mouse model of retinal ischemia	Decreased by day 3 after ischemia	Decreased on day 5 and present on day 7 after ischemia	Yes, at day 3 (axonal degeneration) and 7 (myelin fragmentation) after the injury	(20)
Mouse cuprizone model of experimental demyelination and myelination of corpus callosum	Tendency to decrease, but not reached statistical significance	Increased	Yes, for radial diffusivity (demyelination), only tendency for axial diffusivity (axon damage)	(29)
Mouse cuprizone model of experimental demyelination and myelination of corpus callosum	Decreased	Increased	Yes, for both axial (axon damage) and radial (demyelination)	(33)
Mathematical modeling			No, if the signal-to-noise ratio is low, if crossing fibers are present, or if pathology causes a decrease in anisotropy	(34, 35)
Rat model of liposaccharide injection into the corpus callosum		Increased	No, radial diffusivity increase due to vasogenic edema	(37)
Mouse cuprizone model of experimental demyelination and myelination of corpus callosum	Decreased	Increased	No, axial diffusivity did not correlate with axonal atrophy; did not correlate with myelin loss or astrogliosis	(38)
Mouse model of acute spinal cord injury	Increased	Increased	Good correlation in the epicenter and remotely to the changes, axial and radial diffusivity impacted by vasogenic edema	(39)
Mathematical modeling			Cellularity decrease axon diffusivity, have a limited impact on radial diffusivity; vasogenic edema increases radial diffusivity	(42)

loss, which creates a particularly challenging situation for imaging with axial ($\lambda_{\|}$) and radial ($\lambda_{\perp}$) diffusivity. The timing of inflammation relative to tissue injury is not always known. In addition to the temporal aspect, the pathology in multiple sclerosis is also complex and variable, with axon and myelin injury strongly interlinked. Nevertheless, Oh et al. (44, 45) demonstrated that fractional anisotropy, mean diffusivity, and radial diffusivity ($\lambda_{\perp}$) could efficiently discriminate multiple sclerosis patients with high and low disability levels. Fractional anisotropy was diminished, mean diffusivity increased, and radial diffusivity ($\lambda_{\perp}$) enhanced in subjects with high disability, as compared with low disability, demonstrating good reproducibility.

Kronlage et al. (46) demonstrated that fractional anisotropy and radial diffusivity ($\lambda_{\perp}$) correlated strongly with electrophysiological markers of demyelination, whereas axial diffusivity ($\lambda_{\|}$) did not correlate with markers of axonal neuropathy in subjects with chronic inflammatory demyelinating polyneuropathy. In another study, axial diffusivity ($\lambda_{\|}$) and fractional anisotropy showed a significant correlation with axonal integrity, whereas radial diffusivity ($\lambda_{\perp}$) was related to myelin compactness in an animal model of closed head traumatic brain injury (47). In this study, fractional anisotropy was sensitive to astrogliosis in the gray matter, whereas mean diffusivity was associated with augmented cellularity.

Interestingly, Naismith et al. (48) demonstrated that in remote optic neuritis (commonly one of the first manifestations of multiple sclerosis), radial diffusivity ($\lambda_{\perp}$) may discriminate visual outcomes. White matter tracts consisting of parallel axons tightly packed with myelin are anisotropic, or directional, to the diffusion of water. Chronic injury associated with demyelination and axons loss leads to reduced anisotropy. As a consequence diffusion perpendicular to the white matter tract (analogous to $\lambda_{\perp}$) augments, overall diffusivity (mean diffusivity) increases, and tissue directionality diminishes. At the same time, within the human central nervous system, pathologic changes from the acute to the chronic stage result in axial diffusivity ($\lambda_{\|}$) becoming less informative over time. As myelin debris is cleared, inflammation and edema diminish, demyelinated axons are less tightly packed, and the widening interstitial space dilutes the ability of DTI to detect and measure anisotropic diffusion ($\lambda_{\|}$) within axons. Thus, the correlation between axial diffusivity and visual outcomes in subjects with remote optic neuritis was very modest (48).

To summarize, in cases of axon and myelin injury associated with inflammation and increased cellularity, DTI tends to underestimate the extent of demyelination, while at the same time, may exaggerate the extent of the axonal injury. The final outcome is undervalued radial diffusivity ($\lambda_{\perp}$) and overvalued axial diffusivity ($\lambda_{\|}$). In turn, in chronic diseases associated with intensive axonal loss, the increased isotropic diffusion seems to enhance both radial ($\lambda_{\perp}$) and axial diffusivity ($\lambda_{\|}$). Consequently, DTI can no longer provide sufficient reliability in terms of underlying pathologies when inflammation, axonal loss, axonal injury, and demyelination coexist.

FUTURE PROSPECTS

Song and colleagues have proposed a new methodology called diffusion basis spectrum imaging (DBSI) to address the DTI inaccuracies with respect to radial ($\lambda_\perp$) and axial diffusivity ($\lambda_\parallel$). Phantom tests and *in vivo* experiments using cuprizone-treated mice suggest that DBSI might be capable of quantifying the extent of augmented cellularity and vasogenic edema, constituting a reliable marker of inflammation. Moreover, DBSI seems to improve the quantification of axial ($\lambda_\parallel$) and radial ($\lambda_\perp$) diffusivity, which distinguishes and reflects axonal versus myelin injury (40).

The DBSI model proposed by the Song research group has been validated in several animal and human studies, as reviewed by Cross and Song (49). The possible limitation of the reviewed research describing the interdependencies between axial ($\lambda_\parallel$) versus radial ($\lambda_\perp$) diffusivity, and axonal versus myelin injury (respectively), is that most of the discussed studies originated from one site. In particular, replication of DBSI-derived data is yet to be published. Animal models of neurodegenerative diseases featuring fluorescently labeled axons (50) represent another option to correlate axonal pathology to specific alterations in axial and radial diffusivities. Further development of DTI technology, including DBSI and other concepts (such as specific animal models), may enormously advance our understanding of underlying pathologies in several central nervous disorders.

Diffusion tensor imaging can reveal strategic information with respect to white matter tracts, disconnection mechanisms, and related symptoms. Axial ($\lambda_\parallel$) and radial ($\lambda_\perp$) diffusivity seem to provide quite consistent information in healthy subjects, and in pathological conditions with limited edema and inflammatory changes. DTI remains one of the most promising non-invasive diagnostic tools in medicine.

AUTHOR CONTRIBUTIONS

PW and AS drafted and wrote the manuscript. PN, KJ, ES, and AS commented and revised the manuscript. All authors have read and approved the final version of the manuscript.

ACKNOWLEDGMENTS

We would like to thank Agata Majewska for the excellent technical support, including preparation of figures.

FUNDING

AS and PW are supported by the Polish National Science Centre (NCN) grant numbers 2017/01/X/NZ5/00909 and 2017/01/X/NZ4/00779, respectively.

REFERENCES

1. Alexander AL, Lee JE, Lazar M, Field AS. Diffusion tensor imaging of the brain. *Neurotherapeutics* (2007) 4:316–29. doi:10.1016/j.nurt.2007.05.011
2. Sousa SS, Amaro E Jr, Crego A, Gonçalves ÓF, Sampaio A. Developmental trajectory of the prefrontal cortex: a systematic review of diffusion tensor imaging studies. *Brain Imaging Behav* (2017). doi:10.1007/s11682-017-9761-4
3. Waller R, Dotterer HL, Murray L, Maxwell AM, Hyde LW. White-matter tract abnormalities and antisocial behavior: a systematic review of diffusion tensor imaging studies across development. *Neuroimage Clin* (2017) 14:201–15. doi:10.1016/j.nicl.2017.01.014
4. Asken BM, DeKosky ST, Clugston JR, Jaffee MS, Bauer RM. Diffusion tensor imaging (DTI) findings in adult civilian, military, and sport-related mild traumatic brain injury (mTBI): a systematic critical review. *Brain Imaging Behav* (2017). doi:10.1007/s11682-017-9708-9
5. Khong E, Odenwald N, Hashim E, Cusimano MD. Diffusion tensor imaging findings in post-concussion syndrome patients after mild traumatic brain injury: a systematic review. *Front Neurol* (2016) 7:156. doi:10.3389/fneur.2016.00156
6. Croall ID, Lohner V, Moynihan B, Khan U, Hassan A, O'Brien JT, et al. Using DTI to assess white matter microstructure in cerebral small vessel disease (SVD) in multicentre studies. *Clin Sci* (2017) 131:1361–73. doi:10.1042/CS20170146
7. Merboldt KD, Hanicke W, Frahm J. Self-diffusion NMR imaging using stimulated echoes. *J Magn Reson* (1985) 64:479–86.
8. Taylor DG, Bushell MC. The spatial mapping of translational diffusion coefficients by the NMR imaging technique. *Phys Med Biol* (1985) 30:345–9. doi:10.1088/0031-9155/30/4/009
9. Le Bihan D, Breton E, Lallemand D, Grenier P, Cabanis E, Laval-Jeantet M. MR imaging of intravoxel incoherent motions: application to diffusion and perfusion in neurologic disorders. *Radiology* (1986) 161:401–7. doi:10.1148/radiology.161.2.3763909
10. Stejskal EO, Tanner JE. Spin diffusion measurements: spin echoes in the presence of a time-dependent field gradient. *J Chem Phys* (1965) 42:288–92. doi:10.1063/1.1695690
11. Le Bihan D, Mangin JF, Poupon C, Clark CA, Pappata S, Molko N, et al. Diffusion tensor imaging: concepts and applications. *J Magn Reson Imaging* (2001) 13:534–46. doi:10.1002/jmri.1076
12. Basser PJ, Mattiello J, Le Bihan D. Estimation of the effective self-diffusion tensor from the NMR spin echo. *J Magn Reson* (1994) 103:247–54. doi:10.1006/jmrb.1994.1037
13. Basser PJ, Mattiello J, Le Bihan D. MR diffusion tensor spectroscopy and imaging. *Biophys J* (1994) 66:259–67. doi:10.1016/S0006-3495(94)80775-1
14. Pierpaoli C, Basser PJ. Toward a quantitative assessment of diffusion anisotropy. *Magn Reson Med* (1996) 36:893–906; Erratum in *Magn Reson Med* (1997);37:972. doi:10.1002/mrm.1910360612
15. Basser PJ, Pierpaoli C. A simplified method to measure the diffusion tensor from seven MR images. *Magn Reson Med* (1998) 39:928–34. doi:10.1002/mrm.1910390610
16. Basser PJ. Inferring microstructural features and the physiological state of tissues from diffusion-weighted images. *NMR Biomed* (1995) 8:333–44. doi:10.1002/nbm.1940080707
17. Xue R, van Zijl PC, Crain BJ, Solaiyappan M, Mori S. In vivo three-dimensional reconstruction of rat brain axonal projections by diffusion tensor imaging. *Magn Reson Med* (1999) 42:1123–7. doi:10.1002/(SICI)1522-2594(199912)42:6<1123::AID-MRM17>3.0.CO;2-H
18. Basser PJ, Pajevic S, Pierpaoli C, Duda J, Aldroubi A. In vivo fiber tractography using DT-MRI data. *Magn Reson Med* (2000) 44:625–32. doi:10.1002/1522-2594(200010)44:4<625::AID-MRM17>3.0.CO;2-O
19. Song SK, Sun SW, Ramsbottom MJ, Chang C, Russell J, Cross AH. Dysmyelination revealed through MRI as increased radial (but unchanged axial) diffusion of water. *Neuroimage* (2002) 17:1429–36. doi:10.1006/nimg.2002.1267
20. Song SK, Sun SW, Ju WK, Lin SJ, Cross AH, Neufeld AH. Diffusion tensor imaging detects and differentiates axon and myelin degeneration in mouse optic nerve after retinal ischemia. *Neuroimage* (2003) 20:1714–22. doi:10.1016/j.neuroimage.2003.07.005
21. Scholz J, Tomassini V, Johansen-Berg H. Individual differences in white matter microstructure in the healthy brain. 2nd ed. In: Johansen-Berg H, Behrens TEJ, editors. *Diffusion MRI*. San Diego: Elsevier Inc (2014). p. 301–16.

22. Douek P, Turner R, Pekar J, Patronas NJ, Le Bihan D. MR color mapping of myelin fiber orientation. *J Comput Assist Tomogr* (1991) 15:923–9. doi:10.1097/00004728-199111000-00003
23. McGavern DB, Murray PD, Rodriguez M. Quantitation of spinal cord demyelination, remyelination, atrophy, and axonal loss in a model of progressive neurologic injury. *J Neurosci Res* (1999) 58:492–504. doi:10.1002/(SICI)1097-4547(19991115)58:4<492::AID-JNR3>3.0.CO;2-P
24. Perry VH, Anthony DC. Axon damage and repair in multiple sclerosis. *Philos Trans R Soc Lond B Biol Sci* (1999) 354:1641–7. doi:10.1098/rstb.1999.0509
25. Kawai SI, Vora S, Das S, Gachie E, Becker B, Neufeld AH. Modeling of risk factors for the degeneration of retinal ganglion cells after ischemia/reperfusion in rats: effects of age, caloric restriction, diabetes, pigmentation, and glaucoma. *FASEB J* (2001) 15:1285–7. doi:10.1096/fj.00-0666fje
26. Rosenbaum DM, Rosenbaum PS, Singh M, Gupta G, Gupta H, Li B, et al. Functional and morphologic comparison of two methods to produce transient retinal ischemia in the rat. *J Neuroophthalmol* (2001) 21:62–8. doi:10.1097/00041327-200103000-00015
27. Adachi M, Takahashi K, Nishikawa M, Miki H, Uyama M. High intraocular pressure-induced ischemia and reperfusion injury in the optic nerve and retina in rats. *Graefes Arch Clin Exp Ophthalmol* (1996) 234:445–51. doi:10.1007/BF02539411
28. Kim GM, Xu J, Song SK, Yan P, Ku G, Xu XM, et al. Tumor necrosis factor receptor deletion reduces nuclear factor-kappa B activation, cellular inhibitor of apoptosis protein 2 expression, and functional recovery after traumatic spinal cord injury. *J Neurosci* (2001) 21:6617–25.
29. Song SK, Yoshino J, Le TQ, Lin SJ, Sun SW, Cross AH, et al. Demyelination increases radial diffusivity in corpus callosum of mouse brain. *Neuroimage* (2005) 26:132–40. doi:10.1016/j.neuroimage.2005.01.028
30. Matsushima GK, Morell P. The neurotoxicant, cuprizone, as a model to study demyelination and remyelination in the central nervous system. *Brain Pathol* (2001) 11:107–16. doi:10.1111/j.1750-3639.2001.tb00385.x
31. Armstrong RC, Le TQ, Frost EE, Borke RC, Vana AC. Absence of fibroblast growth factor 2 promotes oligodendroglial repopulation of demyelinated white matter. *J Neurosci* (2002) 22:8574–85.
32. Stidworthy MF, Genoud S, Suter U, Mantei N, Franklin RJ. Quantifying the early stages of remyelination following cuprizoneinduced demyelination. *Brain Pathol* (2003) 13:329–39. doi:10.1111/j.1750-3639.2003.tb00032.x
33. Sun SW, Liang HF, Trinkaus K, Cross AH, Armstrong RC, Song SK. Noninvasive detection of cuprizone induced axonal damage and demyelination in the mouse corpus callosum. *Magn Reson Med* (2006) 55:302–8. doi:10.1002/mrm.20774
34. Wheeler-Kingshott CA, Cercignani M. About "axial" and "radial" diffusivities. *Magn Reson Med* (2009) 61:1255–60. doi:10.1002/mrm.21965
35. Wheeler-Kingshott CA, Ciccarelli O, Schneider T, Alexander DC, Cercignani M. A new approach to structural integrity assessment based on axial and radial diffusivities. *Funct Neurol* (2012) 27:85–90.
36. Rovaris M, Agosta F, Pagani E, Filippi M. Diffusion tensor MR imaging. *Neuroimaging Clin N Am* (2009) 19:37–43. doi:10.1016/j.nic.2008.08.001
37. Lodygensky GA, West T, Stump M, Holtzman DM, Inder TE, Neil JJ. In vivo MRI analysis of an inflammatory injury in the developing brain. *Brain Behav Immun* (2010) 24:759–67. doi:10.1016/j.bbi.2009.11.005
38. Xie M, Tobin JE, Budde MD, Chen CI, Trinkaus K, Cross AH, et al. Rostrocaudal analysis of corpus callosum demyelination and axon damage across disease stages refines diffusion tensor imaging correlations with pathological features. *J Neuropathol Exp Neurol* (2010) 69:704–16. doi:10.1097/NEN.0b013e3181e3de90
39. Kim JH, Loy DN, Liang HF, Trinkaus K, Schmidt RE, Song SK. Noninvasive diffusion tensor imaging of evolving white matter pathology in a mouse model of acute spinal cord injury. *Magn Reson Med* (2007) 58:253–60. doi:10.1002/mrm.21316
40. Wang Y, Wang Q, Haldar JP, Yeh FC, Xie M, Sun P, et al. Quantification of increased cellularity during inflammatory demyelination. *Brain* (2011) 134:3590–601. doi:10.1093/brain/awr307
41. Wang X, Cusick MF, Wang Y, Sun P, Libbey JE, Trinkaus K, et al. Diffusion basis spectrum imaging detects and distinguishes coexisting subclinical inflammation, demyelination and axonal injury in experimental autoimmune encephalomyelitis mice. *NMR Biomed* (2014) 27:843–52. doi:10.1002/nbm.3129
42. Chiang CW, Wang Y, Sun P, Lin TH, Trinkaus K, Cross AH, et al. Quantifying white matter tract diffusion parameters in the presence of increased extra-fiber cellularity and vasogenic edema. *Neuroimage* (2014) 101:310–9. doi:10.1016/j.neuroimage.2014.06.064
43. Cheng YW, Chung HW, Chen CY, Chou MC. Diffusion tensor imaging with cerebrospinal fluid suppression and signal-to-noise preservation using acquisition combining fluid-attenuated inversion recovery and conventional imaging: comparison of fiber tracking. *Eur J Radiol* (2011) 79:113–7. doi:10.1016/j.ejrad.2009.12.032
44. Oh J, Zackowski K, Chen M, Newsome S, Saidha S, Smith SA, et al. Multiparametric MRI correlates of sensorimotor function in the spinal cord in multiple sclerosis. *Mult Scler* (2013) 19:427–35. doi:10.1177/1352458512456614
45. Oh J, Saidha S, Chen M, Smith SA, Prince J, Jones C, et al. Spinal cord quantitative MRI discriminates between disability levels in multiple sclerosis. *Neurology* (2013) 80:540–7. doi:10.1212/WNL.0b013e31828154c5
46. Kronlage M, Pitarokoili K, Schwarz D, Godel T, Heiland S, Yoon MS, et al. Diffusion tensor imaging in chronic inflammatory demyelinating polyneuropathy: diagnostic accuracy and correlation with electrophysiology. *Invest Radiol* (2017) 52:701–7. doi:10.1097/RLI.0000000000000394
47. Tu TW, Williams RA, Lescher JD, Jikaria N, Turtzo LC, Frank JA. Radiological-pathological correlation of diffusion tensor and magnetization transfer imaging in a closed head traumatic brain injury model. *Ann Neurol* (2016) 79:907–20. doi:10.1002/ana.24641
48. Naismith RT, Xu J, Tutlam NT, Trinkaus K, Cross AH, Song SK. Radial diffusivity in remote optic neuritis discriminates visual outcomes. *Neurology* (2010) 74:1702–10. doi:10.1212/WNL.0b013e3181e0434d
49. Cross AH, Song SK. A new imaging modality to non-invasively assess multiple sclerosis pathology. *J Neuroimmunol* (2017) 304:81–5. doi:10.1016/j.jneuroim.2016.10.002
50. Gatto RG, Chu Y, Ye AQ, Price SD, Tavassoli E, Buenaventura A, et al. Analysis of YFP(J16)-R6/2 reporter mice and postmortem brains reveals early pathology and increased vulnerability of callosal axons in Huntington's disease. *Hum Mol Genet* (2015) 24:5285–98. doi:10.1093/hmg/ddv248

2

Disease Specific Autoantibodies in Idiopathic Inflammatory Myopathies

Bruno Stuhlmüller[1], Udo Schneider[1], José-B. González-González[1,2] and Eugen Feist[1*]

[1] Department of Rheumatology and Clinical Immunology, Charité-Universitätsmedizin, Berlin, Germany, [2] Labor Berlin-Charité Vivantes GmbH, Berlin, Germany

***Correspondence:**
Eugen Feist
eugen.feist@charite.de

Idiopathic inflammatory myopathies represent still a diagnostic and therapeutic challenge in different disciplines including neurology, rheumatology, and dermatology. In recent years, the spectrum of idiopathic inflammatory myopathies has been significantly extended and the different manifestations were described in more detail leading to new classification criteria. A major breakthrough has also occurred with respect to new biomarkers especially with the characterization of new autoantibody-antigen systems, which can be separated in myositis specific antibodies and myositis associated antibodies. These markers are detectable in approximately 80% of patients and facilitate not only the diagnostic procedures, but provide also important information on stratification of patients with respect to organ involvement, risk of cancer and overall prognosis of disease. Therefore, it is not only of importance to know the significance of these markers and to be familiar with the optimal diagnostic tests, but also with potential limitations in detection. This article focuses mainly on antibodies which are specific for myositis providing an overview on the targeted antigens, the available detection procedures and clinical association. As major tasks for the near future, the need of an international standardization is discussed for detection methods of autoantibodies in idiopathic inflammatory myopathies. Furthermore, additional investigations are required to improve stratification of patients with idiopathic inflammatory myopathies according to their antibody profile with respect to response to different treatment options.

Keywords: myositis, inflammation, autoantibodies, antigens, biomarker

INTRODUCTION

Idiopathic inflammatory myopathies (IIM) represent a heterogeneous group of acquired muscle diseases with so far unclear etiology. The different entities are associated with diverse clinical symptoms ranging from amyopathic to necrotic inflammatory muscle involvement, typical skin and internal organ involvement. In addition to the clinical picture, histological and serological findings are especially supportive in differentiation and stratification of disease (1). Based on this characteristics, IIM can be classified into different major sub-types: (i) polymyositis (PM), (ii) sporadic inclusion body myositis (sIBM), (iii) dermatomyositis (DM), (iv) immune-mediated necrotizing myopathy (IMNM), and (v) overlap syndromes with myositis (2, 3). Within the spectrum of antibodies two classes have been proposed (4), designated as myositis specific antibodies (MSAs) due to their exclusive association with IIM or as myositis-associated antibodies (MAAs) due to their prevalence in different other connective tissue disorders. This article focuses on an overview on so far identified specific autoantibody-antigen systems in IIM. Furthermore, we discuss the available methods, strategies and pitfalls of autoantibody detection in IIM as well as their diagnostic performance and clinical association.

CHARACTERIZATION OF DISEASE SPECIFIC ANTIGEN-ANTIBODY SYSTEMS IN IIM

As with many other systemic autoimmune diseases, it is unclear so far, whether and how the observed autoantibody formation is directly associated with the pathogenesis of disease or is just an epiphenomenon. However, the striking association between certain autoantibodies with a distinct clinical phenotype, their high disease specificity and their value for stratification and prognosis of disease suggests that they may play a role in disease induction and propagation (5). This section describes in detail the nature and function of so far identified IIM specific antigens. A complete overview on so far identified antigens and the corresponding autoantibodies in adult and in juvenile patients with IIM is given in **Table 1**.

The best-known autoantigen-autoantibody system in IIM is directed against **transport ribonucleoacid (t-RNA) synthetases** and represents a specific finding in patients with so named anti-synthetase syndrome (ASS). The targeted synthetases catalyze the binding of a specific aminoacid to their t-RNA in the cytoplasm of each eukaryotic cell for transportation to the ribosome and subsequent protein synthesis. At least eight t-RNA synthetases have been identified as autoantigens. Anti-Jo1 antibodies are the most common ones and received their designation after the initials of the index patients (44). It is unclear, why not all t-RNA synthetases are targeted by the immune system in ASS, but only the tRNA synthetase for threonyl (PL-7), alanyl (PL-12), isoleucyl (OJ), glycyl (EJ), asparaginyl (KS), phenylalanyl (Zo), tyrosil (Ha), and finally the histidyl synthetase (Jo-1). Even more of interest is the question, whether the antibodies can interfere with the function of the respective t-RNA synthetase as it has been shown for anti-Jo1 antibodies by *in-vitro* experiments (45, 46). This particular antibody specificity belongs mainly to the IgG1 isotype and binds to common epitopes (47).

For the anti-Jo1 antibodies, it was shown that the formation of the major autoepitope is strongly dependent on proper folding of the molecule (46). As a shared risk factor for anti–Jo-1 autoantibody positivity, the HLA–DRB1*0301 allele was identified in European as well as African Americans (48). In the Japanese population, HLA–DRB1*0405 was associated with the formation of an anti-tRNA antibody response (49).

Another specific antigen is **the transcription intermediary factor-1 gamma** (TIF-1γ). This multi-functional protein with a molecular weight (MW) of 140/155 kilo-Dalton (kDa) is mainly involved in gene transcription (27, 50–53). The TIF-1 family is composed of tripartite motif-containing (TRIM) proteins, which are all implicated in cell proliferation, development, apoptosis, and innate immunity (54). All TIF1 proteins share a C-terminal chromatin reading unit consisting of a plant homeodomain finger and a bromo-domain (BROMO) that is highly conserved among TIF1 family members, but which is not present in any of the other TRIM proteins (55, 56). Of note, while the most common target in anti-TIF1-positive CAM (cancer-associated myositis) is TIF1γ, other proteins of the TIF1 family (TIF1α and β) may also be simultaneously targeted by the immune system (53).

The tripartite containing motif (TRIM) allows these proteins also to function as E3-ligases in the ubiquitination pathway to control protein degradation, localization, and function. In this context, it is interesting to mention that TIF1-γ is involved in the regulation of TGF-β signaling via mono-ubiquitination of SMAD-4 leading to suppression of TGF- β. Thus, by stimulating cell growth and differentiation, TIF1-γ could play a pivotal role in promoting or suppressing malignant cell growth and differentiation (57). The known association of anti-TIF1-γ antibodies with a high risk of cancer development in DM suggest that this link could be not random. Of note, anti-TIF antibodies were only rarely detectable in patients with solid cancer (3.1%) or paraneoplastic rheumatic syndrome (3.3%) without DM (58).

Recently, it was recognized that tumors from paraneoplastic anti-TIF1-γ positive patients showed an increased number of genetic alterations, such as mutations and loss of heterozygosity (LOH) in TIF1 genes (59). Compared with type-matched control tumors from non-myositis patients, TIF1-γ staining was also significantly more intense in tumors as well as muscle tissue from anti-TIF1-γ positive patients. This finding could indicate that the co-occurrence of mutations in peptide regions of TIF1 with high affinity for HLA class I and tumors with high-level TIF1 protein expression may initiate a strong adaptive immune response against neoplastic cells with the mutation. Interestingly, LOH is the most frequent way to lose a mutant allele in human cancer and this is key to tumor immune-editing, since tumor cells with mutations producing a neo-antigen may be eliminated by the immune system and replaced by tumor cells with LOH in that region (without the antigenic mutation) (60, 61). Thus, these modifications can induce an immune response, but also cause an escape of the tumor cell from clearance.

It has been described that DM disease increases toward the equator and strongly associate with latitude. Recently, this observation was confirmed by another study showing that relative prevalence of DM and frequency of anti-TIF1-γ autoantibodies were found to be significantly negatively associated with latitude in adult myositis. Furthermore, HLA alleles HLA-DRB1* 07:01 and HLA-DQB1*02 were strongly associated with the DM-specific autoantibodies anti-Mi-2 as well as anti-TIF1-γ (62).

The component of **the nucleosome remodeling deacetylase complex, Mi-2,** is an autoantigen of 240 kDa MW and exists in two isoforms Mi-2α (CHD3) and Mi-2β (CHD4). Mi-2 is responsible for the remodeling of chromatin by de-acetylating histones and plays a role as transcription repressor (63). The role of anti-Mi-2 autoantibodies in the pathogenesis of DM is unclear. However, the autoantigen Mi-2 is found to be up-regulated in the muscle tissue of DM patients. Of note, exposure of keratinocytes to UV radiation has been shown to increase the expression of Mi-2 protein supporting the hypothesis that UV radiation may be associated with the induction of anti-Mi-2 autoantibodies (64). However, a reported increase in the presence of anti-Mi-2 autoantibodies toward the equator was not confirmed by a current study (62, 65). A preferential expression was described in the nucleus of myofibers within fascicles affected by perifascicular atrophy, particularly in the centralized nuclei of small perifascicular muscle fibers expressing

TABLE 1 | Characterization of myositis specific and myositis associated autoantibodies and their respective antigens.

	Autoantigen name and function	Molecular weight in kilodalton	Cellular localization	Disease and associated manifestations	Frequency in adult (A) and juvenile (J) IIM	Conventional and commercial (*) detection systems	References
ANTI-SYNTHETASE SYNDROME (ASS)							
EJ	Glycyl-tRNA synthetase	79	Cy	ASS with mechanic hands, associated with increased risk of interstitial lung disease	(A) <5%	ELISA, IP & WB, *IIFT *Strip test	(6)
Jo-1	Histidyl-tRNA synthetase	60	Cy	ASS with interstitial lung involvement, mechanic hands, Raynaud, arthritis	(A) 20–30%	ELISA, ID, IP & WB, *IIFT, *Strip test	(7–10)
OJ	Isoleucyl-tRNA synthetase	145	Cy	ASS with interstitial lung disease, sometimes also found in RA	(A) 3%	ELISA, IP & WB, IF, *IIFT, *Strip test	(6, 11)
PI-7	Threonyl-tRNA synthetase	83	Cy	ASS with increased risk of interstitial lung disease, Raynaud syndrome,	(A) < 5%	ELISA, ID, IP & WB, *IIFT, *Strip test	(8)
PI-12	Alanyl-tRNA synthetase	108	Cy	ASS associated in 90% with interstitial lung disease	(A) 2–3%	ELISA, ID, IP & WB, *IIFT, *Strip test	(12)
KS	Asparaginyl-tRNA synthetase	51	Cy	ASS	(A) <5%	ELISA, IP & WB	(13, 14)
Ha	Thyrosyl-tRNA synthetase	59	Cy	ASS	(A) < 1%	ELISA, IP & WB	(15)
Zo	Phenylalanyl-t-RNA synthetase	52	Mi	ASS frequently with fever	(A) < 1%	ELISA, IP & WB	(15, 16)
DERMATOMYOSITIS (DM), POLYMYOSITIS (PM) AND IMMUNE MEDIATED NECROTIZING MYOPATHY (IMNM)							
SRP	Signal recognizing particle	72/52	Cy	IMNM, acute und subacute	(A) 5–10% (J) < 3%	WB, IF, *IIFT *Strip test	(7, 17, 18)
MDA-5 / CADM-140	Melanoma differentiation associated Gene 5	140	Cy	Amyopathic dermatomyositis, mostly in relation with progressive interstitial pneumonia	(A) 50–73% in Asian populations	WB, IF, *IIFT	(19, 20)
Mi-2α and β	Nucleosome deacetylase complex; helicase binding protein	240	Nu	DM mild forms	(A) 15–30% (J) 10–15%	WB, IF, *IIFT, *Strip test	(21, 22)
NXP-2 (MJ)	Nuclear matrix protein 2	140	Nu	DM und juvenile DM/PM, mostly associated with calcinosis, in juvenile DM involved with ischemia and in adult PM with cancer	(A) 18–25% (J) 60%	WB, IF, *IIFT, *Strip test	(23, 24)
SAE1/2	Small ubiquitin like modifying and activating enzyme	90/40	Nu	DM, often also found in patients with amyopathic DM	(A) < 5% (J) < 1%	WB, IF, *IIFT, *Strip test	(23, 25, 26)
TIF-1γ	E3-Ligase, transcriptional factor-1γ hetero complex	155/140	Nu	Cancer associated DM in adults, skin ulcerations in juvenile DM	(A) 13–21% (J) 22–29%	IF, WB, *IIFT, *Strip test	(23, 27)
p200/100 HMGCR (HMG-CoA)	3-hydroxy-3-methylglutaryl-CoA reductase	200/100	ER membrane	IMNM frequently associated with prior statin use	(A) 6-10 %	IP and WB	(28–31)
MYOSITIS ASSOCIATED ANTIBODIES (MAA)							
Ku70 / Ku80	DNA-binding protein kinase complex, involved in DNA double strand repair	70/88	Nu	Overlap-Syndrome frequently with pulmonary fibrosis, arthralgia, gastrointestinal involvement,	(A) 7%	WB, IF, *IIFT, *Strip test	(32)

(Continued)

TABLE 1 | Continued

	Autoantigen name and function	Molecular weight in kilodalton	Cellular localization	Disease and associated manifestations	Frequency in adult (A) and juvenile (J) IIM	Conventional and commercial (*) detection systems	References
cN-1A	Enzyme, Cytosolic 5′-nucleotidase	43	Nu	High frequency in sporadic inclusion body myositis (sIBM), but also in Sjogren's syndrome, infrequent in other forms of IIM	(A-) s-IBM 33–44%, PM/DM 5%	ELISA, IF, *IIFT, *Strip test	(33–36)
U1-RNP	U1-ribonuclear Protein	70	Nu	Associated with mixed connective tissue diseases (MCTD)	(A) up to 12%	WB, IF	(32, 37)
SS-B (La)	RNA-metabolism and processing of pre-tRNA; viral RNA binding protein, RNA-chaperone	50	Nu	Associated with Sjogren's syndrome and systemic lupus erythematosus (SLE)	(A) 10%	WB, IF	(38, 39)
SS-A (Ro)	E3-ubiquitine ligase	60/52	Nu / Cy	Associated with Sjogren's syndrome and SLE	(A) 50% (J) 10%	WB, IF, *IIFT, *Strip test	(40–42)
PM/Scl	Exo-ribonuclease	100/75	Nu / Cy	Overlap syndrome with myositis and scleroderma	(A) 5%	IF, WB, *IIFT *Strip test	(7, 43)

ID, Immunodiffusion; IIFT, Indirect Immunofluorescence test; IF, Immunofluorescence; WB, Immunoblotting; IP, Immunoprecipitation; MI, mitochondrium; Cy, cytoplasm; Nu, nucleus; (A), adult IIM; (J), juvenile IIM.

markers of regeneration (66). In a mouse model of muscle injury and repair, Mi-2 levels were dramatically and persistently up-regulated during muscle regeneration *in-vivo*. Of note, premature silencing of Mi-2 with RNA interference *in vitro* resulted in accelerated myoblast differentiation. In summary, these results indicate that this protein may play a role in modulating the kinetics of myoblast differentiation. European and American anti–Mi-2 antibody positive DM patients have a common genetic risk factor DRB1*0701 (67). Furthermore, HLA-DRB1*0302 was identified to be associated with anti–Mi-2 autoantibody positive African American patients (48). Of note, all HLA molecules were found to share a 4–amino-acid sequence motif, which was predicted by comparative homology analyses to have identical 3-dimensional orientations within the peptide-binding groove.

The target antigen of antibodies against **small ubiquitin-like modifier activating enzyme (SAE1/2)** is the SUMO-1 activating enzyme heterodimer with a MW of 40 and 90 kDa, respectively. This antigen is involved in the posttranslational modification of proteins, the so called "sumoylation" (68, 69). Of note, a strong association with the HLA-DRB1*04-DQA1*03-DQB1*03 haplotype has been reported (25). This is another example in IIM, where the association between genotype, serotype and clinical picture suggest a link to the pathogenesis of disease.

Immune reactivity against the **signal recognizing protein hetero-complex (SRP)** is associated with immune-mediated necrotizing myopathy (IMNM). This 72/52 kDa antigen is expressed in the cytoplasm and responsible for transport proteins to the endoplasmic reticulum. SRP consists of six polypeptides (including SRP19 and MIM 182175) as well as seven SL-RNA molecules with partial homology to Alu-DNA (70, 71). Although antibodies against SRP can target each of the different SRP components, a signal peptide-binding 54 kDa subunit (SRP54) represents a major epitope recognized by almost every sera and is, therefore, preferentially used in immunoassays (72–76). Although it is not clear, how the antibodies can interact with the SRP1/2 autoantigen, it was shown that anti-SRP antibodies can inhibit the translocation of secretory proteins into the endoplasmic reticulum *in-vitro* and that a passive transfer of IgG from anti-SRP+ patients with IMNM provoked muscle deficiency through a complement-mediated mechanism in mice model. Interestingly, also active immunization with SRP was able to induce an immune response and provoked disease (76, 77). A correlation between anti-SRP54 antibody titers and disease activity was also shown in a longitudinal follow-up study suggesting a pathogenic role of this antibody entity (78). As a genetic risk factor, HLA- DQA1*0102 was identified in anti–SRP autoantibody positive African American patients (48).

The **melanoma differentiation antigen 5 (MDA-5**, synonym CADM-140) with a MW of 140 kDa belongs to the family of RIG-I-like receptors of adhesion molecules and represents a resistance factor against double stranded RNA viruses (49, 79). The MDA-5 molecule plays an important role in the regulation of the immune response by the innate system. In this context, it was shown that MDA-5 bind virus particles, e.g., picornaviruses such as coxsackievirus, and induce an antiviral responses by producing type-I interferons and tumor necrosis factor (80). It was also reported that hyperferritinemia could be a marker for rapidly progressive ILD in anti–MDA-5 antibody positive DM patients (81, 82). In this context many cytokines regulate the ferritin synthesis, including IL-1β, IL-18, TNF, IFN-γ, and IL-6 and several of these cytokines are considered to be involved in IIM pathogenesis. HLA–DRB1*0101/*0405 was found to be associated with susceptibility to anti–MDA-5 antibody positive DM in the Japanese population (49). Interestingly the same alleles are well-known to play a role in the susceptibility to autoantibody induction in rheumatoid arthritis (83).

Autoantibodies against the **nuclear protein 2 (NXP-2)**, also known as MJ or p140 antibodies, are directed against a nuclear matrix protein complex named NXP2/MORC3, which is involved in regulation of p53-induced cell senescence in the context of oncogenic signals (23). NXP-2 is associated with the small ubiquitin modifier SUMO-2 and represses its expression (84).

The **enzyme 3-hydroxy-3-methylglutaryl-CoA reductase (HMGCR)** was recently identified as a target of autoantibodies induced under treatment with statins. The antigen is expressed in the ER membrane and has a MW of 200/100 kDa. HMGCR catalyzes the conversion of HMG-CoA to mevalonic acid, which is an important step in cholesterol biosynthesis. So far, reports about HMGCR in myositis are rare, however in animal studies it was demonstrated that loss of HMGCR function disrupts vascular stability during developmental processes (4).

DIAGNOSTIC TESTING FOR AUTOANTIBODIES IN IIM

To assess disease activity and as indicators for muscle injury in IIM, basic laboratory diagnostics are used, such as measurements of levels of inflammatory markers as well as serum activity and/or concentration of muscle specific proteins including creatine phosphokinase (CPK) or myoglobin. However, these markers are unspecific and not helpful to distinguish between the different forms of inflammatory muscle damage. In contrast, the reactivity of the described autoantibodies does not sufficiently correlate with disease activity in IIM, but can rather serve for stratification of the disease process and outcome (85). This section focuses on helpful information with respect to routine procedures of autoantibody detection and the recommended diagnostic approaches, since it is of enormous importance to know these basics for appropriate interpretation of results.

Serum is usually used for the detection of autoantibodies, and test procedures are performed according to the manufacturer's validation. From a preanalytical point of view, time point of venepuncture and fasting status of the patient are not relevant. However, hemolytic, lipemic or contaminated blood samples should not be used, since the released proteins and proteinases can interfere with the immunologic method of detection. Especially in case of a prolonged transportation of the blood sample, serum should be separated in advance by centrifugation at 1,300 g. Subsequently, the serum samples can be stored at 2–8°C for up-to 2 weeks before analysis. A longer period requires freezing at minus 20°C, which presumably allows conservation of the autoantibody reactivity for years (86, 87). Furthermore, some treatment procedures including administration of strong immunosuppressive drugs such as B-cell directed therapies as well as plasmapheresis or administration of intravenous immunoglobulins can influence the result of detection by decreasing the concentration of the autoantibodies.

From the methodical point of few, detection of autoantibodies in IIM is not well-standardized and no international reference samples are available so far. In general, immunoprecipitation of radio-labeled proteins or RNA molecules is still considered to represent the "gold standard" (68). However, due to the time-consuming procedure, high amount of required antigens and low sensitivity, this method is not a routine procedure in most clinical laboratories. Therefore, for the detection of IIM specific and/or associated autoantibodies several, more efficient approaches such as immunofluorescence, ELISA and western blotting are widely used (88–90). In general, immunofluorescence requires large experience to interpret patterns and may not be sensitive enough to detect all MSAs/MAA. On the other hand, ELISA methods using recombinant antigens or immunoblotting with denaturated antigens can probably not detect antibodies to certain conformational epitopes. Line-blot assays allow a qualitative detection of many antibodies in one run. In contrast, and in accordance to the manufacturer specification only a limited number of MSAs/MAAs can be detected by commercial available ELISAs so far.

Indirect immunofluorescence (IIF) on HEp-2 cells, a human epithelioma cell line, is commonly be used for detection of anti-nuclear antibodies (ANA), but also enables detection of antibodies against cytoplasmatic antigens. This method allows a screening for a wide range of autoantibodies especially in connective tissue disorders by describing the staining pattern (e.g., nuclear, nucleolar, cytoplamatic), as well as the reactivity titer starting with a serum dilution of usually 1:80. Although no agreement has still been reached on the interpretation and reporting of the ANA titres, results can be considered as weak positive in antibody titer of ≥1:160 and as strong positive in a titres of ≥1:640. In this context, it is important to mention that measured titers often do not correspond with the significance of the results. In other words, a low reactivity should not be considered as irrelevant. Furthermore, it is also important to pay attention to the described pattern of immunofluorescence in the nucleus, but also the cytoplasm. It is helpful to know that IIF on HEp-2 cells shows characteristic patterns of some MSA or MAA antibodies such as those against PM/Scl with prominent homogeneous staining of the nucleous, U1-RNP with coarse speckled staining of the nucleus, Jo-1 or SRP with fine speckled stainings of the cytoplasm (**Figure 1**), but is not sufficiently accurate to be used as the only screening tool for myositis antibodies.

Although most of the targeted antigens in IMM are expressed within HEp-2 cells, their detection by IIF is clearly limited. The reasons for frequent false negative results is diverse including e.g., low expression level of the antigen or low affinity of the antibodies causing a weak staining signal. Furthermore, the intracellular distribution of relevant antigens in IIM is usually diffuse generating an unspecific staining pattern. Thus, week

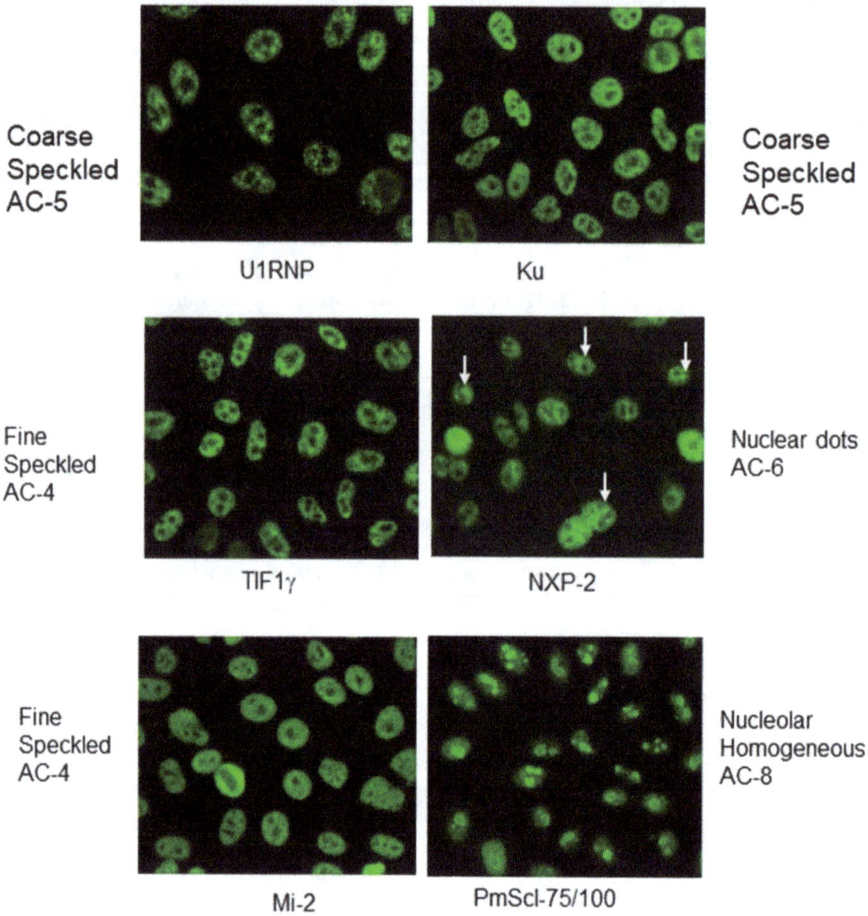

FIGURE 1 | Indirect immunofluorescence with typical nuclear patterns of MSA and MAA. Immunofluorescence patterns are indicated with the terminology of the International Consensus on ANA Patterns (ICAP).

positive results are often not recognized, as it frequently occurs even with anti-tRNA synthetase antibodies. Nevertheless, IIF on HEp-2 cells is an important diagnostic procedure. **Table 1** summarizes frequent staining patterns in conjunction with the respective antibody and, **Figures 1, 2** show representative IIF staining patterns indicating the respective nomenclature for the most frequent MSAs and MAAs by International Consensus on Autoantibody Patterns (ICAP).

For the detection of classical and new myositis antibodies, multi-analyte line blot assays and ELISA are the current routine methods of choice. In contrast to IIF, commercial ELISAs and line-blot assays use purified or recombinant expressed antigens for detection of antibodies. These methods allow the targeted detection or confirmation of respective antibodies in serum samples, which are usually diluted 1:100. In contrast to semi-quantitative results provided by line-blot assays (with negative, weak or strong positive signals, see **Figure 3**), ELISA based methods allow a better quantification of antibody reactivity, especially if international standards will be available. However, the majority of ELISA methods published hitherto to detect novel myositis antibodies are in-house made and most of the commercial ELISAs only report negative or positive results by using a cut-off level of reactivity defined by the providing manufacturer. A multiplex-approach for detection of several antibodies in one immunoassay has also limitations and pitfalls due to the difficult optimization of the cut-off for all investigated antibodies. Therefore, it is always important to check the plausibility of the obtained results, not only in cases of weak or borderline reactivity, but also in case of discordance between the different immunoassays (e.g., negative ANA staining pattern but positive anti-PM/Scl antibodies in ELISA or line-asays). On the solid phase of an immunoassay, the antigen structure can be altered yielding a false positive antibody reactivity, which is not directed against the native antigen. Therefore, it is important, that involved diagnostic laboratories are be informed about the clinical suspected diagnosis and provide high quality assays proven by regular internal and external quality controls.

The major advantage of ELISA and line blot test assays is the option of automation test fastness. In this context, the development of commercial quantitative immunoassays including ELISA, chemiluminescence and immunofluorometry has facilitated the use at large scale in routine laboratories and provided interesting

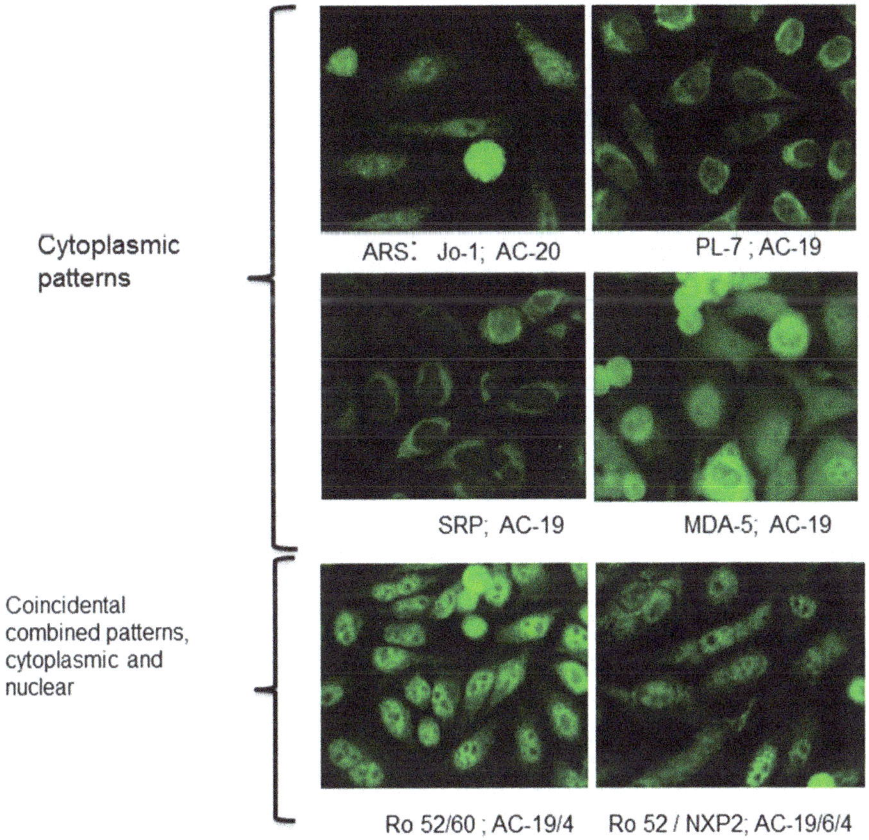

FIGURE 2 | Indirect immunofluorescence with typical cytoplasmic patterns of MSA and MAA. Immunofluorescence patterns are indicated with the terminology of the International Consensus on ANA Patterns (ICAP). AC-19-cytoplasmic dense fine speckled, AC-20-cytoplasmic fine speckled.

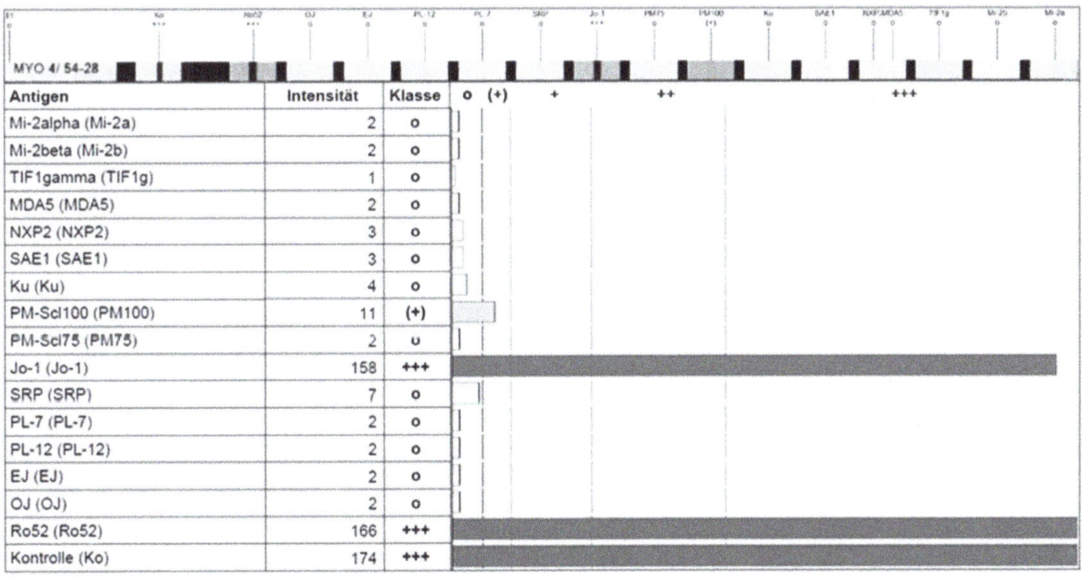

Antigen	Intensität	Klasse
Mi-2alpha (Mi-2a)	2	o
Mi-2beta (Mi-2b)	2	o
TIF1gamma (TIF1g)	1	o
MDA5 (MDA5)	2	o
NXP2 (NXP2)	3	o
SAE1 (SAE1)	3	o
Ku (Ku)	4	o
PM-Scl100 (PM100)	11	(+)
PM-Scl75 (PM75)	2	o
Jo-1 (Jo-1)	158	+++
SRP (SRP)	7	o
PL-7 (PL-7)	2	o
PL-12 (PL-12)	2	o
EJ (EJ)	2	o
OJ (OJ)	2	o
Ro52 (Ro52)	166	+++
Kontrolle (Ko)	174	+++

FIGURE 3 | Detection of anti-Jo-1 and anti Ro-52 antibody reactivity in a line-blot assay showing the reaction intensity by a scan-software of the fabricant (EUROLINE, Euroimmune, Germany).

information on correlation of clinical and serological findings in IIM.

CORRELATION OF MSA WITH CLINICAL FINDINGS

In addition to inflammatory lesions of skeletal muscles, involvement of other organs such as skin, joint, lung and heart is frequent in IIM. Extra-muscular involvement, especially interstitial lung disease (ILD) and underlying malignancy in cancer-associated myositis (CAM) are the two dominating factors contributing to increased mortality in IIM-patients (91, 92). This section gives an overview on the association of MSA with clinical findings and their diagnostic performance. The incidence of most of the so far identified autoantibody activities of European patients is in agreement with similar studies of Japanese and American patients (7).

ANTIBODIES AGAINST T-RNA SYNTHETASES

Patients with antibodies against t-RNA synthetases are prone to develop the so called anti-synthetase syndrome (ASS) characterized by myopathy, interstitial lung disease (ILD), non-erosive arthritis, fever, Raynaud's phenomenon and mechanic's hands. Since not all symptoms are present at disease onset, ASS should be carefully considered in patients presenting with isolated arthritis, even in those with erosive manifestation and RF as well as ACPA-positivity (93, 94). The presence of anti-synthetase antibodies can be suspected if a characteristic cytoplasmic pattern on HEp2 cells is evident (**Figure 1**). However, confirmation is needed using ELISA, immunoblot or line-assays with the isolated antigens. Depending on the diagnostic method anti-Jo-1 antibodies are the most frequent autoantibodies in IIM, they can be detected in 20–30% of patients (7, 95). Titers of Jo-1 antibodies were shown to correlate with disease activity in adults (95). In muscle biopsies of anti-Jo-1 positive myositis patients a specific histologic pattern with peri-fascicular necrosis has been described (96).

The CT- and histomorphologic pattern of ILD in anti-synthetase syndrome can vary between non-specific interstitial and organizing pneumonia (97). Antibodies against PL-7 and PL-12 are positive in up to 5% of IIM patients. Clinically they are associated with less muscle involvement but with a higher proportion of ILD, which might have an acute onset (98). Furthermore, pericarditis was observed in up to 50% of anti-PL7 positive patients (99). Antibodies against OJ, EJ, KS, Zo, and Ha are rare and only present in 1–3% of patients with ARS. The coincidence of anti-Ro52/TRIM21with anti-ASS antibodies was described to be associated with severe myositis and arthropathy as well as with an increased risk of cancer (7, 99, 100). The onset of ILD and myositis, as leading symptoms in ASS, can be subsequently or in parallel, while the course of ILD must not necessarily be progressive.

DM-Specific Antibodies

Anti-Mi-2 antibodies have a high specificity for both adult and juvenile DM (JDM). Mi-2-antibodies produce a fine speckled nuclear pattern in IIF on HEp-2 cells (AC-4 of the ICAP nomenclature) and are detectable in approximately 30% in adult and 10% in juvenile DM (JDM) patients, respectively. Patients with positive anti-Mi-2 antibodies have usually a milder myopathy, lower risk of interstitial lung disease (ILD) and malignancy (101). Skin manifestations, such as Gottron's sign and heliotrope rash, as well, rashes in neck (V rash) and upperback (shawl rash) or cuticular overgrowth are typical. Patients respond well to steroid therapy and have a good prognosis. Furthermore, levels of Mi-2 antibodies were shown to correlate with clinical response to B-cell depletion therapy (102). Although DM with antibodies against Mi2-β can be associated with neoplasia (e.g., colon or mama-carcinoma), anti-Mi-2 antibodies are in general associated with a lower risk of paraneoplastic myositis and hence considered to be a good prognostic factor.

Anti-TIF1γ (anti-155/140) antibodies are detectable in 13–21% of patients with tumor associated adult DM and in approximately 30% of severe juvenile DM patients (23, 27). In fact, these antibodies are the most frequent marker in juvenile IIM (JIIM) and are primarily associated with JDM. They were originally found almost exclusively in JDM, in about of 23–29% of cases using immunoprecipitation and immunoblotting. Interestingly, in recent studies including a total of 374 cases with JIIM, 131 cases (35%) were found to be positive for these antibodies. In detail, the antibodies were detectable in 38% of patients with JDM (123/320) and in 26% of patients with an overlap syndrome with myositis (8/31) (103, 104). TIF-γ-antibodies are known to be very frequently associated with malignancy in adults with a specificity of 89%, sensitivity of 78%, and positive and negative predictive values of 58 and 95%, respectively (105). In contrast to adults, there is no paraneoplastic association in JIIM (106). Skin manifestations are characterized by a usually slowly progressive onset, but are more extensive than in other JDM groups. In fact, skin ulcerations and lipodystrophy were reported to be particularly associated with these antibodies. However, this was not reported uniformly, since recent studies did not observe ulceration or V-rashes significantly more frequent in this group than in others (104). Of note, it has been shown that levels of TIF-γ-antibodies correlate with response to B-cell depletion therapy in pediatric patients (102).

Anti-NXP2 antibodies (MJ or p140) cause a fine speckled ANA pattern on IIF, but this pattern is often misinterpreted as variable nuclear dots (**Figure 1**). These antibodies have been originally described in children with JDM in about 25% of cases (107, 108). In a cohort of 436 patients with JIIM, their prevalence was reported to be approximately 21% in JDM, 9% in JPM and 15% in overlap syndromes (juvenile connective tissue myositis, JCTM) (104). Subsequently, anti-NXP2 antibodies have been also detected in approximately 30% of patients with DM and 8% with PM in a cohort of 58 adult Italian patients (109), but in only 1.6% of 507 adult Japanese patients (110). In the Italian cohort, a good response to therapy was reported for muscle involvement (109). In juvenile

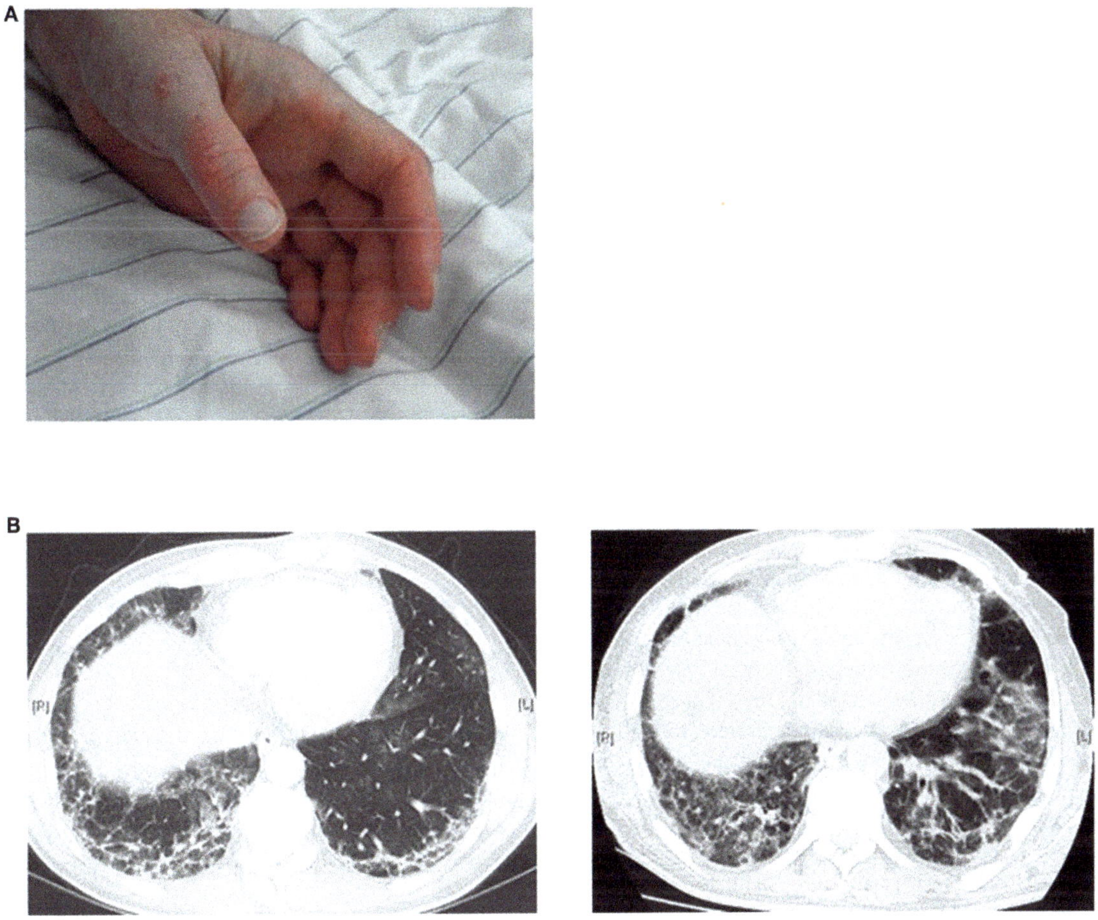

FIGURE 4 | MDA5 positive patient with an amyopathic dermatomyositis **(A)** maculopapular palmar rash and hyperkeratosis, **(B)** rapid progression of ILD manifestations within 5 weeks.

DM, the autoantibodies directed against NXP-2 are frequently associated with calcinosis and ischemic muscle involvement in up to 60% of cases (111). In adults, a possible association was reported with malignancies such as mamma-, uterus- and pancreas-carcinomas.

The ANA pattern of **anti-MDA5 antibodies** on HEp-2 cells in IIF is usually negative. These antibodies were identified for the first time in East-Asian populations. They are more frequently observed in adult DM and were reported in a prevalence of 19–35% (19, 81). In a study with 285 patients with JDM (112), anti-MDA5 antibodies were detectable in 7.4% of patients (21/285) and a recent review reports a prevalence of 0–13% in Europe and USA (113). The typical clinical manifestations of adult IIM patients with anti-MDA5 antibodies were amyopathic myositis with rapidly progressive interstitial lung disease (ILD), which in turn determines a high mortality rate in these patients (**Figure 4**). However, ILD must not be rapidly progressive in every case. In contrast to Asian patients, Caucasian patients often show skin ulcerations and painful palmar papules (114, 115). Furthermore, differences were also reported for Asian compared to Caucasian JDM associated with MDA-5 antibodies. In this context, Japanese patients showed a pulmonary involvement in nearly 50% of patients, whereas the incidence of ILD was much lower in Caucasians. JDM patients with anti-MDA5 antibodies show frequent skin as well as oral ulceration, but no calcinosis and had less severe muscle weakness compared other JDM subtypes. Of note, ILD was found in 4 of 12 cases (19%) on chest X-ray. None of these anti-MDA5 antibodies positive ILD patients was positive for anti-synthetase antibodies suggesting that anti-MDA5 antibodies represent an own subtype of IIM. This study also revealed that more patients with anti-MDA5-antibodies were in remission after 2 years compared to patients without these antibodies. In the follow-up, patients in remission showed a decline in the titer of MDA5 antibodies. These results resemble those of prior studies in which antibodies were shown to disappear during disease remission (20).

The **anti-SAE-antibodies** were originally described in adults with DM exhibiting an amyopathic onset with skin manifestations, but who may develop myositis several months later. Lung involvement was infrequent reported. The antibodies were detected in approximately 7–8% of adult Caucasian patients with DM (25, 116). In a study with 110 Japanese patients with

DM including 13 with JDM, only 2 patients with DM (1,8%) were shown to have SAE-antibodies (117). In a large study with 436 patients with JIIM, only one patient with JDM was positive for **anti-SAE-antibodies** (118). Therefore, the presence of SAE-antibodies in patients with JIIM seems to be extremely rare.

Immune Mediated Necrotizing Myositis (IMNM)

Anti-SRP-Antibodies were detected in about 3 to 7% of adults with IIM (73, 119). In JIIM, these antibodies are even more infrequently observed in only 1.6% of patients exclusively with juvenile polymyositis (JPM) (103, 120). The presence of SRP-antibodies can be suspected by detection of a cytoplasmic staining pattern in ANA IIF (**Figure 1**). Adults with anti-SRP-antibodies develop typically an acute necrotizing myopathy with prominent muscle impairment without skin manifestations. Compared to other myositis forms, a satisfactory response to medicament treatment is difficult to achieve. Pulmonary involvement, Raynaud-symptoms, arthritis or overlap syndromes are infrequent. Similar to adults, juvenile patients have very high levels of CPK as well as often cardiac involvement detectable e.g., by ECG or echocardiography. Of note, adult patients show frequently Raynaud-symptoms, dysphonia and dyspnea under exertion (107). Compared to other forms of JIIM, onset of symptoms is late in patients with anti-SRP-antibodies. However, two unusual cases have been published recently with onset in the first decade of life showing muscular dystrophy and a low degree of inflammation in muscle biopsy (107). The antibody titer against SRP seems to correlate with clinical activity as well as with levels of CPK in adults as well as in JIMM and can be used for monitoring of therapy (78, 121).

Antibodies against the enzyme **3-hydroxy-3-methylglutaryl-CoA reductase** (HMGCR) have been identified initially in patients with immune mediated necrotizing myositis (IMNM) in association with statin treatment. Overall, autoantibodies against HMGCR are detectable in 6–7% of patients with IIM (28–30). Myalgias, as a common side effects under statins, are not associated with this form of myositis and positive HMGCR-antibodies. In fact, only a minority of patients under statin treatment develops myopathy with anti-HMGCR-antibodies (122). Furthermore, even patients without statin treatment can develop necrotizing myositis with positive anti-HMGCR-antibodies (123). Results of a multicenter study show that the majority of patients with anti-HMGCR antibodies have IMNM. In this study, the prevalence of anti-HMGCR antibodies in different subpopulations of IMNM exposed to statins was approximately 70%, and even 75% in patients above the age of 50 years. However, approximately 45% of INMN patients had no exposure to statins and in 5% of cases did not show muscle necrosis (124). In contrast to non-immune statin myopathy, which resolves after stopping statin therapy, patients with anti-HMGCR antibodies have a persistent autoimmune response despite cancelation of treatment with the inducing agent. Similar to SRP antibodies, the titer of anti-HMGCR antibodies correlates with the clinical activity of necrotizing myositis. However, in contrast to SRP antibodies it is not known, whether antibody titres can normalize under effective therapy (125–127). Of note, these antibodies have also been detected in children after statin therapy recently, however, the experience with these cases is very limited (128, 129).

The detection of anti-HMGCR antibodies was performed by only few laboratories using immunoprecipitation so far, since no standardized commercial assay was available. An introduction of other methods such as ELISA or chemiluminescence for the detection of anti-HMGCR antibodies could make this test widely available to facilitate the diagnostic possibilities (130). However, since such immunoassays can yield false positive results due to detection of low avidity antibodies, a confirmatory analysis by immunoprecipitation can be recommended (131). Interestingly, usage of rat hepatocytes in indirect immunofluorescence was proposed (132). However, although some laboratories have adopted this strategy, there are not yet available data from an extended use of this approach (133). Of note, in a French cohort study HMGCR positive IMNM-patients were found to be at higher risk for malignancy (134).

AUTOANTIBODIES IN DM AND THE RISK OF CANCER

A high risk of cancer development is well-described and has led to the sub-categorization of cancer associated myositis (CAM) (135). The overall risk of cancer in myositis is significantly higher than in the age-matched population and approximately 10% of IIM are associated with malignancies (134–138). In DM, the risk is especially increased in the first 5 years after diagnosis (139–144). The most common cancers among the reported cases associated with DM are nasopharyngeal carcinoma and adenocarcinoma of the ovary, lung, pancreas, stomach and colon (139–145). Many studies have claimed the presence or absence of certain antibodies as markers for the risk of cancer in myositis. The autoantibody profile is considered a useful tool to identify patients at risk for CAM (32). In this context, the best established antibodies are directed against TIF1-γ with a high sensitivity and specificity for cancer associated DM in adult patients (27, 52, 53, 105, 146, 147), but not in JDM (50). Furthermore, also NXP-2 positivity in DM patients has been identified as a risk factor for malignancy (148). The association of anti-synthetase and anti-HMGCR antibodies with cancer is less clear and needs further confirmation. To exclude an associated malignancy in clinical practice repetitive examinations can be recommended in DM patients at risk, whereas clear guidelines on the frequency and extension of such diagnostic procedures are missing so far.

SUMMARY

Autoantibodies in IIM are very important diagnostic and prognostic markers, which can help to facilitate our approach to these rare and divers diseases. They correlate closely with the clinical manifestation of disease and allow stratification of patients. However, a laboratory result provides always only a piece of the diagnostic puzzle and should always be questioned if not plausible. For this purpose, a better knowledge on the limitations of the laboratory procedures is necessary and tests should only be performed if indicated according to the clinical picture. To allow comparison and improve reproducibility, the existing assays require uniform standards on an international level, and optimized methods for a broader distribution. If these issues can be solved, antibodies in IIM will play a more prominent role in the classification of disease. Another interesting and important tasks for the future will be to investigate the treatment response in IIM patients according to their antibody profile in more detail. This includes the question, whether different antibodies correlate with disease activity, but can be also used for an individualized approach to predict the response and outcome. Finally, the interaction of the antibodies with the targeted antigens is of major interest especially for the IIM specific entities. A deeper understanding on the mechanisms behind the induction of the respective immune response as well as on the potential role of the targeted antigens in IIM can improve our insight into the pathogenesis of disease.

AUTHOR CONTRIBUTIONS

BS reviewed published articles and contributed to the manuscript on antigen-antibody systems. US reviewed published articles and contributed to the manuscript on clinical aspects. J-BG-G reviewed published articles and contributed to the manuscript on laboratory diagnostic aspects. EF reviewed published articles and contributed to all parts of the manuscript.

REFERENCES

1. Mantegazza R, Bernasconi P, Confalonieri P, Cornelio F. Inflammatory myopathies and systemic disorders: a review of immunopathogenetic mechanisms and clinical features. *J Neurol.* (1997) 244:277–87. doi: 10.1007/s004150050087
2. Nagaraju K, Casciola-Rosen L, Lundberg I, Rawat R, Cutting S, Thapliyal R, et al. Activation of the endoplasmic reticulum stress response in autoimmune myositis: potential role in muscle fiber damage and dysfunction. *Arthritis Rheum.* (2005) 52:1824–35. doi: 10.1002/art.21103
3. Preuße C, Goebel HH, Held J, Wengert O, Scheibe F, Irlbacher K, et al. Immune-mediated necrotizing myopathy is characterized by a specific Th1-M1 polarized immune profile. *Am J Pathol.* (2012) 181:2161–71. doi: 10.1016/j.ajpath.2012.08.033
4. Eisa-Beygi S, Hatch G, Noble S, Ekker M, Moon TW. The 3-hydroxy-3-methylglutaryl-CoA reductase (HMGCR) pathway regulates developmental cerebral-vascular stability via prenylation-dependent signalling pathway. *Dev Biol.* (2013) 373:258–66. doi: 10.1016/j.ydbio.2012.11.024
5. Gunawardena H, Betteridge ZE, McHugh NJ. Myositis-specific autoantibodies: their clinical and pathogenic significance in disease expression. *Rheumatology.* (2009) 48:607–12. doi: 10.1093/rheumatology/kep078
6. Targoff IN. Autoantibodies to aminoacyl-transfer RNA synthetases for isoleucine and glycine. Two additional synthetases are antigenic in myositis. *J Immunol.* (1990) 144:1737–43.
7. Brouwer R, Hengstman GJ, Vree Egberts W, Ehrfeld H, Bozic B, Ghirardello A, et al. Autoantibody profiles in the sera of European patients with myositis. *Ann Rheum Dis.* (2001) 60:116–23. doi: 10.1136/ard.60.2.116
8. Mathews MB, Reichlin M, Hughes GR, Bernstein RM. Anti-threonyl-tRNA synthetase, a second myositis-related autoantibody. *J Exp Med.* (1984) 160:420–34. doi: 10.1084/jem.160.2.420
9. Rutjes SA, Vree Egberts WT, Jongen P, Van Den Hoogen F, Pruijn GJ, Van Venrooij WJ. Anti-Ro52 antibodies frequently co-occur with anti-Jo-1 antibodies in sera from patients with idiopathic inflammatory myopathy. *Clin Exp Immunol.* (1997) 109:32–40. doi: 10.1046/j.1365-2249.1997.4081308.x
10. Mileti LM, Strek ME, Niewold TB, Curran JJ, Sweiss NJ. Clinical characteristics of patients with anti-Jo-1 antibodies: a single center experience. *J Clin Rheumatol.* (2009) 15:254–5. doi: 10.1097/RHU.0b013e3181b0e910
11. Targoff IN, Trieu EP, Miller FW. Reaction of anti-OJ autoantibodies with components of the multi-enzyme complex of aminoacyl-tRNA synthetases in addition to isoleucyl-tRNA synthetase. *J Clin Invest.* (1993) 91:2556–64. doi: 10.1172/JCI116493
12. Bunn CC, Bernstein RM, Mathews MB. Autoantibodies against alanyl-tRNA synthetase and tRNAAla coexist and are associated with myositis. *J Exp Med.* (1986) 163:1281–91. doi: 10.1084/jem.163.5.1281
13. Hirakata M, Suwa A, Nagai S, Kron MA, Trieu EP, Mimori T, et al. Anti-KS: identification of autoantibodies to asparaginyl-transfer RNA synthetase associated with interstitial lung disease. *J Immunol.* (1999) 162:2315–20.
14. Hirakata M, Suwa A, Takada T, Sato S, Nagai S, Genth E, et al. Clinical and immunogenetic features of patients with autoantibodies to asparaginyl-transfer RNA synthetase. *Arthritis Rheum.* (2007) 56:1295–303. doi: 10.1002/art.22506
15. Vartanian OA. Detection of autoantibodies against phenylalanyl-, tyrosyl-, and tryptophanyl-tRNA-synthetase and anti-idiotypic antibodies to it in serum from patients with autoimmune diseases. *Mol Biol.* (1991) 25:1033–9.
16. Betteridge Z, Gunawardena H, North J, Slinn J, McHugh N. Anti-synthetase syndrome: a new autoantibody to phenylalanyl transfer RNA synthetase (anti-Zo) associated with polymyositis and interstitial pneumonia. *Rheumatology.* (2007) 46:1005–8. doi: 10.1093/rheumatology/kem045
17. Vincze M, Molnár PA, Tumpek J, Szollosi L, Gyetvai A, Kapitány A, et al. An unusual association: anti-Jo1 and anti-SRP antibodies in the serum of a patient with polymyositis. *Clin Rheumatol.* (2010) 29:811–4. doi: 10.1007/s10067-010-1394-6
18. Genth E, Mierau R. Diagnostic significance of scleroderma and myositis-associated autoantibodies. *Z Rheumatol.* (1995) 54:39–49.
19. Sato S, Hoshino K, Satoh T, Fujita T, Kawakami Y, Fujita T, et al. RNA helicase encoded by melanoma differentiation-associated gene 5 is a major autoantigen in patients with clinically amyopathic dermatomyositis: association with rapidly progressive interstitial lung disease. *Arthritis Rheum.* (2009) 60:2193–200. doi: 10.1002/art.24621
20. Muro Y, Sugiura K, Hoshino K, Akiyama M. Disappearance of anti-MDA-5 autoantibodies in clinically amyopathic DM/interstitial lung disease during disease remission. *Rheumatology.* (2012) 51:800–4. doi: 10.1093/rheumatology/ker408
21. Targoff IN, Reichlin M. The association between Mi-2 antibodies and dermatomyositis. *Arthritis Rheum.* (1985) 28:796–803. doi: 10.1002/art.1780280711
22. Hirakata M. Autoantibodies and their clinical significance in idiopathic inflammatory myopathies; polymyositis/dermatomyositis and related conditions. *Nihon Rinsho Meneki Gakkai Kaishi.* (2007) 30:444–54. doi: 10.2177/jsci.30.444
23. Gunawardena H, Betteridge ZE, McHugh NJ. Newly identified autoantibodies: relationship to idiopathic inflammatory myopathy subsets and pathogenesis. *Curr Opin Rheumatol.* (2008) 20:675–80. doi: 10.1097/BOR.0b013e328313bff4
24. Aouizerate J, De Antonio M, Bader-Meunier B, Barnerias C, Bodemer C, Isapof A, et al. Muscle ischaemia associated with NXP2 autoantibodies: a severe subtype of juvenile dermatomyositis. *Rheumatology.* (2018) 57:873–9. doi: 10.1093/rheumatology/kex516
25. Betteridge ZE, Gunawardena H, Chinoy H, North J, Ollier WE, Cooper RG, et al. Clinical and human leucocyte antigen class II haplotype associations of

autoantibodies to small ubiquitin-like modifier enzyme, a dermatomyositis-specific autoantigen target, in UK Caucasian adult-onset myositis. *Ann Rheum Dis.* (2009) 68:1621–5. doi: 10.1136/ard.2008.097162

26. Betteridge ZE, Gunawardena H, McHugh NJ. Novel autoantibodies and clinical phenotypes in adult and juvenile myositis. *Arthritis Res Ther.* (2011) 13:209. doi: 10.1186/ar3275
27. Targoff IN, Mamyrova G, Trieu EP, Perurena O, Koneru B, O'Hanlon TP, et al. A novel autoantibody to a 155-kd protein is associated with dermatomyositis. *Arthritis Rheum.* (2006) 54:3682–9. doi: 10.1002/art.22164
28. Mohassel P, Mammen AL. Anti-HMGCR myopathy. *J Neuromuscul Dis.* (2018) 5:11–20. doi: 10.3233/JND-170282
29. Mammen AL, Chung T, Christopher-Stine L, Rosen P, Rosen A, Doering KR, et al. Autoantibodies against 3-hydroxy-3-methylglutaryl-coenzyme A reductase in patients with statin-associated autoimmune myopathy. *Arthritis Rheum.* (2011) 63:713–21. doi: 10.1002/art.30156
30. Padala S, Thompson PD. Statins as a possible cause of inflammatory and necrotizing myopathies. *Atherosclerosis.* (2012) 222:15–21. doi: 10.1016/j.atherosclerosis.2011.11.005
31. Christopher-Stine L, Casciola-Rosen LA, Hong G, Chung T, Corse AM, Mammen AL. A novel autoantibody recognizing 200-kd and 100-kd proteins is associated with an immune-mediated necrotizing myopathy. *Arthritis Rheum.* (2010) 62:2757–66. doi: 10.1002/art.27572
32. Chinoy H, Fertig N, Oddis CV, Ollier WE, Cooper RG. The diagnostic utility of myositis autoantibody testing for predicting the risk of cancer-associated myositis. *Ann Rheum Dis.* (2007) 66:1345–9. doi: 10.1136/ard.2006.068502
33. Ghirardello A, Doria A. New insights in myositis-specific autoantibodies. *Curr Opin Rheumatol.* (2018) 30:614–22. doi: 10.1097/BOR.0000000000000548
34. Tawara N, Yamashita S, Zhang X, Korogi M, Zhang Z, Doki T, et al. Pathomechanisms of anti-cytosolic 5'-nucleotidase 1A autoantibodies in sporadic inclusion body myositis. *Ann Neurol.* (2017) 81:512–25. doi: 10.1002/ana.24919
35. Lilleker JB, Rietveld A, Pye SR, Mariampillai K, Benveniste O, Peeters MT, et al. Cytosolic 5'-nucleotidase 1A autoantibody profile and clinical characteristics in inclusion body myositis. *Ann Rheum Dis.* (2017) 76:862–8. doi: 10.1136/annrheumdis-2016-210282
36. Herbert MK, Stammen-Vogelzangs J, Verbeek MM, Rietveld A, Lundberg IE, Chinoy H, et al. Disease specificity of autoantibodies to cytosolic 5'-nucleotidase 1A in sporadic inclusion body myositis versus known autoimmune diseases. *Ann Rheum Dis.* (2016) 75:696–701. doi: 10.1136/annrheumdis-2014-206691
37. Mimori T, Hinterberger M, Pettersson I, Steitz JA. Autoantibodies to the U2 small nuclear ribonucleoprotein in a patient with scleroderma-polymyositis overlap syndrome. *J Biol Chem.* (1984) 259:560–5.
38. Hilker M, Tröster H, Grölz D, Hake U, Bachmann M. The autoantigen La/SS-B: analysis of the expression of alternatively spliced La mRNA isoforms. *Cell Tissue Res.* (1996) 284:383–9. doi: 10.1007/s004410050599
39. Teppo AM, Gripenberg M, Kurki P, Baklien K, Helve T, Wegelius O. Purification and characterization of a nuclear SS-B antigen. *Scand J Immunol.* (1982) 15:1–7. doi: 10.1111/j.1365-3083.1982.tb00615.x
40. Pakozdi A, Nihtyanova S, Moinzadeh P, Ong VH, Black CM, Denton CP. Clinical and serological hallmarks of systemic sclerosis overlap syndromes. *J Rheumatol.* (2011) 38:2406–9. doi: 10.3899/jrheum.101248
41. Váncsa A, Gergely L, Ponyi A, Lakos G, Németh J, Szodoray P, et al. Myositis-specific and myositis-associated antibodies in overlap myositis in comparison to primary dermatopolymyositis: Relevance for clinical classification: retrospective study of 169 patients. *Joint Bone Spine.* (2010) 77:125–30. doi: 10.1016/j.jbspin.2009.08.008
42. Limaye VS, Cassidy J, Scott G, Roberts-Thomson PJ, Gillis D. Anti-Ro52 antibodies, antisynthetase antibodies, and antisynthetase syndrome. *Clin Rheumatol.* (2008) 27:521–3. doi: 10.1007/s10067-007-0762-3
43. Ghirardello A, Zampieri S, Tarricone E, Iaccarino L, Bendo R, Briani C, et al. Clinical implications of autoantibody screening in patients with autoimmune myositis. *Autoimmunity.* (2006) 39:217–21. doi: 10.1080/08916930600622645
44. Wasicek CA, Reichlin M, Montes M, Raghu G. Polymyositis and interstitial lung disease in a patient with anti-Jo1 prototype. *Am J Med.* (1984) 76:538–44. doi: 10.1016/0002-9343(84)90677-6
45. Yang DC, Dang CV, Arnett FC. Rat liver histidyl-tRNA synthetase. Purification and inhibition by the myositis-specific anti-Jo-1 autoantibody. *Biochem Biophys Res Commun.* (1984) 120:15–21. doi: 10.1016/0006-291X(84)91407-4
46. Brouwer R, Vree Egberts W, Jongen PH, van Engelen BG, van Venrooij WJ. Frequent occurrence of anti-tRNA(His) autoantibodies that recognize a conformational epitope in sera of patients with myositis. *Arthritis Rheum.* (1998) 41:1428–37. doi: 10.1002/1529-0131(199808)41:8<1428::AID-ART12>3.0.CO;2-J
47. Miller FW, Twitty SA, Biswas T, Plotz PH. Origin and regulation of a disease-specific autoantibody response. Antigenic epitopes, spectrotype stability, and isotype restriction of anti-Jo-1 autoantibodies. *J Clin Invest.* (1990) 85:468–75. doi: 10.1172/JCI114461
48. O'Hanlon TP, Rider LG, Mamyrova G, Targoff IN, Arnett FC, Reveille JD, et al. HLA polymorphisms in African Americans with idiopathic inflammatory myopathy: allelic profiles distinguish patients with different clinical phenotypes and myositis autoantibodies. *Arthritis Rheum.* (2006) 54:3670–81. doi: 10.1002/art.22205
49. Gono T, Kawaguchi Y, Kuwana M, Sugiura T, Furuya T, Takagi K, et al. Brief report: association of HLA-DRB1*0101/*0405 with susceptibility to anti-melanoma differentiation-associated gene 5 antibody-positive dermatomyositis in the Japanese population. *Arthritis Rheum.* (2012) 64:3736–40. doi: 10.1002/art.34657
50. Gunawardena H, Wedderburn LR, North J, Betteridge Z, Dunphy J, Chinoy H, et al. Clinical associations of autoantibodies to a p155/140 kDa doublet protein in juvenile dermatomyositis. *Rheumatology.* (2008) 47:324–8. doi: 10.1093/rheumatology/kem359
51. Kaji K, Fujimoto M, Hasegawa M, Kondo M, Saito Y, Komura K, et al. Identification of a novel autoantibody reactive with 155 and 140 kDa nuclear proteins in patients with dermatomyositis: an association with malignancy. *Rheumatology.* (2007) 46:25–8. doi: 10.1093/rheumatology/kel161
52. Fiorentino D, Casciola-Rosen L. TIF1 autoantibodies in dermatomyositis shed insight into the cancer-myositis connection. *Arthritis Rheum.* (2012) 64:346–9. doi: 10.1002/art.33402
53. Fujimoto M, Hamaguchi Y, Kaji K, Matsushita T, Ichimura Y, Kodera M, et al. Myositis-specific anti-155/140 autoantibodies target transcription intermediary factor 1 family proteins. *Arthritis Rheum.* (2012) 64:513–22. doi: 10.1002/art.33403
54. Kawai T, Akira S. Regulation of innate immune signalling pathways by the tripartite motif (TRIM) family proteins. *EMBO Mol Med.* (2011) 3:513–27. doi: 10.1002/emmm.201100160
55. Khetchoumian K, Teletin M, Mark M, Lerouge T, Cerviño M, Oulad-Abdelghani M, et al. TIF1delta, a novel HP1-interacting member of the transcriptional intermediary factor 1 (TIF1) family expressed by elongating spermatids. *J Biol Chem.* (2004) 279:48329–41. doi: 10.1074/jbc.M404779200
56. Venturini L, You J, Stadler M, Galien R, Lallemand V, Koken MH, et al. TIF1gamma, a novel member of the transcriptional intermediary factor 1 family. *Oncogene.* (1999) 18:1209–17. doi: 10.1038/sj.onc.1202655
57. Agricola E, Randall RA, Gaarenstroom T, Dupont S, Hill CS. Recruitment of TIF1γ to chromatin via its PHD finger-bromodomain activates its ubiquitin ligase and transcriptional repressor activities. *Mol Cell.* (2011) 43:85–96. doi: 10.1016/j.molcel.2011.05.020
58. Venalis P, Selickaja S, Lundberg K, Rugiene R, Lundberg IE. Association of anti-transcription intermediary factor 1gamma antibodies with paraneoplastic rheumatic syndromes other than dermatomyositis. *Arthritis Care Res.* (2018) 70:648–51. doi: 10.1002/acr.23325
59. Pinal-Fernandez I, Ferrer-Fabregas B, Trallero-Araguas E, Balada E, Martínez MA, Milisenda JC, et al. Tumour TIF1 mutations and loss of heterozygosity related to cancer-associated myositis. *Rheumatology.* (2018) 57:388–96. doi: 10.1093/rheumatology/kex413
60. Joseph CG, Darrah E, Shah AA, Skora AD, Casciola-Rosen LA, Wigley FM, et al. Association of the autoimmune disease scleroderma with an immunologic response to cancer. *Science.* (2014) 343:152–7. doi: 10.1126/science.1246886

61. Schreiber RD, Old LJ, Smyth MJ. Cancer immunoediting: integrating immunity's roles in cancer suppression and promotion. *Science.* (2011) 331:1565–70. doi: 10.1126/science.1203486
62. Parkes JE, Rothwell S, Oldroyd A, Chinoy H, Lamb JA, Myositis Genetics Consortium (MYOGEN). Genetic background may contribute to the latitude-dependent prevalence of dermatomyositis and anti-TIF1-gamma autoantibodies in adult patients with myositis. *Arthritis Res Ther.* (2018) 20:117. doi: 10.1186/s13075-018-1617-9
63. Wang HB, Zhang Y. Mi2, an auto-antigen for dermatomyositis, is an ATP-dependent nucleosome remodeling factor. *Nucleic Acids Res.* (2001) 29:2517–21. doi: 10.1093/nar/29.12.2517
64. Burd CJ, Kinyamu HK, Miller FW, Archer TK. UV radiation regulates Mi-2 through protein translation and stability. *J Biol Chem.* (2008) 283:34976–82. doi: 10.1074/jbc.M805383200
65. Okada S, Weatherhead E, Targoff IN, Wesley R, Miller FW. Global surface ultraviolet radiation intensity may modulate the clinical and immunologic expression of autoimmune muscle disease. *Arthritis Rheum.* (2003) 48:2285–93. doi: 10.1002/art.11090
66. Mammen AL, Casciola-Rosen LA, Hall JC, Christopher-Stine L, Corse AM, Rosen A. Expression of the dermatomyositis autoantigen Mi-2 in regenerating muscle. *Arthritis Rheum.* (2009) 60:3784–93. doi: 10.1002/art.24977
67. O'Hanlon TP, Carrick DM, Targoff IN, Arnett FC, Reveille JD, Carrington M, et al. Immunogenetic risk and protective factors for the idiopathic inflammatory myopathies: distinct HLA-A, -B, -Cw, -DRB1, and -DQA1 allelic profiles distinguish European American patients with different myositis autoantibodies. *Medicine.* (2006) 85:111–27. doi: 10.1097/01.md.0000217525.82287.eb
68. Ghirardello A, Bassi N, Palma L, Borella E, Domeneghetti M, Punzi L, et al. Autoantibodies in polymyositis and dermatomyositis. *Curr Rheumatol Rep.* (2013) 15:335. doi: 10.1007/s11926-013-0335-1
69. Betteridge Z, Gunawardena H, North J, Slinn J, McHugh N. Identification of a novel autoantibody directed against small ubiquitin-like modifier activating enzyme in dermatomyositis. *Arthritis Rheum.* (2007) 56:3132–7. doi: 10.1002/art.22862
70. Ullu E, Weiner AM. Human genes and pseudogenes for the 7SL RNA component of signal recognition particle. *EMBO J.* (1984) 3:3303–10. doi: 10.1002/j.1460-2075.1984.tb02294.x
71. Targoff IN, Johnson AE, Miller FW. Antibody to signal recognition particle in polymyositis. *Arthritis Rheum.* (1990) 33:1361–70. doi: 10.1002/art.1780330908
72. Janda CY, Li J, Oubridge C, Hernández H, Robinson CV, Nagai K. Recognition of a signal peptide by the signal recognition particle. *Nature.* (2010) 465:507–10. doi: 10.1038/nature08870
73. Satoh T, Okano T, Matsui T, Watabe H, Ogasawara T, Kubo K, et al. Novel autoantibodies against 7SL RNA in patients with polymyositis/dermatomyositis. *J Rheumatol.* (2005) 32:1727–33.
74. Okada N, Mimori T, Mukai R, Kashiwagi H, Hardin JA. Characterization of human autoantibodies that selectively precipitate the 7SL RNA component of the signal recognition particle. *J Immunol.* (1987) 138:3219–23.
75. Reeves WH, Nigam SK, Blobel G. Human autoantibodies reactive with the signal-recognition particle. *Proc Natl Acad Sci USA.* (1986) 83:9507–11. doi: 10.1073/pnas.83.24.9507
76. Römisch K, Miller FW, Dobberstein B, High S. Human autoantibodies against the 54 kDa protein of the signal recognition particle block function at multiple stages. *Arthritis Res Ther.* (2006) 8:R39. doi: 10.1186/ar1895
77. Bergua C, Chiavelli H, Allenbach Y, Arouche-Delaperche L, Arnoult C, Bourdenet G, et al. *In vivo* pathogenicity of IgG from patients with anti-SRP or anti-HMGCR autoantibodies in immune-mediated necrotising myopathy. *Ann Rheum Dis.* (2018) 78:131–9. doi: 10.1136/annrheumdis-2018-213518
78. Benveniste O, Drouot L, Jouen F, Charuel JL, Bloch-Queyrat C, Behin A, et al. Correlation of anti-signal recognition particle autoantibody levels with creatine kinase activity in patients with necrotizing myopathy. *Arthritis Rheum.* (2011) 63:1961–71. doi: 10.1002/art.30344
79. Betteridge ZE, Gunawardena H, McHugh NJ. Pathogenic mechanisms of disease in myositis: autoantigens as clues. *Curr Opin Rheumatol.* (2009) 21:604–9. doi: 10.1097/BOR.0b013e328331638a
80. Takeuchi O, Akira S. MDA5/RIG-I and virus recognition. *Curr Opin Immunol.* (2008) 20:17–22. doi: 10.1016/j.coi.2008.01.002
81. Nakashima R, Imura Y, Kobayashi S, Yukawa N, Yoshifuji H, Nojima T, et al. The RIG-I-like receptor IFIH1/MDA5 is a dermatomyositis-specific autoantigen identified by the anti-CADM-140 antibody. *Rheumatology.* (2010) 49:433–40. doi: 10.1093/rheumatology/kep375
82. Gono T, Kawaguchi Y, Satoh T, Kuwana M, Katsumata Y, Takagi K, et al. Clinical manifestation and prognostic factor in anti-melanoma differentiation-associated gene 5 antibody-associated interstitial lung disease as a complication of dermatomyositis. *Rheumatology.* (2010) 49:1713 9. doi: 10.1093/rheumatology/keq149
83. Szodoray P, Szabó Z, Kapitány A, Gyetvai A, Lakos G, Szántó S, et al. Anti-citrullinated protein/peptide autoantibodies in association with genetic and environmental factors as indicators of disease outcome in rheumatoid arthritis. *Autoimmun Rev.* (2010) 9:140–3. doi: 10.1016/j.autrev.2009.04.006
84. Rosendorff A, Sakakibara S, Lu S, Kieff E, Xuan Y, DiBacco A, et al. NXP-2 association with SUMO-2 depends on lysines required for transcriptional repression. *Proc Natl Acad Sci USA.* (2006) 103:5308–13. doi: 10.1073/pnas.0601066103
85. Targoff IN. Laboratory testing in the diagnosis and management of idiopathic inflammatory myopathies. *Rheum Dis Clin North Am.* (2002) 28:859–90. doi: 10.1016/S0889-857X(02)00032-7
86. Männistö T, Surcel HM, Bloigu A, Ruokonen A, Hartikainen AL, Järvelin MR, et al. The effect of freezing, thawing, and short- and long-term storage on serum thyrotropin, thyroid hormones, and thyroid autoantibodies: implications for analyzing samples stored in serum banks. *Clin Chem.* (2007) 53:1986–7. doi: 10.1373/clinchem.2007.091371
87. Gislefoss RE, Grimsrud TK, Morkrid L. Stability of selected serum proteins after long-term storage in the Janus Serum Bank. *Clin Chem Lab Med.* (2009) 47:596–603. doi: 10.1515/CCLM.2009.121
88. Nakashima R, Hosono Y, Mimori T. Clinical significance and new detection system of autoantibodies in myositis with interstitial lung disease. *Lupus.* (2016) 25:925–33. doi: 10.1177/0961203316651748
89. Aggarwal R, Oddis CV, Goudeau D, Fertig N, Metes I, Stephens C, et al. Anti-transcription intermediary factor 1-gamma autoantibody ELISA development and validation. *Rheumatology.* (2014) 53:433–7. doi: 10.1093/rheumatology/ket383
90. Fujimoto M, Murakami A, Kurei S, Okiyama N, Kawakami A, Mishima M, et al. Enzyme-linked immunosorbent assays for detection of anti-transcriptional intermediary factor-1 gamma and anti-Mi-2 autoantibodies in dermatomyositis. *J Dermatol Sci.* (2016) 84:272–81. doi: 10.1016/j.jdermsci.2016.09.013
91. Johnson C, Pinal-Fernandez I, Parikh R, Paik J, Albayda J, Mammen AL, et al. Assessment of mortality in autoimmune myositis with and without associated interstitial lung disease. *Lung.* (2016) 194:733–7. doi: 10.1007/s00408-016-9896-x
92. Qiang JK, Kim WB, Baibergenova A, Alhusayen R. Risk of malignancy in dermatomyositis and polymyositis. *J Cutan Med Surg.* (2017) 21:131–6. doi: 10.1177/1203475416665601
93. Cavagna L, Nuño L, Scirè CA, Govoni M, Longo FJ, Franceschini F, et al. Serum Jo-1 autoantibody and isolated arthritis in the antisynthetase syndrome: review of the literature and report of the experience of AENEAS collaborative group. *Clin Rev Allergy Immunol.* (2017) 52:71–80. doi: 10.1007/s12016-016-8528-9
94. Klein M, Mann H, Pleštilová L, Betteridge Z, McHugh N, Remáková M, et al. Arthritis in idiopathic inflammatory myopathy: clinical features and autoantibody associations. *J Rheumatol.* (2014) 41:1133–9. doi: 10.3899/jrheum.131223
95. Stone KB, Oddis CV, Fertig N, Katsumata Y, Lucas M, Vogt M, et al. Anti-Jo-1 antibody levels correlate with disease activity in idiopathic inflammatory myopathy. *Arthritis Rheum.* (2007) 56:3125–31. doi: 10.1002/art.22865
96. Mescam-Mancini L, Allenbach Y, Hervier B, Devilliers H, Mariampillay K, Dubourg O, et al. Anti-Jo-1 antibody-positive patients show a characteristic necrotizing perifascicular myositis. *Brain.* (2015) 138:2485–92. doi: 10.1093/brain/awv192
97. Maturu VN, Lakshman A, Bal A, Dhir V, Sharma A, Garg M, et al. Antisynthetase syndrome: an under-recognized cause of interstitial lung disease. *Lung India.* (2016) 33:20–6. doi: 10.4103/0970-2113.173055

98. Shi J, Li S, Yang H, Zhang Y, Peng Q, Lu X, et al. Clinical profiles and prognosis of patients with distinct antisynthetase autoantibodies. *J Rheumatol.* (2017) 44:1051–7. doi: 10.3899/jrheum.161480
99. Labirua-Iturburu A, Selva-O'Callaghan A, Vincze M, Dankó K, Vencovsky J, Fisher B, et al. Anti-PL-7 (anti-threonyl-tRNA synthetase) antisynthetase syndrome: clinical manifestations in a series of patients from a European multicenter study (EUMYONET) and review of the literature. *Medicine.* (2012) 91:206–11. doi: 10.1097/MD.0b013e318260977c
100. Marie I, Hatron PY, Dominique S, Cherin P, Mouthon L, Menard JF, et al. Short-term and long-term outcome of anti-Jo1-positive patients with anti-Ro52 antibody. *Semin Arthritis Rheum.* (2012) 41:890–9. doi: 10.1016/j.semarthrit.2011.09.008
101. Madan V, Chinoy H, Griffiths CEM, Cooper RG. Defining cancer-risk, and assessing diagnostic usefulness of myositis serology, in dermatomyositis- Part 2. *Clin Exp Dermatol.* (2009) 34:561–5. doi: 10.1111/j.1365-2230.2009.03227.x
102. Aggarwal R, Oddis CV, Goudeau D, Koontz D, Qi Z, Reed AM, et al. Autoantibody levels in myositis patients correlate with clinical response during B cell depletion with rituximab. *Rheumatology.* (2016) 55:1710. doi: 10.1093/rheumatology/kew275
103. Rider LG, Shah M, Mamyrova G, Huber AM, Rice MM, Targoff IN, et al. The myositis autoantibody phenotypes of the juvenile idiopathic inflammatory myopathies. *Medicine.* (2013) 92:223–43. doi: 10.1097/MD.0b013e31829d08f9
104. Shah M, Mamyrova G, Targoff IN, Huber AM, Malley JD, Rice MM, et al. The clinical phenotypes of the juvenile idiopathic inflammatory myopathies. *Medicine.* (2013) 92:25–41. doi: 10.1097/MD.0b013e31827f264d
105. Trallero-Araguás E, Rodrigo-Pendás JÁ, Selva-O'Callaghan A, Martínez-Gómez X, Bosch X, Labrador-Horrillo M, et al. Usefulness of anti-p155 autoantibody for diagnosing cancer-associated dermatomyositis: a systematic review and meta-analysis. *Arthritis Rheum.* (2012) 64:523–32. doi: 10.1002/art.33379
106. Chiu YE, Co DO. Juvenile dermatomyositis: immunopathogenesis, role of myositis-specific autoantibodies, and review of rituximab use. *Pediatr Dermatol.* (2011) 28:357–67. doi: 10.1111/j.1525-1470.2011.01501.x
107. Casciola-Rosen L, Mammen AL. Myositis autoantibodies. *Curr Opin Rheumatol.* (2012) 24:602–8. doi: 10.1097/BOR.0b013e328358bd85
108. Espada G, Maldonado Cocco JA, Fertig N, Oddis CV. Clinical and serologic characterization of an Argentine pediatric myositis cohort: identification of a novel autoantibody (anti-MJ) to a 142-kDa protein. *J Rheumatol.* (2009) 36:2547–51. doi: 10.3899/jrheum.090461
109. Ceribelli A, Fredi M, Taraborelli M, Cavazzana I, Franceschini F, Quinzanini M, et al. Anti-MJ/NXP-2 autoantibody specificity in a cohort of adult Italian patients with polymyositis/dermatomyositis. *Arthritis Res Ther.* (2012) 14:R97. doi: 10.1186/ar3822
110. Ichimura Y, Matsushita T, Hamaguchi Y, Kaji K, Hasegawa M, Tanino Y, et al. Anti-NXP2 autoantibodies in adult patients with idiopathic inflammatory myopathies: possible association with malignancy. *Ann Rheum Dis.* (2012) 71:710–3. doi: 10.1136/annrheumdis-2011-200697
111. Chance B, Younkin DP, Kelley R, Bank WJ, Berkowitz HD, Argov Z, et al. Magnetic resonance spectroscopy of normal and diseased muscles. *Am J Med Genet.* (1986) 25:659–79. doi: 10.1002/ajmg.13202 50408
112. Tansley SL, Betteridge ZE, Gunawardena H, Jacques TS, Owens CM, Pilkington C, et al. Anti-MDA5 autoantibodies in juvenile dermatomyositis identify a distinct clinical phenotype: a prospective cohort study. *Arthritis Res Ther.* (2014) 16:R138. doi: 10.1186/ar4600
113. Palterer B, Vitiello G, Carraresi A, Giudizi MG, Cammelli D, Parronchi P. Bench to bedside review of myositis autoantibodies. *Clin Mol Allergy.* (2018) 16:5. doi: 10.1186/s12948-018-0084-9
114. Fiorentino D, Chung L, Zwerner J, Rosen A, Casciola-Rosen L. The mucocutaneous and systemic phenotype of dermatomyositis patients with antibodies to MDA5 (CADM-140): a retrospective study. *J Am Acad Dermatol.* (2011) 65:25–34. doi: 10.1016/j.jaad.2010.09.016
115. Hall JC, Casciola-Rosen L, Samedy LA, Werner J, Owoyemi K, Danoff SK, et al. Anti-melanoma differentiation-associated protein 5-associated dermatomyositis: expanding the clinical spectrum. *Arthritis Care Res.* (2013) 65:1307–15. doi: 10.1002/acr.21992
116. Tarricone E, Ghirardello A, Rampudda M, Bassi N, Punzi L, Doria A. Anti-SAE antibodies in autoimmune myositis: identification by unlabelled protein immunoprecipitation in an Italian patient cohort. *J Immunol Methods.* (2012) 384:128–34. doi: 10.1016/j.jim.2012.07.019
117. Muro Y, Sugiura K, Akiyama M. Low prevalence of anti-small ubiquitin-like modifier activating enzyme antibodies in dermatomyositis patients. *Autoimmunity.* (2013) 46:279–84. doi: 10.3109/08916934.2012.755958
118. Rider LG, Katz JD, Jones OY. Developments in the classification and treatment of the juvenile idiopathic inflammatory myopathies. *Rheum Dis Clin North Am.* (2013) 39:877–904. doi: 10.1016/j.rdc.2013.06.001
119. Hamaguchi Y, Kuwana M, Hoshino K, Hasegawa M, Kaji K, Matsushita T, et al. Clinical correlations with dermatomyositis-specific autoantibodies in adult Japanese patients with dermatomyositis: a multicenter cross-sectional study. *Arch Dermatol.* (2011) 147:391–8. doi: 10.1001/archdermatol.2011.52
120. Rouster-Stevens KA, Pachman LM. Autoantibody to signal recognition particle in African American girls with juvenile polymyositis. *J Rheumatol.* (2008) 35:927–9.
121. Momomura M, Miyamae T, Nozawa T, Kikuchi M, Kizawa T, Imagawa T, et al. Serum levels of anti-SRP54 antibodies reflect disease activity of necrotizing myopathy in a child treated effectively with combinatorial methylprednisolone pulses and plasma exchanges followed by intravenous cyclophosphamide. *Mod Rheumatol.* (2014) 24:529–31. doi: 10.3109/14397595.2013.852852
122. Mammen AL, Pak K, Williams EK, Brisson D, Coresh J, Selvin E, et al. Rarity of anti-3-hydroxy-3-methylglutaryl-coenzyme A reductase antibodies in statin users, including those with self-limited musculoskeletal side effects. *Arthritis Care Res.* (2012) 64:269–72. doi: 10.1002/acr.20662
123. Allenbach Y, Drouot L, Rigolet A, Charuel JL, Jouen F, Romero NB, et al. Anti-HMGCR autoantibodies in European patients with autoimmune necrotizing myopathies: inconstant exposure to statin. *Medicine.* (2014) 93:150–7. doi: 10.1097/MD.0000000000000028
124. Musset L, Allenbach Y, Benveniste O, Boyer O, Bossuyt X, Bentow C, et al. Anti-HMGCR antibodies as a biomarker for immune-mediated necrotizing myopathies: a history of statins and experience from a large international multi-center study. *Autoimmun Rev.* (2016) 15:983–93. doi: 10.1016/j.autrev.2016.07.023
125. Werner JL, Christopher-Stine L, Ghazarian SR, Pak KS, Kus JE, Daya NR, et al. Antibody levels correlate with creatine kinase levels and strength in anti-3-hydroxy-3-methylglutaryl-coenzyme A reductase-associated autoimmune myopathy. *Arthritis Rheum.* (2012) 64:4087–93. doi: 10.1002/art.34673
126. Mohassel P, Mammen AL. Statin-associated autoimmune myopathy and anti-HMGCR autoantibodies. *Muscle Nerve.* (2013) 48:477–83. doi: 10.1002/mus.23854
127. Waters MJ, Limaye V. Clinico-serologic features of statin-induced necrotising autoimmune myopathy in a single-centre cohort. *Clin Rheumatol.* (2018) 37:543–7. doi: 10.1007/s10067-017-3831-2
128. Kishi T, Rider LG, Pak K, Barillas-Arias L, Henrickson M, McCarthy PL, et al. Association of Anti-3-Hydroxy-3-Methylglutaryl-Coenzyme A reductase autoantibodies with DRB1*07:01 and severe myositis in Juvenile myositis patients. *Arthritis Care Res.* (2017) 69:1088–94. doi: 10.1002/acr.23113
129. Liang WC, Uruha A, Suzuki S, Murakami N, Takeshita E, Chen WZ, et al. Pediatric necrotizing myopathy associated with anti-3-hydroxy-3-methylglutaryl-coenzyme A reductase antibodies. *Rheumatology.* (2017) 56:287–93. doi: 10.1093/rheumatology/kew386
130. Shovman O, Gilburd B, Chayat C, Lazar AD, Amital H, Blank M, et al. Anti-HMGCR antibodies demonstrate high diagnostic value in the diagnosis of immune-mediated necrotizing myopathy following statin exposure. *Immunol Res.* (2017) 65:276–81. doi: 10.1007/s12026-016-8867-x
131. Droney L, Gillis D, Wong R. New immunoassays for anti-HMG-CoA reductase antibodies may lead to incorrect diagnosis in inflammatory myositis. *Pathology.* (2017) 49:638–9. doi: 10.1016/j.pathol.2017.04.013
132. Alvarado-Cardenas M, Marin-Sánchez A, Martínez MA, Martínez-Martínez L, Pinal-Fernandez I, Labrador-Horrillo M, et al. Statin-associated autoimmune myopathy: a distinct new IFL pattern can increase the rate of HMGCR antibody detection by clinical laboratories. *Autoimmun Rev.* (2016) 15:1161–6. doi: 10.1016/j.autrev.2016.09.005

133. Palterer B, Cammelli D, Vitiello G, Giudizi MG. Anti-HMGCR and anti-DFS70 antibodies immunofluorescence patterns. *Autoimmun Rev.* (2017) 16:321–2. doi: 10.1016/j.autrev.2017.01.002
134. Allenbach Y, Keraen J, Bouvier AM, Jooste V, Champtiaux N, Hervier B, et al. High risk of cancer in autoimmune necrotizing myopathies: usefulness of myositis specific antibody. *Brain.* (2016) 139:2131–5. doi: 10.1093/brain/aww054
135. Zampieri S, Valente M, Adami N, Biral D, Ghirardello A, Rampudda ME, et al. Polymyositis, dermatomyositis and malignancy: a further intriguing link. *Autoimmun Rev.* (2010) 9:449–53. doi: 10.1016/j.autrev.2009.12.005
136. Buchbinder R, Hill CL. Malignancy in patients with inflammatory myopathy. *Curr Rheumatol Rep.* 4:415–26. doi: 10.1007/s11926-002-0087-9
137. Hill CL, Zhang Y, Sigurgeirsson B, Pukkala E, Mellemkjaer L, Airio A, et al. Frequency of specific cancer types in dermatomyositis and polymyositis: a population-based study. *Lancet.* 357:96–100. doi: 10.1016/S0140-6736(00)03540-6
138. Buchbinder R, Forbes A, Hall S, Dennett X, Giles G. Incidence of malignant disease in biopsy-proven inflammatory myopathy: a population-based Cohort study. *Ann Intern Med.* (2001) 134:1087–95. doi: 10.7326/0003-4819-134-12-200106190-00008
139. Airio A, Pukkala E, Isomäki H. Elevated cancer incidence in patients with dermatomyositis: a population based study. *J Rheumatol.* (1995) 22:1300–3.
140. Barnes BE. Dermatomyositis and malignancya review of the literature. *Ann Intern Med.* (1976) 84:68–76. doi: 10.7326/0003-4819-84-1-68
141. Bonnetblanc JM, Bernard P, Fayol J. Dermatomyositis and malignancy. A multicenter cooperative study. *Dermatologica.* (1990) 180:212–6. doi: 10.1159/000248032
142. Chen YJ, Wu CY, Huang YL, Wang CB, Shen JL, Chang YT. Cancer risks of dermatomyositis and polymyositis: a nationwide cohort study in Taiwan. *Arthritis Res Ther.* (2010) 12:R70. doi: 10.1186/ar2987
143. Chow WH, Gridley G, Mellemkjaer L, McLaughlin JK, Olsen JH, Fraumeni JF. Cancer risk following polymyositis and dermatomyositis: a nationwide cohort study in Denmark. *Cancer Causes Control.* (1995) 6:9–13. doi: 10.1007/BF00051675
144. Maoz CR, Langevitz P, Livneh A, Blumstein Z, Sadeh M, Bank I, et al. High incidence of malignancies in patients with dermatomyositis and polymyositis: an 11-year analysis. *Semin Arthritis Rheum.* (1998) 27:319–24. doi: 10.1016/S0049-0172(98)80052-8
145. Zahr ZA, Baer AN. Malignancy in myositis. *Curr Rheumatol Rep.* (2011) 13:208–15. doi: 10.1007/s11926-011-0169-7
146. Hoshino K, Muro Y, Sugiura K, Tomita Y, Nakashima R, Mimori T. Anti-MDA5 and anti-TIF1-γ antibodies have clinical significance for patients with dermatomyositis. *Rheumatology.* (2010) 49:1726–33. doi: 10.1093/rheumatology/keq153
147. Selva-O'Callaghan A, Trallero-Araguás E, Grau-Junyent JM, Labrador-Horrillo M. Malignancy and myositis: novel autoantibodies and new insights. *Curr Opin Rheumatol.* (2010) 22:627–32. doi: 10.1097/BOR.0b013e32833f1075
148. Fiorentino DF, Chung LS, Christopher-Stine L, Zaba L, Li S, Mammen AL, et al. Most patients with cancer-associated dermatomyositis have antibodies to nuclear matrix protein NXP-2 or transcription intermediary factor 1gamma. *Arthritis Rheum.* (2013) 65:2954–62. doi: 10.1002/art.38093

3

Psychological and Cognitive Markers of Behavioral Variant Frontotemporal Dementia–A Clinical Neuropsychologist's View on Diagnostic Criteria and Beyond

Andreas Johnen[1]* and Maxime Bertoux[2]*

[1] Section for Neuropsychology, Department of Neurology, University Hospital Münster, Münster, Germany, [2] Univ Lille, Inserm UMR 1171 Degenerative and Vascular Cognitive Disorders, CHU Lille, Lille, France

***Correspondence:**
Andreas Johnen
a.johnen@uni-muenster.de
Maxime Bertoux
maxime.bertoux@inserm.fr

Behavioral variant frontotemporal dementia (bvFTD) is the second leading cognitive disorder caused by neurodegeneration in patients under 65 years of age. Characterized by frontal, insular, and/or temporal brain atrophy, patients present with heterogeneous constellations of behavioral and psychological symptoms among which progressive changes in social conduct, lack of empathy, apathy, disinhibited behaviors, and cognitive impairments are frequently observed. Since the histopathology of the disease is heterogeneous and identified genetic mutations only account for ~30% of cases, there are no reliable biomarkers for the diagnosis of bvFTD available in clinical routine as yet. Early detection of bvFTD thus relies on correct application of clinical diagnostic criteria. Their evaluation however, requires expertise and in-depth assessments of cognitive functions, history taking, clinical observations as well as caregiver reports on behavioral and psychological symptoms and their respective changes. With this review, we aim for a critical appraisal of common methods to access the behavioral and psychological symptoms as well as the cognitive alterations presented in the diagnostic criteria for bvFTD. We highlight both, practical difficulties as well as current controversies regarding an overlap of symptoms and particularly cognitive impairments with other neurodegenerative and primary psychiatric diseases. We then review more recent developments and evidence on cognitive, behavioral and psychological symptoms of bvFTD beyond the diagnostic criteria which may prospectively enhance the early detection and differential diagnosis in clinical routine. In particular, evidence on specific impairments in social and emotional processing, praxis abilities as well as interoceptive processing in bvFTD is summarized and potential links with behavior and classic cognitive domains are discussed. We finally outline both, future opportunities and major challenges with regard to the role of clinical neuropsychology in detecting bvFTD and related neurocognitive disorders.

Keywords: bvFTD, cognition, diagnosis, apraxia, social cognition, neuropsychological assessment, interoception, behavior

INTRODUCTION

Behavioral variant frontotemporal dementia (bvFTD) is a neurodegenerative disease characterized by early progressive changes in behavior, social conduct, emotional processing as well as specific cognitive impairments (1, 2). Accounting for this symptomatology is a pronounced and relatively focused neural loss in bilateral frontal, insular, and/or anterior temporal cortices that can typically be found in patients early in the disease.

bvFTD is the most frequent clinical syndrome of FTD (which also includes two other clinical dementia syndromes with predominant language dysfunctions). Fronto-Temporal Lobar Degeneration (FTLD) is the broader pathological disease spectrum also encompassing FTD, motoneuron disease (MND), progressive supranuclear palsy (PSP), and corticobasal degeneration (CBD). Estimated prevalence rates highly vary depending on the employed diagnostic criteria which have been considerably refined during the last two decades (1–3). Prevalence rates are further clouded because bvFTD, FTD, or FTLD patients are not systematically considered separately across studies. The average disease onset of bvFTD is estimated within the early sixth decade of life although patients can also be substantially younger or older as some cases with a disease onset in the 20s and after 85 years of age have been described (4–6). Within the most relevant age range of 45 to 65 years, 10–30 in 100,000 people are estimated to be affected by FTLD (4, 7). Converging evidence then suggests that bvFTD is the second most frequent young-onset (<65 years old) cognitive neurodegenerative disorder following Alzheimer's disease (AD) (4, 7, 8). Due to relatively large symptomatic overlap and the lack of established biomarkers, the prevalence of bvFTD may well be underestimated because of frequent misdiagnoses with either a different neurodegenerative cognitive disorder or a primary psychiatric disorder (9–11). Half of bvFTD patients indeed received a prior primary-psychiatric diagnosis (9, 12).

As FTLD is a heterogenous pathophysiological entity, bvFTD can be caused by different underlying pathologies (13–15). Most of the cases include the abnormal intraneuronal depositions of aberrant forms of specific proteins such as tau (FTLD-tau) and TAR-DNA binding protein 43 (TDP-43; FTLD-TDP) in equal proportion, and less frequently, fused-in-sarcoma (FUS; FTLD-FUS) (16, 17). Currently, no methods allow the detection or prediction of FTLD pathologies during the life of patients and no reliable biomarker exists for the diagnosis of bvFTD, although some associations between genetics and post-mortem histopathological findings have been established (13, 18). While the majority of cases with FTLD are estimated to have a sporadic form, a positive familial history may be found in up to 40% of cases (19, 20), with a suspected autosomal dominant pattern of inheritance found in at least 10% of patients (21, 22). Although other rare genetic variants have been found, mutations in either the MAPT, GRN, or C9orf72 genes account for the vast majority of genetic variants of FTLD. Interestingly, the hexamino acid expansion on the C9orf72 gene is also very frequently associated with families presenting with MND or a combination of FTD and MND (23, 24), suggesting a continuum between both syndromes. Overall, this underlines the importance of a detailed family history during the clinical interview.

On the anatomical level, meta-analyses of the atrophy profile of patients with bvFTD found significant clusters of reduced brain volume in frontomedian areas, in the superior frontal sulcus, parts of the thalamus and insula as well as in striatal regions (25–27). Focal frontal atrophy is a positive marker of bvFTD but can nevertheless be absent or very subtle during the earliest stages of the disease. In those cases, 18-Fluorodeoxyglucose-Positron Emission Tomography (FDG-PET) has shown to enhance diagnostic certainty, by evidencing a regional hypometabolism in similar frontal and anterior temporal brain areas (28, 29). Multimodal imaging approaches simultaneously combining hypometabolism and brain volume loss also showed promising results while being usually not available in clinical routine (30). Interestingly, differential patterns of early brain atrophy have been observed in the genetic forms of bvFTD as well as in asymptomatic mutation carriers, sometimes up to 15 years before the onset of clinical symptoms (31, 32). An atrophy of the hippocampus and amygdala may be observed 15 years before the onset of the disease in asymptomatic MAPT carriers for example (32).

Aims of This Review

As a result of the heterogeneity regarding the underlying pathology of bvFTD, there are currently no reliable, specific, and established biomarkers available to clinicians. A correct and early diagnosis is nevertheless crucial for disease management, initiation of treatment as well as support of the usually highly distressed caregivers (33). Differential diagnosis strongly relies on the correct application of the current FTD Consortium (FTDC) clinical criteria and exclusion of other causes for the symptoms. Recently, however, critics have been raised toward some parts of these criteria, particularly toward their ability to guide the differential diagnosis with AD or primary psychiatric disorders (34, 35). Here, we thus aim for a critical appraisal of the current clinical criteria for the diagnosis of bvFTD. We will highlight strengths, practical difficulties as well as controversies of these criteria, give real-world examples and provide suggestions for their practical evaluation in clinical settings. We then aim to review more recent developments regarding early clinical detection of bvFTD beyond the established diagnostic criteria with an emphasis on in-depth neuropsychological assessment of specific cognitive domains (i.e., social and affective cognition and praxis abilities), physiological alterations (i.e., interoception) and potential links with "classic" behavioral and cognitive symptoms of bvFTD. Finally, we outline current challenges and opportunities for the field of clinical neuropsychology regarding its crucial tasks to develop and establish novel and clinically meaningful "cognitive markers" in order to use them for (i) staging of disease severity, (ii) validating future biomarkers, and (iii) identifying the precise cognitive dysfunctions that will need to be remediated in future disease-modifying strategies for bvFTD.

THE CLINICAL DIAGNOSTIC CRITERIA FOR BVFTD

After an initial paper in 1994, the first comprehensive consensus criteria for bvFTD from the FTDC, an international group of experts on FTD, were released in 1998 (2). These criteria enabled clinicians and researchers to focus on a set of four key criteria for clinical diagnosis, namely a decline in social interpersonal conduct, impairment in regulation of personal conduct, emotional blunting, and loss of insight. Each of these criteria had been standardized by a brief text definition. Key symptoms and definitions have since been consecutively revised and refined and the current set of criteria (1) now reaches high sensitivities and specificities when tested against competing neurodegenerative diseases (by post-mortem pathological confirmation of either of the known underlying FTLD pathologies) as well as good inter-rater reliability (36, 37).

Despite consensus text definitions of the FTDC clinical criteria, clinicians today still face the problem that the criteria have not been standardized by means of "tests" or clinical scales and even the methods of their assessment (e.g., patient anamnesis, clinical judgement, clinical observations, caregiver anamnesis, standardized questionnaires, cognitive performance tests) are not consistently specified and likely differ considerably across centers. In addition, some studies have underlined a substantial overlap between symptoms of specific primary psychiatric diseases (e.g., late-onset unipolar or bipolar affective disorders, schizo-affective disorders) and symptoms of bvFTD. These shared symptoms may explain why bvFTD patients are frequently misdiagnosed with psychiatric disorders as outlined before (9, 12), but they also explain why, on the basis of the FTDC criteria, a significant proportion of psychiatric patients could be misdiagnosed as possible bvFTD (10, 11, 38, 39). Related to the issue of clinical misdiagnoses based on the FTDC criteria and further complicating the picture, a condition mimicking bvFTD has been been described and labeled "bvFTD phenocopy syndrome," implying that patients may display the typical behavioral symptoms of bvFTD but show no progression and no evidence of atrophy or hypometabolism [for a recent systematic review on features of individuals with phenocopy bvFTD, see (40)].

Another important criticism toward the current FTDC criteria for bvFTD is that some exclusion criteria (e.g., the proposed cognitive profile of major executive dysfunction and spared memory functions) seem overly restrictive and may lead to false exclusions (34). In the following, we will first provide an overview on the different sources of information available to clinicians and their respective importance in the process of diagnosing bvFTD. We will then give practical suggestions to assess the proposed behavioral and psychological (section The Clinical Diagnostic Criteria for bvFTD) as well as cognitive (section Cognitive Dysfunctions in bvFTD) criteria (see also **Table 1**).

Sources of Information to Evaluate the FTDC Criteria in a Clinical Setting

Clinical-Neurological Examination

A standardized clinical-neurological examination is critical when an initial suspicion of bvFTD is raised, mainly to exclude alternative causes for the symptoms. For example, ~10% of patients with FTD develop MND and 10–15% of patients with MND also meet criteria for bvFTD (41, 42). Because bvFTD symptomatology may also overlap with CBD and PSP, a standardized neurological assessment of (extrapyramidal) motor functions is particularly important. In most cases of early stage bvFTD, the neurological examination reveals few obvious abnormalities. In particular, reflexes and motor functions are usually not pathological, although primitive "frontal" reflexes (utilization, gripping reflexes) may sometimes be observed (43). Although originally described as a classic sign for PSP, a positive applause sign may also be observed in bvFTD and may be correlated to overall disease severity (44). Another frequently described cognitive-neurological sign of patients with bvFTD is difficulty or failure to perform anti-saccades, most likely reflecting an inability to inhibit the overlearned motor response of a saccade toward a stimulus as compared to its opposing direction (anti-saccade) (45–47). Other clinical signs frequently seen in patients with AD like the "head turning sign," are not particularly indicative of bvFTD (48).

Patient Anamnesis and Clinical Observations of Patients

Patients with bvFTD usually have a diminished or absent sense for the behavioral, cognitive, or psychological changes that are reported by their relatives or co-workers (sometimes referred to as anosognosia). Unlike the lead symptoms of other early neurocognitive disorders, cognitive, or behavioral symptoms are thus rarely spontaneously reported by patients with bvFTD. If they are, reports are usually brief or shallow, in a stereotypical manner and without showing a coherent sense of either suffering from the symptoms or being overly worried about them. During anamnesis, patients with early bvFTD may even remain to be affectively indifferent when directly confronted with reports of negative consequences of their pathological behaviors (e.g., on their family well-being) or with negative feedback (e.g., regarding their poor cognitive test performances). Although an anosognosia or lack of insight into cognitive and behavioral symptoms may sometimes also be observed in patients with AD, a striking difference in patients with bvFTD is a frequent lack of appropriate emotional participation or affective involvement during the clinical assessment and diagnostic procedure (sometimes specifically referred to as anosodiaphoria or in a wider sense as a sign of "emotional blunting"). Such typical clinical observations during anamnesis may be used to develop an initial suspicion of bvFTD but are highly subjective and require clinical expertise. Only few attempts on the other hand have been published to standardize behavioral observations of patients with bvFTD in clinical contexts (49) or in home settings (50). Preliminary validation studies of these scales have shown that

TABLE 1 | Clinical, behavioral, psychological, and cognitive diagnostic domains for bvFTD.

Domain	Suggested method of assessment (scale/test)	Typical results/observation in early bvFTD
Anamnesis/clinical and neurological examination		
Motor-disinhibition	Saccade and anti-saccade test	Fails to perform anti-saccades as compared to saccades.
Speech and language	Clinical observation	Monotonous speech with little tonal modulation, stereotypic utterances, use of "foul" language.
Emotional blunting	Clinical observation	Seems indifferent and without adequate affect toward diagnostic process or toward the suffering of caregivers.
Anosognosia/Lack of insight	Clinical observation and confrontation with deficits	Spontaneously reports little complaints or only in a stereotypic, shallow way. Reacts indifferent toward cognitive deficits or caregiver reports of behavioral changes.
Behavioral and psychological symptoms		
Behavioral disinhibition	Clinical observation, standardized multiple-domain caregiver interview or questionnaire (e.g., FBI, FrSBE)	High total appearance of disinhibited behaviors compared to healthy subjects and compared to premorbid levels. Possible inappropriate comments or actions during the examination, favored by a lack of rigidity in the clinical setting.
Impulsive, disinhibited eating	Caregiver interview, standardized caregiver questionnaire (e.g., APEHQ)	Shows a disinhibited eating pattern and prefers sweets and candy ("sweet tooth"), sometimes increased, impulsive consumption of alcohol or cigarettes.
Apathy	Clinical observation, standardized caregiver questionnaire (e.g., ACL)	High levels of apathy and inertia, few interests, usually little suffering or complaints about affective/mood disturbances. Sometimes there is a need of frequent incentives from the clinicians during non-directive examination and a possible over compliance to the clinician's instructions.
Loss of empathy	Caregiver interview or standardized caregiver questionnaire (e.g., IRI)	Lacks empathy for others, seems irresponsible for others; significant changes in caring compared to premorbid behaviors.
Change of humor or music preference	Clinical observation, caregiver interview	Prefers simple humor (e.g., "slapstick") and less complex types of music as compared to former preferences; sometimes excessive and repetitive consumption of television programs or music.
Rituals and obsessive-compulsive behaviors	Clinical observation, caregiver interview	Excessive collecting or hoarding, sometimes accompanied by deficits in self-care and hygiene (Diogenes syndrome).
Cognitive performance		
Executive Functions	Standardized neuropsychological tests	Subnormal performance specifically in tasks for behavioral inhibition (e.g., Hayling-task) and cognitive flexibility (e.g., letter fluency). Multiple subtest screenings (e.g., FAB, INECO, FRONTIERS) cannot reliably discriminate bvFTD from other neurodegenerative disorders.
Episodic (verbal) memory	Standardized neuropsychological tests (e.g., FCSRT, RAVLT, CVLT-II)	Often subnormal learning curve and deficient free recall compared to healthy controls/normative data. Possible total (cued) recall deficit as well as (free and cued) delayed recall decrease.
Visuospatial processing and navigation	Standardized neuropsychological tests (e.g., RCFT)	Visuoconstruction and drawing usually spared but may nevertheless appear deficient due to planning deficits and visual organization deficits. Use of qualitative strategy scores are recommended
Social Cognition	Standardized neuropsychological tests (e.g., Mini-SEA)	Reduced ability to recognize facial emotions, particularly those with negative valence. Reduced ability to detect and analyse social norms violations and to infer other's intention and feelings (Theory-of-mind abilities).
Reward processing	Standardized neuropsychological tests	Deficit in reward valuation, reinforcement learning, reversal-learning, decreased sensitivity to losses or delayed reward, diminution of normal cognitive/affective bias.
Apraxia	Standardized neuropsychological tests (e.g., DATE)	Deficits in posture/gesture imitation and pantomime of object-use compared to healthy subjects. Relatively more deficits in "buccofacial" praxis tasks (particularly face imitation) as compared to limb imitation.
Staging of disease severity and progression	Standardized interviews with patient and caregiver (e.g., FTLD-CDR, FRS)	Scales are sensitive for clinical disease progression and may guide clinical observations.

bvFTD, behavioral variant frontotemporal dementia; FBI, Frontal Behavioral Inventory; FrSBe, Frontal Systems Behavioral scale; ACL, apathy checklist; IRI, Interpersonal Reactivity Index; FCSRT, free and cued selective reminding test; RAVLT, Rey auditory Verbal Learning test; CVLT-II, California Verbal Learning Test second edition; RCFT, Rey Complex Figure test; Mini-SEA, Mini Social Emotional Assessment; DATE, Dementia Apraxia Test; FTLD-CDR, Clinical Dementia Rating scale for Frontotemporal Lobar Degeneration; FRS, Frontotemporal rating scale.

standardized observations of behavior are a valid method to delineate patients with bvFTD from other diagnoses, however their application require a rigid and time-consuming assessment that is often not feasible in clinical contexts.

Caregiver Interviews and Standardized Questionnaires

Caregiver reports are so far the main source of information for clinicians to detect and diagnose bvFTD in early disease stages. As psychological and behavioral changes are the lead clinical symptoms of patients with bvFTD they should be assessed extensively through caregiver interviewing, as these information principally allow for a diagnostic differentiation against other common neurodegenerative dementia syndromes like AD (51). As pointed out however, patients with bvFTD frequently present with recent diagnoses of depression, bipolar, schizo-affective disorders, or "burn out" syndromes due to an overlap of similar symptoms e.g., reduced activity, apathy, loss of interest, and in some cases euphoria, agitation, and restlessness (52). To enhance diagnostic accuracy for early bvFTD, it is thus particularly crucial to delineate suspicious behavior and psychological alterations from premorbid personality traits or episodic primary psychiatric disorders. Psychological and behavioral symptoms need to be clearly identified as novel, qualitatively different compared to previous behavior and most important, progressively increasing.

Standardized clinical rating scales that aim at staging symptoms severity in patients with FTLD may thus help clinicians to guide and structure the caregiver anamnesis as well as quantify longitudinal changes of symptoms. The well-known Clinical Dementia Rating scale (CDR) is available in a modified version in order to include behavioral and language dysfunctions geared toward patients with FTD (53). The scale and associated structured interview is available in several languages and has proven successful in staging disease progression in bvFTD. An alternative measurement that focuses more on specific symptoms of bvFTD is the semi-standardized interview Frontotemporal dementia Rating Scale (FRS), which allows a fine-grained clinical severity staging (54).

Several other standardized scales to specifically assess behavioral changes in patients with frontal lobe syndromes are also available (see e.g., **Table 1**). These scales differ in terms of administration (e.g., interview, standardized, or semi-standardized questionnaires) and the included sets or domains of behavioral symptoms. In general, standardized scales on behavioral symptoms that focus on the core features of patients with "frontal lobe syndromes" (e.g., behavioral disinhibition, apathy, irritability, emotional blunting etc.) have been found to be more sensitive for the early detection of bvFTD (55) than more general scales that are geared more toward other features (e.g., hallucinations, delusions) commonly seen in specific primary psychiatric disorders [e.g., the Neuropsychiatric Inventory; NPI (56)]. Psychotic symptoms like delusions and (auditory or visual) hallucinations are rarely seen or reported in patients with early bvFTD although particularly bodily delusions (e.g., altered sense of bodily perceptions) might be more frequent in patients that later develop MND and/or have a C9orf72 mutation (57–59). Among the recommendable caregiver scales on specific frontal behavioral changes are the Frontal Behavioral Inventory [FBI (60), also available in a shortened, modified version that may be used as a questionnaire (61)] and the Frontal Systems Behavioral scale [FrSBe (62), similarly available in a shortened, modified questionnaire version (63)]. The DAPHNE scale, specifically adapted from the current FTDC diagnostic criteria for behavioral and psychological symptoms has also demonstrated good psychometric properties (64). Of note, extensive normative data stratified for age and education are usually not provided for any of these scales and translations into languages other than their original ones are rarely available or unofficial. In addition, only a few studies have been conducted to compare caregiver assessments to patients' self-reports or clinicians' evaluations and it is likely that high levels of caregiver distress impact the reporting of symptoms. In that perspective, more education and caregiver interventions are needed in order to both, alleviate the stress/burden and to reduce bias regarding caregiver reports of symptom severity, especially in longitudinal assessments (65). Finally, it seems important to highlight that behavioral symptoms, or the way patients' relatives react to them, may be subject to large variations due to distinct cultural differences (66). Currently however, the field lacks studies that have assessed how such variations may impact behavior in bvFTD or its inception by caregivers.

Behavioral and Psychological Symptoms of the Current FTDC Criteria

Regarding behavioral and psychological symptoms of bvFTD, the FTDC criteria present five core domains of symptoms, which we will briefly summarize in the following, before we will turn to the currently more heavily discussed "neuropsychology item" of the criteria (in section Cognitive Dysfunctions in bvFTD). Importantly, for a new clinical diagnosis of "possible bvFTD," it is sufficient that any three of the following criteria (e.g., two of the five behavioral/psychological criteria plus the cognition item) are fulfilled (i.e., a functional decline in this domain compared to former level of functioning is seen). Moreover, the criteria require that these symptoms are new and develop "early" i.e., within the first three years of the suspected disease onset. For a higher diagnostic level of evidence ("probable bvFTD"), the criteria require focal atrophy on MRI and/or hypometabolism on PET in frontal or anterior temporal cortices or alternatively, a documented decline of behavioral or cognitive symptoms over time (1).

Behavioral Disinhibition

Socially inappropriate behaviors like inappropriate familiarity or a lack of distance (e.g., staring at or touching the clinician, making inappropriate comments or jokes, being inappropriately jovial) during the anamnesis or during the cognitive assessment (e.g., walking out of the room, smiling, shrugging of shoulders) are often subtle signs of early behavioral disinhibition in bvFTD. Difficulties to inhibit irrelevant stimuli from the environment is often considered as a key feature of bvFTD and patients often struggle to focus on a task because of distractors [e.g., (67)], a symptom that has been linked to "environmental dependency" (68) and to increased stimulus-bound thought and behavior

(69). Pathological gambling and personal neglect or reduced self-care (Diogenes syndrome) have been well-described (70, 71), as well as utilization or imitation behaviors (43, 72). Anecdotal evidence also suggests that patients with bvFTD may have early changes regarding their preferred type of humor that may be viewed as a "loss of manners" by others (i.e., patients tend to make crass jokes or prefer "slapstick" humor) (73). In some cases, patients present with more obvious dissocial behavior (e.g., sexists comments, overt aggression) or criminal actions even in early disease stages (74, 75). Law violations as a potential correlate of increased behavioral disinhibition are indeed frequently observed in bvFTD, as indicated by studies conducted in USA, Japan, and Europe. Patients with bvFTD for example commit law violation up to five times more often than AD patients. These could manifest as theft, traffic violations, physical violence, sexual harassment, trespassing, and public urination, thus reflecting mainly disruptive, impulsive actions (74–76). Patients may also exhibit changes in sexual behavior, but usually show diminished sexual drive, intimacy, and display of affection whereas only rarely hypersexual or inappropriate/disinhibited sexual behaviors are reported (77–79). Importantly disruptive symptoms subsumed under early behavioral disinhibition are major predictors for caregiver distress in bvFTD (80).

Apathy and Inertia

As a behavioral syndrome, apathy could manifest itself as a range of concepts, such as emotional blunting, poor initiation or persistence, indifference to choices, reduced curiosity, lack of interest, and activities, difficulties in implementing actions and social withdrawal. Diminished goal-directed behaviors and intellectual activities (such as reading) as well as diminished responsiveness to emotion are however consensually considered as central to apathy and are among the most frequent symptoms of bvFTD (81–83). Along with cognitive impairments, apathy is also fundamentally related to functional disability in terms of impaired instrumental activities of daily-living and it has a profound impact on patients' relatives (83–85). Immobility and reduced levels of daytime activity for example are seen in almost all patients with bvFTD and are a major source of caregiver distress (85). Along with cognitive impairments, apathy is also closely related to functional disability in terms of impaired instrumental activities of daily-living (86). Excessive TV watching, which may be observed more often in bvFTD than in AD may be perceived as a typical symptom of apathy (87), as well as a general reduction of interest toward pre-morbid activities. Importantly, apathy/inertia (i.e., "negative" symptoms) as well as disinhibited, agitated, or impulsive behaviors (i.e., "positive" symptoms) are no contradiction, but are often concomitantly present in patients with bvFTD and may be differentially triggered by certain situational cues (88). Also potentially related to overall levels of apathy, during anamnesis, patients may show a monotonous speech pattern that lacks modulation and prosody (89, 90). To assess specific symptoms in more detail, the Apathy Evaluation Scale [AES (91)] is available to clinicians.

Loss of Empathy or Sympathy

A diminution or lack of empathy is frequently observed in bvFTD in everyday social contexts and often has considerable negative consequences on caregivers (92). Lack of empathy relies on the interaction of several cognitive and sensorimotor processes (93, 94) and thus is a multifaceted symptom (95) that may be grossly defined as a deficit to share other's affective states (e.g., fear, sadness) leading to an absence of affective concern (and subsequently prosocial behaviors like comforting, helping or caring) for them. In its consensual definition, sympathy does not require one to share a specific affective state with someone else but would rather consist in an emotional reaction, such as sorrow or concern, to other's affective experiences (96). These symptoms could manifest as a diminution of projections into fictional situations such as in movies or books but more frequently, caregivers report a decreased spontaneous tendency to react to other's feelings (97). For example, patients could state their thoughts without considering the feelings of their colleagues or relatives (98). This detachment from friends and family go beyond what could be considered as social withdrawal—as observed in depression or apathy—because it also involves an "emotional blunting" about other's feelings, or, more generally, an overall lack of affective involvement. These deficits often lead to unmoderated, tactless, rough, and sometimes aggressive remarks from patients toward others, including their closest family, leading to what is often perceived as a very selfish and egocentric behavior (67). For instance, patients could be disinterested in spending time with their kids (99), they can be indifferent when their next-of-kin are hospitalized due to illness (98) or they may appear unimpressed when their partners cry during anamnesis. Empathy deficits often have a considerable impact on the family environment and are potentially dramatic for relatives and caregivers, especially as patients with bvFTD could overestimate their own empathic abilities (100). Overall, although empathy decrease can be observed in AD as well, it is substantially higher in bvFTD and plays a more important role in caregiver distress (33, 101). For a standardized clinical assessment of empathy deficits, the Interpersonal Reactivity Index [IRI, (102)], a caregiver questionnaire may be used.

Perserverative, Stereotyped, or Compulsive/Ritualistic Behaviors

Patients with bvFTD frequently become rigid and inflexible regarding daily routines, which they want to preserve, and a substantial proportion develops unusual rituals or behaviors such as hoarding or collecting, similarly to what is observed in obsessive-compulsive disorders (103). Other anecdotally reported ritualistic behaviors are inflexible grooming or walking routines, counting and strict timekeeping as well as checking or sorting behaviors (14). However, in contrast to obsessive-compulsive disorder, these rituals are not due to compulsions in bvFTD as neither their expression nor their disruption are related to feelings of anxiety (104). Utterances during anamnesis may thus also appear stereotypic and repetitive and some patients present with additional verbal and/or simple repetitive motor tics (105). A proportion of patients develop a disinhibited drive to listen to music, and some may change their preferred music-style toward less complex music which they may consume in a preserverative manner (106). Creativity abilities have been shown to change during the disease, with patients exhibiting more naïve, stereotypic, and repetitive form of creation (107, 108).

Eating Behavior and Dietary Changes

Patients with bvFTD show significantly stronger changes in stereotypic/altered eating behaviors compared to AD patients (109). A marked hyperphagia (i.e., higher calory intake) has been found as quite specific for bvFTD when compared with other forms of neurodegenerative dementia syndromes, although patients with semantic dementia may also present with similar symptoms (110, 111). A craving for sweet food ("sweet tooth") and a disinhibited, impulsive pattern of eating has been also frequently described as an early and specific sign of bvFTD, with sometimes patients stuffing aliments into their mouth and eating very quickly (binge eating). Patients with bvFTD may also be affected by hyperorality (e.g., Pica-syndrome, i.e., trying to eat inedible things or increased cigarette consumption) and various other dietary changes (112). While this section suggests that cognitive impairments are closely associated with changes in eating beahviors, it is important to highlight that elevated levels of leptin and insulin in bvFTD (as a direct consequence of hypothalamus atrophy) have also been linked to these symptoms (113, 114). The Appetite And Eating Habits Questionnaire [APEHQ (115)] may be used by clinicians to assess specific information on eating habits in a standardized way.

COGNITIVE DYSFUNCTIONS IN BVFTD

Although cognitive dysfunctions are numerically less weighted in the FTDC criteria for bvFTD, representing only 1 out of 6 criteria, the assessment of cognitive performance remains crucial for clinical diagnosis and patient management. Given that the previously described behavioral and psychological changes are often more visible in bvFTD, substantial cognitive impairments (that may account for some of the behavioral symptoms) may easily be overlooked. Recent studies have shown that the vast majority of patients with bvFTD already present with major cognitive dysfunctions in early disease stages when compared with normative data stratified for age and education (116, 117). Presymptomatic mutation carriers (with MAPT mutation) even present with specific (i.e., social cognition and memory) impairments respectively, 2 and 4 years before the diagnosis of bvFTD (118). Critically, commonly used multiple domain screening tests for dementia like the Mini Mental State Examination [MMSE (119)], the Montreal Cognitive Assessment [MoCA (120)] or even the more extensive Addenbrooke's Cognitive Examination [ACE-III (121)] may lack sensitivity to detect bvFTD in early stages and/or specificity to delineate the disease from other conditions, thus clearly warranting a more detailed neuropsychological assessment.

The neuropsychology item in the current criteria requires a cognitive profile of "executive/generation deficits with relative sparing of memory and visuospatial functions" which primarily aims at delineating the cognitive profile of patients with bvFTD from patients with AD (1). An array of recent studies however, revealed a large overlap between early bvFTD and other neurodegenerative diseases (including AD) regarding cognitive performances when using standard neuropsychological test batteries and when examining standard cognitive domains only (117, 122–125). We will thus now summarize the current evidence regarding the cognitive domains mentioned in the criteria (section Cognitive Dysfunctions in bvFTD) and subsequently review newer evidence regarding other cognitive domains (namely social cognition and praxis abilities) that are currently not represented in the criteria (section Promising Cognitive and Psychological Markers for bvFTD Beyond Current Diagnostic Criteria). We finally summarize evidence on impaired processing of interoceptive signals which may constitute a link between a range of cognitive and behavioral deficits in bvFTD.

Executive Functions

Executive functions is an umbrella term for cognitive processes that rely on higher-order cognitive control mechanisms that are proposed to be mainly subserved by a large fronto-parietal network (126, 127). Although the proposed cognitive core deficits in bvFTD are executive dysfunctions, mixed results have been found when evaluating the (differential-) diagnostic properties of performance in neuropsychological tests for executive functions typically used in clinics (116). Executive dysfunction is a common symptom in a range of other neurodegenerative cognitive disorders including Parkinson's disease dementia (128), AD (129), dementia with Lewy-Bodies (130) as well as vascular cognitive impairment (131). When patients reach at least moderate disease severity stages, performances in tests for executive performance becomes strikingly similar across these diagnoses. But even in early stages, assessment of executive functions could not allow to always differentiate bvFTD from AD (116, 122, 125, 129, 132). In addition, executive impairments could be similarly present—or more severe—in a wide range of psychiatric disorders (133–135) and may thus provide only little help for differential diagnosis of bvFTD. Brief screening tools commonly used in clinics and specifically designed to rapidly assess a range of executive functions through a set of commonly employed single tasks [e.g., Frontal Assessment Battery (FAB) (136), INECO Frontal Screening (IFS) (137), FRONTIER Executive Screen (FES) (138)] have shown to effectively detect patients with bvFTD in the general population but have failed to consistently show sharp dissociations between different neurodegenerative dementia syndromes (139). Looking at standard single neuropsychological tasks for executive functions, performances of patients with bvFTD were frequently not unequivocally distinguishable from patients with other neurodegenerative dementia syndromes, including AD (117, 122, 125). This observation remains valid even with the use of more comprehensive evaluation relying on specific neuropsychological batteries such as the Executive Abilities: Measures and Instruments for Neurobehavioral Evaluation and Research (EXAMINER) (129) or the Delis-Kaplan Executive Function System (D-KEFS) (127, 140). When possible, the following part will address the different discriminatory ability of tasks related to classically defined executive domain in the differential diagnosis mainly of bvFTD and AD in early stages.

Response Inhibition and Cognitive Flexibility

Disappointing results in terms of clear discriminative abilities have been shown for the Stroop tests (117, 141, 142), the Wisconsin-Card-Sorting test (143) and graphical sequences (142). Another commonly used test, the Trail-Making-Test part B (TMT-B) may even be more impaired in patients with AD compared to bvFTD (144) although bvFTD patients may be more insensitive to errors in this task (145). Environmental dependency symptoms such as imitation or utilization behavior have been described as more frequently observed in bvFTD than in AD (43, 72) but the variability of their assessment procedures and the probable multidimensionality of these symptoms (68) may have limited the investigations about their clinical relevancy and applicability. Even though saccade or anti-saccade abnormalities are sometimes reported as typical of bvFTD (46, 146), executive-related oculomotor function have been found to be impaired in AD as well (147), although they may be preserved in early disease stages (148). A range of studies have shown that the Hayling test may be a good candidate to more reliably distinguish patients between bvFTD and early AD on the level of individual cases (116, 149) but more research is needed to safely recommend the use of this test in this context test as some contradictory findings have also been reported (142, 150).

Abstract Reasoning

Verbal abstraction deficit as evaluated by categorization/similarities tasks is observed in bvFTD as opposed to AD, during the early stages of the disease (151, 152). These findings are in line with reported increased deficit in proverb interpretation in bvFTD compared to AD (153), although the semantic load of both tasks could also critically impact the performance due to polar temporal involvement (154). On the contrary, clock hand placement in the clock drawing test, hypothesized as involving the ability of abstracting the concept of time and its specific indication, have been shown to be altered preferentially in early AD as compared to bvFTD (155).

Initiation

Design/figural fluency tasks (e.g., 5-point test) are not differentially impaired in bvFTD compared to AD (144) although one study has found a higher number of qualitative repetition errors (156). Patients with bvFTD may score lower compared to AD patients in lexical fluency tasks (129, 157) and may also display a distinct ratio of semantic fluency vs. letter fluency with relatively less impairment in semantic fluency (158, 159).

Strategic Reasoning (Multitasking, Planning Abilities)

The Brixton test did not show any dissociation between bvFTD and AD (160, 161). This is also the case for the Tower of London test (162) although the use of qualitative information has been showed to have the potential to help the discrimination between both diseases (163). The Multiple Errands Test, the Zoo Map (from the Behavioral Assessment of the Dysexecutive Syndrome; BADS) and the Hotel task have all been found to be impaired in bvFTD (149, 164) but the lack of data in AD does not support their use in the context of clinical differential diagnosis. Cognitive estimation has been shown to be impaired in bvFTD as compared to amnestic MCI only (165).

Working Memory and Attentional Control

Auditory attention and verbal working memory deficits have been retrieved through digit span forward and digit span backward tasks respectively, (129, 143, 144) and were neither exclusively nor specifically impaired in bvFTD when compared with AD. Selective attention could be more impaired in bvFTD than in AD as well (141).

Memory, Episodic Future Thinking, and Spatial/Topographical Navigation

Relative sparing of episodic memory remains a diagnostic feature in the neuropsychological criterion for bvFTD and has been historically heralded as one of the clinical gold standards to distinguish bvFTD from AD. However, this notion has been challenged by a study showing that bvFTD could present with severe amnesia, similarly to what is observed in AD (166). The critics that were made to this study (i.e., patients included only received clinical diagnoses and memory storage was only assessed through free recall testing) were addressed in an independent study with diagnoses supported by AD/non-AD biomarkers and memory assessment based on free and cued recall testing that showed similar results and proposed the existence of an amnestic variant of bvFTD following the observation of a bimodal distribution of patients (167). In the next years, several studies showed similar results and helped to further characterize the memory dysfunctions in bvFTD (168–170). A recent meta-analytic review confirmed a 37–62% overlap between bvFTD and AD in learning and recall test performance (171). Independent of the memory test used, the classic profile of bvFTD, i.e., a decreased spontaneous/free recall that can be normalized using recall cues could still be observed in about half of patients with bvFTD, however vast deficits in encoding, storage, and consolidation are present at a similar frequency. Likewise, recognition deficits have been observed in bvFTD (172, 173) further complicating differential diagnosis against AD. Interestingly, longitudinal studies have shown that early bvFTD could already present with severe amnesia (116, 132), in line with a neuropathological study of early FTD (174). While these two longitudinal studies showed a comparable rate of memory decline in bvFTD and AD, another one showed an even faster decline in bvFTD (175). Episodic future thinking, assumed to rely on the same neural mechanisms, has shown to be impaired in bvFTD (176) as well as the emotional enhancement of memory (177), in contrast to mild AD. Prospective memory is also impaired in bvFTD, similarly to AD, in both time-based (the ability to remember and execute an intended action at a future time) and event-based (when a specific event occurs) dimensions (178, 179). Both, recent and remote autobiographical memory were also shown to be impaired in bvFTD as well (180) but only in later stages of the disease (181). The only domain related to memory that seems to be robustly preserved in bvFTD as compared to AD is navigation ability. Topographical short-term memory has been found to be preserved in FTD (182), a finding which has been corroborated by recent studies showing that spatial orientation performance and particularly egocentric orientation (representation of spatial relationships in relation to separate objects) seems better preserved in early bvFTD and could thus allow an effective discrimination against early AD (183–185).

Visuo-Spatial and Visuo-Construction Abilities

Drawing or copying of spatially complex (e.g., three-dimensional) figures and abstract forms (sometimes also referred to as constructional praxis) is a multifactorial process relying on a widespread bilateral neural network from temporo-occipital to parietal and lateral frontal areas (186, 187). From a cognitive stance, visual-perceptual abilities, planning abilities, and more general cognitive control processes are involved in figure-copy performance. Performance in tasks for visuoconstruction, such as drawing and figure copy abilities, has consistently found to be significantly more impaired in patients with AD as compared to bvFTD, and some studies suggest that visuoconstruction and visuoperception may be a specific and unique cognitive marker for preclinical AD (185, 188–191). In two samples (one of which included autopsy-proven FTD patients), patients with FTD had higher scores in the clock drawing test (192, 193). The domain of figure-copy abilities and visuoconstruction has further been shown to be particularly well-preserved in bvFTD over time in comparison to AD and other conditions (175). However, C9orf72 mutation carriers may be more likely to present with visuoconstructional deficits than non-carriers (61, 194). An in-depth assessment of visuospatial processing and visuoconstructional abilities e.g., using tests like the Rey-Osterrieth complex figure test (RCFT) is nevertheless highly recommended for the clinical differentiation between bvFTD and AD (195). Although some patients with bvFTD may still perform bad in some figure copy tasks, this is usually due to a deficit in perceptual organization and planning abilities and not due to a genuine visual-perceptual impairment (196, 197). It is thus recommended to qualitatively take into account the type of errors (e.g., planning deficits vs. spatial deficits) as spatial errors are particularly indicative of AD (198). There are several coding systems available to qualitatively study the types of errors in a visuoconstructive task like the Rey Complex Figure Test (199). Another specific qualitative error in figure-copy tasks that has previously been linked to executive dysfunction in patients with dementia is the phenomenon of "closing in," in which the patient draws the copy very near to the model (200). It will be of particular interest whether qualitative assessment of this and other drawing errors may further enhance differential diagnostic efficiency for bvFTD.

Summary of Cognitive Dysfunctions in bvFTD as Stated in the FTDC Criteria

Taken together, although the majority of studies have confirmed patients with bvFTD to show executive impairment, the proposed prototypical "profile" of pronounced executive dysfunction in bvFTD seems to be of low specificity and the cognitive dysfunctions displayed by patients with bvFTD are more heterogeneous than previously assumed. Although studies conducted in pre-diagnosed genetic bvFTD patients show that attention and executive functions could be early markers of MAPT or GRN mutations (118, 201, 202), they do not seem to precede other early cognitive impairments such as facial emotion recognition deficit or even memory storage impairments (118, 203). Furthermore, not all executive subdomains seem to be impaired in early bvFTD, questioning the notion of a general executive core deficit in bvFTD irrespective of disease stage (116). Small series of cases reports have indeed shown that in the earliest stages of bvFTD, executive functions may be normal (204). Overall, converging evidence rather suggests that only a subset of executive tasks that heavily rely on basic behavioral and motor inhibition abilities are robustly impaired in bvFTD, mostly irrespective of disease stage (116, 139, 142, 205).

PROMISING COGNITIVE AND PSYCHOLOGICAL MARKERS FOR BVFTD BEYOND CURRENT DIAGNOSTIC CRITERIA

In the following section we aim to review newer developments regarding the early detection of bvFTD mainly through cognitive domains currently not mentioned in the FTDC criteria and to give practical suggestions regarding their assessment in clinical routine.

Social and Affective Cognition

Social cognition refers to a set of cognitive processes devoted to, or at least critically involved in, normal social interactions. This conceptual and somewhat arbitrary definition allows disentangling some mechanisms quite specific to the social dimension of cognition from others that may not be considered as specifically "social" despite their importance in interpersonal relationships such as language (206). Affective cognition may be defined as the mechanisms involved in emotional mediation of decision making and judgments, such as valence and reward processing, reinforcement, motivation etc. Both domains overlap widely as in one hand, mechanisms related to affective cognition often underlie social adjustment and in another, group, society, and culture could define or modulate the valence of behaviors. While this field of neurosciences is still emerging, studies that were focused on social and affective cognitive processing in bvFTD have flourished early in the 2000s and have contributed to develop our knowledge on the cognitive domain of social cognition besides helping the characterization of the disease (207, 208). In particular, these early studies showed that bvFTD patients could present a severe and early deficit in facial emotion recognition and theory of mind (or mentalizing), a cognitive ability allowing to infer other people's state of mind, such as what they want, think or feel. These pioneering works were followed by studies aiming to characterize the impairments in bvFTD in contrast to its most frequent differential diagnoses (209–214), to identify the neural correlates of these deficits (215, 216) and to finally enhance the accuracy and earliness of the clinical diagnosis (164, 212). In parallel, the exploration of social and affective cognition in bvFTD also enriched the computational modeling of cognition (217, 218), increased our understanding of the cognitive architecture (219, 220) and provided new theoretical models of social functioning (221). The prototypical social impairments observed in bvFTD have led many to explore social cognition functions in this disease, maybe more than in any other brain disease or neuroatypical functioning, except autism.

Theory of Mind, Mental State-Inference

An impairment in theory of mind abilities has been extensively described in bvFTD (222, 223). Deficits have been observed using different paradigms based on false-belief (224–226), detection of sarcasm (210, 227) or insincere communication (228), agency attribution (229), as well as emotional inference or attribution (209, 230, 231), emotional movement-based inference (232) and social faux pas detection and understanding (207, 209, 212, 213). While similar deficits may be observed in AD as well [e.g., (225, 229) for a review, see (233)], they seem to be variable and to depend on the severity of the disease. In contrast to AD, theory of mind deficits in bvFTD were only sparsely or not associated with other cognitive dysfunctions(209, 225, 232) and only little associations with other cognitive dimensions in bvFTD have been found when cluster-based or regression analyses specifically investing these relationships were employed (219, 220). Considering cases of selective impairment of theory of mind in bvFTD [e.g., (204)], and the vast evidence for theory of mind processing deficits across a wide range of different tasks (i.e., from simple first-order false belief task to more complex test requiring context and social norms processing such as in faux pas detection tasks), a primary deficit of theory of mind in bvFTD, somewhat independent of other cognitive dysfunctions becomes likely. In contrast to that, in AD, a secondary deficit (i.e., impacted by memory or executive dysfunctions) may be assumed (220, 223, 232, 234). However, the primary vs. secondary opposition needs to be refined and may lack of clinical relevancy for single case diagnoses until more reliable measures of theory of mind are available for clinical routine.

Emotion Recognition, Responding, and Expressiveness

Emotion recognition deficits in bvFTD have also been very well described since the earliest studies. Static (208, 235) as well as dynamic (236) facial expression of emotion have been particularly found to be under recognized in bvFTD despite increased eye fixation time being reported (237), with patients over-relying on external contextual information to decode the emotion (238). Emotion responding is also disturbed, with patients showing a diminished self-conscious emotional behavior (embarrassment and amusement) as well as a diminished associated physiological response, particularly toward negative emotional stimuli (239, 240). Similarly, blunted expressiveness in response to emotional stimuli, especially in low-intensity context and decreased autonomic responses such as skin conductance have been observed in bvFTD (241–244). Finally, recent investigations have showed that patients with bvFTD could have difficulties to imitate facial emotion expressions (245). In contrast, independent from the test considered, a systematic review recently conducted has shown that impairment in facial emotion recognition is not a consistent finding in AD and depends on disease severity (246–248).

Self-Related Representations and Agency

Self-related representations are impaired in bvFTD which is sometimes considered as a "prototypical disorder of the self" (249). Patients tend to overestimate their functioning in daily living activities, cognitive, emotional or motivational control, empathic, and social/interpersonal domains (100, 214, 250). As a consequence, they also underestimate their cognitive difficulties and have poor insight about their brain condition and its related management (214, 251). Patients could show inaccurate self-awareness of their current personality (252) and have diminished monitoring abilities and autonomic and emotional reactivity to errors in objective tasks (253, 254). There is also a diminution of the self-reference effect in bvFTD, known to increase performance in controls during memory processing (249).

Social Norms and Rules Processing Deficits

While social norms and rules processing deficits have never been assessed through objective testing in bvFTD unlike in other conditions [e.g., (255)], converging evidence suggest a global deficit in this domain. The differentiation within a culture between proper and improper behaviors that is made through morality mostly provided the most frequent context to assess this domain in the past 20 years. Findings from these studies reported no differences with controls on the evaluation (in terms of right or wrong) of conventional rules such as "how wrong is it if you keep money found on the ground" or in standard moral dilemma such as the Trolley Car Dilemma, in which patients have to adopt a utilitarian choice by deciding between causing the death of either one or five workmen (256). In addition, ratings of responsibility, blameworthiness and punishment were similar between bvFTD, AD and controls in a task involving moral transgressions in low (e.g., cheating for taxes) or high (e.g., murdering one own family) emotional context (257) in a deterministic context (i.e., without free will). However, differences between bvFTD and controls and AD were retrieved in the Footbridge Dilemma that is supposed to illicit empathic concern with a character of the story, as well as in evaluations of social and moral rules that have been considered as being grounded in mutuality and others' respect (256, 258, 259). Interestingly, patients were reported to verbalize less discomfort and also have reduced autonomic response during moral dilemma (256, 260) compared to controls. Lack of empathy, emotional blunting, and cognitive flexibility deficits have been considered as potential explanation for such deficits, as well as an impairment regarding the integration of social contextual information. More recently, the use of more sophisticated tasks to assess moral judgments showed that bvFTD over-rely on outcomes rather than intentions to consider attempted or accidental harms as permissible or not, therefore judging attempted harm as more permissible and accidental harm as less permissible than controls (261).

Reward Processing Deficit and Affective Decision Making

Only a few objective tasks have been used to assess reward processing in bvFTD but they showed that reward processing deficits are also very commonly observed in this disease. Patients could present a general deficit in reward valuation (262, 263) and thus, stimulus-reinforcement learning impairment (264). In patients in earlier stages of the disease who were not impaired in reinforcement learning, difficulties to suppress a previously rewarded behavior when it becomes punishing were observed (215), a lack of "reversal learning" that could prevent the quick adjustments that are needed on a daily basis in the social life. Although social rewards processing itself has been only rarely investigated in bvFTD, one study suggest that patients could be more indifferent to reward in comparison to AD and controls (265). Patients also showed a decreased sensitivity to negative stimuli (266) and delayed reward (267) as well as an absence of some natural decision-making bias such as the certainty effect, leading to a pathologically, albeit more rational, decision-making behavior (268). An innovative, laboratory-based, free-feeding study suggested that binge eating could be partially mediated by reward processing deficit as well, a result coherent with the fact that food is processed as a primary reward in the brain (269). In most of these different tasks, an AD group was included as a pathological control group and showed normal or subnormal performance in comparison to bvFTD. Reward processing deficits could thus be considered as an interesting cognitive marker of bvFTD but more reliable tasks are needed for clinical assessment.

Although the aforementioned tasks could be considered as assessing "decision-making" because they frequently involve binary choices between two items that are modulated by reward or punishment, the concept of decision making has mostly been retained to describe choices based on more complex information processing. In this context, apart from one exception (270), the Iowa Gambling Task has been employed, but revealed controversial results for the diagnosis of bvFTD. While early studies showed a good sensitivity (164) and specificity (209), others reported less clear results (213, 271), revealing a large intra-group variance in patients with bvFTD and AD as well as in controls that was dependent on levels of explicit knowledge individual participants had developed during the task [for a discussion, see (213)].

Symptomatic Behaviors of bvFTD and Social/Affective Cognition Impairments

While direct relationships between specific dysfunctions of social and affective cognition and abnormal behavior in bvFTD still have to be investigated in depth, social cognition assessment offers an objective evaluation of abilities that may drive many aspects of behavior. For example, a deficit in emotion recognition may prevent patients to recognize sadness, fear or anger in others' faces and to adapt their behavior accordingly. An impairment of theory of mind abilities would prevent patients to grasp others' mental states or feelings and thus to predict others' perspectives or actions, leading to behaviors that might appear egocentric or selfish. Similarly, a pathological theory of mind or empathy deficit could lead to commit abuses (223), or to be victim of one. The disintegration of social norms knowledge could also interfere with day-to-day adaptations in new social groups or contexts and may be associated with law violations in bvFTD (272). Alterations in reward processing may have an impact on the motivational aspects of what drives or regulates day-to-day behaviors, and could thus lead to apathy and lack of interest toward others, activities or things (83) and to a decrease of prosocial behavior (273). Likewise disinhibited eating patterns and binge eating has been associated with particular brain circuits involved in reward processing (269). Describing and delineating the different cognitive processes that drive or regulate behavior and that allow a smooth social life is thus among the biggest challenge in modern social and affective neurosciences [e.g., see the recent attempts to delineate apathy into distinct cognitive mechanisms (274, 275)].

Clinical Assessment of Social and Affective Cognition

The identification of social and affective cognition as a distinct cognitive domain [as in the current edition of the Diagnostic And Statistical Manual For Mental Disorders, DSM-5 (276)] allows researchers and clinicians to specifically target its mechanisms for research and clinical assessment. By contrast to behavioral scales or questionnaires such as the IRI, the Social Behavior Observer Checklist or the Social Norms Questionnaire (277), neuropsychological tests of social and affective cognition abilities offer an objective assessment, less impacted by inter-rater variability and by caregivers or clinicians' subjectivity. Thus, although the assessment of social and affective cognition is not mentioned in neuropsychological criteria of bvFTD, we recommend assessing at least one of the aforementioned functions when a social and/or affective cognitive impairment is suspected. Clinically suitable assessment tools differ widely in their length, reliability and norms availability. Clinical validity, i.e., an appropriate sensitivity and specificity for bvFTD is also a key criterion to guide the choice of a clinical tool. Although comparative validity studies are rare, some meta-analyses have been conducted to explore the ability of functions or tests to distinguish bvFTD from AD. For Facial emotion recognition, Ekman faces (278) or dynamic stimuli from the first part of The Awareness of Social Inference Test [TASIT (279)] are among the recommendable assessments in this perspective (280), while the later may not be available in languages other than English. A novel approach to assess emotion processing, which might be more sensitive to slight or subtle impairments is the rating of facial emotion intensity instead of labeling facial emotional expressions (281). For the assessment of theory of mind, Faux pas recognition tests and, to a lesser extent, sarcasm detection appear to be particularly useful to distinguish bvFTD from AD (233). However, particularly faux pas recognition tests are dependent on intact language comprehension, abstract reasoning and patient motivation, limiting their use to early stages of neurodegenerative cognitive disorders (231). Among validated batteries allowing the assessment of both functions (emotion recognition and theory of mind), the TASIT and the mini Social cognition and

Emotional Assessment [mini-SEA; (212)] offer good clinical sensitivity and specificity. Beyond these tools mostly developed for or with patients in neurodegenerative diseases, the Wechsler Advanced Clinical Solutions Social Perception subtest (282), the Edinburgh Social Cognition Test (283) and the EMOTICOM [for Emotion, Motivation, Impulsivity, and Social Cognition (284)] could offer alternative multi-dimensional assessments of social cognitive functions with less language load, but their applicability in neurodegenerative syndromes has not yet been assessed.

Apraxia

Still relatively poorly understood, apraxia is a multifactorial cognitive disorder affecting skilled movement, tool-use and/or gesturing on command despite intact task comprehension and basic sensorimotor functions (285). Impairments in praxis abilities can differentially involve imitation of limb gestures or face postures, the performance of communicative gestures (e.g., pantomiming the use of a common tool) or actual tool-use on command (286). Apraxic movements are qualitatively characterized by slow, insecure, and inaccurate movements which are performed in a halting and erroneous manner including frequent self-corrections (287). Historically, apraxia has been almost exclusively identified and studied in patients with left hemispheric stroke and comorbid aphasia (286, 288, 289). Nonetheless apraxia can also occur in the absence of aphasia, after e.g., right-brain lesions and also in a range of neurodegenerative disorders of which AD has been most extensively studied (290–295).

Apraxia and Impairment of Praxis Domains in Neurodegenerative Diseases

Despite explicit recommendations in consensus diagnostic guidelines for early neurodegenerative dementia syndromes (296) as well as its mentioning as a cognitive subdomain of the visual-perceptual abilities in the DSM-5 (276), the assessment of praxis disorders is currently widely neglected in clinical and neuropsychological diagnostic routine for patients with suspected dementia. Only recently, apraxia has gotten into the focus of clinical research on the early detection and differential diagnosis of neurodegenerative dementia syndromes such as bvFTD and AD (122, 297–300). Although results highly depend on the employed assessment methods and the tested praxis domains, an array of studies has now shown that patients with bvFTD show overall poorer performance in quantitative praxis tasks as well as clinical evaluations of praxis performance (297–301). Regarding the affected dimensions of praxis dysfunction, evidence suggests that performance in the domains imitation of meaningless hand or limb postures, pantomime of common object-use, and particularly imitation of face-postures are each significantly reduced in early stages of bvFTD compared to healthy age-matched controls (299, 302). These results are particularly intriguing as patients with bvFTD show no or only minor comorbid language symptoms in clear contrast to the prototypical apraxic and aphasic patients after left-hemispheric stroke. When compared to patients with AD, bvFTD patients present with a praxis profile of similar or less severe limb apraxia (i.e., imitation of meaningless gestures and pantomime of object-use) but relatively more pronounced buccofacial [or "orofacial," sometimes used synonymously (303)] praxis deficits with a particular impairment regarding the imitation of face postures (122, 297, 299, 301, 302). Across different samples and using diverse apraxia tests such a relative "buccofacial apraxia profile" robustly showed high diagnostic accuracy for the diagnosis of bvFTD and also stood out among several established standard neurocognitive tests and domains (including standard memory and executive tasks) regarding diagnostic accuracy for the discrimination between AD and bvFTD (122, 301). Conversely, a praxis profile that is more indicative of AD (i.e., relatively more deficits in imitation of spatially complex, semantically meaningless limb gestures as compared to facial imitation) successfully predicted ß-amyloid levels (a core biomarker for AD) in the CSF of patients with a wide range of different clinical dementia syndromes (304). Although more research is needed, these results suggest that disease-specific praxis profiles may be related to underlying pathology beyond clinical presentations of neurodegenerative diseases.

Neural Substrates of Praxis Impairments

Regarding neural correlates of praxis impairments, large-scaled lesion studies in patients with stroke imply that limb praxis skills are subserved by densely interconnected but also segregated functional neuroanatomical networks involving parietal, temporal and frontal cortices mainly within the left hemisphere (305–308). More specifically, converging evidence point toward the involvement of at least two segregated neural "streams" for limb praxis [dual-stream model for action (309)]. A "dorsal stream" (leading from occipital visual areas via the parietal cortex into pre-motor areas) is suggested to be involved in gross visuospatial analysis of postures, online-sensorimotor control (e.g., important for the grasping of objects) as well as holding representations of learned skilled movements. For the latter function, neural correlates have been found primarily in the inferior parietal lobe (IPL) so that some authors subdivide this part of the dorsal stream into a "ventro-dorsal stream" (309). The ventral stream (leading from occipital visual areas via the temporo-parietal junction into the anterior temporal lobe) may be more involved with analysis of semantic aspects of gestures and movements including object identification and knowledge about the use and function of tools (307).

To our knowledge, only one study specifically investigated correlations between praxis performance and brain volume in patients with early stage bvFTD and AD so far (310). The authors found significant correlations between performance on the imitation of meaningless limb gestures and volumes of parietal cortices (primarily the IPL and the precuneus), mostly compatible with neural models of limb apraxia derived from patients with stroke. For object-pantomime, the results pointed toward a distinct involvement of the right hemisphere (correlation with middle right temporal gyrus and angular gyrus).

The neural correlates of deficits in buccofacial praxis abilities (as previously mentioned, a domain that is often specifically impaired in bvFTD) are however, mostly unknown regardless of whether investigating patients with stroke or neurodegenerative diseases. Anecdotal evidence however, points toward involvement of (medial) frontal areas and the frontal operculum in buccofacial praxis abilities and/or imitation of face postures (245, 311–313). Interestingly, buccofacial apraxia has also been reported in patients with MND (303).

Clinical Assessment of Praxis Impairments

Praxis dysfunction in bvFTD and other neurodegenerative dementia syndromes may well be tested with standardized assessment tools designed for stroke patients [e.g., Cologne Apraxia Screening (CAS) (314), Test of Upper Limp Apraxia (TULIA-AST) (315)]. However, these tests have not been validated in neurodegenerative dementia samples thus far and it has also not been addressed whether the praxis subdomains included in these tests are similarly relevant or important in neurodegenerative diseases. An exception with that regard is the Dementia Apraxia Test (DATE) (302), which has been constructed using a data-driven approach in order to maximize its utility for the early detection of patients with neurodegenerative dementia and particularly for differential diagnosis between AD and patients with FTD. The test is freely available, offers clinical cut-off scores for dementia (vs. healthy age-matched controls) and has been initially validated in patients with early AD, bvFTD and healthy elderly participants. The test has since also proven valuable for the differential diagnosis of language variants of FTD, showing evidence of disease-specific "apraxia profiles" (301). Data on praxis impairments in other early neurodegenerative patient groups (e.g., Parkinson's disease) as well as more extensive normative data for the DATE involving healthy controls from diverse cultural backgrounds is currently collected.

Interoception and its Potential Links With Social Cognition, Apraxia, and Behavioral Symptoms of bvFTD

Interoception refers to the mechanism allowing us to perceive, infer, and predict our own physiological state through the integration of multimodal sensory input arising from the current state of the body (316). This sense of the body's internal states involves a large-scale brain system among which the insula, the thalamus, the anterior cingulate and the somatosensory cortices play a critical role (317). In bvFTD, interoceptive accuracy, and awareness have been shown to be decreased, notably in relation to fronto-insular gray matter and connectivity decrease (i.e., alterations in functional network connectivity). For example the so-called salience network, functionally connecting the main structures that were identified to be involved in interoceptive processing, has found to be attenuated in bvFTD (318, 319). Deficient processing of internal somatosensory signals in bvFTD has been shown across an array of different modalities including pain, temperature, and heartbeat perception, strengthening the hypothesis that the interoceptive function is a domain-general system supporting or at least strongly overlapping with emotion, motivation/reward processing and affective mental state inference (i.e., theory of mind abilities) (318, 320–324). Compared with healthy subjects, patients with bvFTD for example showed a lower autonomic response toward emotional stimuli (243, 244, 325), even when accuracy of detection was similar (326). Another recent study suggests that interoceptive impairment in different variants of FTD may be related to lower autonomic responses as well as to cognitive aspects of correctly analyzing body state representations (327). Because of the importance of emotion and theory of mind deficits in bvFTD as well as the increasing evidence pointing to interoception deficits and the associations of these deficits with insular damage, bvFTD may represent a prototype to investigate the relationship between these functions and could bring clinical data to understand the generative and predictive nature of the embodied mind.

With regard to links between apraxia, social and affective cognition, and interoception, preliminary data suggest that deficits in the imitation of facial postures may be correlated with facial emotion recognition performance and to a lesser degree also with caregiver reports of social-behavioral abnormalities in bvFTD (301). One reason for these associations and a potential common mechanism for both, facial affect recognition and face imitation may be that an accurate interpretation of internal somatosensory signals (and interoceptive changes) is required to (a) correctly decode and label a facial expression (or a body posture) and (b) to correctly imitate it (328). The broader idea of an "embodied cognition framework" for the perception of action stresses that interoceptive signals (e.g., muscle tonus, perception of spatial body postures) need to be correctly interpreted by the brain in order to then form accurate representations via internal motor simulations [e.g., motor imagery (329, 330)] and subsequently to accurately perform a gesture or posture (331–333). In other words, both accurate interoceptive signals and internal mental simulations (in terms of an accurate interpretation of these signals) may be a necessary and shared prerequisite for the ability to identify and correctly label face postures as well as to imitate them (334). Future research will eventually shed light on the precise associations between (facial) imitation abilities in praxis tasks, facial emotion recognition and processing of interoceptive signals as well as their biological and neural underpinnings in bvFTD and other neurodegenerative syndromes that share an early atrophy of brain regions crucial for interoceptive signal processing (e.g., semantic dementia).

CONCLUSION, CHALLENGES, AND OUTLOOK

Despite refined clinical diagnostic criteria, the early clinical diagnosis of bvFTD is still challenging and requires an in-depth assessment of clinical signs, behavioral and psychological symptoms as well as cognitive performance. Given the typically present anognosia in patients with bvFTD, caregivers are currently the main source of information for the evaluation of disease-typical behavioral and psychological changes. However, a standardized and focused neurocognitive assessment including memory, visuospatial abilities, social cognition, and praxis is crucial for an early differential diagnosis. Although executive dysfunction and preserved episodic memory are required to fulfill the "neuropsychology item" in the current criteria, we have highlighted that a range of studies have shown ambiguous results with more heterogeneous and complex cognitive performance deficits in patients with bvFTD. Neuropsychological assessments of a range of specific functions including aspects of social and affective cognition and praxis abilities have shown to potentially enhance the diagnostic accuracy but are not yet represented in the diagnostic criteria. It is however highly likely that behavioral symptoms e.g., a lack of empathy in bvFTD is mostly a behavioral expression of a social and affective cognitive deficit. Whether behavioral symptoms presented in e.g., psychiatric syndromes or in the phenocopy syndrome of bvFTD could also be captured by specific social and affective cognitive testing remains an open question and a challenge for the field.

In parallel of summarizing behavioral, psychological, and cognitive symptoms of bvFTD, we also presented and critically evaluated common methods of assessment for an early clinical diagnosis of this disease. We came to the conclusion that one of the major challenges of clinical neuropsychology in the coming years will be to fill the current gap of reliable and effective methods to assess cognitive alterations and access the behavioral and psychological symptoms as laid out in the criteria through performance-based testing. Neuropsychologists have to design novel tests that better fit the clinical practice and its requirements. Tools centered on diagnosis, evaluation, and follow-up are critically needed to replace some paper-pencil tests that are in use since several decades. Clinical neuropsychologists need to foster on new theoretical advances (e.g., psychological or neuroscientific models) and concrete (e.g., anatomical or biological) knowledge available in order to design novel ways of assessing cognitive functions and subsequently relate these to the typical behavioral symptoms. The development of new performance-based tasks is necessary to expand our evaluation to the currently over-looked domains of cognition in clinical routine, such as social cognition—a vast domains in itself, as well as reward processing, interoception, decision-making, and praxis abilities. However, in our opinion, there is also a vivid challenge to develop new ways of clinical assessment of the "classic," well-known cognitive functions, such as memory, language, visuospatial processing, or executive functions. Despite the relevance they might have had at a certain time, it is surprising that tests such as the WCST (or its subsequent modified versions), originally published in 1948 (335) and developed to assess abstract reasoning and set-shifting in the normal population, are still used on a daily basis as a clinical test for prefrontal cortex function, despite knowledge about its numerous limits and shortcomings (336) including a lack of validity in non-western cultures (337). Similarly, the typical assessment of "episodic" verbal memory in clinical routine mostly relies on word-list that patients have to remember and recall, despite the lack of ecological value and autonoetic consciousness of this paradigm and the known confounding factor of semantic processing in cue-based recall tests (34). In particular, we believe that the social dimensions of cognitive key domains such as memory need to be taken into account in order to design more ecologically valid tests from which conclusions relevant for both clinical diagnosis and patients' activities of daily living may be drawn. In this perspective, individualized tests that use items specifically relevant to one patient [e.g., presenting faces from colleagues or friends to assess face familiarity (338)] are interesting, although certainly difficult to implement in clinical routine. Digital assessment technologies including computer-games or virtual reality are promising for clinical neuropsychology, however available apps frequently lack data on convergent validity with standard paper-pencil tests and normative data crucial for the interpretation of individual performance is rarely provided. Nevertheless, app-based cognitive research offers promising new opportunities by potentially increasing caregiver's and patient's motivation to participate in cognitive assessments, for example at home and thus with a maximum of comfort. Apps may also provide enormously large data-sets from which normative data and also very early abnormalities may be extracted using statistical "big-data" methods [for a successful example see a recent data analysis involving the app "Sea Hero Quest" (339)].

In the specific case of bvFTD, we believe that a major limitation to include some already well-described novel cognitive markers in the diagnostic criteria is the lack of availability of many current cognitive performance tests and behavioral scales. One of the potential reasons for this is an overall lack of research regarding cross-validation of the existing instruments as well as establishing adequate normative data and evidence of psychometric quality. These approaches require a lot of time and energy while being commonly disregarded in academia and research, as the former often leads to replications or negative-findings and the later will only be published in neuropsychology-specific, often national journals. This might be especially true for neuropsychological tools that are developed within a medical context (such as in neurodegeneration) as the difficulty to convince about the importance of psychometric studies and to conduct such studies in medicine may be higher than in the field of psychology. These shortcomings however, frequently impede a standardized interpretation of a patient's test result (by means of an evaluation of its abnormality) even when standardized performance tests or clinical scales are available for certain symptoms of bvFTD. Particularly, official translations into different languages are rarely provided or have usually not been independently validated in other cultures. In the case of diagnosing bvFTD, this is especially problematic as for example, perceived abnormality of social behaviors is highly culture-dependent. Such cultural variations may directly impact performance-tests as well as, for example, in the commonly used faux pas test: to mistake a young girl for a boy because she has short hair or a man for a waiter because he stands near the checkout in a restaurant may have been considered as rude and as a social faux pas in 1999 in the context of upper-class cantabrigian population in which the test has been originally developed, but may be perceived as simple mistakes without any negative social consequences for a lot of people 20 years later. Although cultural and socio-economical variability may appear as more important for the domain of social cognition, its influence may also be observed in a wide range of neuropsychological measures and "classic" cognitive domains [e.g., (340, 341)]. Finally, the vast majority of the presented standardized performance-tests and scales to differentiate between bvFTD and competing diagnoses (e.g., AD, affective disorders, other neurodegenerative diseases) have so far mainly been shown to function in usually small samples (with specific demographic and cultural characteristics), highlighting the importance of collaborative research and cross-cultural validation studies. Replications and cross-validation studies of tests and scales in larger and more diverse samples including extensive collection of data from healthy controls are needed in order to extrapolate from individual test results onto specific diagnostic decisions (e.g., Which cognitive performance profile or which set of behaviors are both pathological/abnormal and specific for an early diagnosis of bvFTD in a certain age-group, for a specific level of education, and in a certain culture?). In our view, this is currently one of the major challenges in the field of clinical neuropsychology but also a crucial prerequisite for the future establishment of valid and meaningful biomarkers for FTLD. In this perspective, the Social cognition and FTLD network (https://sites.google.com/view/soccogftld) has been created in order to share data on healthy controls and patients allowing large-scale clinical validity and cross-cultural studies—so far using the mini-SEA. If multiplicated, such initiatives may bring important data on both cognitive functions and the tests used to assess them and could later fasten the inclusion of specific cognitive dysfunction into the diagnostic criteria for neurodegenerative diseases.

An important future role of clinical neuropsychology will emerge with the evaluation and comparison of newly developed biomarkers by means of employing the complex assessment methods for behavioral, psychological symptoms as well as cognitive functions in patients with suspected bvFTD and competing diagnoses. Besides its role in cognitive rehabilitation, expertise in clinical neuropsychology will thus continue to play an important role in the detection and diagnosis of early bvFTD even and particularly in the light of emerging biomarkers for the disease.

AUTHOR CONTRIBUTIONS

All authors listed have made a substantial, direct and intellectual contribution to the work, and approved it for publication.

FUNDING

We acknowledge support from the Open Access Publication Fund of the University of Muenster.

REFERENCES

1. Rascovsky K, Hodges JR, Knopman D, Mendez MF, Kramer JH, Neuhaus J, et al. Sensitivity of revised diagnostic criteria for the behavioural variant of frontotemporal dementia. *Brain.* (2011) 134:2456–77. doi: 10.1093/brain/awr179
2. Neary D, Snowden J, Gustafson L. Frontotemporal lobar degeneration A consensus on clinical diagnostic criteria. *Neurology.* (1998) 51:1546–54. doi: 10.1212/WNL.51.6.1546
3. Pressman PS, Miller BL. Diagnosis and management of behavioral variant frontotemporal dementia. *Biol Psychiatry.* (2014) 75:574–81. doi: 10.1016/j.biopsych.2013.11.006
4. Hogan DB, Jetté N, Fiest KM, Roberts JI, Pearson D, Smith EE, et al. The prevalence and incidence of frontotemporal dementia: a systematic review. *Can J Neurol Sci.* (2016) 43:S96–109. doi: 10.1017/cjn.2016.25
5. Onyike CU, Diehl-Schmid J. The epidemiology of frontotemporal dementia. *Int Rev Psychiatry.* (2013) 25:130–7. doi: 10.3109/09540261.2013.776523
6. Gislason TB, Sjögren M, Larsson L, Skoog I. The prevalence of frontal variant frontotemporal dementia and the frontal lobe syndrome in a population based sample of 85 year olds. *J Neurol Neurosurg Psychiatry.* (2003) 74:867–71. doi: 10.1136/jnnp.74.7.867
7. Johnson JK, Diehl J, Mendez MF, Neuhaus J, Shapira JS, Forman M, et al. Frontotemporal lobar degeneration: demographic characteristics of 353 patients. *Arch Neurol.* (2005) 62:925–30. doi: 10.1001/archneur.62.6.925
8. Rosso SM, Kaat LD, Baks T, Joosse M, De Koning I, Pijnenburg Y, et al. Frontotemporal dementia in The Netherlands: patient characteristics and prevalence estimates from a population-based study. *Brain.* (2003) 126:2016–22. doi: 10.1093/brain/awg204
9. Lanata SC, Miller BL. The behavioural variant frontotemporal dementia (bvFTD) syndrome in psychiatry. *J Neurol Neurosurg Psychiatry.* (2016) 87:501–11. doi: 10.1136/jnnp-2015-310697
10. Vijverberg EGB, Dols A, Krudop WA, Peters A, Kerssens CJ, Van Berckel BNM, et al. Diagnostic accuracy of the frontotemporal dementia consensus criteria in the late-onset frontal lobe syndrome. *Dement Geriatr Cogn Disord.* (2016) 41:210–9. doi: 10.1159/000444849
11. Gossink FT, Dols A, Kerssens CJ, Krudop WA, Kerklaan BJ, Scheltens P, et al. Psychiatric diagnoses underlying the phenocopy syndrome of behavioural variant frontotemporal dementia. *J Neurol Neurosurg Psychiatry.* (2016) 87:64–8. doi: 10.1136/jnnp-2014-308284
12. Wooley JD, Khan BK, Murthy NK, Miller BL, Rankin katherine P. The diagnostic challenge of psychiatric symtpoms in neurodegenerative disease; rates of and risk factors for prior psychiatric disgnosis in patients with early neurodegenerative disease. *J Clin Psych.* (2011) 72:126–33. doi: 10.4088/JCP.10m06382oli
13. Perry DC, Brown JA, Possin KL, Datta S, Trujillo A, Radke A, et al. Clinicopathological correlations in behavioural variant frontotemporal dementia. *Brain.* (2017) 2017:1–17. doi: 10.1093/brain/awx254
14. Woollacott IO, Rohrer JD. The clinical spectrum of sporadic and familial forms of frontotemporal dementia. *J Neurochem.* (2016) 138:6–31. doi: 10.1111/jnc.13654
15. Snowden JS, Thompson JC, Stopford CL, Richardson AMT, Gerhard A, Neary D, et al. The clinical diagnosis of early-onset dementias: diagnostic accuracy and clinicopathological relationships. *Brain.* (2011) 134:2478–92. doi: 10.1093/brain/awr189
16. Mackenzie IRA, Neumann M. Molecular neuropathology of frontotemporal dementia: insights into disease mechanisms from postmortem studies. *J Neurochem.* (2016) 138:54–70. doi: 10.1111/jnc.13588
17. Mackenzie IRA, Neumann M, Bigio EH, Cairns NJ, Alafuzoff I, Kril J, et al. Nomenclature for neuropathologic subtypes of frontotemporal lobar degeneration: consensus recommendations. *Acta Neuropathol.* (2009) 117:15–8. doi: 10.1007/s00401-008-0460-5
18. Rohrer JD, Warren JD. Phenotypic signatures of genetic frontotemporal dementia. *Curr Opin Neurol.* (2011) 24:542–9. doi: 10.1097/WCO.0b013e32834cd442
19. Goldman JS, Farmer JM, Van Deerlin VM, Wilhelmsen KC, Miller BL, Grossman M. Frontotemporal dementia: genetics and genetic counseling dilemmas. *Neurologist.* (2004) 10:227–34. doi: 10.1097/01.nrl.0000138735.48533.26
20. Quaid KA. Genetic counseling for frontotemporal dementias. *J Mol Neurosci.* (2011) 45:706–9. doi: 10.1007/s12031-011-9557-8
21. Pottier C, Ravenscroft TA, Sanchez-Contreras M, Rademakers R. Genetics of FTLD: overview and what else we can expect from genetic studies. *J Neurochem.* (2016) 138:32–53. doi: 10.1111/jnc.13622
22. Seelaar H, Rohrer JD, Pijnenburg YL, Fox NC, van Swieten JC. Clinical, genetic and pathological heterogeneity of frontotemporal

dementia: a review. *J Neurol Neurosurg Psychiatry.* (2011) 82:476–86. doi: 10.1136/jnnp.2010.212225

23. Renton AE, Majounie E, Waite A, Simón-Sánchez J, Rollinson S, Gibbs JR, et al. A hexanucleotide repeat expansion in C9ORF72 is the cause of chromosome 9p21-linked ALS-FTD. *Neuron.* (2011) 72:257–68. doi: 10.1016/j.neuron.2011.09.010
24. DeJesus-Hernandez M, Mackenzie IR, Boeve BF, Boxer AL, Baker M, Rutherford NJ, et al. Expanded GGGGCC hexanucleotide repeat in noncoding region of C9ORF72 causes chromosome 9p-linked FTD and ALS. *Neuron.* (2011) 72:245–56. doi: 10.1016/j.neuron.2011.09.011
25. Gordon E, Rohrer JD, Fox NC. Advances in neuroimaging in frontotemporal dementia. *J Neurochem.* (2016) 138:193–210. doi: 10.1111/jnc.13656
26. Pan P, Song W, Yang J. Gray matter atrophy in behavioral variant frontotemporal dementia: a meta-analysis of voxel-based morphometry studies. *Dement Geriatr Cogn Disord.* (2012) 33:141–8. doi: 10.1159/000338176
27. Schroeter ML, Raczka K, Neumann J, Yves von Cramon D. Towards a nosology for frontotemporal lobar degenerations-a meta-analysis involving 267 subjects. *Neuroimage.* (2007) 36:497–510. doi: 10.1016/j.neuroimage.2007.03.024
28. Krämer J, Lueg G, Schiffler P, Vrachimis A, Weckesser M, Wenning C, et al. Diagnostic value of diffusion tensor imaging and positron emission tomography in early stages of frontotemporal dementia. *J Alzheimer's Dis.* (2018) 63:239–53. doi: 10.3233/JAD-170224
29. Kerklaan BJ, van Berckel BNM, Herholz K, Dols A, van der Flier WM, Scheltens P, et al. The added value of 18-fluorodeoxyglucose-positron emission tomography in the diagnosis of the behavioral variant of frontotemporal dementia. *Am J Alzheimer's Dis Other Dementias.* (2014) 29:607–13. doi: 10.1177/1533317514524811
30. Schroeter ML, Laird AR, Chwiesko C, Deuschl C, Schneider E, Bzdok D, et al. Conceptualizing neuropsychiatric diseases with multimodal data-driven meta-analyses - The case of behavioral variant frontotemporal dementia. *Cortex.* (2014) 57:22–37. doi: 10.1016/j.cortex.2014.02.022
31. Whitwell J, Josephs K. Recent advances in the imaging of frontotemporal dementia. *Curr Neurol Neurosci Rep.* (2012) 12:715–23. doi: 10.1007/s11910-012-0317-0
32. Rohrer JD, Nicholas JM, Cash DM, van Swieten J, Dopper E, Jiskoot L, et al. Presymptomatic cognitive and neuroanatomical changes in genetic frontotemporal dementia in the Genetic Frontotemporal dementia Initiative (GENFI) study: a cross-sectional analysis. *Lancet Neurol.* (2015) 14:253–62. doi: 10.1016/S1474-4422(14)70324-2
33. Uflacker A, Edmondson MC, Onyike CU, Appleby BS. Caregiver burden in atypical dementias: comparing frontotemporal dementia, Creutzfeldt-Jakob disease, and Alzheimer's disease. *Int Psychogeriatr.* (2016) 28:269–73. doi: 10.1017/S1041610215001647
34. Hornberger M, Piguet O. Episodic memory in frontotemporal dementia: a critical review. *Brain.* (2012) 135:678–92. doi: 10.1093/brain/aws011
35. Krudop WA, Dols A, Kerssens CJ, Eikelenboom P, Prins ND, Moller C, et al. The pitfall of behavioral variant frontotemporal dementia mimics despite multidisciplinary application of the FTDC criteria. *J Alzheimers Dis.* (2017) 60:959–75. doi: 10.3233/JAD-170608
36. Harris JM, Gall C, Thompson JC, Richardson AMT, Neary D, du Plessis D, et al. Sensitivity and specificity of FTDC criteria for behavioral variant frontotemporal dementia. *Neurology.* (2013) 80:1881–7. doi: 10.1212/WNL.0b013e318292a342
37. La Marre AK, Rascovsky K, Bostrom A, Toofanian P, Wilkins S, Sha SJ, et al. Interrater reliability of the new criteria for behavioral variant frontotemporal dementia. *Neurology.* (2013) 80:1973 7. doi: 10.1212/WNL.0b013e318293e368
38. Dols A, Van Liempt S, Gossink F, Krudop WA, Sikkes S, Pijnenburg YAL, et al. Identifying specific clinical symptoms of behavioral variant frontotemporal dementia versus differential psychiatric disorders in patients presenting with a late-onset frontal lobe syndrome. *J Clin Psychiatry.* (2016) 2016:1391–5. doi: 10.4088/JCP.15m09844
39. Manes F. Psychiatric conditions that can mimic early behavioral variant frontotemporal dementia: the importance of the new diagnostic criteria. *Curr Psychiatry Rep.* (2012) 14:450–2. doi: 10.1007/s11920-012-0294-7
40. Valente ES, Caramelli P, Gambogi LB, Mariano LI, Guimarães HC, Teixeira AL, et al. Phenocopy syndrome of behavioral variant frontotemporal dementia: a systematic review. *Alzheimers Res Ther.* (2019) 2019:11:30. doi: 10.1186/s13195-019-0483-2
41. Lillo P, Mioshi E, Zoing MC, Kiernan MC, Hodges JR. How common are behavioural changes in amyotrophic lateral sclerosis? *Amyotroph Lateral Scler.* (2011) 12:45–51. doi: 10.3109/17482968.2010.520718
42. Burrell JR, Halliday GM, Kril JJ, Ittner LM, Götz J, Kiernan MC, et al. The frontotemporal dementia-motor neuron disease continuum. *Lancet.* (2016) 388:919–31. doi: 10.1016/S0140-6736(16)00737-6
43. Ghosh A, Dutt A, Bhargava P, Snowden J. Environmental dependency behaviours in frontotemporal dementia: have we been underrating them? *J Neurol.* (2013) 260:861–8. doi: 10.1007/s00415-012-6722-0
44. Schönecker S, Hell F, Bötzel K, Wlasich E, Ackl N, Süßmair C, et al. The applause sign in frontotemporal lobar degeneration and related conditions. *J Neurol.* (2019) 266:330–8. doi: 10.1007/s00415-018-9134-y
45. Hellmuth J, Mirsky J, Heuer HW, Matlin A, Jafari A, Garbutt S, et al. Multicenter validation of a bedside antisaccade task as a measure of executive function. *Neurology.* (2012) 78:1824–31. doi: 10.1212/WNL.0b013e318258f785
46. Douglass A, Walterfang M, Velakoulis D, Abel L. Behavioral variant frontotemporal dementia performance on a range of saccadic tasks. *J Alzheimers Dis.* (2018) 65:231–42. doi: 10.3233/JAD-170797
47. Coe BC, Munoz DP. Mechanisms of saccade suppression revealed in the anti-saccade task. *Philos Trans R Soc B Biol Sci.* (2017) 372:192. doi: 10.1098/rstb.2016.0192
48. Durães J, Tábuas-Pereira M, Araújo R, Duro D, Baldeiras I, Santiago B, et al. The head turning sign in dementia and mild cognitive impairment: its relationship to cognition, behavior, and cerebrospinal fluid biomarkers. *Dement Geriatr Cogn Disord.* (2018) 46:42–9. doi: 10.1159/000486531
49. Rankin KP, Santos-Modesitt W, Kramer JH, Pavlic D, Beckman V, Miller BL. Spontaneous social behaviors discriminate behavioral dementias from psychiatric disorders and other dementias. *J Clin Psychiatry.* (2008) 69:60–73. doi: 10.4088/JCP.v69n0109
50. Mendez MF, Fong SS, Shapira JS, Jimenez EE, Kaiser NC, Kremen SA, et al. Observation of social behavior in frontotemporal dementia. *Am J Alzheimers Dis Other Demen.* (2014) 29:215–21. doi: 10.1177/153331751351 7035
51. Mathias JL, Morphett K. Neurobehavioral differences between Alzheimer's disease and frontotemporal dementia : a meta-analysis. *J Clin Exp Neuropsychol.* (2010) 32:682–98. doi: 10.1080/13803390903427414
52. Dols A, Pijnenburg YAL, Wa K, Gossink FT, Stek ML. Late life bipolar disorders evolving into frontotemporal dementia mimic. *Bipolar Disord.* (2015) 17:66–67. doi: 10.2147/NDT.S99229
53. Borroni B, Agosti C, Premi E, Cerini C, Cosseddu M, Paghera B, et al. The FTLD-modified clinical dementia rating scale is a reliable tool for defining disease severity in frontotemporal lobar degeneration: evidence from a brain spect study. *Eur J Neurol.* (2010) 17:703–7. doi: 10.1111/j.1468-1331.2009.02911.x
54. Mioshi E, Hsieh S, Savage S, Hornberger M, Hodges JR. Clinical staging and disease progression in frontotemporal dementia. *Neurology.* (2010) 74:1591–7. doi: 10.1212/WNL.0b013e3181e04070
55. Malloy P, Grace J. A review of rating scales for measuring behavior change due to frontal systems damage background: changes in cognition due to frontal disease or damage. *Cogn Behav Neurol.* (2005) 18:18–27. doi: 10.1097/01.wnn.0000152232.47901.88
56. Cummings JL. The Neuropsychiatric Inventory: assessing psychopathology in dementia patients. *Neurology.* (1997) 48:10–6. doi: 10.1212/WNL.48.5_Suppl_6.10S
57. Snowden JS, Rollinson S, Thompson JC, Harris JM, Stopford CL, Richardson AMT, et al. Distinct clinical and pathological characteristics of frontotemporal dementia associated with C9ORF72 mutations. *Brain.* (2012) 135:693–708. doi: 10.1093/brain/awr355
58. Devenney E, Hornberger M, Irish M, Mioshi E, Burrell J, Tan R, et al. Frontotemporal dementia associated with the C9ORF72 mutation: a unique clinical profile. *JAMA Neurol.* (2014) 71:331–9. doi: 10.1001/jamaneurol.2013.6002

59. Devenney EM, Ahmed RM, Halliday G, Piguet O, Kiernan MC, Hodges JR. Psychiatric disorders in C9orf72 kindreds. *Neurology.* (2018) 91:6344. doi: 10.1212/WNL.0000000000006344
60. Kertesz A, Davidson W, Fox H. Frontal behavioral inventory: diagnostic criteria for frontal lobe dementia. *Can J Neurol Sci.* (1997) 24:29–36. doi: 10.1017/S0317167100021053
61. Suhonen N-M, Hallikainen I, Hanninen T, Jokelainen J, Kruger J, Hall A, et al. The modified frontal behavioral inventory (FBI-mod) for patients with frontotemporal lobar degeneration, alzheimer's disease, and mild cognitive impairment. *J Alzheimer's Dis.* (2017) 56:1241–51. doi: 10.3233/JAD-160983
62. Malloy P, Tremont G, Grace J, Frakey L. The frontal systems behavior scale discriminates frontotemporal dementia from Alzheimer's disease. *Alzheimer's Dement.* (2007) 3:200–3. doi: 10.1016/j.jalz.2007.04.374
63. Duff K, Paulsen JS, Beglinger LJ, Langbehn DR, Wang C, Stout JC, et al. "Frontal" behaviors before the diagnosis of huntington's disease and their relationship to markers of disease progression: evidence of early lack of awareness. *J Neuropsychiatry Clin Neurosci.* (2010) 22:196–207. doi: 10.1176/appi.neuropsych.22.2.196
64. Boutoleau-Bretonnière C, Evrard C, Hardouin JB, Rocher L, Charriau T, Etcharry-Bouyx F, et al. DAPHNE: a new tool for the assessment of the behavioral variant of frontotemporal dementia. *Dement Geriatr Cogn Disord.* (2015) 5:503–16. doi: 10.1159/000440859
65. Wawrziczny E, Larochette C, Papo D, Constant E, Ducharme F, Kergoat MJ, et al. A customized intervention for dementia caregivers: a quasi-experimental design. *J Aging Health.* (2018) 2018:0898264318770056. doi: 10.1177/0898264318770056
66. Ye S, Rosenbohm A, Böhm S, Uttner I, Ji Y, Ludolph AC, et al. Cognitive and behavioral impairments in German and Chinese ALS populations - a *post-hoc* comparison of national study data. *Amyotroph Lateral Scler Frontotemporal Degener.* (2018) 2018:1–9. doi: 10.1080/21678421.2018.1542535
67. Hamdy RC, Kinser A, Kendall-Wilson T, Depelteau A, Whalen K. Impulsive, disinhibited behavior-dining in a restaurant. *Gerontol Geriatr Med.* (2018) 4:2333721418756994. doi: 10.1177/2333721418756994
68. Flanagan EC, Lagarde J, Hahn V, Guichart-Gomez E, Sarazin M, Hornberger M, et al. Executive and social-cognitive determinants of environmental dependency syndrome in behavioral frontotemporal dementia. *Neuropsychology.* (2018) 32:377–84. doi: 10.1037/neu0000433
69. O'Callaghan C, Shine JM, Hodges JR, Andrews-Hanna JR, Irish M. Hippocampal atrophy and intrinsic brain network dysfunction relate to alterations in mind wandering in neurodegeneration. *Proc Natl Acad Sci USA.* (2019) 116:3316–21. doi: 10.1073/pnas.1818523116
70. Finney CM, Mendez MF. Diogenes syndrome in frontotemporal dementia. *Am J Alzheimers Dis Other Demen.* (2017) 32:438–43. doi: 10.1177/1533317517717012
71. Tondo G, De Marchi F, Terazzi E, Sacchetti M, Cantello R. Frontotemporal dementia presenting as gambling disorder: when a psychiatric condition is the clue to a neurodegenerative disease. *Cogn Behav Neurol.* (2017) 30:62–7. doi: 10.1097/WNN.0000000000000122
72. Ghosh A, Dutt A. Utilisation behaviour in frontotemporal dementia. *J Neurol Neurosurg Psychiatry.* (2010) 81:154–6. doi: 10.1136/jnnp.2008.160416
73. Clark CN, Nicholas JM, Gordon E, Golden HL, Cohen MH, Woodward FJ, et al. Altered sense of humor in dementia. *J Alzheimer's Dis.* (2015) 49:111–9. doi: 10.3233/JAD-150413
74. Diehl-Schmid J, Perneczky R, Koch J, Nedopil N, Kurz A. Guilty by suspicion? Criminal behavior in frontotemporal lobar degeneration. *Cogn Behav Neurol.* (2013) 26:73–7. doi: 10.1097/WNN.0b013e31829cff11
75. Liljegren M, Naasan G, Temlett J, Perry DC, Rankin KP, Merrilees J, et al. Criminal behavior in frontotemporal dementia and Alzheimer disease. *JAMA Neurol.* (2015) 72:295–300. doi: 10.1001/jamaneurol.2014.3781
76. Shinagawa S, Shigenobu K, Tagai K, Fukuhara R, Kamimura N, Mori T, et al. Violation of laws in frontotemporal dementia: a multicenter study in Japan. *J Alzheimer's Dis.* (2017) 57:1221–7. doi: 10.3233/JAD-170028
77. Ahmed RM, Goldberg Z, Kaizik C, Kiernan MC, Hodges JR, Piguet O, et al. Neural correlates of changes in sexual function in frontotemporal dementia: implications for reward and physiological functioning. *J Neurol.* (2018) 265:2562–72. doi: 10.1007/s00415-018-9024-3
78. Mendez MF, Shapira JS. Kissing or 'osculation' in frontotemporal dementia. *J Neuropsychiatry Clin Neurosci.* (2014) 26:258–61. doi: 10.1176/appi.neuropsych.13060139
79. Mendez MF, Shapira JS. Hypersexual behavior in frontotemporal dementia: a comparison with early-onset Alzheimer's disease. *Arch Sex Behav.* (2013) 42:501–9. doi: 10.1007/s10508-012-0042-4
80. Cheng ST. Dementia caregiver burden: a research update and critical analysis. *Curr Psychiatry Rep.* (2017) 19:2. doi: 10.1007/s11920-017-0818-2
81. Levy R, Dubois B. Apathy and the functional anatomy of the prefrontal cortex-basal ganglia circuits. *Cereb Cortex.* (2006) 16:916–28. doi: 10.1093/cercor/bhj043
82. Robert P, Onyike CU, Leentjens AFG, Dujardin K, Aalten P, Starkstein S, et al. Proposed diagnostic criteria for apathy in Alzheimer's disease and other neuropsychiatric disorders. *Eur Psychiatry.* (2009) 24:98–104. doi: 10.1016/j.eurpsy.2008.09.001
83. Massimo L, Kales HC, Kolanowski A. State of the science: apathy as a model for investigating behavioral and psychological symptoms in dementia. *J Am Geriatr Soc.* (2018) 66(Suppl 1):S4–12. doi: 10.1111/jgs.15343
84. Massimo L, Powers C, Moore P, Vesely L, Avants B, Gee J, et al. Neuroanatomy of apathy and disinhibition in frontotemporal lobar degeneration. *Dement Geriatr Cogn Disord.* (2009) 27:96–104. doi: 10.1159/000194658
85. Merrilees J, Dowling GA, Hubbard E, Mastick J, Ketelle R, Miller BL. Characterization of apathy in persons with frontotemporal dementia and the impact on family caregivers. *Alzheimer Dis Assoc Disord.* (2013) 27:62–7. doi: 10.1097/WAD.0b013e3182471c54
86. Yassuda MS, Lima da Silva TB, O'Connor CM, Mekala S, Alladi S, Bahia VS, et al. Apathy and functional disability in behavioral variant frontotemporal dementia. *Neurol Clin Pract.* (2018) 8:120–8. doi: 10.1212/CPJ.0000000000000429
87. Shin JS, Kim MS, Kim NS, Kim GH, Seo SW, Kim E-J, et al. Excessive TV watching in patients with frontotemporal dementia. *Neurocase.* (2013) 19:489–96. doi: 10.1080/13554794.2012.701638
88. Lansdall CJ, Coyle-Gilchrist ITS, Jones PS, Rodríguez PV, Wilcox A, Wehmann E, et al. Apathy and impulsivity in frontotemporal lobar degeneration syndromes. *Brain.* (2017) 140:1792–807. doi: 10.1093/brain/awx101
89. Misiewicz S, Brickman AM, Tosto G. Prosodic impairment in dementia: review of the literature. *Curr Alzheimer Res.* (2018) 15:157–63. doi: 10.2174/1567205014666171030115624
90. Nevler N, Ash S, Jester C, Irwin DJ, Liberman M, Grossman M. Automatic measurement of prosody in behavioral variant FTD. *Neurology.* (2017) 89:650–6. doi: 10.1212/WNL.0000000000004236
91. Marin RS, Biedrzycki RC, Firinciogullari S. Reliability and validity of the apathy evaluation scale. *Psychiatry Res.* (1991) 38:143–62. doi: 10.1016/0165-1781(91)90040-V
92. Bartochowski Z, Gatla S, Khoury R, Al-Dahhak R, Grossberg GT. Empathy changes in neurocognitive disorders: a review. *Ann Clin Psychiatry.* (2018) 30:220–32.
93. Shdo SM, Ranasinghe KG, Gola KA, Mielke CJ, Sukhanov PV, Miller BL, et al. Deconstructing empathy: neuroanatomical dissociations between affect sharing and prosocial motivation using a patient lesion model. *Neuropsychologia.* (2018) 116:126–35. doi: 10.1016/j.neuropsychologia.2017.02.010
94. Sturm VE, Sible IJ, Datta S, Hua AY, Perry DC, Kramer JH, et al. Resting parasympathetic dysfunction predicts prosocial helping deficits in behavioral variant frontotemporal dementia. *Cortex.* (2018) 109:141–55. doi: 10.1016/j.cortex.2018.09.006
95. Batson CD. These things called empathy: eight related but distinct phenomena. In: Decety J, William I, editors. *The Social Neuroscience of Empathy.* Cambridge, MA: The MIT Press (2009). doi: 10.7551/mitpress/9780262012973.003.0002
96. Eisenberg N, Eggum ND. Empathic responding: sympathy and personal distress. In: Decety J, William I, editors. *The Social Neuroscience of Empathy.* Cambridge, MA: The MIT Press (2009). doi: 10.7551/mitpress/9780262012973.003.0007

97. Narvid J, Gorno-Tempini ML, Slavotinek A, Dearmond SJ, Cha YH, Miller BL, et al. Of brain and bone: the unusual case of Dr. A. *Neurocase.* (2009) 15:190–205. doi: 10.1080/13554790802632967
98. Cho H, Chin J, Suh MK, Kim HJ, Kim YJ, Ye BS, et al. Postmorbid learning of saxophone playing in a patient with frontotemporal dementia. *Neurocase.* (2015) 21:767–72. doi: 10.1080/13554794.2014.992915
99. Miller BL, Dickerson BC, Lucente DE, Larvie M, Frosch MP. Case records of the Massachusetts General Hospital. Case 9-2015. A 31-year-old man with personality changes and progressive neurologic decline. *N Engl J Med.* (2015) 372:1151–62. doi: 10.1056/NEJMcpc1409839
100. Sollberger M, Rosen HJ, Shany-Ur T, Ullah J, Stanley CM, Laluz V, et al. Neural substrates of socioemotional self-awareness in neurodegenerative disease. *Brain Behav.* (2014) 4:201–14. doi: 10.1002/brb3.211
101. Mioshi E, Foxe D, Leslie F, MClinNeuro SS, Hsieh S, Miller L, et al. The impact of dementia severity on caregiver burden in frontotemporal dementia and alzheimer disease. *Alzheimer Dis Assoc Disord.* (2013) 27:1. doi: 10.1097/WAD.0b013e318247a0bc
102. Davis MH. Measuring individual differences in empathy: evidence for a multidimensional approach. *J Pers Soc Psychol.* (1983) 44:113–26. doi: 10.1037//0022-3514.44.1.113
103. Perry DC, Whitwell JL, Boeve BF, Pankratz VS, Knopman DS, Petersen RC, et al. Voxel-based morphometry in patients with obsessive-compulsive behaviors in behavioral variant frontotemporal dementia. *Eur J Neurol.* (2012) 19:911–7. doi: 10.1111/j.1468-1331.2011.03656.x
104. Moheb N, Charuworn K, Ashla MM, Desarzant R, Chavez D, Mendez MF. Repetitive behaviors in frontotemporal dementia: compulsions or impulsions? *J Neuropsychiatry Clin Neurosci.* (2018) 2018:8060148. doi: 10.1176/appi.neuropsych.18060148
105. Maltete D. Adult-onset stereotypical motor behaviors. *Rev Neurol.* (2016) 172:477–82. doi: 10.1016/j.neurol.2016.07.002
106. Fletcher PD, Downey LE, Witoonpanich P, Warren JD. The brain basis of musicophilia: evidence from frontotemporal lobar degeneration. *Front Psychol.* (2013) 4:1–8. doi: 10.3389/fpsyg.2013.00347
107. De Souza LC, Volle E, Bertoux M, Czernecki V, Funkiewiez A, Allali G, et al. Poor creativity in frontotemporal dementia: a window into the neural bases of the creative mind. *Neuropsychologia.* (2010) 48:3733–42. doi: 10.1016/j.neuropsychologia.2010.09.010
108. de Souza LC, Guimarães HC, Teixeira AL, Caramelli P, Levy R, Dubois B, et al. Frontal lobe neurology and the creative mind. *Front Psychol.* (2014) 5:761. doi: 10.3389/fpsyg.2014.00761
109. Bozeat S, Gregory C, Lambon Ralph MA, Hodges JR. Which neuropsychiatric and behavioural features distinguish frontal and temporal variants of frontotemporal dementia from Alzheimer's disease? *J Neurol Neurosurg Psychiatry.* (2000) 69:178–86. doi: 10.1136/jnnp.69.2.178
110. Ahmed RM, Irish M, Henning E, Dermody N, Bartley L, Kiernan MC, et al. Assessment of eating behavior disturbance and associated neural networks in frontotemporal dementia. *JAMA Neurol.* (2016) 73:282–90. doi: 10.1001/jamaneurol.2015.4478
111. Aiello M, Silani V, Rumiati RI. You stole my food! Eating alterations in frontotemporal dementia. *Neurocase.* (2016) 22:400–9. doi: 10.1080/13554794.2016.1197952
112. Ikeda M, Brown J, Holland AJ, Fukuhara R, Hodges JR. Changes in appetite, food preference, and eating habits in frontotemporal dementia and Alzheimer's disease. *J Neurol Neurosurg Psychiatry.* (2002) 73:371–6. doi: 10.1136/jnnp.73.4.371
113. Woolley JD, Khan BK, Natesan A, Karydas A, Dallman M, Havel P, et al. Satiety-related hormonal dysregulation in behavioral variant frontotemporal dementia. *Neurology.* (2014) 82:512–20. doi: 10.1212/WNL.0000000000000106
114. Ahmed RM, Phan K, Highton-Williamson E, Strikwerda-Brown C, Caga J, Ramsey E, et al. Eating peptides: biomarkers of neurodegeneration in amyotrophic lateral sclerosis and frontotemporal dementia. *Ann Clin Transl Neurol.* (2019) 6:486–95. doi: 10.1002/acn3.721
115. Ahmed RM, Irish M, Kam J, Van Keizerswaard J, Bartley L, Samaras K, et al. Quantifying the eating abnormalities in frontotemporal dementia. *JAMA Neurol.* (2014) 71:1540–6. doi: 10.1001/jamaneurol.2014.1931
116. Ramanan S, Bertoux M, Flanagan E, Irish M, Piguet O, Hodges JR, et al. Longitudinal executive function and episodic memory profiles in behavioral-variant frontotemporal dementia and alzheimer's disease. *J Int Neuropsychol Soc.* (2017) 23:34–43. doi: 10.1017/S1355617716000837
117. Hutchinson AD, Mathias JL. Neuropsychological deficits in frontotemporal dementia and Alzheimer's disease: a meta-analytic review. *J Neurol Neurosurg Psychiatry.* (2007) 78:917–28. doi: 10.1136/jnnp.2006.100669
118. Jiskoot LC, Panman JL, van Asseldonk L, Franzen S, Meeter LHH, Donker Kaat L, et al. Longitudinal cognitive biomarkers predicting symptom onset in presymptomatic frontotemporal dementia. *J Neurol.* (2018) 265:1381–92. doi: 10.1007/s00415-018-8850-7
119. Folstein MF, Folstein SE, McHugh PR, Ingles J. 'Mini-mental state'. A practical method for grading the cognitive state of patients for the clinician. *J Psychiatr Res.* (1975) 12:189–98. doi: 10.1016/0022-3956(75)90026-6
120. Nasreddine ZS, Phillips NA, Bédirian V, Charbonneau S, Whitehead V, Collin I, et al. The montreal cognitive assessment, MoCA: a brief screening tool for mild cognitive impairment. *J Am Geriatr Soc.* (2005) 53:695–9. doi: 10.1111/j.1532-5415.2005.53221.x
121. Hsieh S, Schubert S, Hoon C, Mioshi E, Hodges JR. Validation of the Addenbrooke's cognitive examination III in frontotemporal dementia and alzheimer's disease. *Dement Geriatr Cogn Disord.* (2013) 36:242–50. doi: 10.1159/000351671
122. Reul S, Lohmann H, Wiendl H, Duning T, Johnen A. Can cognitive assessment really discriminate early stages of Alzheimer's and behavioural variant frontotemporal dementia at initial clinical presentation? *Alzheimers Res Ther.* (2017) 9:1–12. doi: 10.1186/s13195-017-0287-1
123. Lagarde J, Valabrègue R, Corvol JC, Pineau F, Le Ber I, Vidailhet M, et al. Are frontal cognitive and atrophy patterns different in PSP and bvFTD? A comparative neuropsychological and VBM study. *PLoS ONE.* (2013) 8:e0080353. doi: 10.1371/journal.pone.0080353
124. Porto CS, Bahia VS, Brucki SMD, Caramelli P, Nitrini R. Neuropsychological differences between frontotemporal lobar degeneration and Alzheimer's disease. *Dement Neuropsychol.* (2008) 2:223–7. doi: 10.1590/S1980-57642009DN20300011
125. Dodich A, Cerami C, Cappa SF, Marcone A, Golzi V, Zamboni M, et al. Combined socio-behavioral evaluation improves the differential diagnosis between the behavioral variant of frontotemporal dementia and Alzheimer's disease: in search of neuropsychological markers. *J Alzheimer's Dis.* (2018) 61:761–72. doi: 10.3233/JAD-170650
126. Stuss DT. Functions of the frontal lobes: relation to executive functions. *J Int Neuropsychol Soc.* (2011) 17:759–65. doi: 10.1017/S1355617711000695
127. Gansler DA, Huey ED, Pan JJ, Wasserman E, Grafman JH. Assessing the dysexecutive syndrome in dementia. *J Neurol Neurosurg Psychiatry.* (2017) 88:254–61. doi: 10.1136/jnnp-2016-313576
128. Kudlicka A, Clare L, Hindle J V. Executive functions in Parkinson's disease: systematic review and meta-analysis. *Mov Disord.* (2011) 26:2305–15. doi: 10.1002/mds.23868
129. Possin KL, Feigenbaum D, Rankin KP, Smith GE, Boxer AL, Wood K, et al. Dissociable executive functions in behavioral variant frontotemporal and Alzheimer dementias. *Neurology.* (2013) 80:2180–5. doi: 10.1212/WNL.0b013e318296e940
130. Gurnani AS, Gavett BE. The differential effects of alzheimer's disease and lewy body pathology on cognitive performance: a meta-analysis. *Neuropsychol Rev.* (2017) 27:9334. doi: 10.1007/s11065-016-9334-0
131. Vasquez BP, Zakzanis KK. The neuropsychological profile of vascular cognitive impairment not demented: a meta-analysis. *J Neuropsychol.* (2015) 9:109–36. doi: 10.1111/jnp.12039
132. Schubert S, Leyton CE, Hodges JR, Piguet O. Longitudinal memory profiles in behavioral-variant frontotemporal dementia and alzheimer's disease. *J Alzheimer's Dis.* (2016) 51:775–82. doi: 10.3233/JAD-150802
133. Fossati P, Ergis AM, Allilaire JF. Problem-solving abilities in unipolar depressed patients: comparison of performance on the modified version of the Wisconsin and the California sorting tests. *Psychiatry Res.* (2001) 104:145–56. doi: 10.1016/S0165-1781(01)00307-9
134. Elderkin-Thompson V, Mintz J, Haroon E, Lavretsky H, Kumar A. Executive dysfunction and memory in older patients with major and minor depression. *Arch Clin Neuropsychol.* (2007) 22:261–70. doi: 10.1016/j.acn.2007.01.021
135. Vijverberg EGB, Schouws S, Meesters PD, Verwijk E, Comijs H, Koene T, et al. Cognitive deficits in patients with neuropsychiatric symptoms:

a comparative study between behavioral variant frontotemporal dementia and primary psychiatric disorders. *J Clin Psychiatry.* (2017) 78:e940–6. doi: 10.4088/JCP.16m11019

136. Dubois B, Slachevsky A, Litvan I, Pillon B. The FAB: a Frontal Assessment Battery at bedside. *Neurology.* (2000) 55:1621–6. doi: 10.1212/WNL.55.11.1621
137. Torralva T, Roca M, Gleichgerrcht E, López P, Manes F. INECO Frontal Screening (IFS): a brief, sensitive, and specific tool to assess executive functions in dementia. *J Int Neuropsychol Soc.* (2009) 15:777–86. doi: 10.1017/S1355617709990415
138. Leslie FVC, Foxe D, Daveson N, Flannagan E, Hodges JR, Piguet O. FRONTIER executive screen: a brief executive battery to differentiate frontotemporal dementia and Alzheimer's disease. *J Neurol Neurosurg Psychiatry.* (2016) 87:831–5. doi: 10.1136/jnnp-2015-311917
139. Moreira HS, Costa AS, Castro SL, Lima CF, Vicente SG. Assessing executive dysfunction in neurodegenerative disorders: a critical review of brief neuropsychological tools. *Front Aging Neurosci.* (2017) 9:369. doi: 10.3389/fnagi.2017.00369
140. Delis D. *Delis-Kaplan Executive Function System (D-KEFS).* The Psychological Corporation: San Antonio, USA, 2001. doi: 10.1037/t15082-000
141. Perry RJ, Hodges JR. Differentiating frontal and temporal variant frontotemporal dementia from Alzheimer's disease. *Neurology.* (2000) 54:2277–84. doi: 10.1212/WNL.54.12.2277
142. Matías-Guiu JA, Cabrera-Martín MN, Valles-Salgado M, Rognoni T, Galán L, Moreno-Ramos T, et al. Inhibition impairment in frontotemporal dementia, amyotrophic lateral sclerosis, and Alzheimer's disease: clinical assessment and metabolic correlates. *Brain Imaging Behav.* (2018) 2018:1–9. doi: 10.1007/s11682-018-9891-3
143. Stopford CL, Thompson JC, Neary D, Richardson AMT, Snowden JS. Working memory, attention, and executive function in Alzheimer's disease and frontotemporal dementia. *Cortex.* (2012) 48:429–46. doi: 10.1016/j.cortex.2010.12.002
144. Ranasinghe KG, Rankin KP, Lobach I V., Kramer JH, Sturm VE, Bettcher BM, et al. Cognition and neuropsychiatry in behavioral variant frontotemporal dementia by disease stage. *Neurology.* (2016) 86:600–10. doi: 10.1212/WNL.0000000000002373
145. Libon DJ, Xie SX, Moore P, Farmer J, Antani S, McCawley G, et al. Patterns of neuropsychological impairment in frontotemporal dementia. *Neurology.* (2007) 68:369–75. doi: 10.1212/01.wnl.0000252820.81313.9b
146. Burrell JR, Hornberger M, Carpenter RHS, Kiernan MC, Hodges JR. Saccadic abnormalities in frontotemporal dementia. *Neurology.* (2012) 78:1816–23. doi: 10.1212/WNL.0b013e318258f75c
147. Garbutt S, Matlin A, Hellmuth J, Schenk AK, Johnson JK, Rosen H, et al. Oculomotor function in frontotemporal lobar degeneration, related disorders and Alzheimer's disease. *Brain.* (2008) 131:1268–81. doi: 10.1093/brain/awn047
148. Heuer WH, Mirsky BJ, Kong LE, Dickerson CB, Miller LB, Kramer HJ, et al. Antisaccade task reflects cortical involvement in mild cognitive impairment. *Neurology.* (2013) 81:1235–43. doi: 10.1212/WNL.0b013e3182a6cbfe
149. Hornberger M, Piguet O, Kipps C, Hodges JR. Executive function in progressive and nonprogressive behavioral variant frontotemporal dementia. *Neurology.* (2008) 71:1481–8. doi: 10.1212/01.wnl.0000334299.72023.c8
150. Buhl C, Stokholm J, Gade A. Clinical utility of short social cognitive tests in early differentiation of behavioral variant frontotemporal dementia from Alzheimer's disease. *Dement Geriatr Cogn Disord.* (2013) 3:376–85. doi: 10.1159/000355123
151. Lagarde J, Valabrégue R, Corvol JC, Garcin B, Volle E, Le Ber I, et al. Why do patients with neurodegenerative frontal syndrome fail to answer: 'in what way are an orange and a banana alike?' *Brain.* (2015) 138:456–71. doi: 10.1093/brain/awu359
152. Garcin B, Volle E, Funkiewiez A, Miller BL, Dubois B, Levy R. A mosquito bites and a butterfly flies: a specific response type of frontal patients in a similarity task. *Neuropsychologia.* (2018) 117:371–8. doi: 10.1016/j.neuropsychologia.2018.06.022
153. Kaiser NC, Lee GJ, Lu PH, Mather MJ, Shapira J, Jimenez E, et al. What dementia reveals about proverb interpretation and its neuroanatomical correlates. *Neuropsychologia.* (2013) 51:1726–33. doi: 10.1016/j.neuropsychologia.2013.05.021
154. Garcin B, Urbanski M, Thiebaut de Schotten M, Levy R, Volle E. Anterior temporal lobe morphometry predicts categorization ability. *Front Hum Neurosci.* (2018) 12:1–12. doi: 10.3389/fnhum.2018.00036
155. Barrows RJ, Barsuglia J, Paholpak P, Eknoyan D, Sabodash V, Lee GJ, et al. Executive abilities as reflected by clock hand placement: frontotemporal dementia versus early-onset alzheimer disease. *J Geriatr Psychiatry Neurol.* (2015) 28:239–48. doi: 10.1177/0891988715598228
156. Possin KL, Chester SK, Laluz V, Bostrom A, Rosen HJ, Miller BL, et al. The frontal-anatomic specificity of design fluency repetitions and their diagnostic relevance for behavioral variant frontotemporal dementia. *J Int Neuropsychol Soc.* (2012) 18:834–44. doi: 10.1017/S1355617712000604
157. Diehl J, Monsch AU, Aebi C, Wagenpfeil S, Krapp S, Grimmer T, et al. Frontotemporal dementia, semantic dementia, and Alzheimer's disease: the contribution of standard neuropsychological tests to differential diagnosis. *J Geriatr Psychiatry Neurol.* (2005) 18:39–44. doi: 10.1177/0891988704272309
158. Rascovsky K, Salmon DP, Hansen LA, Thal LJ, Galasko D. Disparate letter and semantic category fluency deficits in autopsy-confirmed frontotemporal dementia and Alzheimer's disease. *Neuropsychology.* (2007) 21:20–30. doi: 10.1037/0894-4105.21.1.20
159. Libon DJ, McMillan C, Gunawardena D, Powers C, Massimo L, Khan A, et al. Neurocognitive contributions to verbal fluency deficits in frontotemporal lobar degeneration. *Neurology.* (2009) 73:535–42. doi: 10.1212/WNL.0b013e3181b2a4f5
160. Wong S, Flanagan E, Savage G, Hodges JR, Hornberger M. Contrasting prefrontal cortex contributions to episodic memory dysfunction in behavioural variant frontotemporal dementia and Alzheimer's disease. *PLoS ONE.* (2014) 9:e87778. doi: 10.1371/journal.pone.0087778
161. Hornberger M, Savage S, Hsieh S, Mioshi E, Piguet O, Hodges JR. Orbitofrontal dysfunction discriminates behavioral variant frontotemporal dementia from Alzheimer's disease. *Dement Geriatr Cogn Disord.* (2011) 30:547–52. doi: 10.1159/000321670
162. Carey CL, Woods SP, Damon J, Halabi C, Dean D, Delis DC, et al. Discriminant validity and neuroanatomical correlates of rule monitoring in frontotemporal dementia and Alzheimer's disease. *Neuropsychologia.* (2008) 46:1081–7. doi: 10.1016/j.neuropsychologia.2007.11.001
163. Franceschi M, Caffarra P, Savarè R, Cerutti R, Grossi E, Padovani A, et al. Tower of London test: a comparison between conventional statistic approach and modelling based on artificial neural network in differentiating fronto-temporal dementia from Alzheimer's disease. *Behav Neurol.* (2011) 24:149–58. doi: 10.1155/2011/754659
164. Torralva T, Roca M, Gleichgerrcht E, Bekinschtein T, Manes F. A neuropsychological battery to detect specific executive and social cognitive impairments in early frontotemporal dementia. *Brain.* (2009) 132:1299–309. doi: 10.1093/brain/awp041
165. Bisbing TA, Olm CA, McMillan CT, Rascovsky K, Baehr L, Ternes K, et al. Estimating frontal and parietal involvement in cognitive estimation: a study of focal neurodegenerative diseases. *Front Hum Neurosci.* (2015) 9:1–11. doi: 10.3389/fnhum.2015.00317
166. Hornberger M, Piguet O, Graham AJ, Nestor PJ, Hodges JR. How preserved is episodic memory in behavioral variant frontotemporal dementia? *Neurology.* (2010) 74:472–9. doi: 10.1212/WNL.0b013e3181cef85d
167. Bertoux M, De Souza LC, Corlier F, Lamari F, Bottlaender M, Dubois B, et al. Two distinct amnesic profiles in behavioral variant frontotemporal dementia. *Biol Psychiatry.* (2014) 75:582–8. doi: 10.1016/j.biopsych.2013.08.017
168. Fernandez-Matarrubia M, Matias-Guiu JA, Cabrera-Martin MN, Moreno-Ramos T, Valles-Salgado M, Carreras JL, et al. Episodic memory dysfunction in behavioral variant frontotemporal dementia: a clinical and FDG-PET study. *J Alzheimer's Dis.* (2017) 57:1251–64. doi: 10.3233/JAD-160874
169. Wong S, Bertoux M, Savage G, Hodges JR, Piguet O, Hornberger M. Comparison of prefrontal atrophy and episodic memory performance in dysexecutive alzheimer's disease and behavioral-variant frontotemporal dementia. *J Alzheimer's Dis.* (2016) 51:889–903. doi: 10.3233/JAD-151016
170. Bertoux M, Flanagan EC, Hobbs M, Ruiz-Tagle A, Delgado C, Miranda M, et al. Structural anatomical investigation of long-term memory deficit in behavioral frontotemporal dementia. *J Alzheimer's Dis.* (2018) 62:1887–900. doi: 10.3233/JAD-170771

171. Poos JM, Jiskoot LC, Papma JM, van Swieten JC, van den Berg E. Meta-analytic review of memory impairment in behavioral variant frontotemporal dementia. *J Int Neuropsychol Soc.* (2018) 24:593–605. doi: 10.1017/S1355617718000115
172. St. Jacques PL, Grady C, Davidson PSR, Chow TW. Emotional evaluation and memory in behavioral variant frontotemporal dementia. *Neurocase.* (2015) 21:429–37. doi: 10.1080/13554794.2014.917681
173. Flanagan EC, Wong S, Dutt A, Tu S, Bertoux M, Irish M, et al. False recognition in behavioral variant frontotemporal dementia and Alzheimer's disease-disinhibition or amnesia? *Front Aging Neurosci.* (2016) 8:1–11. doi: 10.3389/fnagi.2016.00177
174. Graham A, Davies R, Xuereb J, Halliday G, Kril J, Creasey H, et al. Pathologically proven frontotemporal dementia presenting with severe amnesia. *Brain.* (2005) 128:597–605. doi: 10.1093/brain/awh348
175. Smits LL, Van Harten AC, Pijnenburg YAL, Koedam ELGE, Bouwman FH, Sistermans N, et al. Trajectories of cognitive decline in different types of dementia. *Psychol Med.* (2015) 45:1051–9. doi: 10.1017/S0033291714002153
176. Irish M, Piguet O, Hodges JR, Hornberger M. Common and unique gray matter correlates of episodic memory dysfunction in frontotemporal dementia and alzheimer's disease. *Hum Brain Mapp.* (2014) 35:1422–35. doi: 10.1002/hbm.22263
177. Kumfor F, Irish M, Hodges JR, Piguet O. The orbitofrontal cortex is involved in emotional enhancement of memory: evidence from the dementias. *Brain.* (2013) 136:2992–3003. doi: 10.1093/brain/awt185
178. Kamminga J, Kumfor F, Burrell JR, Piguet O, Hodges JR, Irish M. Differentiating between right-lateralised semantic dementia and behavioural-variant frontotemporal dementia: an examination of clinical characteristics and emotion processing. *J Neurol Neurosurg Psychiatry.* (2015) 86:1082–8. doi: 10.1136/jnnp-2014-309120
179. Dermody N, Hornberger M, Piguet O, Hodges JR, Irish M. Prospective memory impairments in alzheimer's disease and behavioral variant frontotemporal dementia: clinical and neural correlates. *J Alzheimer's Dis.* (2016) 50:425–41. doi: 10.3233/JAD-150871
180. Irish M, Hornberger M, El Wahsh S, Lam BYK, Lah S, Miller L, et al. Grey and white matter correlates of recent and remote autobiographical memory retrieval–insights from the dementias. *PLoS ONE.* (2014) 9:e113081. doi: 10.1371/journal.pone.0113081
181. Irish M, Landin-Romero R, Mothakunnel A, Ramanan S, Hsieh S, Hodges JR, et al. Evolution of autobiographical memory impairments in Alzheimer's disease and frontotemporal dementia - a longitudinal neuroimaging study. *Neuropsychologia.* (2018) 110:14–25. doi: 10.1016/j.neuropsychologia.2017.03.014
182. Bird CM, Chan D, Hartley T, Pijnenburg YA, Rossor MN, Burgess N. Topographical short-term memory differentiates Alzheimer's disease from frontotemporal lobar degeneration. *Hippocampus.* (2010) 20:1154–69. doi: 10.1002/hipo.20715
183. Tu S, Wong S, Hodges JR, Irish M, Piguet O, Hornberger M. Lost in spatial translation - a novel tool to objectively assess spatial disorientation in Alzheimer's disease and frontotemporal dementia. *Cortex.* (2015) 67:83–94. doi: 10.1016/j.cortex.2015.03.016
184. Tu S, Spiers HJ, Hodges JR, Piguet O, Hornberger M. Egocentric versus allocentric spatial memory in behavioral variant frontotemporal dementia and alzheimer's disease. *J Alzheimer's Dis.* (2017) 59:883–92. doi: 10.3233/JAD-160592
185. Coughlan G, Laczó J, Hort J, Minihane AM, Hornberger M. Spatial navigation deficits — overlooked cognitive marker for preclinical Alzheimer disease? *Nat Rev Neurol.* (2018) 14:1–11. doi: 10.1038/s41582-018-0031-x
186. Trojano L, Gainotti G. Drawing disorders in alzheimer's disease and other forms of dementia. *J Alzheimer's Dis.* (2016) 53:31–52. doi: 10.3233/JAD-160009
187. Miall RC, Nam SH, Tchalenko J. The influence of stimulus format on drawing-a functional imaging study of decision making in portrait drawing. *Neuroimage.* (2014) 102:608–19. doi: 10.1016/j.neuroimage.2014.08.015
188. Serra L, Fadda L, Perri R, Spanò B, Marra C, Castelli D, et al. Constructional apraxia as a distinctive cognitive and structural brain feature of pre-senile Alzheimer's disease. *J Alzheimers Dis.* (2014) 38:391–402. doi: 10.3233/JAD-130656
189. Perri R, Koch G, Carlesimo GA, Serra L, Fadda L, Pasqualetti P, et al. Alzheimer's disease and frontal variant of frontotemporal dementia - a very brief battery for cognitive and behavioural distinction. *J Neurol.* (2005) 252:1238–44. doi: 10.1007/s00415-005-0849-1
190. Grossi D, Fragassi NA, Chiacchio L, Valoroso L, Tuccillo R, Perrotta C, et al. Do visuospatial and constructional disturbances differentiate frontal variant of frontotemporal dementia and Alzheimer's disease? An experimental study of a clinical belief. *Int J Geriatr Psychiatry.* (2002) 17:641–8. doi: 10.1002/gps.654
191. Salimi S, Irish M, Foxe D, Hodges JR, Piguet O, Burrell JR. Can visuospatial measures improve the diagnosis of Alzheimer's disease? *Alzheimer's Dement Diagnosis, Assess Dis Monit.* (2018) 10:66–74. doi: 10.1016/j.dadm.2017.10.004
192. Rascovsky K, Salmon DP, Ho GJ, Galasko D, Peavy GM, Hansen LA, et al. Cognitive profiles differ in autopsy-confirmed frontotemporal dementia and AD. *Neurology.* (2002) 58:1801–8. doi: 10.1212/WNL.58.12.1801
193. Blair M, Kertesz A, McMonagle P, Davidson W, Bodi N. Quantitative and qualitative analyses of clock drawing in frontotemporal dementia and Alzheimer's disease. *J Int Neuropsychol Soc.* (2006) 12:159–65. doi: 10.1017/S1355617706060255
194. Floris G, Borghero G, Cannas A, Di Stefano F, Ruiu E, Murru MR, et al. Constructional apraxia in frontotemporal dementia associated with the C9orf72 mutation: broadening the clinical and neuropsychological phenotype. *Amyotroph Lateral Scler Front Degener.* (2015) 16:8–15. doi: 10.3109/21678421.2014.959450
195. Meyers JE, Bayless JD, Meyers KR. Rey complex figure: memory error patterns and functional abilities. *Appl Neuropsychol.* (1996) 3:89–92. doi: 10.1207/s15324826an0302_8
196. Roth HL, Bauer RM, Crucian GP, Heilman KM. Frontal-executive constructional apraxia: when delayed recall is better than copying. *Neurocase.* (2013) 2013:37–41. doi: 10.1080/13554794.2013.770879
197. Possin KL, Laluz VR, Alcantar OZ, Miller BL, Kramer JH. Distinct neuroanatomical substrates and cognitive mechanisms of figure copy performance in Alzheimer's disease and behavioral variant frontotemporal dementia. *Neuropsychologia.* (2011) 49:43–8. doi: 10.1016/j.neuropsychologia.2010.10.026
198. Thompson JC, Stopford CL, Snowden JS, Neary D. Qualitative neuropsychological performance characteristics in frontotemporal dementia and Alzheimer's disease. *J Neurol Neurosurg Psychiatry.* (2005) 76:920–7. doi: 10.1136/jnnp.2003.033779
199. Lezak M, Howieson D, Bigler E, Tranel D. *Neuropsychological Assessment.* New York, NY: Oxford University Press (2012).
200. De Lucia N, Grossi D, Maria Fasanaro A, Carpi S, Trojano L. Frontal defects contribute to the genesis of closing-in in Alzheimer's disease patients. *J Int Neuropsychol Soc.* (2013) 19:802–8. doi: 10.1017/S1355617713000568
201. Hallam BJ, Jacova C, Hsiung GYR, Wittenberg D, Sengdy P, Bouchard-Kerr P, et al. Early neuropsychological characteristics of progranulin mutation carriers. *J Int Neuropsychol Soc.* (2014) 20:694–703. doi: 10.1017/S1355617714000551
202. Cheran G, Wu L, Lee S, Manoochehri M, Cines S, Fallon E, et al. Cognitive indicators of preclinical behavioral variant frontotemporal dementia in MAPT carriers. *J Int Neuropsychol Soc.* (2018) 2018:1–11. doi: 10.1017/S1355617718001005
203. Barandiaran M, Moreno F, de Arriba M, Indakoetxea B, Boda I, Gabilondo A, et al. Longitudinal neuropsychological study of presymptomatic c.709-1G>A progranulin mutation carriers. *J Int Neuropsychol Soc.* (2018) 2018:1–9. doi: 10.1017/S1355617718000735
204. Lough S, Gregory C, Hodges JR. Dissociation of social cognition and executive function in frontal variant frontotemporal dementia. *Neurocase.* (2001) 7:123–30. doi: 10.1093/neucas/7.2.123
205. O'Callaghan C, Hodges JR, Hornberger M. Inhibitory dysfunction in frontotemporal dementia: a review. *Alzheimer Dis Assoc Disord.* (2012) 27:102–8. doi: 10.1097/WAD.0b013e318265bbc9
206. Kennedy DP, Adolphs R. The social brain in psychiatric and neurological disorders. *Trends Cogn Sci.* (2012) 16:559–72. doi: 10.1016/j.tics.2012.09.006
207. Gregory C, Lough S, Stone V, Erzinclioglu S, Martin L, Baron-Cohen S, et al. Theory of mind in patients with frontal variant frontotemporal dementia

and Alzheimer's disease: theoretical and practical implications. *Brain.* (2002) 125:752–64. doi: 10.1093/brain/awf079

208. Lavenu I, Pasquier F, Lebert F, Petit H, Van der Linden M. Perception of emotion in frontotemporal dementia and Alzheimer disease. *Alzheimer Dis Assoc Disord.* (1999) 13:96–101. doi: 10.1097/00002093-199904000-00007
209. Torralva T, Kipps CM, Hodges JR, Clark L, Bekinschtein T, Roca M, et al. The relationship between affective decision-making and theory of mind in the frontal variant of fronto-temporal dementia. *Neuropsychologia.* (2007) 45:342–9. doi: 10.1016/j.neuropsychologia.2006.05.031
210. Rankin KP, Salazar A, Gorno-Tempini ML, Sollberger M, Wilson SM, Pavlic D, et al. Detecting sarcasm from paralinguistic cues: anatomic and cognitive correlates in neurodegenerative disease. *Neuroimage.* (2009) 47:2005–15. doi: 10.1016/j.neuroimage.2009.05.077
211. Kumfor F, Miller L, Lah S, Hsieh S, Savage S, Hodges JR, et al. Are you really angry? The effect of intensity on facial emotion recognition in frontotemporal dementia. *Soc Neurosci.* (2011) 6:502–14. doi: 10.1080/17470919.2011.620779
212. Bertoux M, Delavest M, Cruz De Souza L, Funkiewiez A, Lépine J-P, Fossati P, et al. Social cognition and emotional assessment differentiates frontotemporal dementia from depression. *J Neurol Neurosurg Psychiatry.* (2012) 83:411–6. doi: 10.1136/jnnp-2011-301849
213. Bertoux M, Funkiewiez A, O'Callaghan C, Dubois B, Hornberger M. Sensitivity and specificity of ventromedial prefrontal cortex tests in behavioral variant frontotemporal dementia. *Alzheimer's Dement.* (2012) 9:84–94. doi: 10.1016/j.jalz.2012.09.010
214. Hornberger M, Yew B, Gilardoni S, Mioshi E, Gleichgerrcht E, Manes F, et al. Ventromedial-frontopolar prefrontal cortex atrophy correlates with insight loss in frontotemporal dementia and Alzheimer's disease. *Hum Brain Mapp.* (2014) 35:616–26. doi: 10.1002/hbm.22200
215. Bertoux M, Volle E, Funkiewiez A, de Souza LC, Leclercq D, Dubois B. Social cognition and emotional assessment (SEA) is a marker of medial and orbital frontal functions: a voxel-based morphometry study in behavioral variant of frontotemporal degeneration. *J Int Neuropsychol Soc.* (2012) 18:972–85. doi: 10.1017/S1355617712001300
216. Kumfor F, Irish M, Hodges JR, Piguet O. Discrete neural correlates for the recognition of negative emotions: insights from frontotemporal dementia. *PLoS ONE.* (2013) 8:e67457. doi: 10.1371/journal.pone.0067457
217. O'Callaghan C, Bertoux M, Irish M, Shine JM, Wong S, Spiliopoulos L, et al. Fair play: social norm compliance failures in behavioural variant frontotemporal dementia. *Brain.* (2016) 139:204–16. doi: 10.1093/brain/awv315
218. Melloni M, Billeke P, Baez S, Hesse E, de la Fuente L, Forno G, et al. Your perspective and my benefit: multiple lesion models of self-other integration strategies during social bargaining. *Brain.* (2016) 139:3022–40. doi: 10.1093/brain/aww231
219. Bertoux M, O'Callaghan C, Dubois B, Hornberger M. In two minds: executive functioning versus theory of mind in behavioural variant frontotemporal dementia. *J Neurol Neurosurg Psychiatry.* (2016) 87:231–4. doi: 10.1136/jnnp-2015-311643
220. Ramanan S, de Souza LC, Moreau N, Sarazin M, Teixeira ALL, Allen Z, et al. Determinants of theory of mind performance in Alzheimer's disease: a data-mining study. *Cortex.* (2017) 88:8–18. doi: 10.1016/j.cortex.2016.11.014
221. Ibanez A, Manes F. Contextual social cognition and the behavioral variant of frontotemporal dementia. *Neurology.* (2012) 78:1354–62. doi: 10.1212/WNL.0b013e3182518375
222. Henry JD, Phillips LH, Von Hippel C. A meta-analytic review of theory of mind difficulties in behavioural-variant frontotemporal dementia. *Neuropsychologia.* (2014) 56:53–62. doi: 10.1016/j.neuropsychologia.2013.12.024
223. Strikwerda-Brown C, Ramanan S, Irish M. Neurocognitive mechanisms of theory of mind impairment in neurodegeneration: a transdiagnostic approach. *Neuropsychiatr Dis Treat.* (2019) 15:557–73. doi: 10.2147/NDT.S158996
224. Fernandez-Duque D, Baird JA, Black SE. False-belief understanding in frontotemporal dementia and Alzheimer's disease. *J Clin Exp Neuropsychol.* (2009) 31:489–97. doi: 10.1080/13803390802282688
225. Le Bouc R, Lenfant P, Delbeuck X, Ravasi L, Lebert F, Semah F, et al. My belief or yours? Differential theory of mind deficits in frontotemporal dementia and Alzheimer's disease. *Brain.* (2012) 135:3026–38. doi: 10.1093/brain/aws237
226. Eslinger PJ, Moore P, Troiani V, Antani S, Cross K, Kwok S, et al. Oops! resolving social dilemmas in frontotemporal dementia. *J Neurol Neurosurg Psychiatry.* (2007) 78:457–60. doi: 10.1136/jnnp.2006.098228
227. Kipps CM, Nestor PJ, Acosta-Cabronero J, Arnold R, Hodges JR. Understanding social dysfunction in the behavioural variant of frontotemporal dementia: the role of emotion and sarcasm processing. *Brain.* (2009) 132:592–603. doi: 10.1093/brain/awn314
228. Shany-Ur T, Poorzand P, Grossman SN, Growdon ME, Jang JY, Ketelle RS, et al. Comprehension of insincere communication in neurodegenerative disease: Lies, sarcasm, and theory of mind. *Cortex.* (2012) 48:1329–41. doi: 10.1016/j.cortex.2011.08.003
229. Fong SS, Paholpak P, Daianu M, Deutsch MB, Riedel BC, Carr AR, et al. The attribution of animacy and agency in frontotemporal dementia versus Alzheimer's disease. *Cortex.* (2017) 92:81–94. doi: 10.1016/j.cortex.2017.03.019
230. Schroeter ML, Pawelke S, Bisenius S, Kynast J, Schuemberg K, Polyakova M, et al. A modified reading the mind in the eyes test predicts behavioral variant frontotemporal dementia better than executive function tests. *Front Aging Neurosci.* (2018) 10:1–11. doi: 10.3389/fnagi.2018.00011
231. Dodich A, Cerami C, Crespi C, Canessa N, Lettieri G, Iannaccone S, et al. Differential impairment of cognitive and affective mentalizing abilities in neurodegenerative dementias: evidence from behavioral variant of frontotemporal dementia, alzheimer's disease, and mild cognitive impairment. *J Alzheimer's Dis.* (2016) 50:1011–22. doi: 10.3233/JAD-150605
232. Synn A, Mothakunnel A, Kumfor F, Chen Y, Piguet O, Hodges JR, et al. Mental states in moving shapes: distinct cortical and subcortical contributions to theory of mind impairments in dementia. *J Alzheimers Dis.* (2018) 61:521–35. doi: 10.3233/JAD-170809
233. Bora E, Walterfang M, Velakoulis D. Theory of mind in behavioural-variant frontotemporal dementia and Alzheimer's disease: a meta-analysis. *J Neurol Neurosurg Psychiatry.* (2015) 86:714–9. doi: 10.1136/jnnp-2014-309445
234. Strikwerda-Brown C, Mothakunnel A, Hodges JR, Piguet O, Irish M. External details revisited - a new taxonomy for coding 'non-episodic' content during autobiographical memory retrieval. *J Neuropsychol.* (2018) 2018:12160. doi: 10.1111/jnp.12160
235. Rosen HJ, Pace-Savitsky K, Perry RJ, Kramer JH, Miller BL, Levenson RW. Recognition of emotion in the frontal and temporal variants of frontotemporal dementia. *Dement Geriatr Cogn Disord.* (2004) 17:277–81. doi: 10.1159/000077154
236. Goodkind MS, Sturm VE, Ascher EA, Shdo SM, Miller BL, Rankin KP, et al. Emotion recognition in frontotemporal dementia and Alzheimer's disease: a new film-based assessment. *Emotion.* (2015) 15:416–27. doi: 10.1037/a0039261
237. Hutchings R, Palermo R, Bruggemann J, Hodges JR, Piguet O, Kumfor F. Looking but not seeing: increased eye fixations in behavioural-variant frontotemporal dementia. *Cortex.* (2018) 103:71–81. doi: 10.1016/j.cortex.2018.02.011
238. Kumfor F, Ibanez A, Hutchings R, Hazelton JL, Hodges JR, Piguet O. Beyond the face: how context modulates emotion processing in frontotemporal dementia subtypes. *Brain.* (2018) 141:1172–85. doi: 10.1093/brain/aw y002
239. Sturm VE, Ascher EA, Miller BL, Levenson RW. Diminished self-conscious emotional responding in frontotemporal lobar degeneration patients. *Emotion.* (2008) 8:861–9. doi: 10.1037/a0013765
240. Verstaen A, Eckart JA, Muhtadie L, Otero MC, Sturm VE, Haase CM, et al. Insular atrophy and diminished disgust reactivity. *Emotion.* (2016) 16:903–12. doi: 10.1037/emo0000195
241. Carr AR, Ashla MM, Jimenez EE, Mendez MF. Screening for emotional expression in frontotemporal dementia: a pilot study. *Behav Neurol.* (2018) 2018:1–6. doi: 10.1155/2018/8187457
242. Joshi A, Barsuglia J, Mather M, Jimenez E, Shapira J, Mendez M. Evaluation of emotional blunting in behavioral variant frontotemporal dementia compared to alzheimer's disease. *Dement Geriatr Cogn Disord.* (2011) 193:79–88. doi: 10.1159/000357838
243. Mendez MF, Fong SS, Ashla MM, Jimenez EE, Carr AR. Skin conduction levels differentiate frontotemporal dementia from

alzheimer's disease. *J Neuropsychiatry Clin Neurosci.* (2018) 30:208–13. doi: 10.1176/appi.neuropsych.17080168
244. Kumfor F, Hazelton JL, Rushby JA, Hodges JR, Piguet O. Facial expressiveness and physiological arousal in frontotemporal dementia: phenotypic clinical profiles and neural correlates. *Cogn Affect Behav Neurosci.* (2019) 19:197–210. doi: 10.3758/s13415-018-00658-z
245. Gola KA, Shany-Ur T, Pressman P, Sulman I, Galeana E, Paulsen H, et al. A neural network underlying intentional emotional facial expression in neurodegenerative disease. *NeuroImage Clin.* (2017) 14:672–8. doi: 10.1016/j.nicl.2017.01.016
246. Torres B, Santos RL, Sousa MFBD, Simões Neto JP, Nogueira MML, Belfort TT, et al. Facial expression recognition in Alzheimer's disease: a longitudinal study. *Arq Neuropsiquiatr.* (2015) 73:383–9. doi: 10.1590/0004-282X20150009
247. Lavenu I, Pasquier F. Perception of emotion on faces in frontotemporal dementia and Alzheimer's disease: a longitudinal study. *Dement Geriatr Cogn Disord.* (2005) 19:37–41. doi: 10.1159/000080969
248. Bertoux M, De Souza LC, Sarazin M, Funkiewiez A, Dubois B, Hornberger M. How preserved is emotion recognition in Alzheimer disease compared with behavioral variant frontotemporal dementia? *Alzheimer Dis Assoc Disord.* (2015) 29:154–7. doi: 10.1097/WAD.0000000000000023
249. Wong S, Irish M, Leshikar ED, Duarte A, Bertoux M, Savage G, et al. The self-reference effect in dementia: differential involvement of cortical midline structures in Alzheimer's disease and behavioural-variant frontotemporal dementia. *Cortex.* (2017) 91:169–85. doi: 10.1016/j.cortex.2016.09.013
250. Shany-Ur T, Lin N, Rosen HJ, Sollberger M, Miller BL, Rankin KP. Self-awareness in neurodegenerative disease relies on neural structures mediating reward-driven attention. *Brain.* (2014) 137:2368–81. doi: 10.1093/brain/awu161
251. Arroyo-Anllo EM, Bouston AT, Fargeau M-N, Orgaz Baz B, Gil R. Self-consciousness deficits in alzheimer's disease and frontotemporal dementia. *J Alzheimers Dis.* (2017) 55:1437–43. doi: 10.3233/JAD-160770
252. Rankin KP, Baldwin E, Pace-Savitsky C, Kramer JH, Miller BL. Self awareness and personality change in dementia. *J Neurol Neurosurg Psychiatry.* (2005) 76:632–9. doi: 10.1136/jnnp.2004.042879
253. O'Keeffe FM, Murray B, Coen RF, Dockree PM, Bellgrove MA, Garavan H, et al. Loss of insight in frontotemporal dementia, corticobasal degeneration and progressive supranuclear palsy. *Brain.* (2007) 130:753–64. doi: 10.1093/brain/awl367
254. Scherling CS, Zakrzewski J, Datta S, Levenson RW, Shimamura AP, Sturm VE, et al. Mistakes, too few to mention? Impaired self-conscious emotional processing of errors in the behavioral variant of frontotemporal dementia. *Front Behav Neurosci.* (2017) 11:1–11. doi: 10.3389/fnbeh.2017.00189
255. Duclos H, de La Sayette V, Bonnet A-L, Viard A, Eustache F, Desgranges B, et al. Social cognition in the frontal variant of alzheimer's disease: a case study. *J Alzheimers Dis.* (2017) 55:459–63. doi: 10.3233/JAD-160690
256. Mendez MF, Anderson E, Shapira JS. An investigation of moral judgement in frontotemporal dementia. *Cogn Behav Neurol.* (2005) 18:193–7. doi: 10.1097/01.wnn.0000191292.17964.bb
257. Cova F, Bertoux M, Bourgeois-Gironde S, Dubois B. Judgments about moral responsibility and determinism in patients with behavioural variant of frontotemporal dementia: still compatibilists. *Conscious Cogn.* (2012) 21:851–64. doi: 10.1016/j.concog.2012.02.004
258. Carr AR, Paholpak P, Daianu M, Fong SS, Mather M, Jimenez EE, et al. An investigation of care-based vs. rule-based morality in frontotemporal dementia, Alzheimer's disease, and healthy controls. *Neuropsychologia.* (2015) 78:73–9. doi: 10.1016/j.neuropsychologia.2015.09.033
259. Gleichgerrcht E, Torralva T, Roca M, Pose M, Manes F. The role of social cognition in moral judgment in frontotemporal dementia. *Soc Neurosci.* (2011) 6:113–22. doi: 10.1080/17470919.2010.506751
260. Fong SS, Navarrete CD, Perfecto SE, Carr AR, Jimenez EE, Mendez MF. Behavioral and autonomic reactivity to moral dilemmas in frontotemporal dementia versus Alzheimer's disease. *Soc Neurosci.* (2017) 12:409–18. doi: 10.1080/17470919.2016.1186111
261. Baez S, Couto B, Torralva T, Sposato LA, Huepe D, Montañes P, et al. Comparing moral judgments of patients with frontotemporal dementia and frontal stroke. *JAMA Neurol.* (2014) 71:1172–6. doi: 10.1001/jamaneurol.2014.347
262. Clark CN, Golden HL, McCallion O, Nicholas JM, Cohen MH, Slattery CF, et al. Music models aberrant rule decoding and reward valuation in dementia. *Soc Cogn Affect Neurosci.* (2018) 13:192–202. doi: 10.1093/scan/nsx140
263. Wong S, Irish M, Savage G, Hodges JR, Piguet O, Hornberger M. Strategic value-directed learning and memory in Alzheimer's disease and behavioural-variant frontotemporal dementia. *J Neuropsychol.* (2018) 2018:12152. doi: 10.1111/jnp.12152
264. Strenziok M, Pulaski S, Krueger F, Zamboni G, Clawson D, Grafman J. Regional brain atrophy and impaired decision making on the balloon analog risk task in behavioral variant frontotemporal dementia. *Cogn Behav Neurol.* (2011) 24:59–67. doi: 10.1097/WNN.0b013e3182255a7c
265. Perry DC, Sturm VE, Wood KA, Miller BL, Kramer JH. Divergent processing of monetary and social reward in behavioral variant frontotemporal dementia and Alzheimer disease. *Alzheimer Dis Assoc Disord.* (2015) 29:161–4. doi: 10.1097/WAD.0000000000000012
266. Perry DC, Datta S, Sturm VE, Wood KA, Zakrzewski J, Seeley WW, et al. Reward deficits in behavioural variant frontotemporal dementia include insensitivity to negative stimuli. *Brain.* (2017) 140:3346–56. doi: 10.1093/brain/awx259
267. Bertoux M, de Souza LC, Zamith P, Dubois B, Bourgeois-Gironde S. Discounting of future rewards in behavioural variant frontotemporal dementia and Alzheimer's disease. *Neuropsychology.* (2015) 29:933–9. doi: 10.1037/neu0000197
268. Bertoux M, Cova F, Pessiglione M, Hsu M, Dubois B, Bourgeois-Gironde S. Behavioral variant frontotemporal dementia patients do not succumb to the Allais paradox. *Front Neurosci.* (2014) 8:1–10. doi: 10.3389/fnins.2014.00287
269. Woolley J, Gorno-Tempini M, Seeley W, Rankin K, Lee S, Matthews B, et al. Binge eating is associated with right orbitofrontal-insular-striatal atrophy in frontotemporal dementia. *Neurology.* (2007) 69:1424–33. doi: 10.1212/01.wnl.0000277461.06713.23
270. Rahman S, Sahakian BJ, Hodges JR, Rogers RD, Robbins TW. Specific cognitive deficits in mild frontal variant frontotemporal dementia. *Brain.* (1999) 122(Pt 8):1469–93. doi: 10.1093/brain/122.8.1469
271. Kloeters S, Bertoux M, O'Callaghan C, Hodges JR, Hornberger M. Money for nothing - Atrophy correlates of gambling decision making in behavioural variant frontotemporal dementia and Alzheimer's disease. *NeuroImage Clin.* (2013) 2:263–72. doi: 10.1016/j.nicl.2013.01.011
272. Mendez MF. The unique predisposition to criminal violations in frontotemporal dementia. *J Am Acad Psychiatry Law.* (2010) 38:318–23.
273. Sturm VE, Perry DC, Wood K, Hua AY, Alcantar O, Datta S, et al. Prosocial deficits in behavioral variant frontotemporal dementia relate to reward network atrophy. *Brain Behav.* (2017) 7:e00807. doi: 10.1002/brb3.807
274. Radakovic R, Stephenson L, Newton J, Crockford C, Swingler R, Chandran S, et al. Multidimensional apathy and executive dysfunction in amyotrophic lateral sclerosis. *Cortex.* (2017) 94:142–51. doi: 10.1016/j.cortex.2017.06.023
275. Kumfor F, Zhen A, Hodges JR, Piguet O, Irish M. Apathy in Alzheimer's disease and frontotemporal dementia: distinct clinical profiles and neural correlates. *Cortex.* (2018) 103:350–9. doi: 10.1016/j.cortex.2018.03.019
276. American Psychiatric Association. *Diagnostic and Statistical Manual of Mental Disorders (DSM-5®).* Washington DC: American Psychiatric Association (2013). doi: 10.1176/appi.books.9780890425596
277. Panchal H, Paholpak P, Lee G, Carr A, Barsuglia JP, Mather M, et al. Neuropsychological and neuroanatomical correlates of the social norms questionnaire in frontotemporal dementia versus alzheimer's disease. *Am J Alzheimers Dis Other Demen.* (2015) 31:326–32. doi: 10.1177/1533317515617722
278. Ekman P, Friesen WV. *Pictures of Facial Affect.* Palo Alto: Consulting Psychologists Press (1976).
279. McDonald S, Flanagan S, Rollins J, Kinch J. TASIT: a new clinical tool for assessing social perception after traumatic brain injury. *J Head Trauma Rehabil.* (2003) 18:219–38. doi: 10.1097/00001199-200305000-00001
280. Bora E, Velakoulis D, Walterfang M. Meta-analysis of facial emotion recognition in behavioral variant frontotemporal dementia. *J Geriatr Psychiatry Neurol.* (2016) 29:205–11. doi: 10.1177/0891988716640375

281. Chiu I, Piguet O, Diehl-Schmid J, Riedl L, Beck J, Leyhe T, et al. Dissociation in rating negative facial emotions between behavioral variant frontotemporal dementia and major depressive disorder. *Am J Geriatr Psychiatry.* (2016) 24:1017–27. doi: 10.1016/j.jagp.2016.06.011
282. Kandalaft MR, Didehbani N, Cullum CM, Krawczyk DC, Allen TT, Tamminga CA, et al. The wechsler ACS social perception subtest: a preliminary comparison with other measures of social cognition. *J Psychoeduc Assess.* (2012) 30:455–65. doi: 10.1177/0734282912436411
283. Baksh RA, Abrahams S, Auyeung B, MacPherson SE. The Edinburgh Social Cognition Test (ESCoT): examining the effects of age on a new measure of theory of mind and social norm understanding. *PLoS ONE.* (2018) 13:e0195818. doi: 10.1371/journal.pone.0195818
284. Bland AR, Roiser JP, Mehta MA, Schei T, Boland H, Campbell-Meiklejohn DK, et al. EMOTICOM: a neuropsychological test battery to evaluate emotion, motivation, impulsivity, and social cognition. *Front Behav Neurosci.* (2016) 10:25. doi: 10.3389/fnbeh.2016.00025
285. Gonzalez Rothi LJ, Ochipa C, Heilman KM. A cognitive neuropsychological model of limb praxis. *Cogn Neuropsychol.* (1991) 8:443–58. doi: 10.1080/02643299108253382
286. Goldenberg G. *Apraxia - The Cognitive Side of Motor Control.* New York, NY; Oxford: Elsevier Ltd (2013). doi: 10.1016/j.cortex.2013.07.016
287. Poeck K. The clinical examination for motor apraxia. *Neuropsychologia.* (1986) 24:129–34. doi: 10.1016/0028-3932(86)90046-1
288. Koski L, Iacoboni M, Mazziotta JC. Deconstructing apraxia: understanding disorders of intentional movement after stroke. *Curr Opin Neurol.* (2002) 15:71–7. doi: 10.1097/00019052-200202000-00011
289. Niessen E, Fink GR, Weiss PH. Apraxia, pantomime and the parietal cortex. *NeuroImage Clin.* (2014) 5:42–52. doi: 10.1016/j.nicl.2014.05.017
290. Lesourd M, Le Gall D, Baumard J, Croisile B, Jarry C, Osiurak F. Apraxia and alzheimer's disease: review and perspectives. *Neuropsychol Rev.* (2013) 23:234–56. doi: 10.1007/s11065-013-9235-4
291. Ozkan S, Ozbabalik Adapinar D, Tuncer Elmaci N, Arslantas D. Apraxia for differentiating Alzheimer's disease from subcortical vascular dementia and mild cognitive impairment. *Neuropsychiatr Dis Treat.* (2013) 9:947–51. doi: 10.2147/NDT.S47879
292. Della Sala S, Lucchelli F, Spinnler H. Ideomotor apraxia in patients with dementia of Alzheimer type. *J Neurol.* (1987) 234:91–3. doi: 10.1007/BF00314108
293. Crutch SJ, Rossor MN, Warrington EK. The quantitative assessment of apraxic deficits in Alzheimer's disease. *Cortex.* (2007) 43:976–86. doi: 10.1016/S0010-9452(08)70695-6
294. Parakh R, Roy E, Koo E, Black S. Pantomime and imitation of limb gestures in relation to the severity of Alzheimer's disease. *Brain Cogn.* (2004) 55:272–4. doi: 10.1016/j.bandc.2004.02.049
295. Nagahama Y, Okina T, Suzuki N. Impaired imitation of gestures in mild dementia: comparison of dementia with Lewy bodies, Alzheimer's disease and vascular dementia. *J Neurol Neurosurg Psychiatry.* (2015) 86:1248–52. doi: 10.1136/jnnp-2014-309436
296. Costa A, Bak T, Caffarra P, Caltagirone C, Ceccaldi M, Collette F, et al. The need for harmonisation and innovation of neuropsychological assessment in neurodegenerative dementias in Europe: consensus document of the Joint Program for Neurodegenerative Diseases Working Group. *Alzheimers Res Ther.* (2017) 9:27. doi: 10.1186/s13195-017-0254-x
297. Ahmed S, Baker I, Thompson S, Husain M, Butler CR. Utility of testing for apraxia and associated features in dementia. *J Neurol Neurosurg Psychiatry.* (2016) 87:1158–62. doi: 10.1136/jnnp-2015-312945
298. Chandra SR, Issac TG, Abbas MM. Apraxias in neurodegenerative dementias. *Indian J Psychol Med.* (2015) 37:42–7. doi: 10.4103/0253-7176.150817
299. Johnen A, Tokaj A, Kirschner A, Wiendl H, Lueg G, Duning T, et al. Apraxia profile differentiates behavioural variant frontotemporal from Alzheimer's dementia in mild disease stages. *J Neurol Neurosurg Psychiatry.* (2015) 86:809–15. doi: 10.1136/jnnp-2014-308773
300. Chare L, Hodges JR, Leyton CE, McGinley C, Tan RH, Kril JJ, et al. New criteria for frontotemporal dementia syndromes: clinical and pathological diagnostic implications. *J Neurol Neurosurg Psychiatry.* (2014) 85:865–70. doi: 10.1136/jnnp-2013-306948
301. Johnen A, Reul S, Wiendl H, Meuth SG, Duning T. Apraxia profiles—A single cognitive marker to discriminate all variants of frontotemporal lobar degeneration and Alzheimer's disease. *Alzheimer's Dement Diagn Assess Dis Monit.* (2018) 10:363–71. doi: 10.1016/j.dadm.2018.04.002
302. Johnen A, Frommeyer J, Modes F, Wiendl H, Duning T, Lohmann H. Dementia Apraxia Test (DATE): a brief tool to differentiate behavioral variant frontotemporal dementia from alzheimer's dementia based on apraxia profiles. *J Alzheimer's Dis.* (2015) 49:593–605. doi: 10.3233/JAD-150447
303. Lobo PP, Pinto S, Rocha L, Reimão S, de Carvalho M. Orofacial apraxia in motor neuron disease. *Case Rep Neurol.* (2013) 5:47–51. doi: 10.1159/000349895
304. Pawlowski M, Joksch V, Wiendl H, Meuth SG, Duning T, Johnen A. Apraxia screening predicts Alzheimer pathology in frontotemporal dementia. *J Neurol Neurosurg Psychiatry.* (2018) 2018:1–8. doi: 10.1136/jnnp-2018-318470
305. Buxbaum LJ, Shapiro AD, Coslett HB. Critical brain regions for tool-related and imitative actions: a componential analysis. *Brain.* (2014) 137:1971–85. doi: 10.1093/brain/awu111
306. Hoeren M, Kümmerer D, Bormann T, Beume L, Ludwig VM, Vry M-S, et al. Neural bases of imitation and pantomime in acute stroke patients: distinct streams for praxis. *Brain.* (2014) 137:2796–810. doi: 10.1093/brain/awu203
307. Martin M, Beume L, Kümmerer D, Schmidt CSM, Bormann T, Dressing A, et al. Differential roles of ventral and dorsal streams for conceptual and production-related components of tool use in acute stroke patients. *Cereb Cortex.* (2016) 26:3754–71. doi: 10.1093/cercor/bhv179
308. Manuel AL, Radman N, Mesot D, Chouiter L, Clarke S, Annoni J-M, et al. Inter- and intrahemispheric dissociations in ideomotor apraxia: a large-scale lesion-symptom mapping study in subacute brain-damaged patients. *Cereb Cortex.* (2013) 23:2781–9. doi: 10.1093/cercor/bhs280
309. Binkofski F, Buxbaum LJ. Two action systems in the human brain. *Brain Lang.* (2013) 127:222–9. doi: 10.1016/j.bandl.2012.07.007
310. Johnen A, Brandstetter L, Kärgel C, Wiendl H, Lohmann H, Duning T. Shared neural correlates of limb apraxia in early stages of Alzheimer's dementia and behavioural variant frontotemporal dementia. *Cortex.* (2016) 84:1–14. doi: 10.1016/j.cortex.2016.08.009
311. Leslie KR, Johnson-Frey SH, Grafton ST. Functional imaging of face and hand imitation: towards a motor theory of empathy. *Neuroimage.* (2004) 21:601–7. doi: 10.1016/j.neuroimage.2003.09.038
312. Goldenberg G, Karnath H-O. The neural basis of imitation is body part specific. *J Neurosci.* (2006) 26:6282–7. doi: 10.1523/JNEUROSCI.0638-06.2006
313. Raade A, Ginzalez Rothi L, Heilman K. The relationship between buccofacial and limb apraxia. *Brain Cogn.* (1991) 16:130–46. doi: 10.1016/0278-2626(91)90002-P
314. Weiss P, Kalbe E, Kessler J, Fink G, Binder E, Hesse M, et al. *Kölner Apraxie Screening.* Göttingen: Hogrefe Verlag (2013).
315. Vanbellingen T, Kersten B, Van de Winckel A, Bellion M, Baronti F, Muri R, et al. A new bedside test of gestures in stroke: the apraxia screen of TULIA (AST). *J Neurol Neurosurg Psychiatry.* (2011) 82:389–92. doi: 10.1136/jnnp.2010.213371
316. Cameron OG. Interoception: the inside story - a model for psychosomatic processes. *Psychosom Med.* (2001) 63:697–710. doi: 10.1097/00006842-200109000-00001
317. Kleckner IR, Zhang J, Touroutoglou A, Chanes L, Simmons WK, Quigley KS, et al. Evidence for a large-scale brain system supporting allostasis and interoception in humans. *Nat Hum Behav.* (2017) 1:1–37. doi: 10.1038/s41562-017-0069
318. García-Cordero I, Sedeño L, de la Fuente L, Slachevsky A, Forno G, Klein F, et al. Feeling, learning from and being aware of inner states: interoceptive dimensions in neurodegeneration and stroke. *Philos Trans R Soc B Biol Sci.* (2016) 371:0006. doi: 10.1098/rstb.2016.0006
319. Zhou J, Greicius MD, Gennatas ED, Growdon ME, Jang JY, Rabinovici GD, et al. Divergent network connectivity changes in behavioural variant frontotemporal dementia and Alzheimer's disease. *Brain.* (2010) 133:1352–67. doi: 10.1093/brain/awq075

320. Marshall CR, Hardy CJD, Russell LL, Clark CN, Bond RL, Dick KM, et al. Motor signatures of emotional reactivity in frontotemporal dementia. *Nat Sci Rep*. (2018) 8:1–13. doi: 10.1038/s41598-018-19528-2
321. Fletcher PD, Downey LE, Golden HL, Clark CN, Slattery CF, Paterson RW, et al. Pain and temperature processing in dementia: a clinical and neuroanatomical analysis. *Brain*. (2015) 138:3360–72. doi: 10.1093/brain/awv276
322. Ondobaka S, Kilner J, Friston K. The role of interoceptive inference in theory of mind. *Brain Cogn*. (2017) 112:64–8. doi: 10.1016/j.bandc.2015.08.002
323. Shah P, Catmur C, Bird G. From heart to mind: linking interoception, emotion, and theory of mind. *Cortex*. (2017) 93:220–3. doi: 10.1016/j.cortex.2017.02.010
324. Adolfi F, Couto B, Richter F, Decety J, Lopez J, Sigman M, et al. Convergence of interoception, emotion, and social cognition: a twofold fMRI meta-analysis and lesion approach. *Cortex*. (2017) 88:124–42. doi: 10.1016/j.cortex.2016.12.019
325. Joshi A, Mendez MF, Kaiser N, Jimenez E, Mather M, Shapira JS. Skin conductance levels may reflect emotional blunting in behavioral variant frontotemporal dementia. *J Neuropsychiatry Clin Neurosci*. (2014) 26:227–32. doi: 10.1176/appi.neuropsych.12110332
326. Balconi M, Cotelli M, Brambilla M, Manenti R, Cosseddu M, Premi E, et al. Understanding emotions in frontotemporal dementia: the explicit and implicit emotional cue mismatch. *J Alzheimers Dis*. (2015) 46:211–25. doi: 10.3233/JAD-142826
327. Marshall CR, Hardy CJD, Russell LL, Clark CN, Dick KM, Brotherhood E V., et al. Impaired interoceptive accuracy in semantic variant primary progressive aphasia. *Front Neurol*. (2017) 8:610. doi: 10.3389/fneur.2017.00610
328. Woolley JD. Buccofacial apraxia and the expression of emotion. *Ann N Y Acad Sci*. (2006) 1000:395–401. doi: 10.1196/annals.1280.039
329. Ptak R, Schnider A, Fellrath J. The dorsal frontoparietal network: a core system for emulated action. *Trends Cogn Sci*. (2017) 21:589–99. doi: 10.1016/j.tics.2017.05.002
330. Conson M, Trojano L, Vitale C, Mazzarella E, Allocca R, Barone P, et al. The role of embodied simulation in mental transformation of whole-body images: evidence from Parkinson's disease. *Hum Mov Sci*. (2014) 33:343–53. doi: 10.1016/j.humov.2013.10.006
331. Schwoebel J, Buxbaum LJ, Coslett HB. Representations of the human body in the production and imitation of complex movements. *Cogn Neuropsychol*. (2004) 21:285–98. doi: 10.1080/02643290342000348
332. Buxbaum LJ, Kyle KM, Menon R. On beyond mirror neurons: internal representations subserving imitation and recognition of skilled object-related actions in humans. *Brain Res Cogn Brain Res*. (2005) 25:226–39. doi: 10.1016/j.cogbrainres.2005.05.014
333. Buxbaum LJ, Kalénine S. Action knowledge, visuomotor activation, and embodiment in the two action systems. *Ann N Y Acad Sci*. (2010) 1191:201–18. doi: 10.1111/j.1749-6632.2010.05447.x
334. Rumiati RI, Carmo JC, Corradi-Dell'Acqua C. Neuropsychological perspectives on the mechanisms of imitation. *Philos Trans R Soc Lond B Biol Sci*. (2009) 364:2337–47. doi: 10.1098/rstb.2009.0063
335. Berg E. A simple objective technique for measuring flexibility in thinking. *J Gen Psychol*. (1948) 39:15–22. doi: 10.1080/00221309.1948.9918159
336. Nyhus E, Barcelo F. The wisconsin card sorting test and the cognitive assessment of prefrontal executive functions: a critical update. *Brain Cogn*. (2009) 71:437–51. doi: 10.1016/j.bandc.2009.03.005
337. Kohli A, Kaur M. Wisconsin card sorting test: normative data and experience. *Indian J Psychiatry*. (2006) 48:181–4. doi: 10.4103/0019-5545.31582
338. Ameller A, Picard A, D'Hondt F, Vaiva G, Thomas P, Pins D. Implicit recognition of familiar and unfamiliar faces in schizophrenia: a study of the skin conductance response in familiarity disorders. *Front Psychiatry*. (2017) 8:1–11. doi: 10.3389/fpsyt.2017.00181
339. Coughlan G, Coutrot A, Khondoker M, Minihane A-M, Spiers H, Hornberger M. Toward personalized cognitive diagnostics of at-genetic-risk Alzheimer's disease. *Proc Natl Acad Sci USA*. (2019) 116:9285–92. doi: 10.1073/pnas.1901600116
340. Artiola i Fortuny L, Heaton RK, Hermosillo D. Neuropsychological comparisons of Spanish-speaking participants from the U.S.-Mexico border region versus Spain. *J Int Neuropsychol Soc*. (1998) 4:363–79.
341. Gasquoine PG. Variables moderating cultural and ethnic differences in neuropsychological assessment: the case of Hispanic Americans. *Clin Neuropsychol*. (1999) 13:376–83. doi: 10.1076/clin.13.3.376.1735

4

Fourier-Transform Infrared Imaging Spectroscopy and Laser Ablation-ICPMS New Vistas for Biochemical Analyses of Ischemic Stroke in Rat Brain

Mohamed H. M. Ali[1]*, Fazle Rakib[2], Essam M. Abdelalim[3,4], Andreas Limbeck[5], Raghvendra Mall[6], Ehsan Ullah[6], Nasrin Mesaeli[7], Donald McNaughton[8], Tariq Ahmed[1]* and Khalid Al-Saad[2]*

[1] Neurological Disorders Research Center, Qatar Biomedical Research Institute, Hamad Bin Khalifa University, Qatar Foundation, Doha, Qatar, [2] Department of Chemistry and Earth Sciences, Qatar University, Doha, Qatar, [3] Diabetes Research Center, Qatar Biomedical Research Institute, Hamad Bin Khalifa University, Qatar Foundation, Doha, Qatar, [4] Department of Cytology and Histology, Faculty of Veterinary Medicine, Suez Canal University, Ismailia, Egypt, [5] Institute of Chemical Technologies and Analytics, Vienna University of Technology, Vienna, Austria, [6] Qatar Computing Research Institute, Hamad Bin Khalifa University, Qatar Foundation, Doha, Qatar, [7] Weill Cornell Medicine-Qatar, Qatar Foundation, Doha, Qatar, [8] Centre for Biospectroscopy, School of Chemistry, Monash University, Clayton, VIC, Australia

***Correspondence:**
Mohamed H. M. Ali
mohamali@hbku.edu.qa
Tariq Ahmed
taahmed@hbku.edu.qa
Khalid Al-Saad
kalsaad@qu.edu.qa

Objective: Stroke is the main cause of adult disability in the world, leaving more than half of the patients dependent on daily assistance. Understanding the post-stroke biochemical and molecular changes are critical for patient survival and stroke management. The aim of this work was to investigate the photo-thrombotic ischemic stroke in male rats with particular focus on biochemical and elemental changes in the primary stroke lesion in the somatosensory cortex and surrounding areas, including the corpus callosum.

Materials and Methods: FT-IR imaging spectroscopy and LA-ICPMS techniques examined stroke brain samples, which were compared with standard immunohistochemistry studies.

Results: The FTIR results revealed that in the lesioned gray matter the relative distribution of lipid, lipid acyl and protein contents decreased significantly. Also at this locus, there was a significant increase in aggregated protein as detected by high-levels $A\beta_{1-42}$. Areas close to the stroke focus experienced decrease in the lipid and lipid acyl contents associated with an increase in lipid ester, olefin, and methyl bio-contents with a novel finding of $A\beta_{1-42}$ in the PL-GM and L-WM. Elemental analyses realized major changes in the different brain structures that may underscore functionality.

Conclusion: In conclusion, FTIR bio-spectroscopy is a non-destructive, rapid, and a refined technique to characterize oxidative stress markers associated with lipid degradation and protein denaturation not characterized by routine approaches. This technique may expedite research into stroke and offer new approaches for neurodegenerative disorders. The results suggest that a good therapeutic strategy should include a mechanism that provides protective effect from brain swelling (edema) and neurotoxicity by scavenging the lipid peroxidation end products.

Keywords: photothrombotic, ischemic, brain, stroke model, FTIR imaging spectroscopy, LA-ICPMS, lipid peroxidation, neurodegeneration

INTRODUCTION

Stroke is the leading cause of adult disability in the world, leaving more than half of those affected dependent on daily assistance. Patients are often hospitalized and, or subjected to intensive rehabilitation programs for long periods, with their quality of life severely affected, socially and economically. Hence, a more thorough understanding of the molecular and cellular changes are required for the design of better therapies to treat this debilitating illness (Ramasubbu et al., 1998; Sarti et al., 2000; Snögren and Sunnerhagen, 2009; Lekander et al., 2017).

Ischemic stroke is caused by a reduction in blood circulation in the brain vasculature, resulting in decreased supply of oxygen and nutrients followed by an ischemic cascade, and if not reversed results in neurodegeneration and ultimately cell death (Deb et al., 2010; Xing et al., 2012; Hu et al., 2017). Acute ischemic stroke causes unregulated cation influx, mainly Na^{+}, which initiates the cytotoxic edema (Liang et al., 2007). Also, accumulation of Ca^{2+} inside forebrain neurons initiates glutamate mediated excitotoxicity (Lai et al., 2014; Prentice et al., 2015). This enhanced intra-cellular calcium-levels activates numerous pathways including proteases which can degrade proteins and membrane lipids and promote the generation of free radicals and reactive oxygen species (ROS) which can lead to neuronal damage, particularly of the cell membrane (Lee et al., 2000; Bretón and Rodríguez, 2012). Furthermore, mitochondria dysfunction can also result in apoptosis (Broughton et al., 2009; Xing et al., 2012). Stroke insult, also weakens and disturbs the blood–brain barrier (BBB) which can result in the development of vasogenic edema (Dostovic et al., 2016). Vasogenic edema causes disturbances in brain function, mass-effect (displacing surrounding brain tissues) with distortion, tissue shift and increased intracranial pressure and damage (Simard et al., 2007; Michinaga and Koyama, 2015).

Tissue in adjacent regions also undergo morphological, cellular and sub-cellular changes (Dirnagl et al., 1999; Lo et al., 2003; Shichita et al., 2014; Hu et al., 2017), such as gliosis (Garcia, 1984; Li et al., 2005; Huang et al., 2014), lipid peroxidation (Yamamoto et al., 1983; Yildirim et al., 2007; Zeiger et al., 2009) and protein malformation (Brouns et al., 2010; Zhao and Bateman, 2015). Perilesional changes are not necessarily detrimental, as neuronal plasticity and tissue reorganization in GM and WM may compensate and contribute to recovery post ischemic stroke (Carmichael, 2003; Cheatwood et al., 2008; Murphy and Corbett, 2009). Delay and ongoing tissue damage post ischemic stroke results in impeding brain tissue repair and recovery and contributes to brain dysfunctions. A model to study ischemic stroke is the photo-thrombotic model of focal ischemia, where photosensitive dye is excited by fluorescence causing a blood clot (Pevsner et al., 2001). Conventional techniques, such as magnetic resonance imaging (MRI) (Van Bruggen et al., 1992; Pevsner et al., 2001), auto-radiography (Dietrich et al., 1986), routine histology (Van Bruggen et al., 1992; Pevsner et al., 2001; Kuroiwa et al., 2009), and IHC (Van Bruggen et al., 1992) have been applied to characterize the biochemical and anatomical alterations after stroke in many studies (Dietrich et al., 1986; Pevsner et al., 2001; Kuroiwa et al., 2009). These techniques provide important data, but for example, MRI is not sufficient to study bio-chemical and bio-molecular changes at cellular and sub-cellular levels. Whereas, histology and IHC give high spatial resolution but again, only limited to certain biochemical markers as well as disrupting the tissue morphology.

Spectroscopic techniques such as FT-IR imaging spectroscopy and laser ablation inductively coupled plasma mass spectrometry (LA-ICP-MS) are potentially attractive bio-imaging platforms that can provide molecular (Kazarian and Chan, 2006; Petibois and Desbat, 2010) and elemental images (Becker et al., 2014), respectively. Both techniques offer high resolution (in the range of 5–10 μm), yielding detailed information about bio-chemical and chemical features at the cellular and/or sub-cellular level (Lasch et al., 2002; Kumar et al., 2014; Harrison and Berry, 2017) related to pathology. In contrast to standard histological staining methods, FTIR imaging has the ability to detect, simultaneously, discrete changes in molecular structure and composition of tissues. Direct biochemical analyses of all macromolecular components within tissue samples can be obtained from a single data acquisition, without the addition of chemical stains or reagents and without disrupting the tissue morphology (Petibois et al., 2009; Miller et al., 2013). Infrared (IR) spectra are dominated by macromolecular building blocks, such as proteins, lipids, cholesterols, phospholipids, carbohydrates, and nucleic acids (Carter et al., 2010; Srinivasan, 2010; Ami et al., 2013). The IR spectral absorptions provide readouts about these bio-molecules and produce a specific biochemical fingerprint of the sample (Ami et al., 2013; Baker et al., 2014; Kohler et al., 2015). FT-IR based techniques have been used to image molecular alterations associated with neuro-degeneration in animal models of Alzheimer's disease (AD) (Miller et al., 2006; Leskovjan et al., 2010; Liao et al., 2013; Benseny-Cases et al., 2014), Parkinson's disease (PD) (Szczerbowska-Boruchowska et al., 2007), amyotrophic lateral sclerosis (Kastyak et al., 2010), multiple sclerosis (Heraud et al., 2010), cerebral malaria (Hackett et al., 2015b), epilepsy (Turker, 2012; Turker et al., 2014) and hemorrhagic stroke (Ali et al., 2016; Caine et al., 2016; Balbekova et al., 2017). These studies have shown the potential of FTIR to assess molecular and neurochemical changes associated with brain pathology.

Laser ablation inductively coupled plasma mass spectrometry (LA-ICP-MS) has been developed and established as a technique in the generation of quantitative images of metal distributions in thin brain tissue sections with applications in research related to neurological disorders. This technique detects trace elements that are essential for brain function, such as zinc (Zn), copper (Cu), and iron (Fe) (Becker et al., 2014). Simultaneous analysis of these trace elements in brain can yield important information on the processes of neuronal (dys) function for example after PD (Hare et al., 2009; Hare et al., 2010; Matusch et al., 2010, 2012), AD (Matusch and Becker, 2012), stroke (Becker et al., 2011) and

Abbreviations: CC, corpus callosum; CL-GM, contra-lesioned gray matter; CL-WM, contra-lesioned white matter; FTIR, Fourier transform Infrared; GM, gray matter; IHC, immunohistochemistry; LA-ICPMS, laser-ablation inductively-coupled-plasma mass-spectrometry; L-WM, lesioned white matter; PL-GM, perilesioned gray matter; PS-GM, primary stroke lesion gray matter; ROI, regions of interest; TC-GM, time control gray matter; WM, white matter.

brain tumor (Becker et al., 2011). LA-ICP-MS is suitable for the imaging of metals in thin cross sections of soft and hard biological tissues with very low concentrations such as sub μg/g level (Hare et al., 2009; Becker et al., 2011; Matusch and Becker, 2012; Becker et al., 2014). The advantages of LA-ICP-MS is that it is highly sensitivity, accurate, precise as well as being a unique technique to scan the elemental distribution in the whole brain section.

In the present study, we combined FTIR and LA-ICP-MS with routine histological/IHC to characterize the bio-chemical and elemental changes in PS-GM, PL-GM, L-WM, CL-WM, CL-GM, and CC following 1-week photothrombotic stroke in rat brain sections. Our goal was to use FTIR and LA-ICPMS imaging techniques with conventional histological studies to identify alterations of specific bio-molecules and elements associated with ischemic stroke. In addition, this study will advance stroke bio-diagnostics and treatment and provide links between tissue injury, plasticity and repair, as well as identifying novel therapeutic targets and interventions.

MATERIALS AND METHODS

Animal Model

All experimental protocols and animal handling procedures were in accordance with the National Institutes of Health (NIH) recommendations and with guidelines of the European Communities Council Directive. The experimental animals protocol was approved by the by the University of Utrecht Animal Research Ethics Board (DEC 2013.I.08.063), and adhered to the Netherlands Council on Animal Care guidelines for humane animal use (Ali et al., 2016; Balbekova et al., 2017). A total of 12 male (11 week-old, Sprague-Dawley rats; Charles River Laboratories International, Wilmington, MA, United States), from which six animals were used in the Photothrombotic stroke, which was induced in the right sensorimotor cortex (Ali et al., 2016) and remainder six rats served as age-matched controls. Data were analyzed by comparing the lesioned generated values with the unlesioned (contralateral) hemisphere.

Block and Tissue Preparation

One week after stroke induction, the animals were sacrificed with an overdose of isoflurane followed by transcardial perfusion. Brains were extracted, fixed in 4% paraformaldehyde (PFA) for 24 h and embedded in paraffin (Balbekova et al., 2017). Paraffin embedded tissue blocks were serially cut into 5 μm slices using a microtome (Leica RM 2155 semi-automated rotary microtome, Germany). Thin coronal sections of brain were taken from central location of the lesion (Bregma 1.20 mm). Serial and consecutive sections were obtained for FTIR measurements, LA-ICPMS, and hematoxylin and eosin (H&E) staining and IHC studies. The brain sections for FTIR imaging were mounted on a CaF_2 window and a transflective slide. The brain sections used for the histology and IHC were mounted on Flex IHC microscopic slides (Dako, Fisher Scientific, United States). Routine histology was performed on control healthy rats to confirm normal tissue morphology (Ali et al., 2016).

Immunohistochemistry

Slides of brain sections 5 μm sections were washed with phosphate buffered saline (PBS) and maintained in 0.1 M PBS with 0.2% Triton X-100, pH 7.4 (PBST) for 2 days at 4°C. For antigen retrieval, the slides were incubated in 10 mM sodium citrate containing 0.05% Tween 20, pH 6.0 for 1 h at room temperature. To block non-specific protein binding, sections were incubated in 6% bovine serum albumin (BSA) in PBST for 2 h at room temperature, then incubated for 3 days at 4°C with the primary antibodies. The primary antibodies (all Abcam, Ltd., Cambridge, United Kingdom, unless stated) were rabbit polyclonal anti-amyloid precursor protein (APP) (1:1000 dilution; ab2072), rabbit polyclonal anti-Tau (1:1000 dilution, ab47579), rabbit anti-GFAP (1:2000 dilution; ab7260), rabbit anti-MAP2 (1:2000 dilution; ab5622), or mouse anti-myelin basic protein (MBP) (1:2000 dilution; ab62631), or chicken anti-beta amyloid (1:2000 dilution; ab134022). The primary antibodies were diluted in 2% BSA in PBST. After the sections had been rinsed three times with PBST (10 min each), sections were incubated for 2 h at room temperature with Alexa Fluor 488-conjugated donkey anti-chicken IgG, Alexa Fluor 647-conjugated donkey anti-rabbit IgG, or Alexa Fluor 647-conjugated donkey anti-mouse IgG (1:500; Thermo Fisher Scientific, United States). Negative controls were subjected to the same protocol without primary antibodies. After three rinses with PBST, the mounting media containing DAPI (nuclear stain) were added to the slides and then overlayed with cover slips. The slides were kept away from light and examined using a fluorescence microscope.

Fourier Transform Infrared Spectroscopy (FTIR)

Fourier transform infrared spectroscopy (FTIR) spectra were recorded using an Agilent FTIR Cary 620 micro-spectrometer in reflection mode within the range of 4000–700 cm^{-1} with 64 scans per spectrum, 4 cm^{-1} spectral resolution and spatial resolution 80 μm. Background single beam spectra were measured on a substrate without biological tissue by co-adding 64 scans. FTIR chemical images were recorded using a 64 × 64 Mercury Cadmium Telluride (MCT) Focal Plane Array (FPA) liquid nitrogen cooled detector in mosaic mode. FTIR imaging was performed with a 15× objective (numerical aperture = 0.62), yielding a pixel size of 5.5 μm × 5.5 μm. The average size of the brain is 1 cm × 1.2 cm. Three sections of the same anatomy per animal were examined. From each region of interest an area of 200 μm × 200 μm were analyzed. To ensure consistency in the data and negate technical errors, exemplar samples were mounted on CaF_2 slides and measured in transmission mode as well as in the *trans*-reflective mode using transflective slides. In both modes, we obtained very similar results. To circumvent the electric field standing wave effect (EFSW) reported for variations in section thickness, we repeated exemplar sections at 8 and 10 μm thickness, and here again, we obtained very similar spectral profiles as the measured samples. **Supplementary Table S1** (Stable 1) shows the FTIR assignments used in the medical and biomedical fields (Goormaghtigh, 2016).

Data Pre-processing and Analysis

All data processing and image generation were using either Resolution Pro. Software, (version 5.0), or Cytospec, (version 2.00.03) and Origin software (version 8). The representative FTIR spectrum acquired from brain WM region of a control rat brain in the spectral range of 4000–800 cm^{-1} is shown in **Supplementary Figure S1** and the detailed spectral band assignments are given in **Supplementary Table S1** in which different contribution to each band were presented (Kneipp et al., 2000; Cakmak et al., 2012). Baseline correction was performed on the full range of wavelengths for the spectra. FTIR images of the functional groups were calculated using the baseline areas under the FTIR absorption bands based on the assignments in (**Supplementary Table S1**) (Kneipp et al., 2000; Cakmak et al., 2012). In this study, the area under the curve from specific bands were calculated in order to measure different bio-chemical contents after photothrombotic ischemic stroke induction and values were normalized to the contralateral (unlesioned) hemisphere values. For example the total lipid was represented by (C–H stretching region) in the spectral range of 3000–2800 cm^{-1}; lipid acyl $\nu_s(CH_2)$ groups at 2860–2840 cm^{-1}; lipid ester ν(C = O) at 1755–1715 cm^{-1}; olefinic = CH band at 3027–3000 cm^{-1}; CH_3 asymmetric stretching $\nu_{as}(CH_3)$ (methyl concentration) at 2960–2950 cm^{-1}; amide I band (total protein) at 1700–1600 cm^{-1}; β-sheet aggregate at 1630 cm^{-1} and α-helix structures at 1655 cm^{-1} as detailed in **Table 1** and **Supplementary Table S1** (Kneipp et al., 2000; Cakmak et al., 2012).

The C-H spectral region is dominated by lipid contribution and a small contribution from proteins, carbohydrates and nucleic acids (Kneipp et al., 2000). Based on this understanding, the following CH_2 asymmetric, CH_3 asymmetric; olefinic = CH and lipid ester (C = O) lipid assignment were all good approximate values. Lipid molecular and structural alterations were investigated by evaluating the integrated area under specific lipid spectral bands as follows: CH_2 asymmetric (chain lipid length); CH_3 asymmetric (methyl concentration); olefinic = CH (unsaturated lipid) and lipid ester (C = O) (oxidative stress by-products) as shown in **Table 1**. Raw spectra were vector normalized and second derivative was computed by calculating forward difference twice and smoothed using spline fitting. The spline fitting used cubic spline interpolation of the second derivative to smoothen spectra. Resonance Mie scattering can affect the spectra from the border between a brain tissue and a substrate which is commonly existing in biological samples and spectra acquired from a substrate apart from brain tissue area were eliminated from analysis (Bassan et al., 2010). The contribution of different types of proteins was calculated by fitting a linear mixed model of Gaussian bands centered at the wavenumbers of the protein types. Relative distribution of β-sheet aggregate protein were determined at 1625 cm^{-1} from the second-derivative intensity spectrum (Pribic, 1994; Hackett et al., 2015b; Caine et al., 2016). The relative amount of the protein aggregation content was quantified from the curve fitting of original absorbance spectra (Hackett et al., 2015b). Curve fitting was performed with MATLAB (version 2014a, United States) over the spectral range 1700-1600 cm^{-1}.

TABLE 1 | The spectral regions used for analytical purposes.

Infrared band	Integrated spectral range (cm^{-1})
Lipid components	
CH_2 symmetric stretching	2852–2800
CH_2 asymmetric stretching	2915–2930
CH_3 asymmetric stretching	2950–2960
*C-H stretching	2994–2800
Olefin = CH	3000–3027
Carbonyl ester (C = O) stretching	1745–1731
Protein components	
Amide I	1700–1600
Amide II	1555–1535
β-sheet aggregate	1630
α-helix structures	1655

**Total lipid regions.*

Chemometric Data Pre-processing and Analysis

Chemometric analyses, incorporating principal component analysis (PCA) and hierarchical cluster analysis (HCA), were used to differentiate the spectral types with the FTIR spectra of the brain pre-processed prior to analysis using shape-preserving piece-wise cubic interpolation (Pribic, 1994). The infrared spectra were converted from Agilent system format to comma separated values (CSV) to create data sets that were suitable for PCA analysis using the "prcomp" function in the "stats" package in R (Becker et al., 1988; Sanchez, 2011). Three principal components (PCs) were used for analysis since they explained the highest percentage of variations. The 3D scores plot of the PCs that explain the majority of the variance in the dataset enabled spectra to be grouped according to the chemical information they contained (Pribic, 1994).

Hierarchical cluster analysis was applied using the A2R package in R to compare the three brain regions (PS-GM, PL-GM, and CL-GM) based on their PCA projections in the 3D score space (Becker et al., 1988; Pribic, 1994; Sanchez, 2011). HCA was used to group spectra that displayed the same degree of similarity by calculating the Euclidean distance between all the data sets using Ward's algorithm. The result was visualized in a dendrogram and the grouping of the three brain regions were presented as images consisting of colors clusters according to the heterogeneity scale (Becker et al., 1988; Sanchez, 2011).

Laser Ablation ICPMS

An ICPQMS (Agilent 7700) laser ablation system (CETAC Technologies, Omaha, NE, United States) with a Nd:YAG laser at wavelength 266 nm was used throughout this work. **Table 2** shows the laser ablation and ICP triggering operational conditions. The data were processed to generate elemental images using a macro, and image processing software 'ImageJ.' The scan speed of each line was 120 μms^{-1}, and the ICP-MS was

TABLE 2 | Parameters for measuring a brain samples by LA-ICPMS.

Parameters	Condition
Spot size	100 microns
Space between lines	4 micron
Laser energy	15%
Laser shot frequency	20 Hz
Shutter delay	10 s
Scan rate	160
Number of lines	120
Integration time	Varies from 0.02–0.06 s
Total integration time	0.614 s
Total acquisition time	67 s

configured in data-only mode to collect 185 readings per line scan at a rate of 2 s^{-1} (Hare et al., 2010; Matusch and Becker, 2012).

Statistical Analysis

A paired *t*-test was performed to assess significant differences between the molecular content of the PS-GM and PL-GM; PS-GM and CL-GM and PL-GM and the CL-GM tissue. For each group, a mean and standard deviation was generated for each animal. Then the individual animal values were averaged for each group. Mann–Whitney-*U* test was performed on all data to test for significant differences ($p < 0.05$) between control and treated groups. All *t*-tests were two tailed and the 95% confidence limit was used to test for significance.

RESULTS

Histological and Immunohistochemical Changes After Photo-Thrombotic Stroke

One of the major aims of this study was to correlate molecular alterations after ischemic photo-thrombotic stroke, by using FTIR spectroscopy and elemental distribution changes (LA-ICPMS bio-imaging) and complement these results with immunostaining analyses of specific biomarkers. Hematoxylin and eosin (H&E) staining of the brain sections from unlesioned rats (native time-matched controls) is presented in **Figure 1A**. The locus of the photo-thrombotic ischemic stroke was confirmed using H&E staining (**Figure 1B**). The image clearly depicts loss of brain structure and integrity at the stroke focus and results in an absence of H&E staining within the ischemic infarct. The rim of the stroke region is the characteristic pale expression of the H&E staining due to brain edema (see inset **Figure 1B**). The contralateral hemisphere of the affected brain shows H&E strong staining expression. The six ROI for this study were: (a) the PS-GM; (b) PL-GM; (c) L-WM; (d) CL-WM; (e) CL-GM; and (f) CC (**Figure 1C**).

To gain insights into the effects of stroke on nerve cells in the lesion as well as the healthy areas of the brain, IHC analyses using specific biomarkers was carried out. Immunohistochemical analysis of lesioned tissue sections (ipsilateral side) established neuronal degeneration in the infarct region with immunofluorescence analyses highlighting GFAP expression, the astrocyte marker, strongly localized within the PL-GM, indicating astrogliosis post stroke (**Figures 1D,E**). The infract region experienced neuronal loss, sections were tested for the principal neuronal marker proteins: MAP2 and Tau (**Figures 1F–I**). In both instances, we failed to detect these proteins within the infarct region- validating neuronal loss. Comparing the contralesion sections with the ischemic brain sections, we documented APP (**Figures 2A–D**) and aggregated $A\beta_{1-42}$ (**Figures 2C–H**) in the GM and the PL-GM. Mis-processed APP, ($A\beta_{1-42}$) its extracellular aggregation is one neuropathological marker used to classify Alzheimer's disease (AD) (Paul Murphy and LeVine, 2010; Esparza et al., 2016; Wildburger et al., 2017). Surprisingly in the L-WM there was an increase in $A\beta_{1-42}$ aggregates (**Figure 2G**). Examination of MBP showed loss in integrity and significant disorganization of the myelin sheaths in the WM, at the ipsilateral side, below the stroke point (**Figure 2G**). Interesting to note, that the contra-lesioned white matter (CL-WM, **Figure 2H**) shows uniform MBP staining throughout WM tracts as seen with the native control (**Figure 2E**).

Molecular and Elemental Changes Due to Stroke

FTIR Spectra and Images

Fourier transform Infrared bands assignments in this study were based on the specific spectral bands as defined in the Section "Materials and Methods" (**Supplementary Figure S1** and **Supplementary Table S1**). As an example, the FTIR spectrum for the WM we observed that spectral bands corresponding to lipid, protein, ester, nucleic acids, and carbohydrates dominate the spectra (**Supplementary Figure S1**). All samples were prepared, treated and processed in the same manner, it should be noted that lipid, protein and other biochemical component values from the lesioned (ipsilateral side) were normalized to the contra-lateral side. Again, the contralateral hemisphere bio-chemical components values were used as a base line values indicating the stroke induced changes to the cortical region and the surrounding WM.

In Hematoxylin and Eosin section captured by digital scanning microscope, a parallel-unstained image of a control brain section, captured by FTIR microscope bright field is depicted together with the corresponding chemical FTIR spectroscopic image (**Figures 3A–C**). Lipid and protein distribution, as found in native healthy rat brain sections,was represented in **Figures 3D,E**. In contrast to the even distribution of protein and lipid in the control, the lesioned brain lipid and protein show distinct distribution patterns (**Figures 3F,G**). For example, in the PS-GM both lipid and protein levels were greatly reduced and associated with increasing aggregated protein. The PL-GM and L-WM regions experienced decrease in the lipid and protein components associated with protein aggregation (**Figures 3F,G** and see also **Figure 3M**). **Figures 3H,I** depict the average FTIR spectra for different tissue regions and the analysis of these spectra were performed on $n = 6$ animals. In the stroke PS-GM region, the FTIR spectra revealed that the lipid, protein, lipid acyl bands $\nu_s(CH_2)$,

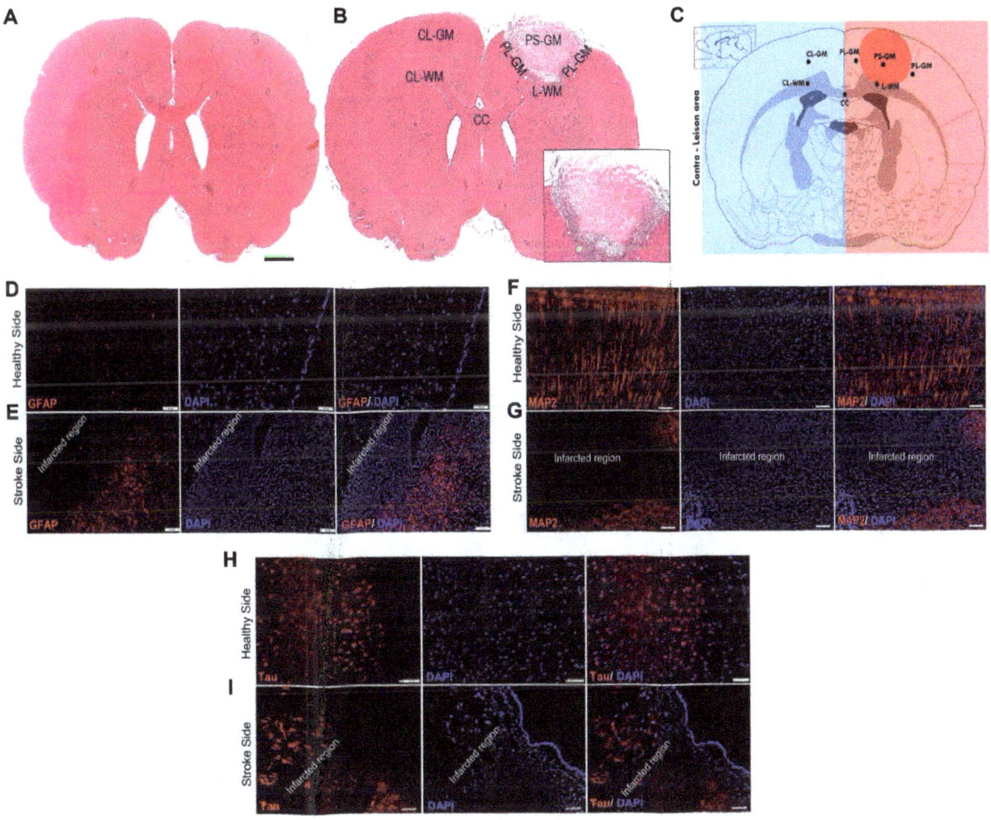

FIGURE 1 | Photothrombotic lesion in rat somatosensory cortex results in cell death and astrigliosis. **(A)** Hematoxylin and Eosin (H&E) staining brain section of native control brain (magnification 5×). **(B)** H&E stained image 1-week post-stroke brain (magnification 5×). **(C)** Brain section scheme for the six regions of interest (ROI): primary stroke lesion gray matter (PS-GM), perilesional gray matter (PL-GM), lesioned white matter (L-WM) and contra-lesioned white matter (CL-WM), contra-lesioned gray matter (CL-GM), and corpus callosum white matter (CC). **(D,E)** Healthy control and lesioned brain sections labeled with GFAP and DAPI: primary lesion gray matter (PS), perilesional gray matter (PL) indicated activated astrocytes (GFAP, red stain) around the ischemic region (peri-infarct region) and degenerated neurons with shrunken nuclei (DAPI, blue stain). Infiltration of the astrocytes around the primary lesion PS-GM region with GFAP (red). The DAPI labels (blue) degenerated cells. **(F,G)** Healthy control and affected stroke rat brains sections were labeled with MAP2 and DAPI. **(H,I)** Healthy control and affected stroke rat brains sections labeled with Tau and DAPI to assist in comparisons. Scale bar = 100 μm.

the lipid ester band ν(C = O) decrease compared with the PL-GM and CL-GM (**Figures 3H,I**). The stroke PS-GM FTIR spectrum had a significant reduction in the absorption band centered at 1227 cm^{-1} which arises from the P = O symmetric stretching vibrations of the phosphodiester bonds in DNA/RNA polysaccharide backbones (Carter et al., 2010; Srinivasan, 2010; Ami et al., 2013).

A more detailed representation of the average FTIR spectra of the PS-GM, CL-GM, CL-WM, and L-WM shown in **Figure 3H**. This highlights that lipid acyl bands were severely reduced in PS-GM and L-WM compared with CL-GM and CL-WM, respectively. The CH_3 (methyl concentration), olefinic = CH (unsaturated lipid) and the lipid ester (CO) (oxidative stress) were significantly increased while that of the CH_2 (chain lipid length) was decreased in the L-WM spectrum. The average FTIR spectra collected from the PS-GM, PL-GM, CL-GM and native control GM revealed marked reduction in lipid, lipid-acyl and protein in the ipsilateral compared with contralateral hemisphere; which were reduced when compared with the native control (**Figure 3I**).

Fourier transform Infrared analysis revealed that lipid content (n = 6 animals) was markedly reduced in the primary PS-GM (0.21 ± 0.010) when compared to the PL-GM (0.55 ± 0.028) and L-WM (0.89 ± 0.045) in the ipsilesional hemisphere. The amount of the lipid in PS-GM, PL-GM and L-WM were greatly reduced when compared with the contra-lesioned white matter (CL-WM) (1.1 ± 0.055) and contra-lesioned gray matter (CL-GM) (0.72 ± 0.036). These results were further compared with the healthy native control GM (0.79 ± 0.040) and WM (1.32 ± 0.066), where higher lipid content in comparison with the ipsilateral and contralateral hemisphere of the experimental animals (**Figures 3D,F** and see also **Figure 4L**). The results also revealed that the lipid acyl content (CH_2) concentration in the PS-GM (0.264 ± 0.019), PL-GM (0.522 ± 0.026), and L-WM (0.563 ± 0.028) decreased compared to the contralateral region (0.6012 ± 0.030) of the ischemic brain, and all values were less than the healthy native animal (0.649 ± 0.035) as presented in (**Figures 4C,D,M**).

In converse, the degree of unsaturated components olefinic = CH increased, in the PL-GM (0.0049 ± 0.0002) and L-WM (0.0062 ± 0.0003), compared to the contralateral

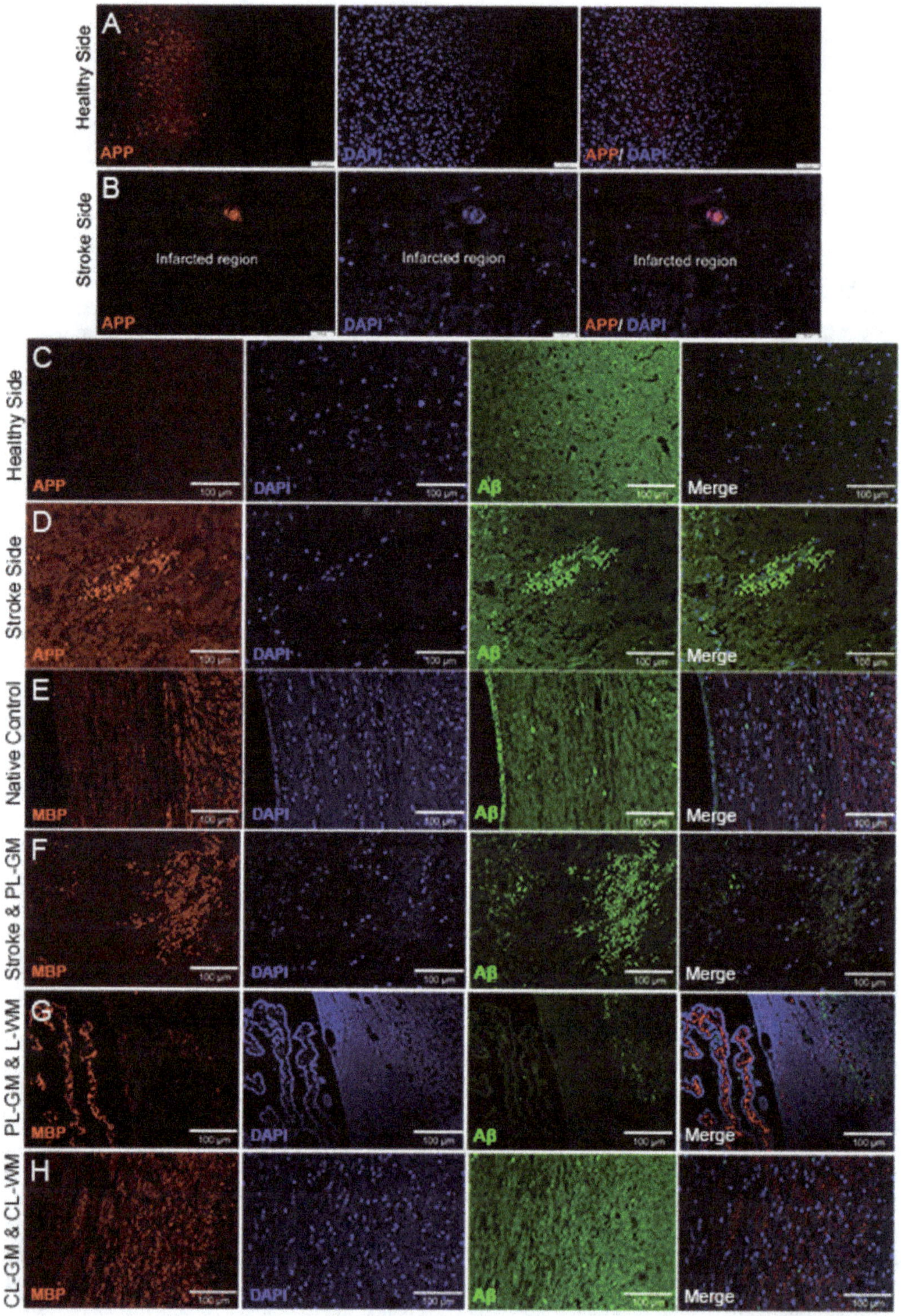

FIGURE 2 | Immunohistochemistry staining identifying altered APP and $A\beta_{1-42}$ in infarcted brain sections. **(A,B)** Contra-lesioned and lesioned hemispheres labeled with APP and DAPI: primary lesion gray matter (PS) shows amyloid precursor protein (APP) and contra-lesioned gray matter (CL-GM) with normal homogenous distribution of APP (red). **(C,D)** Contra-lesioned and affected stroke hemispheres were labeled with APP (red), DAPI (Blue) and $A\beta_{1-42}$ (green). **(E–H)** Native control and 1-week affected stroke rat brains sections labeled with myelin basic protein (MBP, red), DAPI (blue), and $A\beta_{1-42}$ (green). **(F,G)** Primary lesion gray matter (PS-GM) contains degenerated neurons (DAPI, blue) and disorganization of the myelin sheath (MBP, red) of the axonal neurons in the lesioned white matter (L-WM) scale bar = 100 μm for **(A–H)**.

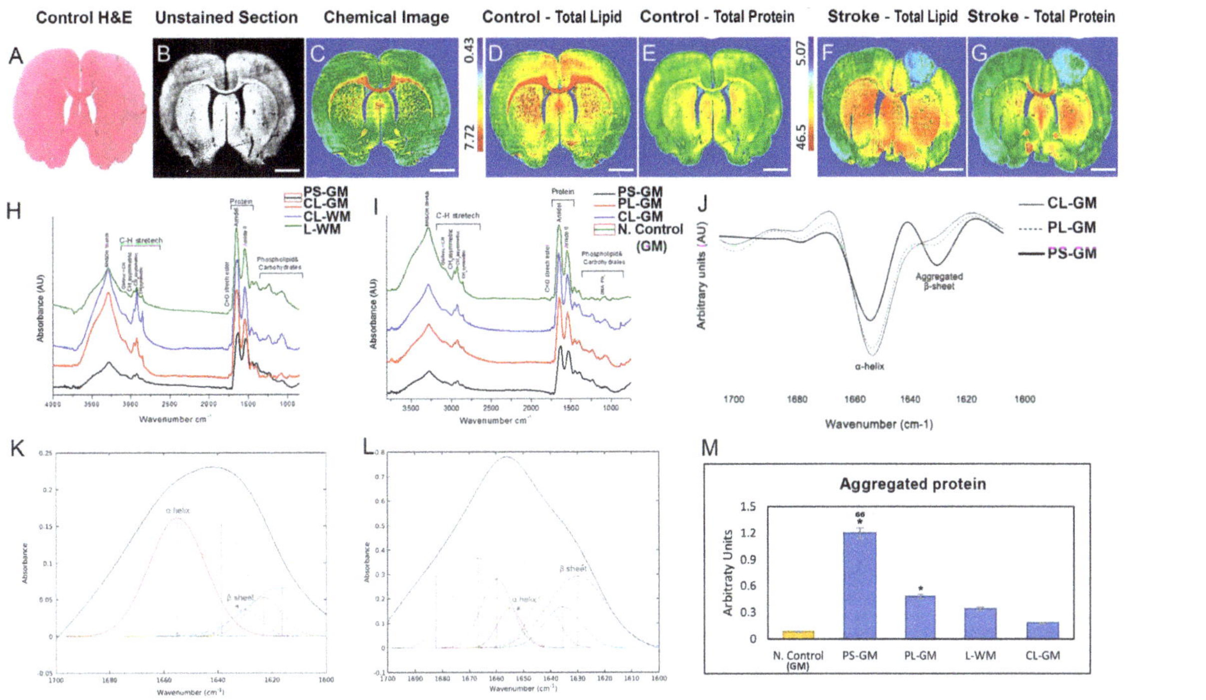

FIGURE 3 | Whole brain section-FTIR imaging of biochemical changes within contralateral and ipsilateral hemispheres following photothrombotic focal ischemic insult to the somatosensory cortex. **(A)** H&E stained brain section captured by Digital Scanning Microscope Bright field (20×). **(B)**. Representative unstained FTIR light microscopic image of the healthy control rat brain (10×). **(C)**. Representative FTIR chemical image of the unstained brain section showing main biochemical components: lipid, phospholipid, protein, carbohydrates and nucleic acids. **(D,E)** FTIR image that represent the total lipid and total protein distribution in the healthy control rat brain. **(F,G)** FTIR image that represent the total lipid and total protein distribution in the stroke affected rat brain. Scale bars = 100 μm. **(H)** Representative FTIR averaged spectra in the range of 4000–400 cm^{-1} acquired from the cortical region of the PS-GM, L-WM, CL-GM, and CL-WM. **(I)** Representative FTIR averaged spectra in the range of 4000–400 cm^{-1} acquired from the cortical region of the PS-GM, PL-GM, CL-GM and native control GM. **(J)** Representative average second-derivative spectra of the amide I band in the spectral range of 1700–1600 cm^{-1} acquired from the primary lesion gray matter (PS-GM), perilesional gray matter (PL-GM), and contra-lesioned gray matter (CL-GM) regions post ischemic. The spectra show α- helical secondary protein structure at 1655 cm^{-1} and β-sheets protein conformation at 1630 cm^{-1}. **(K,L)** Representative curve fitting of the amide I band in the spectral range of 1700-1600 cm^{-1} of the CL-GM and PS-GM, respectively, to quantify the aggregated protein relatively. **(M)** Histogram of the aggregated protein comparing different regions of interest: native control, PS-GM, PL-GM, L-WM with CL-GM. The FTIR images were colored-coded: red color corresponds to the highest content and blue color corresponds to the lowest content as shown on the color bars in the figures. Statistical significance was determined from six animals with a paired *t*-test and the 95% confidence interval. Bars represent mean ± SD. $^{*}p > 0.05$, $^{**}p > 0.01$ relative to CL-GM. $^{\sigma}p > 0.05$, $^{\sigma\sigma}p > 0.01$ relative to PL-GM.

hemisphere (0.0026 ± 0.0002) and the healthy native animal (0.0014 ± 0.0001) as shown in **Figures 4E,F,N**. These results also indicated that the CH_3 (methyl concentration) is severely reduced within the PS-GM (0.0048 ± 0.0002). On the other hand, the methyl concentration increased in the PL-GM (0.0494 ± 0.003) and L-WM (0.0627 ± 0.003) in the ipsilateral hemisphere in comparison to the contralateral hemisphere (0.0276 ± 0.0014) and the healthy native brain (0.0111 ± 0.0005) as represented in **Figures 4G,H,O**, respectively. Also documented was that the value of lipid ester (C = O) in the PS-GM region (0.11 ± 0.0055) was markedly reduced compared to PL-GM (0.64 ± 0.032) and L-WM (0.75 ± 0.0375) regions. Interestingly, lipid ester (C = O) amount in the contralateral hemisphere (0.28 ± 0.014) and native healthy brain (0.15 ± 0.0075) was lower than the PL-GM and L-WM as shown in **Figures 4I,J,P**.

The FTIR spectra revealed that total protein distribution in the cortex, especially in the PS-GM and PL-GM was greatly affected, due to stroke and, in the focal point of the stroke, there was protein aggregation. These analyses revealed that the protein level in the PS-GM (3.2 ± 0.16) was lower compared to PL-GM (12 ± 0.61). PS-GM and PL-GM experience severe reduction in protein in comparison to contralateral hemisphere (14.6 ± 0.73) and native healthy brain (17.8 ± 0.89) as presented in **Figures 3E,G** and see also **Figure 4K**. Moreover, the second derivative of the FTIR, range 1700–1600 cm^{-1}, specifically protein band at the spectral range of 1630–1625 cm^{-1}, indicates protein aggregation in the affected stroke region (**Figure 3J**), i.e., an increase in β-sheet and decrease in α-helix structures at 1660–1655 cm^{-1} as shown in the CL-GM and PS-GM spectra curve fitting (**Figures 3K,L**, respectively). The results indicate that the PS-GM (1.2 ± 0.06) region had increased aggregated protein content in comparison with the PL-GM (0.48 ± 0.024) and contralateral hemisphere (0.18 ± 0.009) and these two regions were having higher value than the native control (0.08 ± 0.004) (**Figure 3M**). (These findings correlate well with the histochemistry results see **Figure 2**). Here the results identified a decrease in the relative amount of lipid and protein bio-content in the PL-GM region of the ischemic brain

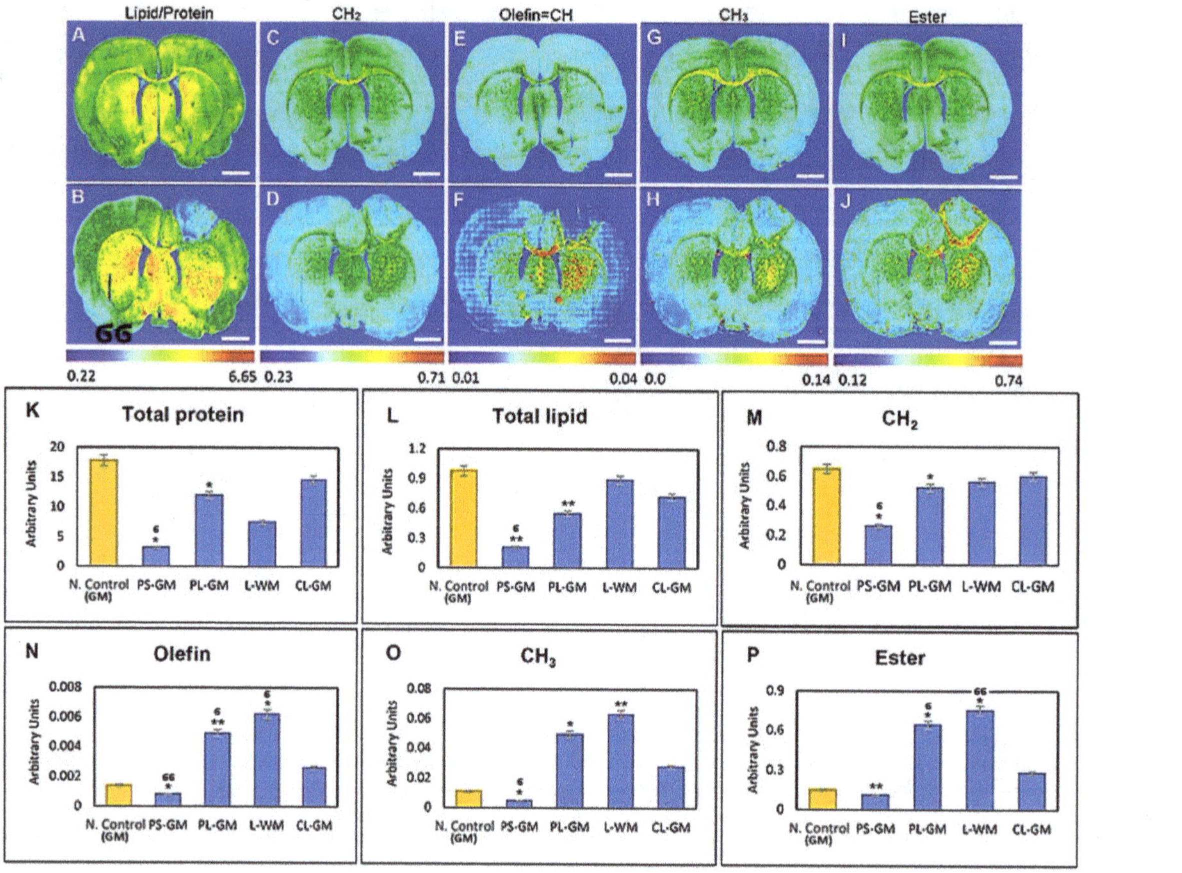

FIGURE 4 | Functional group (macromolecular/sub-cellular/biochemical) images obtained of the native control ischemic stroke brain sections. **(A–I)**. Representative FTIR images of lipid/protein, lipid acyl group (CH_2), olefin = CH, methyl (CH_3) and lipid ester (C = O) distribution in the native healthy control brain tissue sections, respectively. **(B–J)** The same function groups (above) obtained from the ischemic stroke brain sections. **(K–P)** Histogram of specific bio-molecules content such as total protein, total lipid, lipid acyl group (CH_2), olefin = CH, methyl (CH_3), and lipid ester (C = O), respectively. The regions of interest were native control rat brain GM and ischemic brain PS-GM, PL-GM, L-WM, and CL-GM. The FTIR images were color coded, red color corresponds to the highest content and blue color corresponds to the lowest content as shown on the color bars in the figures. Statistical significance was determined from six animals. Statistical significance was determined from six animals with a paired *t*-test and the 95% confidence interval. Bars represent mean ± SD. $^{*}p > 0.05$, $^{**}p > 0.01$ relative to CL-GM. $^{\sigma}p > 0.05$, $^{\sigma\sigma}p > 0.01$ relative to PL-GM.

in comparison to the native healthy control brain. Changes in the lipid/protein ratio (**Figures 4A,B**) suggest that these biochemical alterations associated with the stroke are due to triggering and initiating specific mechanisms of neurodegeneration.

The FTIR assays identified that the CC in the experimental animal (lesioned) brain, experienced reduction in lipid content (0.91 ± 0.0455) in comparison to the native healthy control animal (1.34 ± 0.067) (**Figures 3D,G**). The results also showed that that the lipid acyl (CH_2) amounts in the lesioned CC (0.582 ± 0.0291) decreased compared to the native animal (0.661 ± 0.033) (**Figures 4C,D**). There is also an increase in the unsaturated components olefinic = CH (0.0058 ± 0.0003) compared to the healthy animal (0.0040 ± 0.0002) (**Figures 4E,F**). These results also indicated that the CH_3 (methyl group) concentration in the lesioned CC (0.0574 ± 0.00278) increased compared to the native animal (0.0439 ± 0.0022) (**Figures 4G,H**). The lipid ester (C = O) concentration in the lesioned brain CC (0.64 ± 0.032) also experienced an increase in comparison to native animal (0.52 ± 0.026) ($p = 0.73$, $n = 6$) as shown in **Figures 4I,J**.

As a further analysis of the FTIR data, PCA was performed on the spectral second derivatives in the range of 4000–700 cm^{-1} (with the range of 2500–2000 cm^{-1} removed) for the native control and lesioned rat brain sections (**Figure 5A**). The differences were mainly significant in the region of 3994–2800 cm^{-1}, which correlates to the lipid bio-molecular changes in the primary lesion. Also, there were molecular changes in the spectral region of 1530–1680 cm^{-1} which is related to protein structure in the tissue section. The scores plot revealed that the spectral data collected from the rat cortices were clustered into two distinct groups that correlate with healthy (native) and stroke affected. The clear segregation between the two groups in the PCA plots revealed that the molecular makeup of the cortical tissue has changed due to ischemic stroke with the first 3PCs accounting for ~98.5% of the total variation as shown in **Figure 5B**. The PCA analysis also resulted in clustering of the

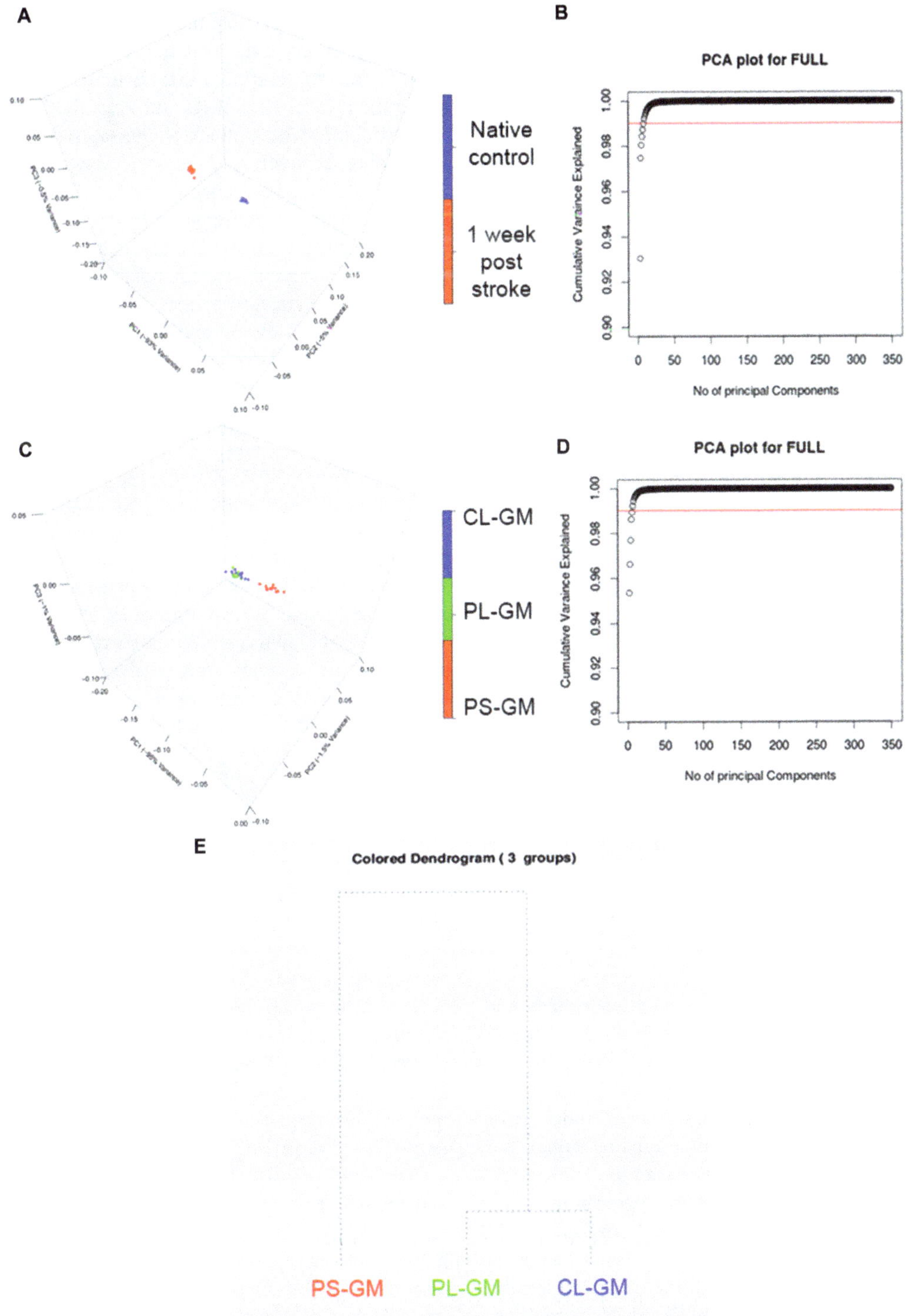

FIGURE 5 | Principle component analysis (PCA) analyses of averaged FTIR spectroscopic studies. **(A)** Representative 3D score plot for PCA analysis based on the average FTIR spectral data in the region of 4000–700 cm^{-1} (with the range of 2500–2000 cm^{-1} removed) collected from the time point of native healthy control and stroke affected rat brain. **(B)**. The score plot of the PCA shows that there are three main PCs that separate the time point native control healthy and the affected stroke rat brains and are accounted for PC1 (93%), PC2 (4%), and PC3 (1%). **(C)** Represents the PCs plot that shows that there are the three main PCs that separate PS-GM, PL-GM, and CL-GM spectra. **(D)** The score plot of the PCA and shows that there are three main PCs that separate the PS-GM, PL-GM, and CL-GM spectra are counted for PC1 (95%), PC2 (1.5%), and PC3 (1%). **(E)** Represents the hierarchical dendrogram that shows a clear separation PS-GM, PL-GM, and CL-GM regions in the ipsilateral side of 1-week post ischemic stroke. The hierarchical dendrogram shows that PS-GM is located in one group while the PL-GM and CL-GM regions are located in the second group.

PS-GM, PL-GM, and CL-GM (**Figure 5C**) from the scores plot of the three significant components: PC1 (95%), PC2 (1.5%), and PC3 (1%) as shown in **Figure 5D**. The first cluster contains the spectra from the PS-GM region, while the second group contains the spectra from PL-GM and CL-GM with this separation clearly shown in the hierarchical dendrogram (**Figure 5E**). The advantage of PCA is to allow the rat brain cortices to be clearly distinguished into healthy (control) and stroke region. Moreover, **Figure 5B** outlines an estimate that more than ~98.5% of the variance in the spectra can be captured by the first three PCs. Furthermore, the PCA result makes it feasible to perform hierarchical clustering, thereby, combining PS-GM region with PL-GM and CL-GM regions using a dendrogram.

Elemental Analysis by Laser Ablation (LA-ICPMS)

Employing LA-ICP-MS can be used to assess the elemental distributions of C, P, S, Cu, Fe, Zn, and Ca in the rat brain section 1-week post-stroke (**Figures 6A–G**). Here element values from the ipsilateral cortex (lesioned hemisphere) were compared with those of the contralateral cortex. The LA-ICPMS results provide three main observations: (a) a reduction in all element concentrations (Ca, C, Fe, Cu, S, P, and Zn) inside the stroke focus point (PS-GM) region; (b) Ca, Cu, and Zn were mainly accumulated at the edge of the injured brain hemisphere; and (c) significant and high accumulation of Fe around the PS-GM and in the lesion rim, shown in detail in **Figures 6H–N**. Further, the results indicate that the distribution of the brain elements were greatly affected by the ischemic stroke. This abnormal distribution might also effect brain functions involved in muscle control, movement and memory (Prashanth et al., 2015; Chen et al., 2016).

DISCUSSION

In this study diverse techniques were applied to delineate bio-chemical and elemental alterations 1-week post-stroke in the PS-GM, PL-GM, L-WM, CL-WM, CL-GM, and CC. A combination of FTIR and LA-ICPMS with PCA analysis, yielded novel results: significant changes in lipid values; protein conformation and in elemental distribution in multiple regions, which may correlate with morphological changes. For example, FTIR studies identified significantly enhanced protein aggregation, which included $A\beta_{1-42}$ – one of the pathological markers of AD (Prashanth et al., 2015; Baldassarre et al., 2016; Chen et al., 2016). Moreover, we detected $A\beta_{1-42}$ in the ipsilateral lesioned WM – further proof that the site of stroke is more global than originally thought. It should be noted that we do not detect $A\beta_{1-42}$ aggregates in the contra-lateral WM indicative that the lesion induces APP/Aβ aggregation in the ipsilateral side. Furthermore, the breakdown of MBP and decrease in the myelin sheath thickness, post-ischemic stroke, which increases the vulnerability of exposed axons and leads to a decline in functional connectivity and behavioral deficits (Li et al., 2014; Baldassarre et al., 2016). Notably, other studies have reported that MBP dysfunction(s) were associated with physiological response to stress and emotional states, including anxiety and depression in adulthood, all possible indicators for commonalities in brain traumas (Drevets et al., 2008; Edgar and Sibille, 2012).

Ischemic stroke causes extensive brain damage through the generation of free radicals such as ROS O_2^- (Olmez and Ozyurt, 2012) which attack polyunsaturated fatty acid (PUFA) containing structures (Allen and Bayraktutan, 2009). FTIR imaging identified a change in the lipid/protein ratio in the PL-GM region an event triggered by specific processes that lead to bio-chemical changes. The histological data revealed that the insulted brain experienced edema. Previous studies reported that edema initiates oxidative stress and increased protein oxidation and protein mis-folding and cell degeneration (Hackett et al., 2015a). Edema and oxidative stress may be the driving factors in lipid fragmentation, protein aggregation (mis-folding) (Hackett et al., 2015a), neurodegeneration (Klein and Ackerman, 2003; Uttara et al., 2009) and cell death (Ryter et al., 2007). Current bio-diagnostic techniques, such as MRI and biochemical assays are not sensitive enough to detect oxidative stress. Whereas, FTIR imaging spectroscopy is, to our knowledge, the only technique sensitive enough to detect these molecular changes associated with oxidative stress (Kneipp et al., 2000; Wang et al., 2005; Ozek et al., 2010; Caine et al., 2016). Thus, in order to understand the lipid alteration associated with ischemic stroke, FTIR spectra of lipids were analyzed. In the brain sections, we found significant alteration in the lipid acyl (CH_2), lipid ester (C = O); olefinic = CH and methyl group (CH_3). When double bond sites of PUFA are attacked by free radicals this leads to degradation of lipids into smaller fragments (Allen and Bayraktutan, 2009; Olmez and Ozyurt, 2012; Caine et al., 2016). Lipid peroxidation is associated with increased methyl (CH_3) concentration and the formation of degradation products such as alkanes, carbonyl compounds, lipid aldehydes and alkyl radicals (Lamba et al., 1994; de Zwart et al., 1999; Manda et al., 2007; Yin et al., 2011).

Ischemic stroke caused reduction in the total lipid and lipid acyl contents at stroke focal PS-GM, PL-GM, and L-WM in the ipsilateral hemisphere. In PS-GM, total lipid decreased, as expected, due to tissue loss, evidenced also as protein loss. Hence, lipid acyl (CH_2), lipid ester (C = O), olefinic = CH, and methyl (CH_3) all declined significantly. However, in contrast to the PS-GM in the PL-GM, L-WM, and CC we observed a significant increase in lipid ester (C = O), olefinic = CH and methyl (CH_3). An increase in the olefinic = CH content at the ipsilateral hemisphere compared with contralateral and native controls suggests that stroke induced an increase in the unsaturated fatty acids. Although, lipid peroxidation should result in loss of olefinic = CH bonds, but interestingly in our study we observed an increase in the olefinic = CH bio-content, which can be due to accumulation of double bond end products through lipid peroxidation compensation mechanisms (Liu et al., 2002; Severcan et al., 2005). Our results are in good agreement with previous studies on the effect of the lipid peroxidation on diabetic rat liver microsomal membranes and diabetic patients' platelets (Liu et al., 2002; Severcan et al., 2005). These studies highlighted that lipid peroxidation induced an increase in the olefinic = CH content, which originated mainly from double

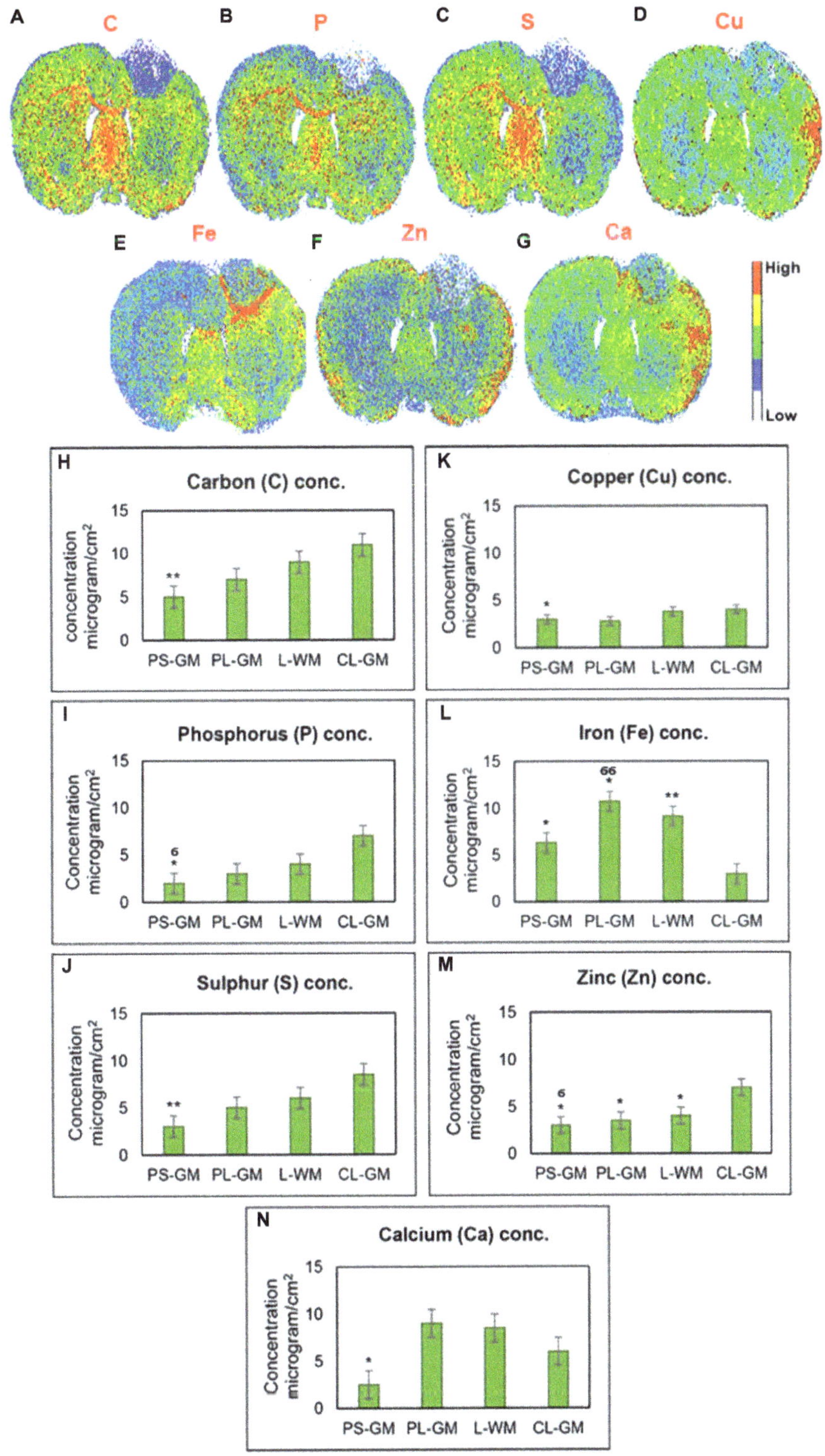

FIGURE 6 | Qualitative elemental maps for whole rat brain sections. **(A–G)** Represent images of the elemental distributions of C, P, S, Cu, Fe, Zn, and Ca, respectively, in the rat brain section 1-week post-ischemic stroke measured by LA-ICP-QMS. **(H–N)** Elemental concentration of C, P, S, Cu, Fe, Zn, and Ca, respectively, from four regions of interest such as PS-GM, PL-GM, L-GM, and CL-GM. These LA images were color-labeled according to the calculated concentration values, where red corresponds to the highest concentration and white corresponds to the lowest concentration as shown on the color bars in the figures. Statistical significance was determined from six animals with a paired *t*-test and the 95% confidence interval. Bars represent mean ± SD. $^{*}p > 0.05$, $^{**}p > 0.01$ relative to CL-GM. $^{\sigma}p > 0.05$, $^{\sigma\sigma}p > 0.01$ relative to PL-GM.

bond lipid peroxidation products (Kar et al., 2004; Gouras et al., 2010). Our results also show an increase in the lipid ester (C = O) post stroke. Thus, our results emphasize that ischemic stroke induced lipid peroxidation which results in marked decreases in the total lipid and lipid CH_2 contents associated with increases in the lipid ester (C = O), olefinic = CH and CH_3 bio-contents (Lamba et al., 1994; de Zwart et al., 1999; Manda et al., 2007; Cakmak et al., 2011). These bio-chemical alterations occurs at the PL-GM, L-WM and the CC but were prominent at L-WM and the CC due to higher lipid content.

From immunohistochemical studies we noted high GFAP expression, an indicator for astrogliosis, and from elemental data enhanced Fe levels-a possible marker for increased mitochondria; in all, a likelihood that glia are metabolizing lipids esters and olefins, including removing necrotic tissue. In the WM, below the site of the lesion, we again noted a decrease in total lipid content, which was associated with significant increase in lipid ester, olefin, and CH_3 indicative that possibly degradation of long chain fats was occurring, including cell membranes. Intriguingly at this locus, we detected only $A\beta_{1-42}$, which is thought to be formed due to exposure to reactive oxygen species.

Protein exposure to reactive oxygen results in protein cross-linking, aggregation, fragmentation, and denaturation, resulting in loss of function. The levels of the total protein and aggregated protein were calculated from the amide I band at 1700–1600 cm^{-1} and curve fitting at 1630 cm^{-1}, respectively. As expected from histological data the FTIR amide I data indicated a loss of protein from the lesioned GM (PS-GM) compared with the control samples. Interestingly, we observed that there is an increase in the band absorption of β-sheets at 1630 cm^{-1} and associated decrease of α- helical protein band absorption at 1655 cm^{-1} indicating protein aggregation. This protein conformational change was not detected on the contra-lateral side, which indicate that stroke induces protein alterations. The PS-GM and PL-GM regions experienced a decrease in total protein levels (amide values), with the most surprising and dramatic change in aggregated protein in these areas. Histochemical studies identified significant changes in APP in the infarcted area (closely associated with glial cells) and tests for $A\beta_{1-42}$- which has been previously reported to increase, not only in stroke, but also in other neurodegenerative disorders (Paul Murphy and LeVine, 2010; Esparza et al., 2016; Wildburger et al., 2017). It should be noted no Tau protein was detected in the lesioned area, thus it was inferred that the protein aggregation was exclusively APP derived and was $A\beta_{1-42}$. Moreover, it is tempting to speculate that $A\beta_{1-42}$ accumulation due to ischemic stroke might also trigger other neurological deficits and subsequent neurodegeneration (Kar et al., 2004; Gouras et al., 2010).

Elemental studies clearly defined significant loss of C, P, and S from the PS-GM, PL-GM, and the L-WM as these are the major components of nucleic acids, protein and lipids that make up cells. Sulfur concentration were greatly reduced in the ipsilateral hemisphere. Sulfur is a constituent of the anti-oxidant enzymes glutathione peroxidases (GP) and thioredoxin reductases (TR) and of the metabolic enzyme S-adenosylhomocysteine (S-ACH) (Zima et al., 1996; Birben et al., 2012; Li et al., 2013). In several neurodegenerative disorders loss of these enzymes has been postulated as a corollary of enhanced cell pathology (Zima et al., 1996; Birben et al., 2012; Li et al., 2013). Surprisingly, in the cortices we identified significantly high levels of Ca and Fe. From studies in the hippocampus, high Ca^{2+} levels were found to be excitotoxic (Dong et al., 2009) and in the brain Fe ions can increase the formation of reactive radicals and thus lipid peroxidation (Halliwell and Gutteridge, 1986). This change can also be attributed to an increase in to astroglial cells that metabolizing necrotic tissue. In our study, a small change in Cu values was found, but this could be linked to the fact that Cu and Zn are bound to synaptic termini and regulate exocytosis (Sadiq et al., 2012), thus the possibility is that release of these metals into the micro-environment may account for the increased neuronal excitability that has been reported by others after stroke (Li and Zhang, 2012). Our results indicate that ischemic stroke can induce significant changes in the stroke focus point, the GM, as well as in the adjacent WM of the affected hemisphere. Furthermore, the enriched lipid brain regions, especially brain WM are vulnerable to ischemic stroke and can be highly affected by the production of free radicals and bi-products of oxidation.

The chemometric analyses, PCA in the spectral range of 3500–900 cm^{-1} and the hierarchy dendrogram from HCA, delineated a clear separation between the control and the lesioned sections. From the PCA plot, it was clear that the primary stroke PS-GM clustered in one group while both PL-GM and CL-GM clustered together. This clear separation reveals that the stroke focus region PS-GM has significant molecular changes in its bio-chemical makeup. One of these major bio-molecular alterations was found by curve fitting of the second derivative of the protein bands in the PS-GM spectrum. It revealed an increase in the β-sheet content and an associated decrease in α-helical secondary structure- again the interpretation being that protein aggregation, a marker for neurodegeneration, occurred. The data also indicate that the effects of stroke are much more global on the ipsilateral side than originally thought. Thus, newer or more improved ischemic stroke management in the sub-acute phase should prioritize treating edema and the oxidative stress damage in order to have a successful outcome to maintain and improve the PL-GM and L-WM brain tissue.

Our findings suggest that edema and oxidative stress are the major factors that affect the integrity, structure and functionality of the brain as well as leading to bio-molecular and elemental alterations 1 week post-stroke. However, it has been found that 24 h post stroke, the molecular and elemental alterations are mainly due to tissue swelling following edema but oxidative-damage is not responsible for the these alterations especially at perilesional gray matter (PL-GM) region (Caine et al., 2016). Our results show that FTIR bio-spectroscopy is a non-destructive, rapid, and a refined technique to characterize oxidative stress bio-markers not obtained by routine approaches for lipid degradation. Also, we can detect secondary structure protein changes such as β-sheet formation. Normally, detection of these changes requires biochemical methods that include tissue homogenization and, or treatment for immunoblotting or IHC, destroying the spatial-temporal integrity of the brain. In summary, these results suggest that a good therapeutic strategy should include a mechanism that provides protective effect from brain swelling (edema) and neurotoxicity by scavenging the lipid peroxidation end products. This strategy can include the protection of the blood–brain barrier (BBB) endothelial cells. Thus, we conclude that FTIR can complement and expedite research into stroke.

AUTHOR CONTRIBUTIONS

MA and FR performed all the FTIR and LA measurements in this study. MA, TA, KA-S, and EA were involved in data interpretation, drafting and editing the manuscript. AL was involved in elemental analysis studies. EA and NM were involved in IHC studies. RM and EU were involved in processing the experimental data and performing the multivariate and statistical analysis. All authors discussed the results and commented on the manuscript and in critical revision of this manuscript.

FUNDING

This study was made possible by a NPRP Award [5-381-3-101] from the Qatar National Research Fund (a member of The Qatar Foundation). The statements made herein are solely the responsibility of the authors.

ACKNOWLEDGMENTS

We would like to thank Drs. Geralda van Tilborg, Rick M. Dijkhuizen (Biomedical MR Imaging and Spectroscopy Group, Center for Image Sciences, University Medical Center Utrecht, Utrecht, Netherlands) for providing us the brain samples for this study. We would like to thank Drs. Omar M. A. El-Agnaf, Stephen Ogg, Mohamed M. Emara, Sara Abdulla, and Wesal Habbab and Hamda S. Al Mutawa from QBRI for advice and technical support. Also, Divya Viswanathan from WCM-Q and Dr. Mohamed Yousef, Qatar University for their technical assistance.

SUPPLEMENTARY MATERIAL

FIGURE S1 | The representative FTIR spectrum of white matter (WM) in a native control rat brain in the spectral range of 4000–700 cm^{-1} and mechanical properties of the native and lesioned brain sections. Representative FTIR spectra of WM in the native control rat brain from region 4000–700 cm^{-1}.

TABLE S1 | Fourier transform Infrared (FTIR) spectral bands and their corresponding bio-chemical assignment.

REFERENCES

1. Ali, M. H., Al-Saad, K., Popelka, A., van Tilborg, G., and Goormaghtigh, E. (2016). Application of Fourier transform infrared (FTIR) spectroscopy and atomic force microscopy in stroke-affected brain tissue. *Swift J. Med. Med. Sci.* 2, 011–024.
2. Allen, C. L., and Bayraktutan, U. (2009). Oxidative stress and its role in the pathogenesis of ischaemic stroke. *Int. J. Stroke* 4, 461–470. doi: 10.1111/j.1747- 4949.2009.00387.x
3. Ami, D., Mereghetti, P., and Doglia, S. M. (2013). "Multivariate analysis for Fourier transform infrared spectra of complex biological systems and processes," in *Multivariate Analysis in Management, Engineering and the Sciences*, ed. B. Akselsen (London: InTech).
4. Baker, M. J., Trevisan, J., Bassan, P., Bhargava, R., Butler, H. J., Dorling, K. M., et al. (2014). Using Fourier transform IR spectroscopy to analyze biological materials. *Nat. Protoc.* 9, 1771–1791. doi: 10.1038/nprot.2014.110
5. Balbekova, A., Lohninger, H., van Tilborg, G. A., Dijkhuizen, R. M., Bonta, M., Limbeck, A., et al. (2017). Fourier transform infrared (FT-IR) and laser ablation inductively coupled plasma-mass spectrometry (LA-ICP-MS) imaging of cerebral ischemia: combined analysis of rat brain thin cuts toward improved tissue classification. *Appl. Spectrosc.* 72, 241–250. doi: 10.1177/ 0003702817734618
6. Baldassarre, A., Ramsey, L. E., Siegel, J. S., Shulman, G. L., and Corbetta, M. (2016). Brain connectivity and neurological disorders after stroke. *Curr. Opin. Neurol.* 29, 706–713. doi: 10.1097/WCO.0000000000000396
7. Bassan, P., Kohler, A., Martens, H., Lee, J., Byrne, H. J., Dumas, P., et al. (2010). "Resonant MIE scattering (RMieS) correction of infrared spectra from highly scattering biological samples". *Analyst* 135, 268–277. doi: 10.1039/b921056c
8. Becker, J. S., Matusch, A., Becker, J. S., Wu, B., Palm, C., Becker, A. J., et al. (2011). Mass spectrometric imaging (MSI) of metals using advanced BrainMet techniques for biomedical research. *Int. J. Mass Spectrom.* 307, 3–15. doi: 10.1016/j.ijms.2011.01.015
9. Becker, J. S., Matusch, A., and Wu, B. (2014). Bioimaging mass spectrometry of trace elements–recent advance and applications of LA-ICP-MS: a review. *Anal. Chim. Acta* 835, 1–18. doi: 10.1016/j.aca.2014.04.048
10. Becker, R. A., Chambers, J. M., and Wilks, A. R. (1988). *The New S Language*. Monterey, CA: Wadsworth & Brooks/Cole.
11. Benseny-Cases, N., Klementieva, O., Cotte, M., Ferrer, I., and Cladera, J. (2014). Microspectroscopy (μFTIR) reveals co-localization of lipid oxidation and amyloid plaques in human Alzheimer disease brains. *Anal. Chem.* 86, 12047–12054. doi: 10.1021/ac502667b
12. Birben, E., Sahiner, U. M., Sackesen, C., Erzurum, S., and Kalayci, O. (2012). Oxidative stress and antioxidant defense. *World Allergy Organ. J.* 5, 9–19. doi: 10.1097/WOX.0b013e3182439613
13. Bretón, R. R., and Rodríguez, J. C. G. (2012). "Excitotoxicity and oxidative stress in acute ischemic stroke," in *Acute Ischemic Stroke*, ed. J. C. G. Rodríguez (London: InTech).
14. Broughton, B. R., Reutens, D. C., and Sobey, C. G. (2009). Apoptotic mechanisms after cerebral ischemia. *Stroke* 40, e331–e339. doi: 10.1161/STROKEAHA.108. 531632
15. Brouns, R., De Vil, B., Cras, P., De Surgeloose, D., Mariën, P., and De Deyn, P. P. (2010). Neurobiochemical markers of brain damage in cerebrospinal fluid of acute ischemic stroke patients. *Clin. Chem.* 56, 451–458. doi: 10.1373/clinchem. 2009.134122
16. Caine, S., Hackett, M. J., Hou, H., Kumar, S., Maley, J., Ivanishvili, Z., et al. (2016). A novel multi-modal platform to image molecular and elemental alterations in ischemic stroke. *Neurobiol. Dis.* 91, 132–142. doi: 10.1016/j.nbd.2016.03.006
17. Cakmak, G., Miller, L. M., Zorlu, F., and Severcan, F. (2012). Amifostine, a radioprotectant agent, protects rat brain tissue lipids against ionizing radiation induced damage: an FTIR microspectroscopic imaging study. *Arch. Biochem. Biophys.* 520, 67–73. doi: 10.1016/j.abb.2012. 02.012
18. Cakmak, G., Zorlu, F., Severcan, M., and Severcan, F. (2011). Screening of protective effect of amifostine on radiation-induced structural and functional variations in rat liver microsomal membranes by FT-IR spectroscopy. *Anal. Chem.* 83, 2438–2444. doi: 10.1021/ac102043p
19. Carmichael, S. T. (2003). Plasticity of cortical projections after stroke. *Neuroscientist* 9, 64–75. doi: 10.1177/1073858402239592
20. Carter, E. A., Rayner, B. S., McLeod, A. I., Wu, L. E., Marshall, C. P., Levina, A., et al. (2010). Silicon nitride as a versatile growth substrate for

microspectroscopic imaging and mapping of individual cells. *Mol. Biosyst.* 6, 1316–1322. doi: 10.1039/c001499k

21. Cheatwood, J. L., Emerick, A. J., and Kartje, G. L. (2008). Neuronal plasticity and functional recovery after ischemic stroke. *Top. Stroke Rehabil.* 15, 42–50. doi: 10.1310/tsr1501-42
22. Chen, P., Miah, M. R., and Aschner, M. (2016). Metals and neurodegeneration. *F1000Res.* 5:F1000FacultyRev-366. doi: 10.12688/f1000research.7431.1
23. de Zwart, L. L., Meerman, J. H., Commandeur, J. N., and Vermeulen, N. P. (1999). Biomarkers of free radical damage: applications in experimental animals and in humans. *Free Radic. Biol. Med.* 26, 202–226. doi: 10.1016/S0891-5849(98) 00196-8
24. Deb, P., Sharma, S., and Hassan, K. M. (2010). Pathophysiologic mechanisms of acute ischemic stroke: an overview with emphasis on therapeutic significance beyond thrombolysis. *Pathophysiology* 17, 197–218. doi: 10.1016/j.pathophys. 2009.12.001
25. Dietrich, W. D., Ginsberg, M. D., Busto, R., and Watson, B. D. (1986). Photochemically induced cortical infarction in the rat. Acute and subacute alterations in local glucose utilization. *J. Cereb. Blood Flow Metab.* 6, 195–202. doi: 10.1038/jcbfm.1986.32
26. Dirnagl, U., Iadecola, C., and Moskowitz, M. A. (1999). Pathobiology of ischaemic stroke: an integrated view. *Trends Neurosci.* 22, 391–397. doi: 10.1016/S0166- 2236(99)01401-0
27. Dong, X. X., Wang, Y., and Qin, Z. H. (2009). Molecular mechanisms of excitotoxicity and their relevance to pathogenesis of neurodegenerative diseases. *Acta Pharmacol. Sin.* 30, 379–387. doi: 10.1038/aps.2009.24
28. Dostovic, Z., Dostovic, E., Smajlovic, D., Ibrahimagic, O. C., and Avdic, L. (2016). Brain edema after ischaemic stroke. *Med. Arch.* 70, 339–341. doi: 10.5455/ medarh.2016.70.339-341
29. Drevets, W. C., Price, J. L., and Furey, M. L. (2008). Brain structural and functional abnormalities in mood disorders: implications for neurocircuitry models of depression. *Brain Struct. Funct.* 213, 93–118. doi: 10.1007/s00429-008-0189-x
30. Edgar, N., and Sibille, E. (2012). A putative functional role for oligodendrocytes in mood regulation. *Transl. Psychiatry* 2:e109. doi: 10.1038/tp.2012.34
31. Esparza, T. J., Wildburger, N. C., Jiang, H., Gangolli, M., Cairns, N. J., Bateman, R. J., et al. (2016). Soluble amyloid-beta aggregates from human Alzheimer's disease brains. *Sci. Rep.* 6:38187. doi: 10.1038/srep38187
32. Garcia, J. H. (1984). Experimental ischemic stroke: a review. *Stroke* 15, 5–14. doi: 10.1161/01.STR.15.1.5
33. Goormaghtigh, E. (2016). Infrared imaging in histopathology: is a unified approach possible? *Biomed. Spectrosc. Imaging* 5, 325–346. doi: 10.3233/BSI-160151
34. Gouras, G. K., Tampellini, D., Takahashi, R. H., and Capetillo-Zarate, E. (2010). Intraneuronal β-amyloid accumulation and synapse pathology in Alzheimer's disease. *Acta Neuropathol.* 119, 523–541. doi: 10.1007/s00401-010-0679-9
35. Hackett, M. J., DeSouza, M., Caine, S., Bewer, B., Nichol, H., Paterson, P. G., et al. (2015a). A new method to image heme-Fe, total Fe, and aggregated protein levels after intracerebral hemorrhage. *ACS Chem. Neurosci.* 6, 761–770. doi: 10.1021/acschemneuro.5b00037
36. Hackett, M. J., Lee, J., El-Assaad, F., McQuillan, J. A., Carter, E. A., Grau, G. E., et al. (2015b). A new method to image heme-Fe, total Fe, and aggregated protein levels after intracerebral hemorrhage. *ACS Chem. Neurosci.* 6, 761–770. doi: 10.1021/acschemneuro.5b00037
37. Halliwell, B., and Gutteridge, J. M. (1986). Iron and free radical reactions: two aspects of antioxidant protection. *Trends Biochem. Sci.* 11, 372–375. doi: 10.1016/0968-0004(86)90207-0
38. Hare, D., Reedy, B., Grimm, R., Wilkins, S., Volitakis, I., George, J. L., et al. (2009). Quantitative elemental bio-imaging of Mn, Fe, Cu and Zn in 6-hydroxydopamine induced Parkinsonism mouse models. *Metallomics* 1, 53– 58. doi: 10.1039/c0mt00039f
39. Hare, D. J., George, J. L., Grimm, R., Wilkins, S., Adlard, P. A., Cherny, R. A., et al. (2010). Three-dimensional elemental bio-imaging of Fe, Zn, Cu, Mn and P in a 6-hydroxydopamine lesioned mouse brain. *Metallomics* 2, 745–753. doi: 10.1039/c0mt00039f
40. Harrison, J. P., and Berry, D. (2017). Vibrational spectroscopy for imaging single microbial cells in complex biological samples. *Front. Microbiol.* 8:675. doi: 10.3389/fmicb.2017.00675
41. Heraud, P., Caine, S., Campanale, N., Karnezis, T., McNaughton, D., Wood, B. R., et al. (2010). Early detection of the chemical changes occurring during the induction and prevention of autoimmune-mediated demyelination detected by FT-IR imaging. *Neuroimage* 49, 1180–1189. doi: 10.1016/j.neuroimage.2009. 09.053
42. Hu, X., De Silva, T. M., Chen, J., and Faraci, F. M. (2017). Cerebral vascular disease and neurovascular injury in ischemic stroke. *Circ. Res.* 120, 449–471. doi: 10.1161/CIRCRESAHA.116.308427
43. Huang, L., Wu, Z. B., ZhuGe, Q., Zheng, W., Shao, B., Wang, B., et al. (2014). Glial scar formation occurs in the human brain after ischemic stroke. *Int. J. Med. Sci.* 11, 344–348. doi: 10.7150/ijms.8140
44. Kar, S., Slowikowski, S. P., Westaway, D., and Mount, H. T. (2004). Interactions between β-amyloid and central cholinergic neurons: implications for Alzheimer's disease. *J. Psychiatry Neurosci.* 29, 427–441.
45. Kastyak, M. Z., Szczerbowska-Boruchowska, M., Adamek, D., Tomik, B., Lankosz, M., and Gough, K. M. (2010). Pigmented creatine deposits in Amyotrophic Lateral Sclerosis central nervous system tissues identified by synchrotron Fourier Transform Infrared microspectroscopy and X-ray fluorescence spectromicroscopy. *Neuroscience* 166, 1119–1128. doi: 10.1016/j.neuroscience.2010. 01.017
46. Kazarian, S. G., and Chan, K. L. A. (2006). Applications of ATR-FTIR spectroscopic imaging to biomedical samples. *Biochim. Biophys. Acta* 1758, 858–867. doi: 10.1016/j.bbamem.2006.02.011
47. Klein, J. A., and Ackerman, S. L. (2003). Oxidative stress, cell cycle, and neurodegeneration. *J. Clin. Invest.* 111, 785–793. doi: 10.1172/JCI200318182 Kneipp, J., Lasch, P., Baldauf, E., Beekes, M., and Naumann, D. (2000). Detection of pathological molecular alterations in scrapie-infected hamster brain by Fourier transform infrared (FT-IR) spectroscopy. *Biochim. Biophys. Acta* 1501, 189–199. doi: 10.1016/S0925-4439(00)00021-1
48. Kohler, A., Böcker, U., Shapaval, V., Forsmark, A., Andersson, M., Warringer, J., et al. (2015). High-throughput biochemical fingerprinting of *Saccharomyces cerevisiae* by Fourier transform infrared spectroscopy. *PLoS One* 10:e0118052. doi: 10.1371/journal.pone.0118052
49. Kumar, S., Shabi, T. S., and Goormaghtigh, E. (2014). A FTIR imaging characterization of fibroblasts stimulated by various breast cancer cell lines. *PLoS One* 9:e111137. doi: 10.1371/journal.pone.0111137
50. Kuroiwa, T., Xi, G., Hua, Y., Nagaraja, T. N., Fenstermacher, J. D., and Keep, R. F. (2009). Development of a rat model of photothrombotic ischemia and infarction within the caudoputamen. *Stroke* 40, 248–253. doi: 10.1161/STROKEAHA.108.527853
51. Lai, T. W., Zhang, S., and Wang, Y. T. (2014). Excitotoxicity and stroke: identifying novel targets for neuroprotection. *Prog. Neurobiol.* 115, 157–188. doi: 10.1016/ j.pneurobio.2013.11.006
52. Lamba, O. P., Borchman, D., and Garner, W. H. (1994). Spectral characterization of lipid peroxidation in rabbit lens membranes induced by hydrogen peroxide in the presence of $Fe2^+$ $Fe3^+$ cations: a site-specific catalyzed oxidation. *Free Radic. Biol. Med.* 16, 591–601. doi: 10.1016/0891-5849(94) 90059-0
53. Lasch, P., Boese, M., Pacifico, A., and Diem, M. (2002). FT-IR spectroscopic investigations of single cells on the subcellular level. *Vib. Spectrosc.* 28, 147–157. doi: 10.1016/S0924-2031(01)00153-9
54. Lee, J. M., Grabb, M. C., Zipfel, G. J., and Choi, D. W. (2000). Brain tissue responses to ischemia. *J. Clin. Invest.* 106, 723–731. doi: 10.1172/JCI11003
55. Lekander, I., Willers, C., Von Euler, M., Lilja, M., Sunnerhagen, K. S., Pessah- Rasmussen, H., et al. (2017). Relationship between functional disability and costs one and two years post stroke. *PLoS One* 12:e0174861. doi: 10.1371/ journal.pone.0174861
56. Leskovjan, A. C., Kretlow, A., and Miller, L. M. (2010). Fourier transform infrared imaging showing reduced unsaturated lipid content in the hippocampus of a mouse model of Alzheimer's disease. *Anal. Chem.* 82, 2711–2716. doi: 10.1021/ ac1002728
57. Li, J., Li, W., Jiang, Z. G., and Ghanbari, H. A. (2013). Oxidative stress and neurodegenerative disorders. *Int. J. Mol. Sci.* 14, 24438–24475. doi: 10.3390/ijms141224438
58. Li, W., Li, Y., Zhu, W., and Chen, X. (2014). Changes in brain functional network connectivity after stroke. *Neural Regen. Res.* 9, 51–60. doi: 10.4103/1673-5374. 125330
59. Li, Y. I., Chen, J., Zhang, C. L., Wang, L., Lu, D., Katakowski, M., et al. (2005). Gliosis and brain remodeling after treatment of stroke in rats with marrow stromal cells. *Glia* 49, 407–417. doi: 10.1002/glia.20126

60. Li, Y. V., and Zhang, J. H. (eds). (2012). "Metal ions in stroke pathophysiology," in *Metal Ion in Stroke*, (New York, NY: Springer), 1–12. doi: 10.1007/978-1-4419- 9663-3_1
61. Liang, D., Bhatta, S., Gerzanich, V., and Simard, J. M. (2007). Cytotoxic edema: mechanisms of pathological cell swelling. *Neurosurg. Focus* 22, 1–9. doi: 10.3171/foc.2007.22.5.3
62. Liao, C. R., Rak, M., Lund, J., Unger, M., Platt, E., Albensi, B. C., et al. (2013). Synchrotron FTIR reveals lipid around and within amyloid plaques in transgenic mice and Alzheimer's disease brain. *Analyst* 138, 3991–3997. doi: 10.1039/c3an00295k
63. Liu, K. Z., Bose, R., and Mantsch, H. H. (2002). Infrared spectroscopic study of diabetic platelets. *Vib. Spectrosc.* 28, 131–136. doi: 10.1016/S0924-2031(01) 00163-1
64. Lo, E. H., Dalkara, T., and Moskowitz, M. A. (2003). Neurological diseases: mechanisms, challenges and opportunities in stroke. *Nat. Rev. Neurosci.* 4, 399–414. doi: 10.1016/j.smim.2016.03.015
65. Manda, K., Ueno, M., Moritake, T., and Anzai, K. (2007). α-Lipoic acid attenuates x-irradiation-induced oxidative stress in mice. *Cell Biol. Toxicol.* 23, 129–137. doi: 10.1007/s10565-006-0137-6
66. Matusch, A., and Becker, J. S. (2012). Bio-imaging of metals in a mouse model of Alzheimer's disease by laser ablation inductively coupled plasma mass spectrometry. *Biomed. Spectrosc. Imaging* 1, 57–65.
67. Matusch, A., Depboylu, C., Palm, C., Wu, B., Höglinger, G. U., Schäfer, M. K. H., et al. (2010). Cerebral bioimaging of Cu, Fe, Zn, and Mn in the MPTP mouse model of Parkinson's disease using laser ablation inductively coupled plasma mass spectrometry (LA-ICP-MS). *J. Am. Soc. Mass Spectrom.* 21, 161–171. doi: 10.1016/j.jasms.2009.09.022
68. Matusch, A., Fenn, L. S., Depboylu, C., Klietz, M., Strohmer, S., McLean, J. A., et al. (2012). Combined elemental and biomolecular mass spectrometry imaging for probing the inventory of tissue at a micrometer scale. *Anal. Chem.* 84, 3170–3178. doi: 10.1021/ac203112c
69. Michinaga, S., and Koyama, Y. (2015). Pathogenesis of brain edema and investigation into anti-edema drugs. *Int. J. Mol. Sci.* 16, 9949–9975. doi: 10.3390/ijms16059949
70. Miller, L. M., Bourassa, M. W., and Smith, R. J. (2013). FTIR spectroscopic imaging of protein aggregation in living cells. *Biochim. Biophys. Acta* 1828, 2339–2346. doi: 10.1016/j.bbamem.2013.01.014
71. Miller, L. M., Wang, Q., Telivala, T. P., Smith, R. J., Lanzirotti, A., and Miklossy, J. (2006). Synchrotron-based infrared and X-ray imaging shows focalized accumulation of Cu and Zn co-localized with β-amyloid deposits in Alzheimer's disease. *J. Struct. Biol.* 155, 30–37. doi: 10.1016/j.jsb.2005.09.004
72. Murphy, T. H., and Corbett, D. (2009). Plasticity during stroke recovery: from synapse to behaviour. *Nat. Rev. Neurosci.* 10, 861–872. doi: 10.1038/nrn2735 Olmez, I., and Ozyurt, H. (2012). Reactive oxygen species and ischemic cerebrovascular disease. *Neurochem. Int.* 60, 208–212. doi: 10.1016/j.neuint. 2011.11.009
73. Ozek, N. S., Tuna, S., Erson-Bensan, A. E., and Severcan, F. (2010). Characterization of microRNA-125b expression in MCF7 breast cancer cells by ATR-FTIR spectroscopy. *Analyst* 135, 3094–3102. doi: 10.1039/c0an00543f
74. Paul Murphy, M., and LeVine, H. I. I. I. (2010). Alzheimer's disease and the β-amyloid peptide. *J. Alzheimers Dis.* 19, 311–323. doi: 10.3233/JAD-2010-1221 Petibois, C., and Desbat, B. (2010). Clinical application of FTIR imaging: new reasons for hope. *Trends Biotechnol.* 28, 495–500. doi: 10.1016/j.tibtech.2010. 07.003
75. Petibois, C., Wehbe, K., Belbachır, K., Noreen, R., and Déléris, G. (2009). Current trends in the development of FTIR imaging for the quantitative analysis of biological samples. *Acta Phys. Pol. A Gen. Phys.* 115:507. doi: 10.12693/ APhysPolA.115.507
76. Pevsner, P. H., Eichenbaum, J. W., Miller, D. C., Pivawer, G., Eichenbaum, K. D., Stern, A., et al. (2001). A photothrombotic model of small early ischemic infarcts in the rat brain with histologic and MRI correlation. *J. Pharmacol. Toxicol. Methods* 45, 227–233. doi: 10.1016/S1056-8719(01) 00153-8
77. Prashanth, L., Kattapagari, K. K., Chitturi, R. T., Baddam, V. R. R., and Prasad, L. K. (2015). A review on role of essential trace elements in health and disease. *J. NTR Univ. Health Sci.* 4, 75–85. doi: 10.4103/2277-8632.158577
78. Prentice, H., Modi, J. P., and Wu, J. Y. (2015). Mechanisms of neuronal protection against excitotoxicity, endoplasmic reticulum stress, and mitochondrial dysfunction in stroke and neurodegenerative diseases. *Oxid. Med. Cell. Longev.* 2015:964518. doi: 10.1155/2015/964518
79. Pribic, R. (1994). Principal component analysis of Fourier transform infrared and/or circular dichroism spectra of proteins applied in a calibration of protein secondary structure. *Anal. Biochem.* 223, 26–34. doi: 10.1006/abio.1994.1541
80. Ramasubbu, R., Robinson, R. G., Flint, A. J., Kosier, T., and Price, T. R. (1998). Functional impairment associated with acute post stroke depression: the Stroke Data Bank Study. *J. Neuropsychiatry Clin. Neurosci.* 10, 26–33. doi: 10.1176/jnp. 10.1.26
81. Ryter, S. W., Kim, H. P., Hoetzel, A., Park, J. W., Nakahira, K., Wang, X., et al. (2007). Mechanisms of cell death in oxidative stress. *Antioxid. Redox Signal.* 9, 49–89. doi: 10.1089/ars.2007.9.49
82. Sadiq, S., Ghazala, Z., Chowdhury, A., and Büsselberg, D. (2012). Metal toxicity at the synapse: presynaptic, postsynaptic, and long-term effects. *J. Toxicol.* 2012:132671. doi: 10.1155/2012/132671
83. Sanchez, G. (2011). *Visualizing Dendrograms in R.* Available at: http://rpubs.com/ gaston/dendrograms Sarti, C., Rastenyte, D., Cepaitis, Z., and Tuomilehto, J. (2000). International trends in mortality from stroke, 1968 to 1994. *Stroke* 31, 1588–1601. doi: 10.1161/01. STR.31.7.1588
84. Severcan, F., Gorgulu, G., Gorgulu, S. T., and Guray, T. (2005). Rapid monitoring of diabetes-induced lipid peroxidation by Fourier transform infrared spectroscopy: evidence from rat liver microsomal membranes. *Anal. Biochem.* 339, 36–40. doi: 10.1016/j.ab.2005.01.011
85. Shichita, T., Ito, M., and Yoshimura, A. (2014). Post-ischemic inflammation regulates neural damage and protection. *Front. Cell. Neurosci.* 8:319. doi: 10.3389/fncel.2014.00319
86. Simard, J. M., Kent, T. A., Chen, M., Tarasov, K. V., and Gerzanich, V. (2007). Brain oedema in focal ischaemia: molecular pathophysiology and theoretical implications. *Lancet Neurol.* 6, 258–268. doi: 10.1016/S1474-4422(07)70055-8
87. Snögren, M., and Sunnerhagen, K. S. (2009). Description of functional disability among younger stroke patients: exploration of activity and participation and environmental factors. *Int. J. Rehabil. Res.* 32, 124–131. doi: 10.1097/MRR. 0b013e328325a5be
88. Srinivasan, G. (2010). *Vibrational Spectroscopic Imaging for Biomedical Applications*. New York, NY: McGraw Hill Professional.
89. Szczerbowska-Boruchowska, M., Dumas, P., Kastyak, M. Z., Chwiej, J., Lankosz, M., Adamek, D., et al. (2007). Biomolecular investigation of human *Substantia nigra* in Parkinson's disease by synchrotron radiation Fourier transform infrared microspectroscopy. *Arch. Biochem. Biophys.* 459, 241–248. doi: 10.1016/j.abb.2006.12.027
90. Turker, S. (2012). Application of infrared spectroscopy in the study of neurological diseases. *Biomed. Spectrosc. Imaging* 1, 303–323.
91. Turker, S., Severcan, M., Ilbay, G., and Severcan, F. (2014). Epileptic seizures induce structural and functional alterations on brain tissue membranes. *Biochim. Biophys. Acta* 1838, 3088–3096. doi: 10.1016/j.bbamem.2014.08.025
92. Uttara, B., Singh, A. V., Zamboni, P., and Mahajan, R. T. (2009). Oxidative stress and neurodegenerative diseases: a review of upstream and downstream antioxidant therapeutic options. *Curr. Neuropharmacol.* 7, 65–74. doi: 10.2174/ 157015909787602823
93. Van Bruggen, N., Cullen, B. M., King, M. D., Doran, M., Williams, S. R., Gadian, D. G., et al. (1992). T2-and diffusion-weighted magnetic resonance imaging of a focal ischemic lesion in rat brain. *Stroke* 23, 576–582. doi: 10.1161/01.STR.23. 4.576
94. Wang, Q., Kretlow, A., Beekes, M., Naumann, D., and Miller, L. (2005). In situ characterization of prion protein structure and metal accumulation in scrapie- infected cells by synchrotron infrared and X-ray imaging. *Vib. Spectrosc.* 38, 61–69.
95. Wildburger, N. C., Esparza, T. J., LeDuc, R. D., Fellers, R. T., Thomas, P. M., Cairns, N. J., et al. (2017). Diversity of amyloid-beta proteoforms in the Alzheimer's disease brain. *Sci. Rep.* 7:9520. doi: 10.1038/s41598-017-10422-x
96. Xing, C., Arai, K., Lo, E. H., and Hommel, M. (2012). Pathophysiologic cascades in ischemic stroke. *Int. J. Stroke* 7, 378–385. doi: 10.1111/j.1747-4949.2012.00839.x Yamamoto, M., Shima, T., Uozumi, T., Sogabe, T., Yamada, K., and Kawasaki, T. (1983). A possible role of lipid peroxidation in cellular damages caused by cerebral ischemia and the protective effect of alpha-tocopherol administration. *Stroke* 14, 977–982. doi: 10.1161/01. STR.14.6.977

97. Yildirim, A., Kotan, D., Yildirim, S., Ayguel, R., and Akçay, F. (2007). Increased lipid peroxidation and decreased antioxidant response in serum and cerebrospinal fluid in acute ischemic stroke. *Turk. J. Med. Sci.* 37, 75–81.
98. Yin, H., Xu, L., and Porter, N. A. (2011). Free radical lipid peroxidation: mechanisms and analysis. *Chem. Rev.* 111, 5944–5972. doi: 10.1021/cr200084z Zeiger, S. L., Musiek, E. S., Zanoni, G., Vidari, G., Morrow, J. D., Milne,
99. G. J., et al. (2009). Neurotoxic lipid peroxidation species formed by ischemic stroke increase injury. *Free Radic. Biol. Med.* 47, 1422–1431. doi: 10.1016/j.freeradbiomed.2009.08.011
100. Zhao, C., and Bateman, A. (2015). Progranulin protects against the tissue damage of acute ischaemic stroke. *Brain* 138, 1770–1773. doi: 10.1093/brain/awv123 Zima, T., Štípek, S., Crkovská, J., Ne˘mec˘ek, K., Pláteník, J., Bártová, V., et al. (1996).
101. Antioxidant enzymes-superoxide dismutase and glutathione peroxidase-in haemodialyzed patients. *Blood Purif.* 14, 257–261. doi: 10.1159/000170269

5

Apolipoprotein E Homozygous ε4 Allele Status: A Deteriorating Effect on Visuospatial Working Memory and Global Brain Structure

Janik Goltermann[1], Ronny Redlich[1], Katharina Dohm[1], Dario Zaremba[1], Jonathan Repple[1], Claas Kaehler[1,2], Dominik Grotegerd[1], Katharina Förster[1], Susanne Meinert[1], Verena Enneking[1], Emily Schlaghecken[1], Lara Fleischer[1], Tim Hahn[1], Harald Kugel[3], Andreas Jansen[4,5,6], Axel Krug[4], Katharina Brosch[4], Igor Nenadic[4], Simon Schmitt[4], Frederike Stein[4], Tina Meller[4], Dilara Yüksel[4], Elena Fischer[4], Marcella Rietschel[7], Stephanie H. Witt[7], Andreas J. Forstner[8,9,10], Markus M. Nöthen[8], Tilo Kircher[4], Anbupalam Thalamuthu[11], Bernhard T. Baune[1,12,13], Udo Dannlowski[1†] and Nils Opel[1†]*

[1] Department of Psychiatry, University of Münster, Münster, Germany, [2] Department of Mathematics and Computer Science, University of Münster, Münster, Germany, [3] Institute of Clinical Radiology, University of Münster, Münster, Germany, [4] Department of Psychiatry, University of Marburg, Marburg, Germany, [5] Core-Facility BrainImaging, Faculty of Medicine, University of Marburg, Marburg, Germany, [6] Center for Mind, Brain and Behavior, University of Marburg, Marburg, Germany, [7] Department of Genetic Epidemiology, Central Institute of Mental Health, University of Heidelberg, Mannheim, Germany, [8] School of Medicine & University Hospital Bonn, Institute of Human Genetics, University of Bonn, Bonn, Germany, [9] Centre for Human Genetics, University of Marburg, Marburg, Germany, [10] Department of Biomedicine, University of Basel, Basel, Switzerland, [11] Centre for Healthy Brain Ageing, School of Psychiatry, University of New South Wales Sydney, Sydney, NSW, Australia, [12] Department of Psychiatry, Melbourne Medical School, The University of Melbourne, Melbourne, VIC, Australia, [13] The Florey Institute of Neuroscience and Mental Health, The University of Melbourne, Parkville, VIC, Australia

***Correspondence:**
Udo Dannlowski
dannlow@uni-muenster.de

† These authors have contributed equally to this work and are senior authors

Theoretical background: The Apolipoprotein E (APOE) ε4 genotype is known to be one of the strongest single-gene predictors for Alzheimer disease, which is characterized by widespread brain structural degeneration progressing along with cognitive impairment. The ε4 allele status has been associated with brain structural alterations and lower cognitive ability in non-demented subjects. However, it remains unclear to what extent the visuospatial cognitive domain is affected, from what age onward changes are detectable and if alterations may interact with cognitive deficits in major depressive disorder (MDD). The current work investigated the effect of APOE ε4 homozygosity on visuospatial working memory (vWM) capacity, and on hippocampal morphometry. Furthermore, potential moderating roles of age and MDD were assessed.

Methods: A sample of $n = 31$ homozygous ε4 carriers was contrasted with $n = 31$ non-ε4 carriers in a cross-sectional design. The sample consisted of non-demented, young to mid-age participants (mean age = 34.47; $SD = 13.48$; 51.6% female). Among them were $n = 12$ homozygous ε4 carriers and $n = 12$ non-ε4 carriers suffering from MDD (39%). VWM was assessed using the Corsi block-tapping task. Region of interest analyses of hippocampal gray matter density and volume were conducted using voxel-based morphometry (CAT12), and Freesurfer, respectively.

Results: Homozygous ε4 carriers showed significantly lower Corsi span capacity than non-ε4 carriers did, and Corsi span capacity was associated with higher gray matter density of the hippocampus. APOE group differences in hippocampal volume could be detected but were no longer present when controlling for total intracranial volume. Hippocampal gray matter density did not differ between APOE groups. We did not find any interaction effects of age and MDD diagnosis on hippocampal morphometry.

Conclusion: Our results point toward a negative association of homozygous ε4 allele status with vWM capacity already during mid-adulthood, which emerges independently of MDD diagnosis and age. APOE genotype seems to be associated with global brain structural rather than hippocampus specific alterations in young- to mid-age participants.

Keywords: apolipoprotein E, visuospatial working memory, cognitive deficits, hippocampus, structural MRI, Alzheimer, major depression

INTRODUCTION

Alzheimer disease (AD) is a leading cause of dementia and associated with major cognitive and daily life impairments as well as psychiatric symptoms, such as depressed affect, agitation, and delusions (1). AD is a neurodegenerative disease that can be linked to extensive cerebral atrophy typically affecting structures involved in memory and cognition (2–4). Degenerations caused by AD are typically progressive, and mild cognitive impairment (MCI) can be found years before the outbreak of clinically relevant symptoms and constitutes a risk factor for AD (3). Both MCI and AD have been repeatedly associated with a deterioration of the hippocampus and the entorhinal cortex (4). Evidence from longitudinal studies suggests that these regions are the first to be affected by observable structural alterations in the course of AD (5, 6). Cerebral atrophies in these areas are accompanied by neurocognitive decline in several domains (7) as associative verbal memory (8), visuospatial memory (9, 10), and reasoning (11).

Brain structural changes associated with AD have also been shown to play a role in major depressive disorder (MDD) (12). Furthermore, a lifetime history of MDD poses a risk factor for developing AD later in life (13). However, the exact interplay between AD, MDD and brain structural alterations remains unclear.

The Apolipoprotein E (APOE) genotype is the strongest known single predictor of AD. APOE ε4 allele dose has been associated with higher risk and earlier onset of AD (14, 15). Heterozygous ε4 allele carriers are estimated to have a three-fold, and ε4 homozygotes an eight- to fifteen-fold increased risk to develop AD compared to subjects without an ε4 allele (14, 15). The risk effect of the APOE genotype has been replicated numerous times (16) and there is evidence that it is stronger in female compared to male (17).

The APOE genotype has further been associated with cognitive ability in elderly, non-demented samples. Evidence from studies contrasting healthy ε4 allele carriers with non-ε4 carriers suggests better performance in episodic memory (18, 19), working memory (20) and global cognitive functioning (21) in favor of non-ε4 carriers. However, empirical evidence is inconclusive with a considerable number of contradicting findings (21). Heterogeneity of findings may reflect methodological differences in ε4 allele status categorization (coding of zygosity), in the selection and operationalization of cognitive domains, as well as varying sample characteristics regarding age (21). Strongest effects of the APOE genotype have been found in elderly samples above 60 years and for APOE ε4 homozygotes (21). The role of the APOE status for the visuospatial domain has been discussed particularly controversially. There is some evidence for a visuospatial deficit in non-demented ε4 carriers that are mid-adult age (22) and elderly (23), however with no deficit found in a subgroup of age 80 and older (24). Although most studies investigating the APOE effect on cognition examine elderly samples deteriorating genotype effects on visuospatial performance can also be found in children (25) with some evidence for stronger deficits in girls (26). Contrasting findings exist (19) and a meta-analysis concluded that there is little evidence for group differences for the visuospatial domain between ε4 carriers and non-carriers (21). However, due to insufficient available sample sizes this meta-analysis did not carry out analyses comparing homozygous ε4 carriers with non-ε4 carriers, which might be an important biasing factor.

The effect of APOE status on cognitive ability appears to come along with functional and structural brain alterations. Evidence from an early PET study suggests inhibited glucose metabolism in ε4 homozygotes in temporal, frontal, and parietal regions, as well as the posterior cingulum already in a non-demented mid-elderly sample with normal cognitive functioning (27). Further, findings of hippocampal volume reductions are reported in healthy elderly ε4 homozygotes (28) as well as structural alterations in the temporal lobe in heterozygous ε4 carriers in a sample of healthy adults with a wide range of age (29).

A review (30) and a meta-analysis (31) further support these findings of structural alterations particularly in the hippocampal region in healthy elderly subjects as a function of the APOE genotype. However, evidence seems to be inconclusive regarding the role of heterozygous ε4 carriers as some studies find an ε4 dose effect, some find a similar degree and rate of cerebral atrophy for heterozygotes as for homozygotes while other studies find heterozygotes to be indifferent from non-ε4 carriers in respect to brain structural alterations (30). The degree to which studies differentiate the APOE genotype, and what genotypes are categorized as ε4 carriers vary. This has direct implications for methodological considerations of studies investigating APOE effects in that designs should differentiate ε4 allele dosage.

The evidence for a detrimental effect of the APOE ε4 allele on hippocampal structure as well as on vWM task performance raises the question if the hippocampal region might be the neuronal locus of the APOE genotype affecting the vWM. Although the visuospatial cognitive domain is commonly associated with the frontoparietal network (32) there are also studies linking it to the hippocampus. Performance in the Corsi block tapping task has been shown to be impaired in subjects with lesions in the right temporal lobe (33), and to be associated with augmented activation in the hippocampus in addition to frontoparietal regions (34). Other studies report that lower vWM capacity is associated with structural characteristics of the hippocampus, as lesions (35) and atrophy (36).

Brain structures and cognitive domains affected by the APOE genotype (as outlined above) are also closely related to detrimental processes involved in MDD (37, 38). There are studies linking MDD to a two-fold increased risk of AD (13) as well as at least one study suggesting that APOE genotype moderates this risk (39) and evidence linking APOE genotype to an increased risk for depressive symptoms (40). However, the exact interplay between the APOE gene, MDD, cognitive decline, and AD remain largely unresolved. Taylor et al. (41) investigated a sample containing MDD and healthy subjects and found no differences in various cognitive domains and structural MRI in function of ε4 presence (not differentiating between ε4 zygosities) regardless of diagnosis.

Small sample sizes of homozygous ε4 carriers are a common problem in APOE research due to the rare co-occurrence of two ε4 alleles [prevalence 2.9% (42)]. Only few studies exist that include sufficient sample sizes of ε4 homozygotes and further provide structural brain imaging data, and behavioral cognition measures. Despite the potential importance of MDD for APOE effects even fewer studies include mid-age subjects with MDD subsamples. Most studies including these aspects investigate elderly samples, while not differentiating ε4 zygosity (43, 44). To our knowledge only one study exists that included mid-age MDD subjects, however also not differentiating ε4 zygosity (41). We know of no study that has been published combining structural MRI data, and neuropsychological data in mid-age subjects, that includes homozygous ε4, and MDD subsamples.

The goal of the current work was to investigate the relationship of the APOE genotype with visuospatial working memory (vWM) and brain structural alterations first and foremost in the hippocampus in a young- to mid-age, non-demented sample. Further objectives were to identify potential moderators of these relationships, namely age and MDD diagnosis. Importantly homozygous ε4 carriers were operationalized as the genetic risk group and contrasted with a sample without ε4 allele as the literature outlined above suggests effects of the APOE genotype to be most pronounced for homozygotes. We hypothesized that 1) ε4 homozygotes show on average lower vWM performance compared to non-ε4 carriers, 2) vWM performance correlates positively

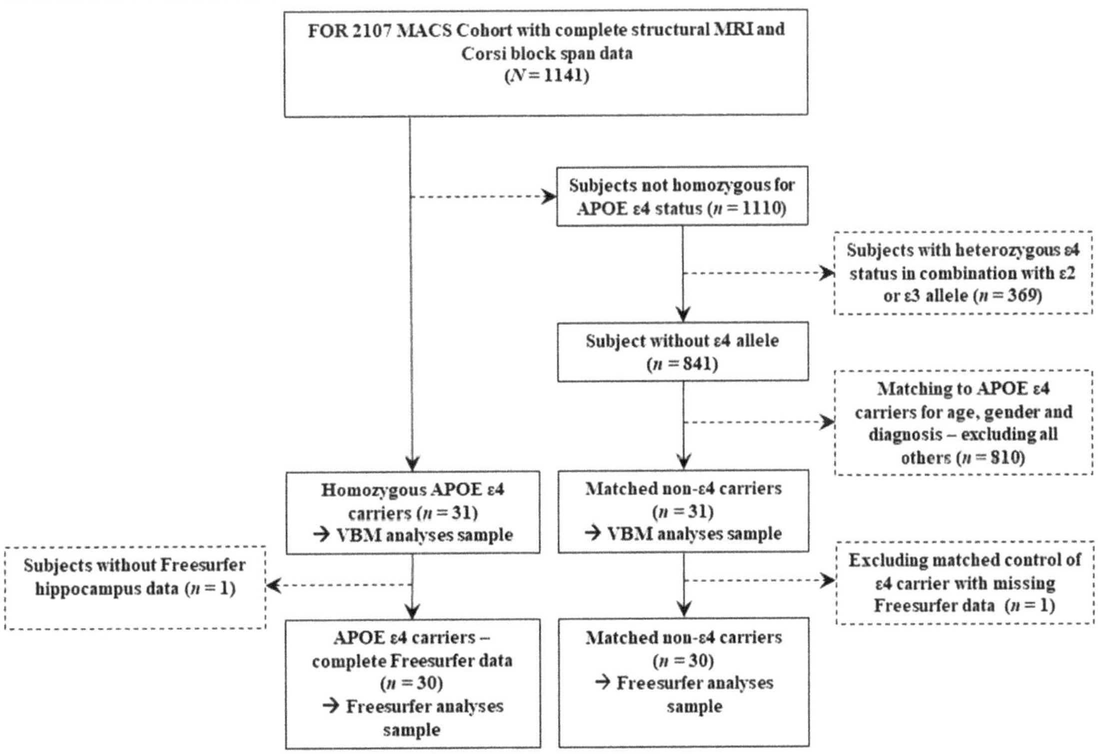

FIGURE 1 | Sample flowchart showing all data exclusion steps for both genotype groups.

with hippocampal volume and gray matter density, and 3) homozygous ε4 carriers exhibit smaller volume and gray matter density in the hippocampal area compared to non-ε4 carriers.

METHODS

Participants

A sample of $N = 1,141$ adult subjects with complete cross-sectional MRI and neuropsychological data was available from the FOR2107 Marburg-Münster Affective Cohort Study (MACS) (45) which includes subjects with MDD and healthy control (HC) subjects. Exclusion criteria were any history of neurological (e.g., concussion, stroke, tumor, neuro-inflammatory diseases) and medical (e.g., cancer, chronic inflammatory or autoimmune diseases, heart diseases) conditions as well as substance-related addiction, and MRI contraindications. The study sample was selected based on the genotype of the APOE gene. Within the FOR2107 MACS cohort a study sample of $n = 31$ homozygous ε4 carriers was available which was contrasted with $n = 31$ non-ε4 carriers that were matched for age, sex, and diagnosis. For Freesurfer (FS) analyses a sample of $N = 60$ ($n = 30$ ε4 homozygotes; $n = 30$ matched controls) was available due to missing data for one of the ε4 homozygotes. The sample selection process is depicted in **Figure 1**.

The final sample of $N = 62$ included $n = 24$ MDD patients and $n = 38$ HC subjects. The mean age of the sample was 34.47 ($SD = 13.48$), ranging from 19 to 63 with 51.6% of the sample being female. A more detailed description of the distribution of demographic characteristics can be found in **Table 1**.

Subjects from the MACS cohort were recruited using advertisement in psychiatric hospitals, and outpatient therapeutic offices as well as advertisement in other public places and newspapers. Data were collected at the Departments of Psychiatry either at the University of Marburg or at the University of Münster. Before study participation, all subjects gave written and informed consent. All participants received a financial compensation.

TABLE 1 | Demographic characteristics of the final study sample.

	ε4 homozygotes		Non-ε4 carriers	
	n	Mean age (*SD*)	*n*	Mean age (*SD*)
MDD				
Male	7	41.86 (15.25)	7	41.71 (15.13)
Female	5	35.40 (18.12)	5	35.40 (18.12)
Total	12	39.17 (16.03)	12	39.08 (15.96)
HC				
Male	8	24.50 (2.78)	8	24.50 (2.78)
Female	11	36.64 (12.49)	11	36.64 (12.49)
Total	19	31.53 (11.30)	19	31.53 (11.30)

Materials and Procedure

Neuropsychological Assessment

The Corsi block tapping task (33) was administered in a forward and a backward version. This task is a well-established measure of vWM that has shown to be sensitive for cognitive decline associated with AD (46–48). A mean individual block span capacity was calculated over both version scores regarding a lack of evidence for conceptual differences between both version performances (49).

Clinical Assessment

A structured clinical interview for DSM-IV (SCID-I) was conducted with each participant in order to assess current and lifetime psychopathological diagnoses (50). All subjects allocated to the MDD group in this study either fulfilled the DSM-IV criteria for an acute major depressive episode or had a lifetime history of a major depressive episode. All HC subjects were ensured to be free from presence or any history of psychiatric disorders according to DSM-IV criteria.

Structural Image Acquisition and Processing

T1-weighted high-resolution anatomical images were acquired for all participants. Two MRI scanners were used for data acquisition located at the sites in Marburg and Münster with different hardware and software configurations. In Marburg, a 3T MRI scanner (Tim Trio, Siemens, Erlangen, Germany) was used combined with a 12-channel head matrix Rx-coil. In Münster, data were acquired at a 3T MRI scanner (Prisma, Siemens, Erlangen, Germany) using a 20-channel head matrix Rx-coil. Pulse sequence parameters were standardized across both sites to the extent permitted by each platform. Further details of the imaging procedures and implemented quality assurance protocol have been extensively described elsewhere (51).

Image preprocessing has been conducted using two complementary approaches that have frequently been described in our previous work: voxel-based morphometry (VBM) (52–54) using CAT12 (http://dbm.neuro.uni-jena.de/cat/) and FS (53, 55) based automatic segmentation (Version 5.3) with default parameters (https://surfer.nmr.mgh.harvard.edu/).

CAT12 preprocessing was done using default parameters: Briefly, images were bias-corrected, tissue classified, and normalized to MNI-space using linear (12-parameter affine) and non-linear transformations, within a unified model including high-dimensional DARTEL-normalization. The modulated gray matter images were smoothed with a Gaussian kernel of 8 mm FWHM. Absolute threshold masking with a threshold value of 0.1 was used for all second level analyses as recommended for VBM analyses (http://www.neuro.uni-jena.de/cat/). Image quality was assessed by visual inspection as well as by using the check for homogeneity function implemented in the CAT12 toolbox.

For all analyses using FS based segmentations, volumetric measures of the hippocampal region were used (56). Quality checks of segmentations were done visually and based on a statistical outlier analysis following a standardized protocol provided by the ENIGMA consortium (http://enigma.ini.usc.edu/protocols/imaging-protocols).

Genotyping and Quality Control

DNA was extracted from EDTA blood samples using the chemagic 360 instrument (PerkinElmer, Waltham, MA, USA). Individuals were genotyped using the Infinium PsychArray BeadChip (Illumina, San Diego, CA, USA) and standard protocols. Genotyping was performed at the Institute of Human Genetics, University Hospital Bonn, Germany. Clustering and initial quality control were conducted using GenomeStudio v.2011.1 (Illumina, San Diego, CA, USA) and the Genotyping Module v.1.9.4. Quality control procedures were implemented using PLINK (57) on the FOR2107 dataset. Samples with low genotype rates <95%, sex inconsistencies (X-chromosome heterozygosity), and genetically related individuals were not included in the present study. We also excluded SNPs that had a poor genotyping rate (<95%), strand ambiguity (A/T and C/G SNPs), a minor allele frequency (MAF) <1%, or that showed deviation from Hardy-Weinberg Equilibrium ($p < 10^{-6}$). The quality controlled genotype data was imputed in the Michigan imputation server (https://imputationserver.sph.umich.edu) (58) using the Haplotype Reference Consortium reference panel (v3.20101123). The hard called genotypes for the single nucleotide polymorphisms (SNPs) rs7412 and rs429358 in APOE were extracted from the imputed dosage using PLINK. Both the SNPs were imputed with high accuracy ($R^2 > 0.99$). Participants homozygous for the ε4 allele (ε4/ε4) were contrasted with subjects without an ε4 allele (genotypes ε2/ε2, ε2/ε3, or ε3/ε3).

Statistical Analyses

APOE Status and Visuospatial Working Memory

In order to test our first hypothesis (expecting reduced vWM performance in ε4 homozygotes), APOE genotype was entered as a predicting factor for Corsi block span in a general linear model. Age, sex, and presence of MDD diagnosis were included as covariates in the model.

Visuospatial Working Memory and Hippocampus

The second hypothesis (positive correlation between vWM performance and hippocampus morphometry) was similarly tested using a general linear model. Total intracranial volume (TIV) and scanner site were used as covariates in addition to the covariates age, sex, and MDD diagnosis, while Corsi block span was used as the predictor variable. For this analysis step both (a) FS based analysis using hippocampal volumes as dependent variable (including hippocampal laterality as a within-subject factor in the model) and (b) VBM region of interest analysis of the hippocampus were conducted.

APOE Status and Hippocampus

Identical analyses as for the second hypothesis were used for the investigation of our third hypothesis (negative relationship between homozygous ε4 status and hippocampal morphometry), except that APOE status was used as a predictor instead of Corsi block span. Again the model was used for the prediction of (a) hippocampal volume, and (b) gray matter density (VBM) in two separate analyses in accordance with analyses testing the second hypothesis.

General Aspects and Exploratory Analyses

Generally, all analyses were based on a significance threshold of $p < 0.05$, unless noted differently. However, as all hypotheses were clearly one-sided, halved p-values are reported regarding the main hypotheses (effect of APOE status on vWM, effect of vWM on hippocampal morphometry, and effect of APOE status on hippocampal morphometry) if not specified otherwise. Any interaction terms, and whole brain effects tested for significance were regarded as exploratory and thereby tested two-sided.

VBM analyses were carried out using SPM12 (https://www.fil.ion.ucl.ac.uk/spm/). The hippocampal mask for VBM analyses was created by means of the WFU PickAtlas (59) according to the AAL-Atlas (60) and dilated 2 mm.

To control for multiple comparisons, threshold-free cluster enhancement (TFCE) corrections were applied for all VBM analyses using $N = 1{,}000$ permutations and a cluster size weighting of $E = 0.5$.

All further analyses were conducted with SPSS (version 25.0). Partial η^2 values are reported as effect size measure for significant effects. Reported effect sizes of VBM analyses are based on extracted eigenvariates on cluster level.

RESULTS

APOE Status and Visuospatial Working Memory

In order to test our first hypothesis vWM was predicted with APOE genotype in the above described model. Results yielded a significant main effect of APOE status [$F_{[1,57]} = 6.21, p = 0.02, \eta^2 = 0.10$] with lower Corsi block span in APOE ε4 carriers. Further, a main effect of diagnosis emerged [$F_{[1,57]} = 4.21, p = 0.05, \eta^2 = 0.07$] with lower mean block span in MDD subjects. The model yielded no further main effects (all other $p > 0.53$).

When adding an interaction term between APOE status and age it turned out non-significant [$F_{[1,56]} = 0.21, p = 0.65$], as was the interaction effect between APOE genotype and sex [$F_{[1,56]} = 2.22$, $p = 0.14$]. Descriptively mean differences as a function of APOE status were more pronounced for MDD compared to HC subjects. However, testing an interaction term between APOE status and diagnosis also yielded a non-significant effect [$F_{[1,5]} = 0.93$, $p = 0.34$]. Mean differences in Corsi span over APOE and diagnosis groups are depicted in **Figure 2**.

Visuospatial Working Memory and Hippocampus

For our second hypothesis the general linear model described above was fitted with Corsi block span predicting hippocampal volume. Results yielded a non-significant effect of block span on FS derived hippocampal volume [$F_{[1,53]} = 0.34$, $p = 0.56$]. The main effect of diagnosis was significant [$F_{[1,53]} = 6.63, p = 0.01$, $\eta^2 = 0.11$], with lower hippocampal volume in MDD compared to HC subjects. No significant effect of hippocampal laterality [$F_{[1,53]} = 0.01$, $p = 0.94$], and no other significant main effect of interest was found (all other $p > 0.47$).

When interaction terms were added to the model, results yielded a non-significant interaction effects between Corsi block

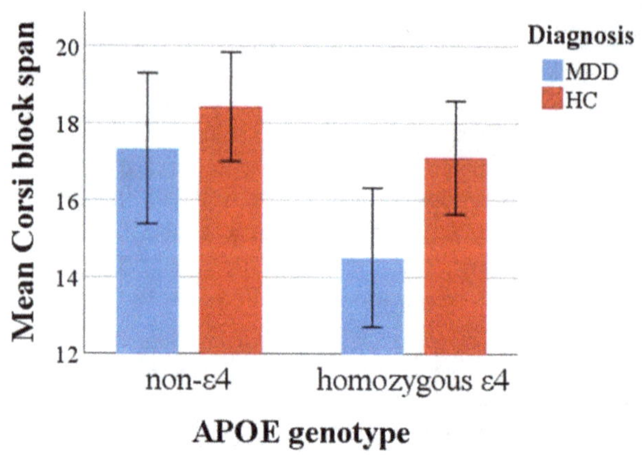

FIGURE 2 | Mean Corsi block span capacity over APOE genotype and diagnosis groups. Error bars represent 95% confidence intervals.

span and age [$F_{[1,52]} = 0.03$, $p = 0.86$], and between Corsi block span and sex [$F_{[1,52]} = 0.69$, $p = 0.41$]. Testing an interaction term between Corsi block span and MDD diagnosis also yielded a non-significant interaction effect [$F_{[1,52]} = 1.76$, $p = 0.19$]. Exploratory analyses revealed that when removing TIV from the model, the main effect of Corsi block span on hippocampal volume becomes significant [$F_{[1,52]} = 3.49$, $p = 0.03$, $\eta^2 = 0.06$]. Further, when substituting hippocampal volume with TIV as the criterion variable the main effect of Corsi block span was significant [$F_{[1,54]} = 5.49$, $p = 0.02$, $\eta^2 = 0.09$], with higher Corsi block span being associated with higher TIV.

In order to further investigate our second hypothesis, model estimation was repeated within a VBM analysis. For the hypothesized main effect of vWM on hippocampal gray matter density the analysis yielded two marginally significant clusters just above a TFCE-corrected significance threshold of $p < 0.05$ (left: $k = 132$, $p = 0.05$, $x = -38$, $y = -28$, $z = -15$, TFCE = 203.05, $\eta^2_{cluster} = 0.18$; right: $k = 50$, $p = 0.07$, $x = 38$, $y = -24$, $z = -18$, TFCE = 181.78, $\eta^2_{cluster} = 0.23$).

Exploratory whole brain analysis for the main effect of vWM revealed three clusters below the exploratory uncorrected threshold of $p < 0.001$ with a minimum cluster size of 20 voxels ($k = 31$, $p < 0.001$, $x = 36$, $y = -14$, $z = -28$; $k = 21$, $p < 0.001$, $x = 38$, $y = -22$, $z = -20$; $k = 20$, $p < 0.001$, $x = -38$, $y = -28$, $z = -15$). Clusters were located in the right parahippocampus, fusiform gyrus, and hippocampus, as well as left temporal inferior and fusiform gyrus, and left hippocampus but not in any other region (see **Figure 3**).

APOE Status and Hippocampus

No significant main effect of APOE status on hippocampal volume using the general linear model outlined above could be detected [$F_{[1,53]} = 0.67$, $p = 0.42$]. However, a significant main effect of MDD diagnosis [$F_{[1,53]} = 7.87$, $p = 0.01$, $\eta^2 = 0.13$] was found, with smaller hippocampal volume in the MDD group compared to the HC group. No within-subject effect of hippocampus laterality [$F_{[1,53]} = 0.33$, $p = 0.57$], and no other main effects of interest emerged (all other $p > 0.41$).

When adding an interaction term between APOE status and age to the model this yielded a non-significant interaction effect [$F_{[1,52]} = 0.12$, $p = 0.73$]. Adding an interaction term between APOE status and sex also yielded a non-significant effect [$F_{[1,52]} = 0.03$, $p = 0.86$]. The interaction between APOE status and diagnosis was also non-significant [$F_{[1,53]} = 0.05$, $p = 0.82$]. Exploratory analyses revealed that when removing TIV from the model, hippocampal volume was significantly predicted by APOE genotype [$F_{[1,54]} = 11.64$, $p = 0.001$, $\eta^2 = 0.18$]. In order to further explore the role of TIV, the same model as described above was applied to predict TIV instead of hippocampal volume in a subsequent analysis. This yielded a significant main effect of APOE status [$F_{[1,54]} = 25.59$, $p < 0.001$, $\eta^2 = 0.32$], with lower mean TIV in ε4 homozygotes. Mean TIV and hippocampal volume over APOE genotype is depicted in **Figure 4**.

VBM model estimation yielded no clusters beyond significance threshold for the APOE genotype contrast at a TFCE-corrected significance level of $p < 0.05$. Exploratory whole brain VBM analysis using the same model yielded eight clusters beyond an exploratory uncorrected threshold of $p < 0.001$ and a minimum cluster size of 20 voxels (see **Table 2**). No clusters remained significant when applying TFCE corrections on whole brain level. When using the exploratory uncorrected threshold at $p < 0.001$ with a minimum cluster size of 20 voxels no clusters emerged for the inverted contrast of greater gray matter density in the ε4 homozygotes on whole brain level.

DISCUSSION

The main finding of the present study is that APOE ε4 homozygosity is associated with lower vWM ability already in young to mid-age, non-demented subjects. Effect size estimates indicate a medium sized effect. This effect seems to be age-independent within the age range of our sample (19–63 years) and is of comparable magnitude in the MDD subsample as in the HC sample. Similarly, we found lower vWM capacity in people with MDD diagnosis compared to HC subjects. Although some evidence was found that hippocampal gray matter density was associated with vWM, no specific relationship was detected between vWM and hippocampal volume when including TIV as a covariate. Furthermore, both measures of hippocampal structure (gray matter density and volume) did not significantly differ between genotypes in our sample when controlling for global brain structural measures. In addition, a specific effect of MDD diagnosis on hippocampal volume was found which appeared to be independent from APOE genotype.

Previous work investigating the influence of APOE genotype on cognitive abilities present a general trend of lower abilities in various cognitive domains for ε4 carriers (18, 20, 21, 24, 41, 61). Although some studies also find differences regarding the visuospatial domain (24, 25) the evidence is more inconsistent in this field and a meta-analysis even concluded that there is little evidence for an impact on the visuospatial domain by the APOE gene (21). This may hold true for heterozygous ε4 carriers compared to non-ε4 carriers (as most studies compare these groups). However, little research exists including valid sample sizes of ε4 homozygotes. The current study provides a comparatively large sample size of ε4 homozygotes. It revealed

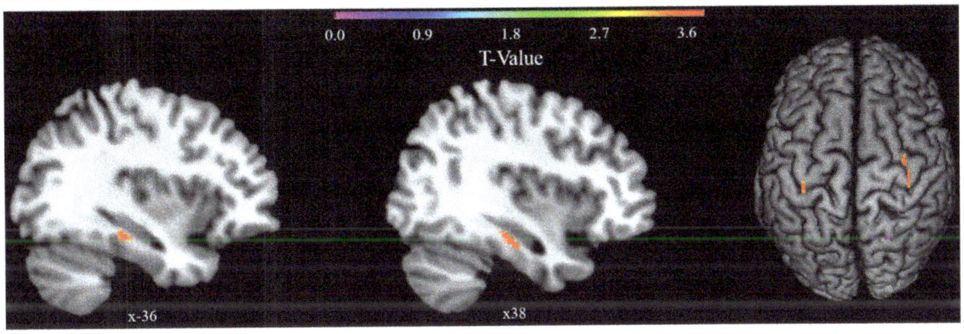

FIGURE 3 | VBM whole brain results showing clusters with a positive correlation of gray matter density with Corsi span in the general linear model. Results are presented below an exploratory uncorrected significance threshold of $p < 0.001$ with a minimum cluster size of 20 voxels. Clusters are located in the left temporal inferior and fusiform gyrus and left hippocampus, and in the right parahippocampus, hippocampus, and fusiform gyrus.

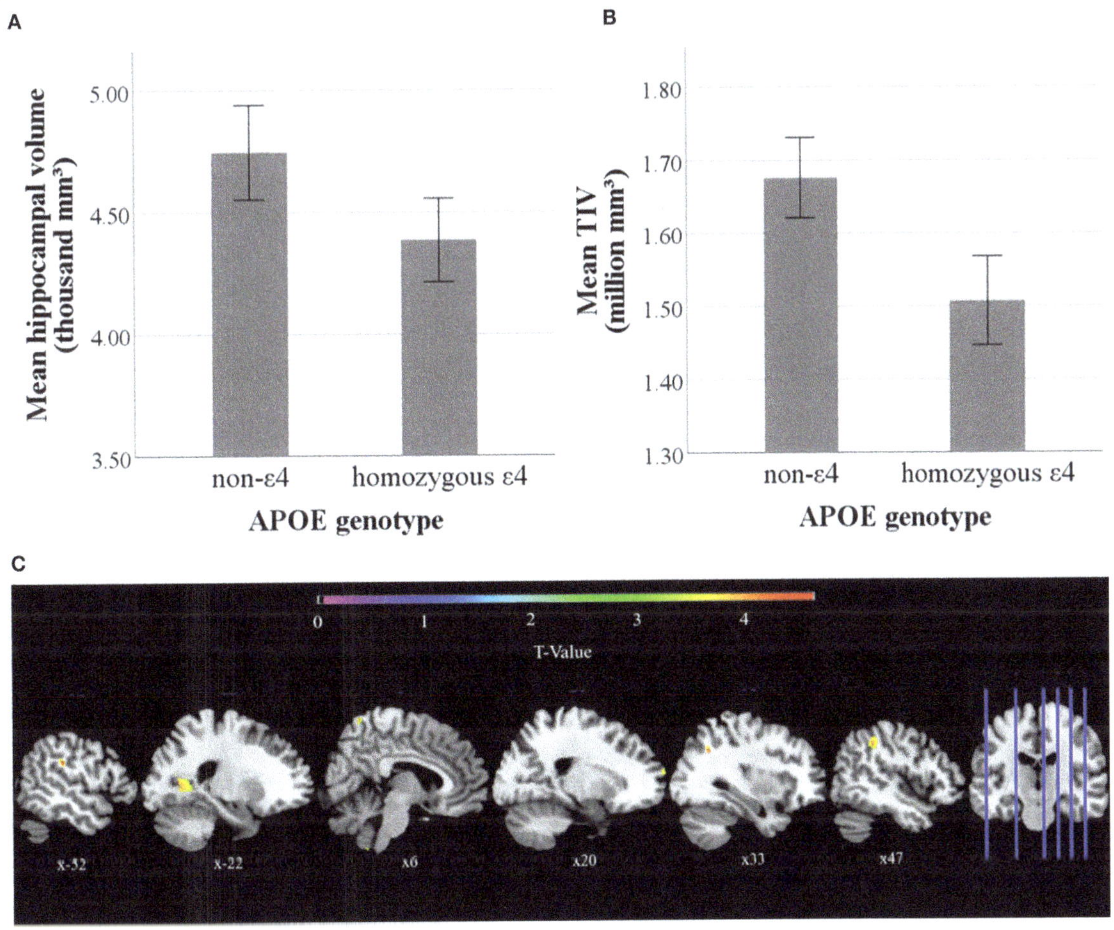

FIGURE 4 | Mean hippocampal volume **(A)**, and mean total intracranial volume (TIV) volume **(B)** differences over APOE genotypes. Depicted hippocampal volumes were calculated as mean volumes between left and right laterality. Error bars represent 95% confidence intervals. VBM results of the contrast that ε4 homozygotes have lower gray matter density than non-ε4 carriers are depicted at the bottom **(C)**. Presented clusters correspond to the clusters described in **Table 2**.

medium sized group differences for the Corsi block-tapping task performance. As measures of visuospatial ability vary between studies it cannot be ruled out that the effect shows more in the Corsi task than other tasks of visuospatial performance that might tax domain components differently (for example more or less taxing of executive components of working memory).

The findings of the current study suggest that both APOE status and MDD diagnosis have deteriorating effects on vWM,

TABLE 2 | Clusters above exploratory uncorrected significance threshold $p < 0.001$ with minimum voxel number of 20 for the contrast of lower gray matter density in homozygous APOE ε4 carriers.

Main area	k_E	Peak voxel coordinates			Peak voxel coefficients	
		x	*y*	*z*	*t*	*p*
Supramarginal gyrus	51	−52	−30	30	4.62	0.000
Angular gyrus	26	33	−57	34	4.24	0.000
Supramarginal gyrus	119	48	−40	42	3.74	0.000
Precuneus	20	6	−58	68	3.70	0.000
Superior frontal gyrus	31	20	69	15	3.66	0.000
Calcarine	311	−24	−62	8	3.64	0.000
Cerebellum	46	2	−50	−58	3.40	0.000
Middle temporal gyrus	26	−63	−22	0	3.24	0.001

Uncorrected p-values of peak voxel differences are reported.

which appear to be of an additive nature. In contrast a longitudinal study investigating the interplay between depression and APOE status on AD risk, proposes an interactional relationship, as that depression constitutes a risk factor only in ε4 carriers (39). Regarding cross-sectional effects in mid-life, our results are in line with other evidence proposing that MDD and ε4 effects on cognitive ability are rather additive (41, 62) suggesting that interactional effects might only show later in life and/or in combination with demential processes.

The literature addressing interaction effects between APOE genotype and age on cognitive ability is very heterogeneous depending on cognitive measures and age span under investigation. Most studies finding cognitive decline effects in APOE ε4 carriers have investigated elderly samples from 60 years upwards (63). Evidence is mixed for mid-age samples (61) while a meta-analysis regarding children and young adults suggest no cognitive differences dependent on APOE status (64). For the sample investigated in the current study no moderating influence of age on APOE effects on cognition became evident. Genotype effects were further not found to be moderated by sex.

Regarding the relationship between vWM and brain structural measures the results found here hold several important insights. Two measures of hippocampal morphometry were used in the current study and findings varied depending on the measure. While hippocampal volume was not associated with vWM capacity, gray matter density was marginally significantly increased in higher vWM capacity individuals. Furthermore, exploratory additional analyses indicated that the effect on hippocampal volume was masked by the covariate TIV (possibly suggesting a more unspecific, global association), while the exploratory whole brain VBM analysis suggested a specific effect located in the hippocampal and parahippocampal area (as no other areas were associated with vWM capacity). Findings suggest a global correlate of vWM regarding volumetric measures, while gray matter density seems to be associated with vWM specifically in the hippocampal and parahippocampal regions. Other findings suggesting a local link between the hippocampus and vWM capacity have used different measures of brain function (9, 34) and structure, as lesions (10, 35), gray matter density (9), and volume (36).

The pattern of results found in the current study suggests that although the ε4 allele may be associated with lower vWM capacity, the neuronal locus of this effect is not the hippocampal region specifically. Previous findings suggest a robust deteriorating APOE ε4 effect on hippocampal structure that supposedly is most pronounced for ε4 homozygotes (30, 31). However, in the current study we were unable to replicate group differences of hippocampal morphometry in dependence of APOE status (neither for a volumetric, nor for a gray matter density measure) after controlling for global brain measures. This finding is particularly surprising since we contrasted ε4 homozygotes with non-ε4 carriers. One possible explanation is given by Cherbuin et al. (30): the authors reviewed studies showing an effect and studies with contradicting findings, and propose that a potential effect of APOE genotype on hippocampal alterations may show only in a narrow age range around ~70 years. It is suggested that samples below the age of 60 years may not be affected yet, while an APOE effect may be masked by more general age-related alterations in samples over 80 years (30). This interpretation would be in line with our findings as most participants of our sample are considerably younger. A different explanatory approach arises from our exploratory analyses that revealed that the relationship between APOE status and hippocampus is covered by the covariate TIV that may have too much explanatory variance in common with the hippocampal volume. One interpretation of this finding is that the APOE genotype affects the cerebral morphometry on a more global level. This interpretation is in line with a brain reserve hypothesis that implies that a globally increased brain volume serves as a protective factor regarding demential processes (65). Although this hypothesis has been discussed controversially (66, 67) our findings suggest that a protective effect of the APOE genotype (not having an ε4 allele) regarding AD might be mediated by global TIV. Further, it is also possible that the smaller TIV of ε4 homozygotes does not constitute a causal link between genotype and AD risk but is a byproduct of other neuronal processes. Either way, although the rational of controlling for TIV in brain morphology analyses seems straight forward, one should be aware that controlling for TIV variance might also covert morphometric effects of interest (68).

Causality of a genotype on an associated present phenotype cannot be definitely concluded as linkage disequilibrium with other causal factors cannot be ruled out (69). However, there is some evidence for a causal effect of the APOE genotype on visuospatial ability coming from animal models showing a reduced performance in a water maze task in APOE knockout mice with synthetic human APOE ε4 compared to APOE ε3 (70). Even though the translation to humans is not certain this finding supports the notion of a causal effect of APOE genotype on cognition in the current study. Owing to the cross-sectional nature of our data the reported link between brain structure and vWM cannot be interpreted regarding to its causal direction.

Major strengths of the current work comprise the relatively large sample of ε4 homozygotes compared to previous studies (bearing in mind that this cohort was obtained from a total of *N*

= 1,141). Another major strength lies in the inclusion of cognitive as well as brain structural data.

The results of the current study underlie several limitations which have been addressed in part. Firstly, only homozygous ε4 carriers were compared to non-ε4 carriers. Consequently, no conclusions can be derived regarding a potential dose effect of the ε4 allele status, and also no differential conclusions can be made about subgroups of different non-ε4 genotypes. Further, despite the availability of a large initial sample only a relatively small study sample of ε4 homozygotes could be included due to a naturally low occurrence rate of the ε4 allele. Thus, small effects are more difficult to detect and it cannot be ruled out that associations with small effect sizes can be found in higher-powered studies that were not significant in the current study. This could for example concern a potential interaction effect of MDD diagnosis and APOE status that was descriptively looming in the current study but did not become significant. A potential interaction of age and APOE status could particularly be affected by small sample sizes because samples have to be sufficiently powered across the whole age-range under investigation. The current study does not allow conclusions about age effects below the age of 19 and above the age of 63. Further, interactions of small effect sizes may be present within this range.

Furthermore, conclusions derived regarding the vWM capacity are to be interpreted with caution as the concept of vWM is rather heterogeneous and results may vary over different measures of vWM.

CONCLUSIONS

Combined results suggest that a detrimental effect of APOE genotype on vWM capacity exists and might be mediated by global volumetric measures rather than by region-specific volumetric or gray matter density measures. More specific hippocampus alterations as a function of APOE status may occur later in life but do not become evident in our young- to mid-age sample.

More longitudinal high-powered studies investigating the interplay between the APOE genotype, MDD and cognitive deficits, as well as neuronal processes involved are needed. It is important that future studies include sufficient sample sizes of ε4 homozygotes. Large multi-centered studies constitute a promising approach for achieving this goal.

AUTHOR CONTRIBUTIONS

JG, RR, NO, UD, BB, TK, MN, MR, IN, AK, and AJ: study concept and design. JG, NO, RR, UD, KD, KF, DZ, SM, VE, ES, LF, KB, DG, AT, SS, FS, TM, DY, and EF: acquisition, analysis, or interpretation of data. JG, NO, and UD: drafting of the manuscript. RR, TK, AJ, BB, AF, VE, SW, AK, TH, KF, JR, DZ, KD, CK, DG, SM, ES, LF, TH, AK, IN, SM, FS, TM, DY, EF and MR: critical revision of the manuscript for important intellectual content. JG, NO, RR, and UD: statistical analysis. UD, NO, RR, and TK: obtained funding. RR, KF, KD, DZ, SM, VE, ES, LF, KB, JG, CK, HK, DG, TH, AT, SS, FS, TM, DY and EF: administrative, technical, or material support. UD, NO, BB, TK, MN, MR, IN, AK, and AJ: study supervision. All authors read and approved the submitted version of the manuscript.

FUNDING

The FOR 2107 consortium is supported by the German Research Council (Deutsche Forschungsgemeinschaft, DFG, Grant nos. KI 588/14-1, KI 588/14-2, KR 3822/7-1, KR 3822/7-2, NE 2254/1-2, DA 1151/5-1, DA 1151/5-2, SCHW 559/14-1, 545/7-2, RI 908/11-2, WI 3439/3-2, NO 246/10-2, DE 1614/3-2, HA 7070/2-2, JA 1890/7-1, JA 1890/7-2, MU 1315/8-2, RE 737/20-2, KI 588/17-1).

This work was furthermore funded by the German Research Foundation (DFG, grant FOR2107 DA1151/5-1 and DA1151/5-2 to UD; SFB-TRR58, Projects C09 and Z02 to UD) and the Interdisciplinary Center for Clinical Research (IZKF) of the Medical Faculty of Münster (grant Dan3/012/17 to UD).

We further acknowledge support from the Open Access Publication Fund of the University of Münster.

ACKNOWLEDGMENTS

We are deeply indebted to all participants of this study, the recruitment sites, and their staff.

REFERENCES

1. Burns A, Iliffe S. Alzheimer's disease. *Br Med J.* (2009) 338:471. doi: 10.1136/bmj.b158
2. Nestor PJ, Scheltens P, Hodges JR. Advances in the early detection of Alzheimer's disease. *Nat Med.* (2004) 10:34–41. doi: 10.1038/nm1433
3. Ries ML, Carlsson CM, Rowley HA, Sager MA, Gleason CE, Asthana S, et al. Magnetic resonance imaging characterization of brain structure and function in mild cognitive impairment: a review. *J Am Geriatr Soc.* (2008) 56:920–34. doi: 10.1111/j.1532-5415.2008.01684.x
4. Chandra A, Dervenoulas G, Politis M. Magnetic resonance imaging in Alzheimer's disease and mild cognitive impairment. *J Neurol.* (2019). 266:1293–302. doi: 10.1007/s00415-018-9016-3
5. Li X, Coyle D, Maguire L, Watson DR, McGinnity TM. Gray matter concentration and effective connectivity changes in Alzheimer's disease: a longitudinal structural MRI study. *Neuroradiology.* (2011) 53:733–48. doi: 10.1007/s00234-010-0795-1
6. Thompson PM, Hayashi KM, Zubicaray G, Janke AL, Rose SE, Semple J. Dynamics of gray matter loss in Alzheimer's disease. *J Neurosci.* (2003) 23:994–1005. doi: 10.1523/JNEUROSCI.23-03-00994.2003
7. Jack CR Jr., Shiung MM, Gunter JL, O'Brien PC, Weigand SD, Knopman DS, et al. Comparison of different MRI brain atrophy rate measures with clinical disease progression in AD. *Neurology.* (2004) 62:591–600. doi: 10.1021/nl061786n
8. Giovanello KS, Schnyer DM, Verfaellie M. A critical role of the anterior hippocampus in relational memory: evidence from an fMRI study comparing associative and item recognition. *Hippocampus.* (2004) 14:5–8. doi: 10.1002/hipo.10182
9. De Rover M, Pironti VA, McCabe JA, Acosta-Cabronero J, Arana FS, Morein-Zamir S, et al. Hippocampal dysfunction in patients with mild cognitive impairment: a functional neuroimaging study of a visuospatial paired associates learning task. *Neuropsychologia.* (2011) 49:2060–70. doi: 10.1016/j.neuropsychologia.2011.03.037
10. Moses SN, Cole C, Ryan JD. Relational memory for object identity and spatial

location in rats with lesions of perirhinal cortex, amygdala and hippocampus. *Brain Res Bull.* (2005) 65:501–12. doi: 10.1016/j.brainresbull.2005.02.029

11. Schott JM, Crutch SJ, Frost C, Warrington EK, Rossor MN, Fox NC. Neuropsychological correlates of whole brain atrophy in Alzheimer's disease. *Neuropsychologia.* (2008) 46:1732–7. doi: 10.1016/j.neuropsychologia.2008.02.015
12. Dohm K, Redlich R, Zwitserlood P, Dannlowski U. Trajectories of major depression disorders: a systematic review of longitudinal neuroimaging findings. *Aust N Z J Psychiatry.* (2017) 51:441–54. doi: 10.1177/0004867416661426
13. Ownby RL, Crocco E, Acevedo A, John V, Loewenstein D. Depression and risk for Alzheimer disease: systematic review, meta-analysis, and metaregression analysis. *Arch Gen Psychiatry.* (2006) 63:530–8. doi: 10.1111/j.1743-6109.2008.01122.x.Endothelial
14. Corder E, Saunders A, Strittmatter W, Schmechel D, Gaskell P, Small G, et al. Gene dose of apolipoprotein E type 4 Allele and the risk of Alzheimer's disease in late onset families. *Science.* (1993) 261:921–3.
15. Farrer LA. Effects of age, sex, and ethnicity on the association between apolipoprotein E genotype and Alzheimer disease. *J Am Med Assoc.* (1997) 278:1349. doi: 10.1001/jama.1997.03550160069041
16. Bu G. Apolipoprotein E and its receptors in Alzheimer's disease: pathways, pathogenesis and therapy. *Nat Rev Neurosci.* (2009) 10:333–44. doi: 10.1038/nrn2620
17. Altmann A, Tian L, Victor WH, Greicius MD. Sex modifies the APOE-related risk of developing Alzheimer's disease. *Ann Neurol.* (2014) 75:563–73. doi: 10.1016/j.asieco.2008.09.006.EAST
18. Baxter LC, Caselli RJ, Johnson SC, Reiman E, Osborne D. Apolipoprotein E ε4 affects new learning in cognitively normal individuals at risk for Alzheimer's disease. *Neurobiol Aging.* (2003) 24:947–52. doi: 10.1016/S0197-4580(03)00006-X
19. Caselli RJ, Reiman EM, Osborne D, Hentz JG, Baxter LC, Hernandez JL, et al. Longitudinal changes in cognition and behavior in asymptomatic carriers of the APOE e4 allele. *Neurology.* (2004) 62:1990–5. doi: 10.1212/01.WNL.0000129533.26544.BF
20. Reinvang I, Winjevoll IL, Rootwelt H, Espeseth T. Working memory deficits in healthy APOE epsilon 4 carriers. *Neuropsychologia.* (2010) 48:566–73. doi: 10.1016/j.neuropsychologia.2009.10.018
21. Small BJ, Rosnick CB, Fratiglioni L, Bäckman L. Apolipoprotein E and cognitive performance: a meta-analysis. *Psychol Aging.* (2004) 19:592–600. doi: 10.1037/0882-7974.19.4.592
22. Flory JD, Manuck SB, Ferrell RE, Ryan CM, Muldoon MF. Memory performance and the apolipoprotein E polymorphism in a community sample of middle-aged adults. *Am J Med Genet.* (2000) 96:707–11. doi: 10.1002/1096-8628(20001204)96:6<707::AID-AJMG1>3.0.CO;2-V
23. Berteau-Pavy F, Park B, Raber J. Effects of sex and APOE ε4 on object recognition and spatial navigation in the elderly. *Neuroscience.* (2007) 147:6–17. doi: 10.1016/j.neuroscience.2007.03.005
24. Negash S, Greenwood PM, Sunderland T, Parasuraman R, Geda YE, Knopman DS, et al. The influence of apolipoprotein E genotype on visuospatial attention dissipates after age 80. *Neuropsychology.* (2009) 23:81–9. doi: 10.1037/a0014014.The
25. Bloss CS, Delis DC, Salmon DP, Bondi MW. Decreased cognition in children with risk factors for Alzheimer's disease. *Biol Psychiatry.* (2008) 64:904–6. doi: 10.1016/j.biopsych.2008.07.004
26. Acevedo SF, Piper BJ, Craytor MJ, Benice TEDS, Raber J, Neuroscience B, et al. Apolipoprotein E4 and sex affect neurobehavioral performance in primary school children. *Pediatr Res.* (2010) 67:293–9. doi: 10.1203/PDR.0b013e3181cb8e68
27. Reiman EM, Caselli RJ, Yun LS, Chen K, Bandy D, Minoshima S, et al. Preclinical evidence of Alzheimer's disease in persons homozygous for the ε4 Allele for apolipoprotein E. *N Engl J Med.* (1996) 334:752–8. doi: 10.1056/NEJM199603213341202
28. Lemaître H, Crivello F, Dufouil C, Grassiot B, Tzourio C, Alpérovitch A, et al. No ε4 gene dose effect on hippocampal atrophy in a large MRI database of healthy elderly subjects. *Neuroimage.* (2005) 24:1205–13. doi: 10.1016/j.neuroimage.2004.10.016
29. Wishart HA, Saykin AJ, McAllister TW, Rabin LA, McDonald BC, Flashman LA, et al. Regional brain atrophy in cognitively intact adults with a single APOE epsilon 4 allele. *Neurology.* (2006) 67:1221–4. doi: 10.1212/01.wnl.0000238079.00472.3a
30. Cherbuin N, Leach LS, Christensen H, Anstey KJ. Neuroimaging and APOE genotype: a systematic qualitative review. *Dement Geriatr Cogn Disord.* (2007) 24:348–62. doi: 10.1159/000109150
31. Liu Y, Yu J-T, Wang H-F, Han P-R, Tan C-C, Wang C, et al. APOE genotype and neuroimaging markers of Alzheimer's disease: systematic review and meta-analysis. *J Neurol Neurosurg Psychiatry.* (2015) 86:127–34. doi: 10.1136/jnnp-2014-307719
32. Owen AM, McMillan KM, Laird AR, Bullmore E. N-back working memory paradigm: a meta-analysis of normative functional neuroimaging studies. *Hum Brain Mapp.* (2005) 25:46–59. doi: 10.1002/hbm.20131
33. Corsi PM. *Human Memory and the Medial Temporal Region of the Brain.* Montreal, QC: McGill University (1972).
34. Toepper M, Markowitsch HJ, Gebhardt H, Beblo T, Thomas C, Gallhofer B, et al. Hippocampal involvement in working memory encoding of changing locations: an fMRI study. *Brain Res.* (2010) 1354:91–9. doi: 10.1016/j.brainres.2010.07.065
35. Piekema C, Fernández G, Postma A, Hendriks MPH, Wester AJ, Kessels RPC. Spatial and non-spatial contextual working memory in patients with diencephalic or hippocampal dysfunction. *Brain Res.* (2007) 1172:103–9. doi: 10.1016/j.brainres.2007.07.066
36. Longoni G, Rocca MA, Pagani E, Riccitelli GC, Colombo B, Rodegher M, et al. Deficits in memory and visuospatial learning correlate with regional hippocampal atrophy in MS. *Brain Struct Funct.* (2015) 220:435–44. doi: 10.1007/s00429-013-0665-9
37. Arnone D, McIntosh AM, Ebmeier KP, Munafò MR, Anderson IM. Magnetic resonance imaging studies in unipolar depression: systematic review and meta-regression analyses. *Eur Neuropsychopharmacol.* (2012) 22:1–16. doi: 10.1016/j.euroneuro.2011.05.003
38. Lee RSC, Hermens DF, Porter MA, Redoblado-Hodge MA. A meta-analysis of cognitive deficits in first-episode major depressive disorder. *J Affect Disord.* (2012) 140:113–24. doi: 10.1016/j.jad.2011.10.023
39. Karlsson IK, Bennet AM, Ploner A, Andersson TM-L, Reynolds CA, Gatzc M, et al. Apolipoprotein E ε4 genotype and the temporal relationship between depression and dementia. *Neurobiol Aging.* (2015) 36:1751–6. doi: 10.1016/j.neurobiolaging.2015.01.008
40. Lavretsky H, Ercoli L, Siddarth P, Bookheimer S, Miller K, Small G. Apolipoprotein ε4 Allele status, depressive symptoms, and cognitive decline in middle-aged and elderly persons without dementia. *Am J Geriatr Psychiatry.* (2003) 11:667–73. doi: 10.2217/nnm.12.167
41. Taylor WD, Boyd B, Turner R, McQuoid DR, Ashley-Koch A, MacFall JR, et al. APOE ε4 associated with preserved executive function performance and maintenance of temporal and cingulate brain volumes in younger adults. *Brain Imaging Behav.* (2017) 11:194–204. doi: 10.1007/s11682-016-9522-9
42. Meyer MR, Tschanz JT, Norton MC, Welsh-Bohmer KA, Steffens DC, Wyse BW, et al. APOE genotype predicts when — not whether — one is predisposed to develop Alzheimer disease. *Nat Genet.* (1998) 19:321–2.
43. O'Brien JT, Lloyd A, McKeith I, Gholkar A, Ferrier N. A longitudinal study of hippocampal volume, cortisol levels, and cognition in older depressed subjects. *Am J Psychiatry.* (2004) 161:2081–90. doi: 10.1176/appi.ajp.161.11.2081
44. Egger K, Schocke M, Weiss E, Auffinger S, Esterhammer R, Goebel G, et al. Pattern of brain atrophy in elderly patients with depression revealed by voxel-based morphometry. *Psychiatry Res.* (2008) 164:237–44. doi: 10.1016/j.pscychresns.2007.12.018
45. Kircher T, Wöhr M, Nenadić I, Schwarting R, Schratt G, Alferink J, et al. Neurobiology of the major psychoses. A translational perspective on brain structure and function: the FOR2107 consortium. *Eur Arch Psychiatry Clin Neurosci.* (2018). doi: 10.1007/s00406-018-0943-x. [Epub ahead of print].
46. Carlesimo GA, Fadda L, Lorusso S, Caltagirone C. Verbal and spatial memory spans in Alzheimer's and multi-infarct dementia. *Acta Neurol Scand.* (1994) 89:132–8. doi: 10.1111/j.1600-0404.1994.tb01648.x
47. Trojano L, Chiacchio L, De Luca G, Fragassi NA, Grossi D. Effect of testing procedure on Corsi's block-tapping task in normal subjects and Alzheimer-type dementia. *PerceptMotSkills.* (1994) 78:859–63. doi: 10.2466/pms.1994.78.3.859
48. Grossi D, Becker JT, Smith C, Trojano L. Memory for visuospatial patterns in Alzheimer's disease. *Psychol Med.* (1993) 23:65–70. doi: 10.1017/S003329170003885X

49. Donolato E, Giofrè D, Mammarella IC. Differences in verbal and visuospatial forward and backward order recall: a review of the literature. *Front Psychol.* (2017) 8:663. doi: 10.3389/fpsyg.2017.00663
50. Wittchen H-U, Wunderlich U, Gruschwitz S, Zaudig M. *SKID-I. Strukturiertes Klinisches Interview für DSM-IV*. Göttingen: Hogrefe (1997).
51. Vogelbacher C, Möbius TWD, Sommer J, Schuster V, Dannlowski U, Kircher T, et al. The Marburg-Münster Affective Disorders Cohort Study (MACS): a quality assurance protocol for MR neuroimaging data. *Neuroimage.* (2018) 172:450–60. doi: 10.1016/j.neuroimage.2018.01.079
52. Dannlowski U, Grabe HJ, Wittfeld K, Klaus J, Konrad C, Grotegerd D, et al. Multimodal imaging of a tescalcin (TESC) regulating polymorphism (rs7294919)-specific effects on hippocampal gray matter structure. *Mol Psychiatry.* (2015) 20:398–404. doi: 10.1038/mp.2014.39
53. Opel N, Amare AT, Redlich R, Repple J, Kaehler C, Grotegerd D, et al. Cortical surface area alterations shaped by genetic load for neuroticism. *Mol Psychiatry.* (2018). doi: 10.1038/s41380-018-0236-9. [Epub ahead of print].
54. Redlich R, Opel N, Grotegerd D, Dohm K, Zaremba D, Burger C, et al. Prediction of individual response to electroconvulsive therapy via machine learning on structural magnetic resonance imaging data. *JAMA Psychiatry.* (2016) 73:557–64. doi: 10.1001/jamapsychiatry.2016.0316
55. Opel N, Redlich R, Repple J, Kaehler C, Grotegerd D, Dohm K, et al. Childhood maltreatment moderates the influence of genetic load for obesity on reward related brain structure and function in major depression. *Psychoneuroendocrinology.* (2019) 100:18–26. doi: 10.1016/j.psyneuen.2018.09.027
56. Fischl B, Salat DH, Busa E, Albert M, Dieterich M, Haselgrove C, et al. Whole brain segmentation: automated labeling of neuroanatomical structures in the human brain. *Neuron.* (2002) 33:341–55. doi: 10.1016/S0896-6273(02)00569-X
57. Chang CC, Chow CC, Tellier LC, Vattikuti S, Purcell SM, Lee JJ. Second-generation PLINK: rising to the challenge of larger and richer datasets. *Gigascience.* (2015) 4:7. doi: 10.1186/s13742-015-0047-8
58. Das S, Forer L, Schönherr S, Sidore C, Locke AE, Kwong A, et al. Next-generation genotype imputation service and methods. *Nat Genet.* (2016) 48:1284–7. doi: 10.1038/ng.3656
59. Maldjian JA, Laurienti PJ, Kraft RA, Burdette JH. An automated method for neuroanatomic and cytoarchitectonic atlas-based interrogation of fMRI data sets. *Neuroimage.* (2003) 19:1233–9. doi: 10.1016/S1053-8119(03)00169-1
60. Tzourio-Mazoyer N, Landeau B, Papathanassiou D, Crivello F, Etard O, Delcroix N, et al. Automated anatomical labeling of activations in SPM using a macroscopic anatomical parcellation of the MNI MRI single-subject brain. *Neuroimage.* (2002) 15:273–89. doi: 10.1006/nimg.2001.0978
61. Greenwood PM, Espesetz T, Lin M-K, Reinvang I, Prasuraman R. Longitudinal change in working memory as a function of APOE genotype in midlife and old age. *Scand J Psychol.* (2014) 55:268–77. doi: 10.1111/j.1743-6109.2008.01122.x
62. Luciano M, Pujals AMF, Marioni RE, Campbell A, Hayward C, MacIntyre DJ, et al. Current versus lifetime depression, APOE variation, and their interaction on cognitive performance in younger and older adults. *Psychosom Med.* (2015) 77:480–92. doi: 10.1097/PSY.0000000000000190
63. Wisdom NM, Callahan JL, Hawkins KA. The effects of apolipoprotein E on non-impaired cognitive functioning: a meta-analysis. *Neurobiol Aging.* (2011) 32:63–74. doi: 10.1016/j.neurobiolaging.2009.02.003
64. Ihle A, Bunce D, Kliegel M. APOE epsilon 4 and cognitive function in early life: a meta-analysis. *Neuropsychology.* (2012) 26:267–77. doi: 10.1037/a0026769
65. Perneczky R, Wagenpfeil S, Lunetta KL, Cupples LA, Green RC, Decarli C, et al. Head circumference, atrophy, and cognition: Implications for brain reserve in Alzheimer disease. *Neurology.* (2010) 75:137–42. doi: 10.1212/WNL.0b013e3181e7ca97
66. Jenkins R, Fox NC, Rossor AM, Harvey RJ, Rossor MN. Intracranial volume and Alzheimer disease. *Arch Neurol.* (2014) 57:220–4. doi: 10.1001/archneur.57.2.220
67. Christensen H, Anstey KJ, Parslow RA, Maller J, Mackinnon A, Sachdev P. The brain reserve hypothesis, brain atrophy and aging. *Gerontology.* (2007) 53:82–95. doi: 10.1159/000096482
68. Voevodskaya O. The effects of intracranial volume adjustment approaches on multiple regional MRI volumes in healthy aging and Alzheimer's disease. *Front Aging Neurosci.* (2014) 6:264. doi: 10.3389/fnagi.2014.00264
69. Marian AJ. Causality in genetics: the gradient of genetic effects and back to Koch's postulates of causality. *Circ Res.* (2014) 114:e18–21. doi: 10.1161/CIRCRESAHA.114.302904
70. Raber J, Wong D, Buttini M, Orth M, Bellosta S, Pitas RE, et al. Isoform-specific effects of human apolipoprotein E on brain function revealed in ApoE knockout mice: increased susceptibility of females. *PNAS.* (1998) 95: 10914–9.

6

Basal Forebrain Volume, but not Hippocampal Volume, is a Predictor of Global Cognitive Decline in Patients with Alzheimer's Disease Treated with Cholinesterase Inhibitors

Stefan J. Teipel[1,2], Enrica Cavedo[3,4,5,6,7], Harald Hampel[3,4,5,6] and Michel J. Grothe[1] for the Alzheimer's Disease Neuroimaging Initiative† and Alzheimer Precision Medicine Initiative (APMI)*

[1] German Center for Neurodegenerative Diseases-Rostock/Greifswald, Rostock, Germany, [2] Department of Psychosomatic Medicine, University of Rostock, Rostock, Germany, [3] AXA Research Fund and Sorbonne University Chair, Paris, France, [4] Sorbonne University, GRC n° 21, Alzheimer Precision Medicine, AP-HP, Pitié-Salpêtrière Hospital, Boulevard de l'Hôpital, Paris, France, [5] Brain and Spine Institute (ICM), INSERM U 1127, CNRS UMR 7225, Boulevard de l'Hôpital, Paris, France, [6] Department of Neurology, Institute of Memory and Alzheimer's Disease (IM2A), Pitié-Salpêtrière Hospital, AP-HP, Boulevard de l'Hôpital, Paris, France, [7] IRCCS Istituto Centro San Giovanni di Dio-Fatebenefratelli, Brescia, Italy

***Correspondence:**
Stefan J. Teipel
stefan.teipel@med.uni-rostock.de

† Data used in preparation of this article were obtained from the Alzheimer's Disease Neuroimaging Initiative (ADNI) database (adni.loni.usc.edu/). As such, the investigators within the ADNI contributed to the design and implementation of ADNI and/or provided data but did not participate in analysis or writing of this report. A complete listing of ADNI investigators can be found at: http://adni.loni.usc.edu/wp-content/uploads/how_to_apply/ADNI_Acknowledgement_List.pdf

Background: Predicting the progression of cognitive decline in Alzheimer's disease (AD) is important for treatment selection and patient counseling. Structural MRI markers such as hippocampus or basal forebrain volumes might represent useful instruments for the prediction of cognitive decline. The primary objective was to determine the predictive value of hippocampus and basal forebrain volumes for global and domain specific cognitive decline in AD dementia during cholinergic treatment.

Methods: We used MRI and cognitive data from 124 patients with the clinical diagnosis of AD dementia, derived from the ADNI-1 cohort, who were on standard of care cholinesterase inhibitor treatment during a follow-up period between 0.4 and 3.1 years. We used linear mixed effects models with cognitive function as outcome to assess the main effects as well as two-way interactions between baseline volumes and time controlling for age, sex, and total intracranial volume. This model accounts for individual variation in follow-up times.

Results: Basal forebrain volume, but not hippocampus volume, was a significant predictor of rates of global cognitive decline. Larger volumes were associated with smaller rates of cognitive decline. Left hippocampus volume had a modest association with rates of episodic memory decline. Baseline performance in global cognition and memory was significantly associated with hippocampus and basal forebrain volumes; in addition, basal forebrain volume was associated with baseline performance in executive function.

Conclusions: Our findings indicate that in AD dementia patients, basal forebrain volume may be a useful marker to predict subsequent cognitive decline during cholinergic treatment.

Keywords: cholinergic treatment, MRI, prediction, memory, executive function, basal forebrain, hippocampus

INTRODUCTION

A prediction of the individual course of cognitive change in Alzheimer's disease (AD) would help adequate resource allocation, patient care, and counseling. Evidence suggests that the hippocampus supports the consolidation of long-term declarative memory (1, 2), showing neurodegeneration in autopsy data and atrophy in *in vivo* MRI scans as early as in predementia stages of AD (3, 4). Its measurement is standardized, robust, accessible and feasible for *in vivo* studies using established volumetric protocols, with the most recent advance being an internationally harmonized protocol for a consistent delineation of the hippocampus' anatomical borders on MRI scans (5). The cholinergic basal forebrain is the main source of neocortical acetylcholine (6), and is involved in attentional processes, such as immediate recall and executive function (7). Autopsy studies found degeneration of cholinergic basal forebrain neurons in early clinical stages of AD (8, 9), and the resulting reduction of cholinergic cortical activity represents the rationale for the use of cholinergic treatment in AD dementia. The hippocampus represents a key input area of cholinergic projections from the basal forebrain (10). In recent years, MRI based protocols for an automated measurement of cholinergic basal forebrain volumes have been established that make use of stereotactic information derived from combined post mortem MRI and histology (11–13). Based on these protocols, several MRI volumetric studies have shown consistent pattern of hippocampus and cholinergic basal forebrain atrophy in AD dementia (11, 14) and prodromal at-risk stages of AD dementia, such as amnestic mild cognitive impairment (MCI) (15, 16) or individuals with amyloid positive MCI (17).

Based on these findings, hippocampus and cholinergic basal forebrain volumes may help to predict cognitive change and response to cholinergic treatment in patients with AD dementia or prodromal AD. A previous study found that the thickness of the substantia innominata, a potential proxy of cholinergic basal forebrain integrity (18), was associated with rates of cognitive change in 82 AD dementia patients during 9 months of treatment with a cholinesterase inhibitor, with smaller rates of cognitive decline in people with a lower thickness of the substantia innominata (19). In people with MCI, hippocampus volume was associated with rates of cognitive decline with a moderate effect size (20–24). In 37 AD dementia cases, smaller hippocampus volume was associated with faster global cognitive decline during cholinergic treatment (25). In a recent randomized controlled trial of donepezil, we found that hippocampus volume, but not basal forebrain volume, was a predictor of subsequent cognitive decline in 216 MCI cases (26); this effect, however, was independent of treatment. In summary, in MCI cases hippocampus volume, but not basal forebrain volume, was found to be a significant predictor of cognitive decline, irrespective of treatment. In studies on AD dementia cases, hippocampus volume and a proxy for basal forebrain volume were found significant predictors of cognitive decline during cholinergic treatment.

Here, we used longitudinal cognitive data of 124 AD dementia cases retrieved from the Alzheimer's Disease Neuroimaging Initiative (ADNI-1) database, all receiving cholinergic treatment. Based on the previous evidence on the potential predictive value of these brain regions in AD, we determined the association of hippocampus and basal forebrain volume with rates of global and domain-specific cognitive decline during cholinergic treatment. We expected that lower basal forebrain (hippocampus) volume would predict a faster rate of global and executive (global and episodic memory) function. Secondly, we determined the predictive use of basal forebrain and hippocampus volumes for the identification of cognitively stable vs. cognitively declining patients, where we expected that cognitively stable patients would have larger basal forebrain and hippocampus volumes at baseline. These data help to assess the potential usefulness of volumetric MRI to identify people with a more rapid disease progression; such data would support clinical decision making on allocation of treatment resources and care.

METHODS

Study Population

Data used in the preparation of this article were obtained from the Alzheimer's Disease Neuroimaging Initiative (ADNI) database (adni.loni.usc.edu). The ADNI was launched in 2003 as a public-private partnership, led by Principal Investigator Michael W. Weiner, MD. The primary goal of ADNI has been to test whether serial magnetic resonance imaging (MRI), positron emission tomography (PET), other biological markers, and clinical and neuropsychological assessment can be combined to measure the progression of mild cognitive impairment (MCI) and early Alzheimer's disease (AD). A fuller description of ADNI and up-to-date information is available at www.adni-info.org. We retrieved data of participants of the ADNI-1 study who had a clinical diagnosis of AD dementia at baseline, a baseline MRI scan, neuropsychological testing at baseline and follow-up and documented treatment with any cholinesterase inhibitor during follow-up time. We retrieved 124 cases, 56 women, fulfilling these conditions. We included only people with a clinical diagnosis of AD dementia, because cholinesterase inhibitor treatment is only approved for this diagnosis, but not for MCI or other diagnoses.

Neuropsychological Tests

We used ADAScog11 as measure of global cognitive decline (27–29). ADAScog 11 has frequently been used in clinical efficacy trials of cholinesterase inhibitors in AD as primary endpoint (30, 31). In addition, we used composite measures for memory and executive function, respectively, to account for the different versions of the word lists of neuropsychological tests employed in the ADNI psychometric assessment. The ADNI composite scores have been previously defined and they appear to: (i) have good validity, (ii) include additional information, incorporating all of the domain-specific information available from the neuropsychological battery administered in ADNI, and (iii) be strongly associated with a priori specified neuroimaging parameters selected on the basis of their known association with the respective cognitive domain (32, 33).

MRI Acquisition

ADNI MRI data were acquired on multiple 1.5 Tesla MRI scanners using phantom-calibrated scanner-specific T1-weighted sagittal 3D MPRAGE sequences. In order to increase signal uniformity across the multicenter scanner platforms, original MPRAGE acquisitions in ADNI undergo standardized image pre-processing correction steps. Standardization of MRI sequences across ADNI sites and centralized image pre-processing steps have been described in detail previously (34) and are documented on the ADNI website (http://adni.loni.usc.edu/methods/).

MRI Data Processing

The processing of structural MRI scans was implemented through statistical parametric mapping, SPM8 (Wellcome Dept. of Imaging Neuroscience, London), and the VBM8-toolbox (http://dbm.neuro.uni-jena.de/vbm/) implemented in MATLAB 7.1 (Mathworks, Natwick), and has been described in detail previously (35, 36). Briefly, MRI scans were automatically segmented into gray matter (GM), white matter (WM), and cerebrospinal fluid (CSF) partitions of 1.5 mm isotropic voxel-size, using the segmentation routine of the VBM8-toolbox. The resulting GM and white matter partitions of each subject in native space were then high-dimensionally registered to an aging/AD-specific reference template based on a completely independent cohort (37) using the Diffeomorphic Anatomic Registration using Exponentiated Lie algebra (DARTEL) algorithm (38). Individual flow-fields obtained from the DARTEL registration to the reference template were used to warp the GM segments and voxel-values were modulated for volumetric changes introduced by the high-dimensional normalization, such that the total amount of GM volume present before warping was preserved. All preprocessed GM maps passed a visual inspection for overall segmentation and registration accuracy.

The total intracranial volume (TIV) was calculated as the sum of the total segmented GM, WM, and CSF volumes (38). GM volumes of the hippocampus and basal forebrain cholinergic nuclei were automatically extracted by summing up the modulated GM voxel values within respective regions of interest (ROI) in the reference space. The basal forebrain ROI was based on a recently published cytoarchitectonic map of basal forebrain cholinergic nuclei in MNI space, derived from combined histology, and in cranio MRI of a post-mortem brain (13). This cytoarchitectonic map matches standard MNI space and was projected into the aging-AD specific template space using non-linear warping parameters obtained from a DARTEL registration. Although the cytoarchitectonic basal forebrain map comprises detailed outlines of different cholinergic subdivisions within the basal forebrain, including cell clusters corresponding to the medial septum, diagonal band, nucleus subputaminalis, and nucleus basalis Meynert, in the current study we only considered the entire volume of the map, including all cholinergic subdivisions, as a proxy for overall basal forebrain cholinergic system integrity. The ROI mask for the hippocampus was obtained by manual delineation of the hippocampus in the reference template of aging-AD specific anatomy (37) using the interactive software package Display (McConnell Brain Imaging Centre at the Montreal Neurological Institute) and a previously described protocol for segmentation of the medial temporal lobe (39). An illustration of both ROIs in the gray matter fraction of the reference space template employed in our current study can be found in the previous publications (15, 40, 41).

Statistical Analysis

We conducted two types of analysis. The first analysis determined associations of volumetric markers with rates of change in cognitive scores as continuous outcomes. The second analysis determined the accuracy of response prediction in cognitive scores as binary outcome.

Association With Rates of Change

We determined the main effects and the two-way interactions of baseline volumes by time on neuropsychological performance as dependent variable using linear mixed effects models with subject-related random effects for intercept and time, controlling for age, sex, and TIV. The model fit was compared between nested models (random intercept vs. uncorrelated random intercept and slope vs. correlated random intercept and slope) using Akaike's information criterion (AIC) (42). Significance of parameters was determined using t-statistics with degrees of freedom determined according to the Satterthwaite approximation. Mixed effect model analyses were calculated in R, including the libraries "lme4" and "lmerTest," available at http://cran.r-project.org/web/packages.

Response Prediction

We originally had planned to determine response prediction. Similarly to previous studies (43), we defined response as more than 4 points improvement (i.e., at least 4 points decline) in ADAScog11 over one year. This criterion, however, yielded only three responders so that an analysis was not feasible. Consequently, we relaxed the response criterion and discriminated between non-decliners (zero change or better) vs. decliners in the cognitive endpoints. Rates of change in cognitive scores were derived from the coefficients of the subject-related random effect for time on the cognitive scores, controlling for age and sex. We determined logistic regression models regressing the binary endpoint of decline vs. non-decline on those volumetric markers that had shown a significant association with the continuous rates of cognitive decline in the previous models.

We used block-wise cross validation with repeated random sampling, based on Gaussian-distributed random numbers generated in R. We repeatedly split the data set into 63.2% of training data and 36.8% of test data. For each of the repeatedly drawn training samples, the logistic regression parameters were estimated and subsequently applied to the remaining test data set. Bootstrapping aimed to assess levels of predictive accuracy in the test data so to avoid overestimation of accuracy levels that occurs when assessment is based on the training data. We recorded areas under the receiver operating characteristic curves (AUC) for each test data set; different to the rate of correctly identified cases, the AUC is insensitive to an uneven distribution of outcomes. The entire cross-validation process was iterated 100 times to determine the variability of the estimates of accuracy

TABLE 1 | Baseline demographic characteristics.

N (women)	124 (56)
Age, mean (*SD*) in years	75.3 (7.4)
MMSE, mean (*SD*)	23.5 (1.9)
ADAScog11, mean (*SD*)	19.0 (6.4)
ADNI-MEM, mean (*SD*)	−0.9 (0.5)
ADNI-EXE, mean (*SD*)	−0.9 (0.8)
L. hippocampus volume (*SD*) in mm^3	2,038 (337)
R. hippocampus volume (*SD*) in mm^3	2,212 (374)
Basal forebrain volume (*SD*) in mm^3	481 (85)

ADAScog11 - 11-items version of the Alzheimer's Disease Assessment Scale–Cognitive subscale, higher values indicate worse performance.
ADNI-MEM - ADNI memory score (32); this scale provides z-standardized performance scores, lower values indicate worse performance.
ANDI-EXE - ADNI executive function score (33); this scale provides z-standardized performance scores, lower values indicate worse performance.

across runs. We determined nonparametric bootstrap confidence intervals with the 2.5 and 97.5 percentiles defining the lower and upper limits of the confidence interval [(44), Chapter 13]. Logistic regression analysis was calculated in R, using function glm with the parameter family = binary.

All analyses were performed with RStudio, version 0.98.1102, a user interface of R Project for Statistical Computing Analyses.

RESULTS

Sample

We retrieved 124 (56 women) cases with AD dementia fulfilling the inclusion criteria. Follow-up times ranged between 0.4 and 3.1 years, number of follow-up time points ranged between 1 and 5. Baseline demographic characteristics and hippocampus and basal forebrain volumes are given in **Table 1.**

Association With Global and Domain-Specific Cognitive Rates of Change

For **ADAScog11,** the best fit was achieved with a model allowing for a correlated random intercept and slope. Detailed results are shown in **Table 2.** ADAScog11 showed a significant worsening over time with 4.3 points increase per year. Left and right hippocampus and basal forebrain volumes were significantly correlated with ADAScog11 baseline performance, with better performance with higher volume. In addition, basal forebrain volume was associated with less worsening in ADAScog11 performance over time ($t = -2.9$, 115 df, $p < 0.005$) with the effect amounting to 1.6 points less increase in ADAScog11 per year when the volume of basal forebrain was one standard deviation higher (**Figure 1**). The partial correlation coefficient (controlling for TIV) between slopes of ADAScog11 change from the mixed effects model and basal forebrain baseline volume was $r = -0.23$, $p < 0.01$. Left and right hippocampus volumes had no significant effects on the ADAScog11 rates of change over time ($p > 0.22$ for all comparisons).

For **ADNI memory score,** the best fit was achieved with a model allowing for an uncorrelated random intercept and slope. Detailed results are shown in **Table 2.** On average, patients lost 0.21 z-score points per year. Left and right hippocampus and basal forebrain volumes were significantly associated with baseline memory performance, with higher performance associated with higher volume. In addition, left hippocampus volume was associated with less worsening in the ADNI memory score over time ($t = -2.0$, 109 df, $p < 0.05$) with the effect amounting to 0.04 less z-score points lost per year when the volume was one standard deviation higher (**Figure 2**). The partial correlation coefficient (controlling for TIV) between slopes of ADNI memory rates of change from the mixed effects model and left hippocampus baseline volume was −0.15, $p < 0.1$. Right hippocampus and basal forebrain volumes had no significant effects on the ADNI memory rates of change over time ($p > 0.16$ for all comparisons).

For **ADNI executive function score** the best fit was achieved with a model allowing for an uncorrelated random intercept and slope. Detailed results are shown in **Table 2.** On average, patients lost 0.29 z-score points per year ($t = -10.1$, 98 df, $p < 0.001$). Basal forebrain was significantly associated with baseline executive function performance ($t = 3.2$, 123 df, $p < 0.002$), with better performance associated with higher volume; there was no effect for left or right hippocampus volume. Neither bilateral hippocampus nor basal forebrain volumes had a significant effect on the executive function rates of change over time ($p > 0.20$ for all comparisons).

The covariates that were used in the model showed no effect of age, sex or total intracranial volume on ADAScog; age had a significant effect on ADNI memory and executive function scores ($p < 0.05$), but sex and TIV had no significant effects on these scores.

Response Prediction

Basal forebrain volume was significantly associated with the outcome of non-decline in ADAScog11 with an odds ratio of 2.5 ($p < 0.05$), i.e., a one standard deviation higher basal forebrain volume increased the odds of non-decline by a factor of 2.5. The corresponding bootstrapped AUC in the test data was 0.78, the 2.5/97.5 percentile confidence interval was 0.50 to 0.98. For the ADNI memory score there were no non-decliners, rendering further analysis infeasible.

DISCUSSION

We found significant decline of global cognitive function as well as memory and executive function in AD dementia cases during follow-up. Higher basal forebrain volume was associated with slower global cognitive decline, and higher left hippocampus volume was associated with slower memory decline. The prognostic use of basal forebrain volume to discriminate between cognitive decliners and cognitive stable persons based on the global ADAScog11 score reached a cross-validated area under the ROC curve of 0.78, indicating a fair accuracy, however with a broad bootstrapped confidence interval including the random guessing level of AUC = 0.5.

The clear decline of global cognitive function as assessed by ADAScog11 is consistent with previous studies on the course of

TABLE 2 | Summary of predictor effects.

		Left Hp t(df); *p*	Right Hp t(df); *p*	BF t(df); *p*
ADAScog11	Volume	−2.1(120); <0.04	−3.6 (120); <0.001	−3.0(119); <0.004
	Time	8.0(109); 10^{-11}	8.0(109); 10^{-11}	8.0(109); 10^{-11}
	Time*Volume	n.s.	n.s.	−2.9(115); <0.005
ADNI-MEM	Volume	2.3(129); <0.03	3.3(128); <0.002	3.9(128); <0.001
	Time	−10.7(112); 10^{-14}	−10.7(112); 10^{-14}	−10.7(112); 10^{-14}
	Time*Volume	−2.0(109); <0.05	n.s.	n.s.
ADNI-EXE	Volume	n.s.	n.s.	3.2(123); <0.002
	Time	−10.1(98); 10^{-14}	−10.1(98); 10^{-14}	−10.1(98); 10^{-14}
	Time*Volume	n.s.	n.s.	n.s.

Reported are the main effect of time and volume and the interaction effects of volume by time. All models were controlled for age, sex, and total intracranial volume.
Data are given as: t-values (t); number of degrees of freedom (df); p-value (p).
Please note: the sign of the t-value gives the direction of the effect, i.e., a positive t-value indicates that test scores were higher with higher volume and vice versa.
Hp, hippocampus.
BF, basal forebrain.
ADAScog11, 11-items version of the Alzheimer's Disease Assessment Scale–Cognitive subscale.
ADNI-MEM, ADNI memory score (32).
ANDI-EXE, ADNI executive function score (33).

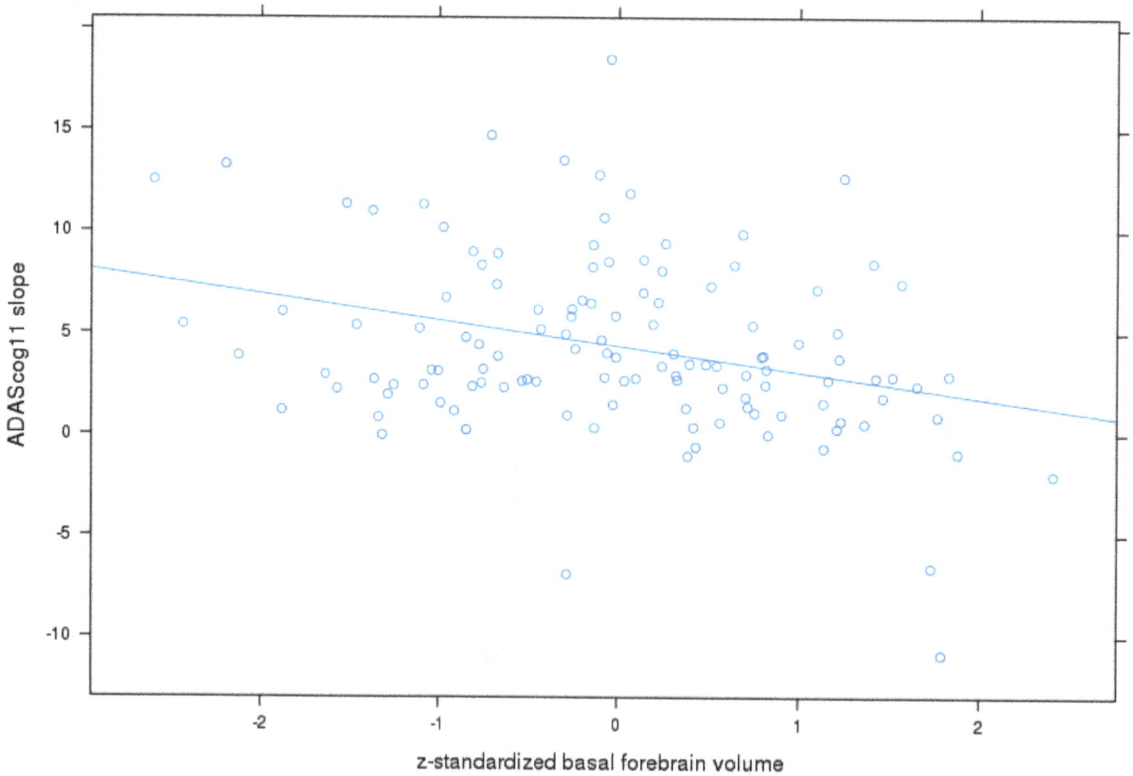

FIGURE 1 | Basal forebrain volume and rates of change in ADAScog11. Plot of z-standardized basal forebrain volume on mixed effects linear model estimates of rates of change in ADAScog score controlling for age and sex, with linear regression line.

cognitive decline in dementia stages of AD (45). A large cohort study of 622 cases with cholinesterase inhibitor treatment and paired assessments of MMSE at baseline and after 3 to 4 months showed a response rate of 37%, when defining response by at least 2 points MMSE increase (46). The findings in this large cohort study agree with findings in randomized controlled trials with cholinesterase inhibitors showing an increase of MMSE or decrease in ADAScog scores in the first 3 to 6 months of treatment with subsequent decline (47, 48). Here, we assessed longer term follow-up, between 0.4 and 3.1 years, accounting for

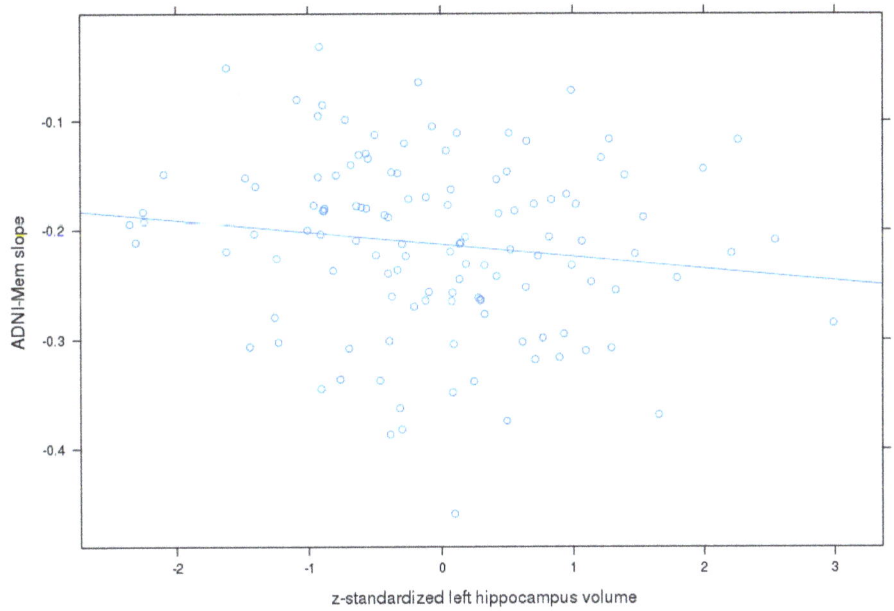

FIGURE 2 | Left hippocampus volume and rates of change in ADNI memory score. Plot of z-standardized left hippocampus volume on mixed effects linear model estimates of rates of change in ADNI memory (ADNI-Mem) score controlling for age and sex, with linear regression line.

the low number of cases fulfilling response criteria (only 10 of 124 cases, even when defining response as non-decline).

In the cross-sectional analyses, baseline volumes of basal forebrain, and left and right hippocampus were associated with global cognitive function as well as memory performance, as assessed by the ADNI memory composite score. These findings agree with previous studies showing that hippocampus volume was associated with episodic memory (49) and global cognitive (50) performance in AD patients. Similarly, previous studies have described associations of basal forebrain volume with global cognitive and episodic memory performance in AD dementia and MCI cases in cross-sectional analysis (15, 40, 41). In addition, in the current study, basal forebrain volume was associated with the executive function composite score. This agrees with the observation that cholinergic activity subserves executive function and attention that is supported by the adverse effects of anticholinergic treatment on executive function and attention (51–53), and by findings of similar associations in independent cohorts (15, 40, 41).

Cholinergic basal forebrain volume was significantly associated with subsequent global cognitive decline as assessed by ADAScog11. AD dementia cases with a one standard deviation higher basal forebrain volume had 1.6 points less worsening in ADAScog11 per year, accounting for 37% of the annual overall rate of ADAScog11 worsening. Basal forebrain volume allowed correct discrimination between cognitive non-decliners and cognitive decliners with an AUC of 0.78. We used the AUC as measure of accuracy, because this measure is less sensitive to the proportion of non-decliners; in contrast, the level of correct case identification would have been uninformative, because with only 10 non-decliners simply predicting non-conversion in all cases would already yield correct classification in 114 out of 124 cases. Our findings indicate that in the presence of cholinergic treatment, a high cholinergic basal forebrain volume is associated with more benign global cognitive decline. Our findings agree with a previous exploratory study, where response to cholinergic treatment over 9 months as measured by the MMSE score was significantly associated with gray matter volume in basal forebrain regions from a voxel based regression analysis in 23 AD cases (54). Our findings disagree with a study in 82 AD dementia patients using the substantia innominata thickness as a proxy of cholinergic basal forebrain integrity (18); here smaller rate of cognitive decline was found associated with a smaller thickness of the substantia innominata during 9 months cholinergic treatment (19). The number of subjects was higher and the average follow-up time was longer in our study compared to the previous study. In addition, manual measurement of the thickness of the substantia innominata is prone to intra- and inter-rater variability, and assesses only a small subsection of the cholinergic basal forebrain compared to the automated measurement of basal forebrain volume based on a post mortem reference map (11).

Hippocampus volume was not associated with the subsequent rate of global cognitive decline. In a small sample of 37 AD patients, a previous study found a higher hippocampus volume associated with less worsening of ADAScog score over 0.5 to 2 years of follow-up (25). A part of these 37 individuals had been classified as very mild AD, resembling rather the prodromal MCI than the dementia stage of AD. This outcome therefore agrees with the results of our previous study on 216 MCI cases, where we found that higher hippocampus volume, rather than basal forebrain volume, was associated with more benign rates of global cognitive and memory decline (26). Taken together these findings suggest that hippocampus volume may be a proxy of reserve capacity in MCI individuals, but no more in AD dementia patients. This interpretation would agree with the notion that hippocampus atrophy begins to degenerate earlier than basal forebrain and reaches a plateau in the dementia stage of AD so that the functional relevance of hippocampus volume variation would be limited in the dementia stage of the disease. In contrast, changes in basal forebrain volume may still dynamically progress during AD dementia and may thus serve as a better predictor of disease progression in more advanced disease stages (37).

In contrast to global cognitive decline, left hippocampus volume was significantly associated with the rate of episodic memory score decline, consistent with previous evidence in subjects with MCI (26, 55). Different to global cognitive decline we could not determine the predictive accuracy of hippocampus volume for non-decline, as non-decline did not occur in our sample. The partial r of −0.15, however, points to a small effect size for left hippocampus volume on subsequent rate of memory decline, consistent with a limited role of hippocampus volume for predicting subsequent cognitive decline in the AD dementia stage, even when considering the hippocampus-specific functional measure of episodic memory performance.

Beyond structural markers, such as hippocampus or basal forebrain volumes, a previous study found cortical network functional integrity in functional MRI as a significant predictor of cholinergic treatment response, but the study included only 18 cases (56).

Several limitations have to be considered with our study. First, similar to previous studies in AD dementia (19, 25) we determined the predictive value of hippocampus and basal forebrain volumes for cognitive decline in patients who all received treatment. Therefore, we can only derive conclusions on prediction of cognitive decline during treatment, but not on prediction of treatment effects; in our view this distinction is sometimes not made explicit enough in the literature (19, 25). We had decided to exclude AD dementia cases without documentation of cholinergic treatment since the lack of documentation of treatment may not be a reliable indicator for the lack of treatment in the ADNI cohort. In addition, the lack of treatment in a cohort like ADNI will likely be related to selection bias; the ADNI cohort by design features no random allocation to treatment. Furthermore, information on the duration of treatment before inclusion in the ADNI cohort was not available so that stratification according to duration of treatment was not possible. Our findings encourage the analysis of prospective controlled clinical trials in AD dementia for a potential association of basal forebrain and hippocampus volumes with rates of subsequent cognitive change in dependency of treatment. Secondly, observation periods were very heterogeneous in the ADNI cohort. We used a mixed effects model to explicitly model variability in observation periods. Indeed, the models including a random effects term for time provided a better fit than models excluding such term. Thirdly, it would have been interesting following previous evidence on the corticotopic organization of the cholinergic basal forebrain to analyze a differential involvement of antero-medial vs. postero-lateral basal forebrain subregions. Anterior-medial basal forebrain nuclei project mainly to the hippocampus and ventromedial cortical regions, whereas posterior-lateral nuclei project more densely to lateral neocortical areas (6, 57, 58), which may also be related to different functional representation of these subnuclei. However, the overall small size of the basal forebrain volume restricts the accuracy of subregional assessments so that we did not include such an analysis. Fourthly, we had selected the ADNI memory and executive function composite scores to reduce the dimensionality of our analyses. Previous studies had shown that both composite measures exhibited more consistent rates of change in MCI and AD dementia individuals than the respective single tests (32, 33). Finally, we aimed to determine odds ratios of volumes for predicting clinically significant response to treatment. Such response has previously been defined to equal at least 4 points decrease in ADAScog11 (43). Since only 3 cases fulfilled this response criterion, we could not conduct the intended analysis. When we used a more liberal criterion of no cognitive decline, i.e., ≤ 0 points change in ADAScog11, we found a significant odds ratio of 2.5. This indicates that a person with a one standard deviation higher basal forebrain volume has a 2.5 higher chance of no decline, all other variables kept constant. However, this analysis detects a clinically potentially less relevant endpoint than the originally planned analysis of 4 points change.

In summary, we found significant decline of global cognitive function as well as memory and executive function in AD dementia patients treated with cholinesterase inhibitors. Basal forebrain volume, but not hippocampus volume, was a predictor of global cognitive decline with a cross-validated accuracy of approximately 78% to discriminate between non-decliners and decliners, albeit based on a small sample of non-decliners. In contrast, left hippocampus volume showed only a modest association with subsequent rates of memory decline during cholinergic treatment. Our data suggest that with the transition from prodromal MCI to AD dementia the brain areas with biologically meaningful dynamic variation and ensuing predictive value may shift from the hippocampus to the basal forebrain region. The use of hippocampus and basal forebrain volumes to predict response to cholinergic treatment in AD dementia needs to be studied in cohorts with controlled treatment.

ETHICS APPROVAL AND CONSENT TO PARTICIPATE

All procedures performed in the ADNI studies involving human participants were in accordance with the ethical standards of the institutional research committees and with the 1964 Helsinki declaration and its later amendments. Written informed consent was obtained from all participants or their authorized representatives.

The study procedures were approved by the institutional review boards of all participating centers (https://adni.loni.usc.edu/wp-content/uploads/how_to_apply/ADNI_Acknowledgement_List.pdf:) Oregon Health and Science University; University of Southern California; University of California—San Diego; University of Michigan; Mayo Clinic, Rochester; Baylor College of Medicine; Columbia University Medical Center; Washington University, St. Louis; University of Alabama at Birmingham; Mount Sinai School of Medicine; Rush University Medical Center; Wien Center; Johns Hopkins University; New York University; Duke University Medical Center; University of Pennsylvania; University of Kentucky; University of Pittsburgh; University of Rochester Medical Center; University of California, Irvine; University of Texas Southwestern Medical School; Emory University; University of Kansas, Medical Center; University of California, Los Angeles; Mayo Clinic, Jacksonville; Indiana University; Yale University School of Medicine; McGill University, Montreal-Jewish General Hospital; Sunnybrook Health Sciences, Ontario; U.B.C. Clinic for AD & Related Disorders; Cognitive Neurology—St. Joseph's, Ontario; Cleveland Clinic Lou Ruvo Center for Brain Health; Northwestern University; Premiere Research Inst (Palm Beach Neurology); Georgetown University Medical Center; Brigham and Women's Hospital; Stanford University; Banner Sun Health Research Institute; Boston University; Howard University; Case Western Reserve University; University of California, Davis—Sacramento; Neurological Care of CNY; Parkwood Hospital; University of Wisconsin; University of California, Irvine—BIC; Banner Alzheimer's Institute; Dent Neurologic Institute; Ohio State University; Albany Medical College; Hartford Hospital, Olin Neuropsychiatry Research Center; Dartmouth-Hitchcock Medical Center; Wake Forest University Health Sciences; Rhode Island Hospital; Butler Hospital; UC San Francisco; Medical University South Carolina; St. Joseph's Health Care Nathan Kline Institute; University of Iowa College of Medicine; Cornell University and University of South Florida: USF Health Byrd Alzheimer's Institute.

AUTHOR CONTRIBUTIONS

ST and MG have made substantial contributions to conception and design of the study, and the analysis and interpretation of data, drafted the manuscript, given final approval of the version to be published, agreed to be accountable for all aspects of the work in ensuring that questions related to the accuracy or integrity of any part of the work are appropriately investigated and resolved. EC and HH have made substantial contributions to analysis and interpretation of data, been involved in revising the manuscript critically for important intellectual content, given final approval of the version to be published, agreed to be accountable for all aspects of the work in ensuring that questions related to the accuracy or integrity of any part of the work are appropriately investigated and resolved.

FUNDING

Data collection and sharing for this project was funded by the Alzheimer's Disease Neuroimaging Initiative (ADNI) (National Institutes of Health Grant U01 AG024904) and DOD ADNI (Department of Defense award number W81XWH-12-2-0012). ADNI is funded by the National Institute on Aging, the National Institute of Biomedical Imaging and Bioengineering, and through generous contributions from the following: AbbVie,Alzheimer's Association; Alzheimer's Drug Discovery Foundation; Araclon Biotech; BioClinica, Inc.; Biogen;Bristol-Myers Squibb Company; CereSpir, Inc.; Cogstate; Eisai Inc.; Elan Pharmaceuticals, Inc.; Eli Lilly and Company; EuroImmun; F. Hoffmann-La Roche Ltd and its affiliated company Genentech, Inc.; Fujirebio; GE Healthcare; IXICO Ltd.; Janssen Alzheimer Immunotherapy Research & Development, LLC.; Johnson & Johnson Pharmaceutical Research & Development LLC.; Lumosity; Lundbeck; Merck & Co., Inc.; Meso Scale Diagnostics, LLC.; NeuroRx Research; Neurotrack Technologies; Novartis Pharmaceuticals Corporation; Pfizer Inc.; Piramal Imaging; Servier; Takeda Pharmaceutical Company; and Transition Therapeutics. The Canadian Institutes of Health Research is providing funds to support ADNI clinical sites in Canada. Private sector contributions are facilitated by the Foundation for the National Institutes of Health (www.fnih.org). The grantee organization is the Northern California Institute for Research and Education, and the study is coordinated by the Alzheimer's Therapeutic Research Institute at the University of Southern California. ADNI data are disseminated by the Laboratory for Neuro Imaging at the University of Southern California. HH is supported by the AXA Research Fund, the Fondation Partenariale Sorbonne Université and the Fondation pour la Recherche sur Alzheimer, Paris, France. The research leading to these results has received funding from the program Investissements d'Avenir ANR-10-IAIHU-06 (Agence Nationale de la Recherche-10-IA Agence Institut Hospitalo-Universitaire-6). This publication benefited from the support of the Program PHOENIX® led by the Sorbonne University Foundation and sponsored by la Fondation pour la Recherche sur Alzheimer.

ACKNOWLEDGMENTS

Data used in the preparation of this article were obtained from the Alzheimer's Disease Neuroimaging Initiative (ADNI) database (adni.loni.usc.edu). The ADNI was launched in 2003 by the National Institute on Aging (NIA), the National Institute of Biomedical Imaging and Bioengineering (NIBIB), the Food and Drug Administration (FDA), private pharmaceutical companies and non-profit organizations, as a $60 million, 5-year public-private partnership. The primary goal of ADNI has been to test whether serial magnetic resonance imaging (MRI), positron emission tomography (PET), other biological markers, and clinical and neuropsychological assessment can be combined to measure the progression of mild cognitive impairment (MCI) and early Alzheimer's disease (AD). Determination of sensitive and specific markers of very early AD progression is intended to aid researchers and clinicians to develop new treatments and monitor their effectiveness, as well as lessen the time and cost of clinical trials.

The Principal Investigator of this initiative is Michael W. Weiner, MD, VA Medical Center and University of California—San Francisco. ADNI is the result of efforts of many co-investigators from a broad range of academic institutions and private corporations, and subjects have been recruited from over 50 sites across the U.S. and Canada. The initial goal of ADNI was to recruit 800 subjects but ADNI has been followed by ADNI-GO and ADNI-2. To date these three protocols have recruited over 1500 adults, ages 55 to 90, to participate in the research, consisting of cognitively normal older individuals, people with early or late MCI, and people with early AD. The follow up duration of each group is specified in the protocols for ADNI-1, ADNI-2, and ADNI-GO. Subjects originally recruited for ADNI-1 and ADNI-GO had the option to be followed in ADNI-2. For up-to-date information, see www.adni-info.org.

Contributors to the Alzheimer precision medicine initiative - working group (APMI-WG): Lisi Flores Aguilar (Montréal), Claudio Babiloni (Rome), Filippo Baldacci (Pisa), Norbert Benda (Bonn), Keith L. Black (Los Angeles), Arun L. W. Bokde (Dublin), Ubaldo Bonuccelli (Pisa), Karl Broich (Bonn), René S. Bun (Paris), Francesco Cacciola (Siena), Juan Castrillo† (Derio), Enrica Cavedo (Paris), Roberto Ceravolo (Pisa), Patrizia A. chiesa (Paris), Olivier Colliot (Paris), Cristina-Maria Coman (Paris), Jean-Christophe Corvol (Paris), Augusto Claudio Cuello (Montréal), Jeffrey L. Cummings (Las Vegas), Herman Depypere (Gent), Bruno Dubois (Paris), Andrea Duggento (Rome), Stanley Durrleman (Paris), Valentina Escott-price (Cardiff), Howard Federoff (Irvine), Maria Teresa Ferretti (Zürich), Massimo Fiandaca (Irvine), Richard A. Frank (Malvern), Francesco Garaci (Rome), Remy Genthon (Paris), Nathalie George (Paris), Filippo S. Giorgi (Pisa), Manuela Graziani (Roma), Marion Haberkamp (Bonn), Marie-Odile Habert (Paris), Harald Hampel (Paris), Karl Herholz (Manchester), Eric Karran (Cambridge), Seung H. KIM (Seoul), Yosef Koronyo (Los Angeles), Maya Koronyo-Hamaoui (Los Angeles), Foudil Lamari (Paris), Todd Langevin (Minneapolis-Saint Paul), Stéphane Lehéricy (Paris), Simone Lista (Paris), Jean Lorenceau (Paris), Mark Mapstone (Irvine), Christian Neri (Paris), Robert Nisticò (Rome), Francis Nyasse-Messene (Paris), Sid E. O'Bryant (Fort Worth), George Perry (San Antonio), Craig Ritchie (Edinburgh), Katrine Rojkova (Paris), Simone Rossi (Siena), Amira Saidi (Rome), Emiliano Santarnecchi (Siena), Lon S. Schneider (Los Angeles), Olaf Sporns (Bloomington), Nicola Toschi (Rome), Steven R. Verdooner (Sacramento), Andrea Vergallo (Paris), Nicolas Villain (Paris), Lindsay A. Welikovitch (Montréal), Janet Woodcock (Silver Spring), Erfan Younesi (Esch-sur-Alzette).

REFERENCES

1. Carr VA, Viskontas IV, Engel SA, Knowlton BJ. Neural activity in the hippocampus and perirhinal cortex during encoding is associated with the durability of episodic memory. *J Cogn Neurosci.* (2010) 22:2652–62. doi: 10.1162/jocn.2009.21381
2. Deweer B, Pillon B, Pochon JB, Dubois B. Is the HM story only a "remote memory"? Some facts about hippocampus and memory in humans. *Behav Brain Res.* (2001) 127:209–24. doi: 10.1016/S0166-4328(01)00366-7
3. Price JL, Morris JC. Tangles and plaques in nondemented aging and "preclinical" Alzheimer's disease. *Ann Neurol.* (1999) 45:358–68. doi: 10.1002/1531-8249(199903)45:3<358::AID-ANA12>3.0.CO;2-X
4. Kaye JA, Swihart T, Howieson D, Dame A, Moore MM, Karnos T, et al. Volume loss of the hippocampus and temporal lobe in healthy elderly persons destined to develop dementia. *Neurology* (1997) 48:1297–304.
5. Frisoni GB, Jack CR Jr, Bocchetta M, Bauer C, Frederiksen KS, Liu Y, et al. The EADC-ADNI Harmonized Protocol for manual hippocampal segmentation on magnetic resonance: evidence of validity. *Alzheimers Dement* (2015) 11:111–25. doi: 10.1016/j.jalz.2014.05.1756
6. Mesulam MM, Mufson EJ, Levey AI, Wainer BH. Cholinergic innervation of cortex by the basal forebrain: cytochemistry and cortical connections of the septal area, diagonal band nuclei, nucleus basalis (substantia innominata), and hypothalamus in the rhesus monkey. *J Comp Neurol.* (1983) 214:170–97. doi: 10.1002/cne.902140206
7. Bracco L, Bessi V, Padiglioni S, Marini S, Pepeu G. Do cholinesterase inhibitors act primarily on attention deficit? A naturalistic study in Alzheimer's disease patients. *J Alzheimers Dis.* (2014) 40:737–42. doi: 10.3233/JAD-131154
8. Mesulam M, Shaw P, Mash D, Weintraub S. Cholinergic nucleus basalis tauopathy emerges early in the aging-MCI-AD continuum. *Ann Neurol.* (2004) 55:815–28. doi: 10.1002/ana.20100
9. Sassin I, Schultz C, Thal DR, Rub U, Arai K, Braak E, et al. Evolution of Alzheimer's disease-related cytoskeletal changes in the basal nucleus of Meynert. *Acta Neuropathol.* (2000) 100:259–69. doi: 10.1007/s0040199 00178
10. Mesulam MM. Cholinergic circuitry of the human nucleus basalis and its fate in Alzheimer's disease. *J Comp Neurol.* (2013) 521:4124–44. doi: 10.1002/cne.23415
11. Teipel SJ, Flatz WH, Heinsen H, Bokde AL, Schoenberg SO, Stockel S, et al. Measurement of basal forebrain atrophy in Alzheimer's disease using MRI. *Brain* (2005) 128(Pt 11):2626–44. doi: 10.1093/brain/awh589
12. Zaborszky L, Hoemke L, Mohlberg H, Schleicher A, Amunts K, Zilles K. Stereotaxic probabilistic maps of the magnocellular cell groups in human basal forebrain. *NeuroImage* (2008) 42:1127–41. doi: 10.1016/j.neuroimage.2008.05.055
13. Kilimann I, Grothe M, Heinsen H, Alho EJ, Grinberg L, Amaro Jr E, et al. Subregional basal forebrain atrophy in Alzheimer's Disease: a multicenter study. *J Alzheimers Dis.* (2014) 40:687–700. doi: 10.3233/JAD-132345
14. Teipel SJ, Meindl T, Grinberg L, Grothe M, Cantero JL, Reiser MF, et al. The cholinergic system in mild cognitive impairment and Alzheimer's disease: an *in vivo* MRI and DTI study. *Human Brain Mapp.* (2011) 32:1349–62. doi: 10.1002/hbm.21111
15. Grothe M, Zaborszky L, Atienza M, Gil-Neciga E, Rodriguez-Romero R, Teipel SJ, et al. Reduction of basal forebrain cholinergic system parallels cognitive impairment in patients at high risk of developing Alzheimer's disease. *Cereb Cortex* (2010) 20:1685–95. doi: 10.1093/cercor/bhp232
16. Muth K, Schonmeyer R, Matura S, Haenschel C, Schroder J, Pantel J. Mild cognitive impairment in the elderly is associated with volume loss of the cholinergic basal forebrain region. *Biol Psychiatry* (2010) 67:588–91. doi: 10.1016/j.biopsych.2009.02.026
17. Teipel S, Heinsen H, Amaro E, Jr., Grinberg LT, Krause B, Grothe M, et al. Cholinergic basal forebrain atrophy predicts amyloid burden in Alzheimer's disease. *Neurobiol Aging* (2013) 35:482–91. doi: 10.1016/j.neurobiolaging.2013.09.029
18. Hanyu H, Asano T, Sakurai H, Tanaka Y, Takasaki M, Abe K. MR analysis of the substantia innominata in normal aging, Alzheimer disease, and other types of dementia. *Am J Neuroradiol.* (2002) 23:27–32.
19. Tanaka Y, Hanyu H, Sakurai H, Takasaki M, Abe K. Atrophy of the substantia innominata on magnetic resonance imaging predicts response to donepezil

treatment in Alzheimer's disease patients. *Dement Geriatr Cogn Disord.* (2003) 16:119–25. doi: 10.1159/000070998
20. Jack CR, Jr., Petersen RC, Xu YC, O'Brien PC, Smith GE, Ivnik RJ, et al. Prediction of AD with MRI-based hippocampal volume in mild cognitive impairment. *Neurology* (1999) 52:1397–403.
21. Erten-Lyons D, Howieson D, Moore MM, Quinn J, Sexton G, Silbert L, et al. Brain volume loss in MCI predicts dementia. *Neurology* (2006) 66:233–5. doi: 10.1212/01.wnl.0000194213.50222.1a
22. Apostolova LG, Dutton RA, Dinov ID, Hayashi KM, Toga AW, Cummings JL, et al. Conversion of mild cognitive impairment to Alzheimer disease predicted by hippocampal atrophy maps. *Arch Neurol* (2006) 63:693–9. doi: 10.1001/archneur.63.5.693
23. Macdonald KE, Bartlett JW, Leung KK, Ourselin S, Barnes J, investigators A. The value of hippocampal and temporal horn volumes and rates of change in predicting future conversion to AD. *Alzheimer Disease Assoc Disord.* (2013) 27:168–73. doi: 10.1097/WAD.0b013e318260a79a
24. Ewers M, Walsh C, Trojanowski JQ, Shaw LM, Petersen RC, Jack CR Jr, et al. Prediction of conversion from mild cognitive impairment to Alzheimer's disease dementia based upon biomarkers and neuropsychological test performance. *Neurobiol Aging* (2012) 33:1203–14. doi: 10.1016/j.neurobiolaging.2010.10.019
25. Csernansky JG, Wang L, Miller JP, Galvin JE, Morris JC. Neuroanatomical predictors of response to donepezil therapy in patients with dementia. *Arch Neurol.* (2005) 62:1718–22. doi: 10.1001/archneur.62.11.1718
26. Teipel SJ, Cavedo E, Grothe MJ, Lista S, Galluzzi S, Colliot O, et al. Predictors of cognitive decline and treatment response in a clinical trial on suspected prodromal Alzheimer's disease. *Neuropharmacology* (2016) 108:128–35. doi: 10.1016/j.neuropharm.2016.02.005
27. Wessels AM, Dowsett SA, Sims JR. Detecting Treatment Group Differences in Alzheimer's disease clinical trials: a comparison of alzheimer's disease assessment scale - Cognitive Subscale (ADAS-Cog) and the Clinical Dementia Rating - Sum of Boxes (CDR-SB). *J Prev Alzheimers Dis.* (2018) 5:15–20. doi: 10.14283/jpad.2018.2
28. Sevigny JJ, Peng Y, Liu L, Lines CR. Item analysis of ADAS-Cog: effect of baseline cognitive impairment in a clinical AD trial. *Am J Alzheimers Dis Other Demen.* (2010) 25:119–24. doi: 10.1177/1533317509350298
29. Wouters H, van Gool WA, Schmand B, Zwinderman AH, Lindeboom R. Three sides of the same coin: measuring global cognitive impairment with the MMSE, ADAS-cog and CAMCOG. *Int J Geriatr Psychiatry* (2010) 25:770–9. doi: 10.1002/gps.2402
30. Birks JS, Grimley Evans J. Rivastigmine for Alzheimer's disease. *Cochrane Database Syst Rev.* (2015) 4:CD001191. doi: 10.1002/14651858.CD001191.pub3
31. Loy C, Schneider L. Galantamine for Alzheimer's disease. *Cochrane Database Syst Rev.* (2004) 4:CD001747. doi: 10.1002/14651858.CD001747.pub2
32. Crane PK, Carle A, Gibbons LE, Insel P, Mackin RS, Gross A, et al. Development and assessment of a composite score for memory in the Alzheimer's Disease Neuroimaging Initiative (ADNI). *Brain Imaging Behav.* (2012) 6:502–16. doi: 10.1007/s11682-012-9186-z
33. Gibbons LE, Carle AC, Mackin RS, Harvey D, Mukherjee S, Insel P, et al. A composite score for executive functioning, validated in Alzheimer's Disease Neuroimaging Initiative (ADNI) participants with baseline mild cognitive impairment. *Brain Imaging Behav.* (2012) 6:517–27. doi: 10.1007/s11682-012-9176-1
34. Jack CR Jr., Bernstein MA, Fox NC, Thompson P, Alexander G, Harvey D, et al. The Alzheimer's Disease Neuroimaging Initiative (ADNI): MRI methods. *J Magn Reson Imaging* (2008) 27:685–91. doi: 10.1002/jmri.21049
35. Teipel SJ, Flatz W, Ackl N, Grothe M, Kilimann I, Bokde AL, et al. Brain atrophy in primary progressive aphasia involves the cholinergic basal forebrain and Ayala's nucleus. *Psychiatry Res.* (2014) 221:187–94. doi: 10.1016/j.pscychresns.2013.10.003
36. Grothe MJ, Schuster C, Bauer F, Heinsen H, Prudlo J, Teipel SJ. Atrophy of the cholinergic basal forebrain in dementia with Lewy bodies and Alzheimer's disease dementia. *J Neurol.* (2014) 261:1939–48. doi: 10.1007/s00415-014-7439-z
37. Grothe M, Heinsen H, Teipel S. Longitudinal measures of cholinergic forebrain atrophy in the transition from healthy aging to Alzheimer's disease. *Neurobiol Aging* (2013) 34:1210–20. doi: 10.1016/j.neurobiolaging.2012.10.018
38. Ashburner J. A fast diffeomorphic image registration algorithm. *NeuroImage* (2007) 38:95–113. doi: 10.1016/j.neuroimage.2007.07.007
39. Pruessner JC, Li LM, Serles W, Pruessner M, Collins DL, Kabani N, et al. Volumetry of hippocampus and amygdala with high-resolution MRI and three-dimensional analysis software: minimizing the discrepancies between laboratories. *Cerebral Cortex* (2000) 10:433–42. doi: 10.1093/cercor/10.4.433
40. Grothe MJ, Ewers M, Krause B, Heinsen H, Teipel SJ. Basal forebrain atrophy and cortical amyloid deposition in nondemented elderly subjects. *Alzheimers Dement* (2014) 10(5 Suppl.):S344–53. doi: 10.1016/j.jalz.2013.09.011
41. Grothe MJ, Heinsen H, Amaro E, Jr., Grinberg LT, Teipel SJ, Alzheimer's disease neuroimaging i. cognitive correlates of basal forebrain atrophy and associated cortical hypometabolism in mild cognitive impairment. *Cereb Cortex* (2016) 26:2411–26. doi: 10.1093/cercor/bhv062
42. Sakamoto Y, Ishiguro M, Kitagawa G. *Akaike Information Criterion Statistics.* Boston: D. Reidel Publishing Company (1986).
43. Ohnishi T, Sakiyama Y, Okuri Y, Kimura Y, Sugiyama N, Saito T, et al. The prediction of response to galantamine treatment in patients with mild to moderate Alzheimer's disease. *Curr Alzheimer Res.* (2014) 11:110–8. doi: 10.2174/156720501131066601 67
44. Efron B, Tibshirani RJ. *An Introduction to the Bootstrap.* New York, NY: Chapman & Hall/CRC (1994). Available online at: https://www.crcpress.com/An-Introduction-to-the-Bootstrap/Efron-Tibshirani/p/book/9780412042317
45. Raghavan N, Samtani MN, Farnum M, Yang E, Novak G, Grundman M, et al. The ADAS-Cog revisited: novel composite scales based on ADAS-Cog to improve efficiency in MCI and early AD trials. *Alzheimers Dement* (2013) 9(1 Suppl):S21–31. doi: 10.1016/j.jalz.2012.05.2187
46. Van Der Putt R, Dineen C, Janes D, Series H, McShane R. Effectiveness of acetylcholinesterase inhibitors: diagnosis and severity as predictors of response in routine practice. *Int J Geriatr Psychiatry* (2006) 21:755–60. doi: 10.1002/gps.1557
47. Birks J, Grimley Evans J, Iakovidou V, Tsolaki M, Holt FE. Rivastigmine for Alzheimer's disease. *Cochrane Database Syst Rev.* (2009) 2:CD001191. doi: 10.1002/14651858.CD001191.pub2
48. Birks J, Harvey RJ. Donepezil for dementia due to Alzheimer's disease. *Cochrane Database Syst Rev.* (2006) 1:CD001190. doi: 10.1002/14651858.CD001190.pub2
49. Kasper E, Brueggen K, Grothe MJ, Bruno D, Pomara N, Unterauer E, et al. Neuronal correlates of serial position performance in amnestic mild cognitive impairment. *Neuropsychology* (2016) 30:906–14. doi: 10.1037/neu0000287
50. Colliot O, Chetelat G, Chupin M, Desgranges B, Magnin B, Benali H, et al. Discrimination between Alzheimer disease, mild cognitive impairment, and normal aging by using automated segmentation of the hippocampus. *Radiology* (2008) 248:194–201. doi: 10.1148/radiol.2481070876
51. Pomara N, Nolan K, Halpern G. Scopolamine-induced impairment as a potential predictor of Alzheimer's disease in individuals with Apolipoprotein E type 4 alleles. *Neurochem Res.* (1995) 20:1519–20. doi: 10.1007/BF00970602
52. Snyder PJ, Lim YY, Schindler R, Ott BR, Salloway S, Daiello L, et al. Microdosing of scopolamine as a "cognitive stress test": rationale and test of a very low dose in an at-risk cohort of older adults. *Alzheimers Dement* (2014) 10:262–7. doi: 10.1016/j.jalz.2014.01.009
53. Dumas JA, Newhouse PA. The cholinergic hypothesis of cognitive aging revisited again: cholinergic functional compensation. *Pharmacol Biochem Behav.* (2011) 99:254–61. doi: 10.1016/j.pbb.2011.02.022
54. Bottini G, Berlingeri M, Basilico S, Passoni S, Danelli L, Colombo N, et al. GOOD or BAD responder? Behavioural and neuroanatomical markers of clinical response to donepezil in dementia. *Behav Neurol.* (2012) 25:61–72. doi: 10.1155/2012/538542
55. Mielke MM, Okonkwo OC, Oishi K, Mori S, Tighe S, Miller MI, et al. Fornix integrity and hippocampal volume predict memory decline and progression to Alzheimer's disease. *Alzheimers Dement* (2012) 8:105–13. doi: 10.1016/j.jalz.2011.05.2416

56. Miettinen PS, Jauhiainen AM, Tarkka IM, Pihlajamaki M, Grohn H, Niskanen E, et al. Long-Term Response to Cholinesterase Inhibitor Treatment Is Related to Functional MRI Response in Alzheimer's Disease. *Dement Geriat Cogn Disord.* (2015) 40:243–55. doi: 10.1159/000435948
57. Zaborszky L, Csordas A, Mosca K, Kim J, Gielow MR, Vadasz C, et al. Neurons in the basal forebrain project to the cortex in a complex topographic organization that reflects corticocortical connectivity patterns: an experimental study based on retrograde tracing and 3D reconstruction. *Cereb Cortex* (2015) 25:118–37. doi: 10.1093/cercor/bht210
58. Ghashghaei HT, Barbas H. Neural interaction between the basal forebrain and functionally distinct prefrontal cortices in the rhesus monkey. *Neuroscience* (2001) 103:593–614. doi: 10.1016/S0306-4522(00)00585-6

7

Dysphagia as Isolated Manifestation of Jo-1 Associated Myositis?

Bendix Labeit, Paul Muhle, Sonja Suntrup-Krueger, Sigrid Ahring, Tobias Ruck, Rainer Dziewas and Tobias Warnecke*

Department of Neurology, University Hospital Muenster, Muenster, Germany

***Correspondence:** *Bendix Labeit* *benlabeit@wwu.de*

Dysphagia can be predominant or sole symptom of myositis. However, diagnostic evaluation is difficult in such cases. Here, we present evidence for dysphagia as sole manifestation of Jo-1 associated myositis. A 77-year-old patient suffering from isolated dysphagia was assessed by flexible endoscopic evaluation of swallowing, videofluoroscopy, high resolution esophageal manometry, whole body muscle MRI, electroneurographic and electromyographic examination, cerebrospinal fluid analysis, screening for autoantibodies, and body plethysmography. We detected isolated oropharyngeal dysphagia including a decreased pressure of the upper esophageal sphincter leading to cachexia in an anti-Jo-1 positive patient without any abnormalities in the other diagnostics. Immunosuppressive therapy with cortisone and azathioprine led to long-term improvement of dysphagia. This is the first report of isolated dysphagia as manifestation of Jo-1 associated myositis. Therefore, Jo-1 associated myositis should be considered as a possible differential diagnosis for isolated dysphagia. Typical signs for myositis in instrumental dysphagia assessment are presented.

Keywords: dysphagia, myositis, antisynthetase syndrome, antisynthetase antibody, Jo-1, Jo-1 autoantibody, diagnostic algorithm, idiopathic inflamed myopathy

INTRODUCTION

Dysphagia is frequently reported in patients with myositis (1–6) with prevalence rates ranging from 30 to 72% (5, 6). Typical symptoms of myositis related dysphagia are coughing, choking, bolus-sticking in the pharynx and swallowing problems with dry and solid food consistencies (1, 5). Early diagnosis and specific therapeutic management of dysphagia is crucial as it can lead to aspiration pneumonia with respiratory failure, which is the leading cause of mortality in patients with myositis (1, 7). Dysphagia can occur as predominant or sole symptom of myositis: Oh et al. described dysphagia as the only manifestation of inclusion body myositis (8). Shapiro et al. reported 3 cases of isolated pharyngeal dysphagia with biopsies of the omohyoid and cricopharyngeus muscles showing inflammatory myopathy (9). In such cases, diagnostic evaluation is particularly difficult, as myositis-related dysphagia may also be present if laboratory or electrophysiological diagnostics remain unremarkable (10). The role of autoantibodies in the diagnosis of myositis is steadily increasing. Jo-1 antibodies are now part of the current EULAR diagnostic criteria alongside clinical criteria, CK blood level, and histological signs (11). Further, autoantibodies can be helpful in the classification of myositis (12). This biomarker driven development might also be beneficial in patients with unclear dysphagia. In this case-report we present evidence for dysphagia as isolated manifestation of Jo-1 associated myositis, which to the best of our knowledge has not been reported so far. In addition, we give an overview of the literature on the pathophysiology of dysphagia in myositis.

CASE REPORT

Patient History

A 77-year-old patient was presented to our outpatient clinic due to progressive dysphagia. About 10 years ago, he noticed taste disturbances and discomfort in the mouth region, hindering his speech. During the last 3 years, he predominantly suffered from swallowing impairment. He reported of choking and hiccups in particular when eating solid food. In addition, he needed increasingly longer to finish a normal meal and had to extraordinarily concentrate on the eating process. As a consequence, he avoided eating in public. Recently, he was hospitalized due to an aspiration pneumonia. The patient did not take any medication. The detailed clinical examination revealed no fasciculations, muscle weakness, double vision, raynaud's phenomenon, mechanic's hands, skin rash or dyspnea, only a cachectic nutritional status due to dysphagia (size 1.8 m, weight 53 kg, BMI 16.4) was remarkable. There were no relevant pre-existing diseases. Cerebral MRI that had been performed before the presentation in our department showed no pathological findings.

Diagnostic Procedures

Flexible endoscopic evaluation of swallowing (FEES) revealed severe oropharyngeal dysphagia with intradeglutitive aspiration and postdeglutitive residue in the vallecula und pyriform sinus (graded as severe for semisolid and solid consistencies according to the Yale Pharyngeal Residue Severity Scale (13) as a sign of weak pharyngeal constriction (**Figure 1**). The FEES tensilon test (14, 15) showed no improvement of dysphagia upon application of edrophonium. Videoflouroscopy of swallowing (VFSS) confirmed severe pharyngeal dysphagia with markedly restricted pharyngeal contraction and consecutive nasopharyngeal reflux as well as postdeglutitive aspiration due to considerable retention. Furthermore, there was a markedly delayed triggering of swallowing reflex with reduced hyolaryngeal elevation and predeglutitive aspiration, Rosenbek grade 7 (16, 17). High resolution esophageal manometry (HRM) showed a markedly reduced pressure of the upper esophageal sphincter with extended relaxation and recovery time and an amotile tubular esophagus. Functional dysphagia severity according to the FOIS-Score was 1 (18). Basic laboratory and CSF diagnostics were normal (no cytalbuminary dissociation, normal CK-blood level). CSF-screening for ganglioside antibodies was negative (Ganglioside Profile 2 IgG and IgM Euroline, Euroimmun; Lübeck, Germany). Whole body muscle MRI was unremarkable without edema or atrophy. The electroneurographic examination detected a length-dependent, axonal, sensitive polyneuropathy as incidental finding. Repetitive stimulation of the n. facialis on both sides with recording from the m. nasalis revealed no decrement. Repetitive stimulation of the n. ulnaris on the left side with recording from the m. abductor digiti minimi before and after 1-min maximum arbitrary innervation revealed no increment. In the electromyographic examination, isolated chronic neurological changes of the right hand muscles, but otherwise inconspicuous findings were observed (m. deltoideus on both sides: no pathological spontaneous activity, motor unit potential normally configurated, regular recruitment, dense interference; m. abductor pollicis brevis on both sides: no pathological spontaneous activity, motor unit potential on the right side partly with high amplitude, recruitment and interference on the right side slightly reduced; m. abductor digiti minimi on both sides: no pathological spontaneous activity, motor unit potential on the right side partly with high amplitude, recruitment and interference on the right side slightly reduced; m. vastus on both sides: no pathological spontaneous activity, motor unit potential normally configurated, regular recruitment, dense interference; m. tibialis anterior on both sides: no pathological spontaneous activity, motor unit potential normally configurated, regular recruitment, dense interference; paravertebral T8 on both sides: no pathological spontaneous activity; m. glossus on the left side: no pathological spontaneous activity). The antibody screening was positive for Jo-1 IgG (++) and negative for the other screened autoantibodies (ANA, Mi-2a, Mi-2b, TIF1g, MDA5, NXP2, SAE1, Ku, PM100, PM75, SRP, PL-7, PL-12, EJ, OJ, Ro52, Euroline, Euroimmun, Lübeck, Germany, and anti-HMG-CoA, MVZ Labor Volkmann, Karlsruhe, Germany). Also, no myasthenia antibodies could be detected (negative for AChR, titin, MuSK, and VGCC, Euroline, Euroimmun, Lübeck, Germany). Although the role of Jo-1-IgG in the pathophysiology of myositis is poorly understood, it is a highly reliable marker for idiopathic inflammatory myopathies (19). In the absence of signs for other diseases, this led to the diagnosis of Jo-1 associated myositis as underlying disease. Body plethysmography and x-ray-chest revealed no indication of pulmonary involvement.

Therapy

A PEG tube was placed to ensure sufficient enteral nutrition. In addition, an intravenous cortisone therapy with 1 g methylprednisolone per day for 5 days followed by oral therapy with prednisolone and azathioprine was performed. After 4 months of therapy the swallowing function improved, and FEES showed a reduction in penetration and aspiration frequency and severity, lower levels of penetration and aspiration volume, and a more effective bolus clearance. The FOIS-scale had improved from 1 on admission to 3, so that a reinstitution of oral feeding parallel to the PEG nutrition was recommended (18). This improvement sustained in the long term (currently 12 months after beginning of therapy).

DISCUSSION

There are only few studies that investigated the pathophysiological characteristics of myositis related dysphagia. Ebert et al. claimed that myositis mainly affects the proximal esophageal skeletal muscle. They reported decreased upper sphincter pressure and absent pharyngeal contractions in manometry (3). Casal-Dominguez et al. also reported decreased upper esophageal sphincter pressure and failed waves in patients with polymyositis (20). Ertekin et al. showed that myositis mainly leads to pharyngeal dysphagia with prolonged phase of pharyngeal swallowing and weakness of the striated oropharyngeal muscles. Contrary to other manometry studies, they found that the cricopharyngeal sphincter was affected less frequently and showed both

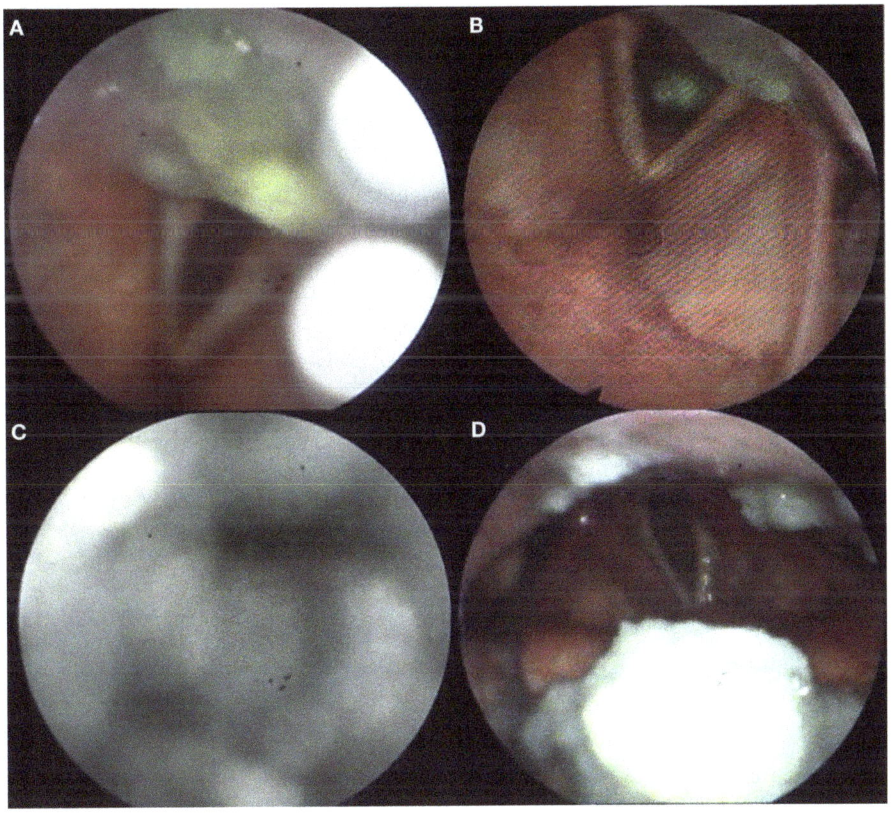

FIGURE 1 | **(A)** Postdeglutitive residue of pudding; **(B)** Aspiration of pudding; **(C)** Weak white-out as sign for reduced pharyngeal contractility; **(D)** Postdeglutitive residue of bread.

hyporeflexic and hyperreflexic states in myositis (2). In a study using VFSS, Langdon et al. reported delayed swallowing initiation, decreased hyolaryngeal excursion, pyriform residue and penetration (5). Consistent with these findings, Oh et al. also described impaired laryngeal elevation, pharyngeal pooling, disturbed tongue retraction and abnormal cricopharyngeal function (1).

Whether inflammatory myopathies constitute a homogeneous pathophysiological pathophysiological dysphagia entity or specific sub forms e.g., inclusion body myositis, dermatomyositis, and antisynthetase syndrome show their own specific pathophysiological characteristics largely remains an open question. Oh et al. did not find differences between inclusion body myositis, dermatomyositis, and polymyositis in VFSS findings (1). Casal-Dominguez et al. report that antisynthetase syndrome is associated with decreased and hypotonic lower esophageal sphincter pressure and conclude that the autoimmune reaction of this specific myositis entity may affect the smooth muscle of the esophageal body in particular and cause impairment in the lower esophageal sphincter (20). Inclusion body myositis seems to be rather associated with an increased pressure of the upper esophagus sphincter due to a relaxation deficit (21, 22) which manifests as pharyngeal muscle propulsion between C3 and C7 in VFSS (21). Typical findings of instrumental dysphagia assessment that may indicate myositis are shown in **Table 1**.

TABLE 1 | Typical signs for myositis in instrumental dysphagia assessment.

Flexible Endoscopic Evaluation of Swallowing:
- *Reduced pharyngeal contractility (pharyngeal squeeze maneuver)*
- *Weak white-out*
- Pharyngeal residue
- Postdeglutitive penetration/aspiration

Videofluoroscopy:
- *Decreased hyolaryngeal elevation*
- *Pharyngeal muscle propulsions at C3-C7*
- Impairment of the upper or lower esophagus sphincter
- Pharyngeal residue
- Postdeglutitive penetration/aspiration

High Resolution Manometry:
- Impairment of the upper or lower esophagus sphincter

Signs that are specific to one diagnostic procedure are printed in italics.

Here, to our knowledge we present the first ever reported case of isolated dysphagia due to Jo-1 associated myositis: we found pharyngeal dysphagia with impairment of the upper esophagus similar to the impairment pattern commonly described in myositis. This case demonstrates that not only the smooth esophageal muscle (20) but also the striated muscle of the pharynx and upper esophagus can be affected by the Jo-1 associated autoimmune reaction. Based on our case report, we therefore recommend that myositis focused diagnostics including an autoantibody panel should be done in patients with unclear dysphagia that show typical sings for myositis in the instrumental dysphagia assessment.

LIMITATIONS

There are only few studies that investigated the pathophysiological characteristics of myositis related dysphagia. The pathophysiological conclusions in this study must therefore be considered cautiously. According to the EULAR criteria, the probability of myositis in a patient with dysphagia and detection of Jo-1 antibodies is 80% (11). Myositis is therefore only the probable underlying disease. Since no muscle biopsy was performed, other diseases e.g., atypical IBM cannot be ruled out with certainty.

AUTHOR CONTRIBUTIONS

BL and TW were responsible for the preparation and conceptual design of the manuscript. TR was responsible for advising on antibody diagnostics. SA was responsible for the coordination and realization of the FEES examination. All other authors (PM, SS-K, and RD) were involved in the preparation and editing of the manuscript.

FUNDING

We acknowledge support from the Open Access Publication Fund of the University of Muenster.

ACKNOWLEDGMENTS

We are very grateful to the patient for giving his consent to the publication of this case report.

REFERENCES

1. Oh TH, Brumfield KA, Hoskin TL, Stolp KA, Murray JA, Bassford JR. Dysphagia in inflammatory myopathy: Clinical characteristics, treatment strategies, and outcome in 62 patients. *Mayo Clin Proc.* (2007) 82:441–7. doi: 10.4065/82.4.441
2. Ertekin C, Secil Y, Yuceyar N, Aydogdu I. Oropharyngeal dysphagia in polymyositis/dermatomyositis. *Clin Neurol Neurosurg.* (2004) 107:32–7. doi: 10.1016/j.clineuro.2004.02.024
3. Ebert EC. Review article: the gastrointestinal complications of myositis. *Aliment Pharmacol Ther.* (2010) 31:359–65. doi: 10.1111/j.1365-2036.2009.04190.x
4. Marie I, Hatron PY, Levesque H, Hachulla E, Hellot MF, Michon-Pasturel U, et al. Influence of age on characteristics of polymyositis and dermatomyositis in adults. *Medicine.* (1999) 78:139–47.
5. Langdon PC, Mulcahy K, Shepherd KL, Low VH, Mastaglia FL. Pharyngeal dysphagia in inflammatory muscle diseases resulting from impaired suprahyoid musculature. *Dysphagia.* (2012) 27:408–17. doi: 10.1007/s00455-011-9384-7
6. Mulcahy KP, Langdon PC, Mastaglia F. *Dysphagia* in inflammatory myopathy: self-report, incidence, and prevalence. *Dysphagia.* (2012) 27:64–9. doi: 10.1007/s00455-011-9338-0
7. Lynn SJ, Sawyers SM, Moller PW, O'Donnell JL, Chapman PT. Adult-onset inflammatory myopathy: North Canterbury experience 1989-2001. *Intern Med J.* (2005) 35:170–3. doi: 10.1111/j.1445-5994.2004.00764.x
8. Olive M, Villanueva P, Ferrer I, Montero J, Martinez-Matos JA. Dysphagia as the only manifestation of inclusion body myositis. *Neurologia.* (1994) 9:202–3.
9. Shapiro J, Martin S, DeGirolami U, Goyal R. Inflammatory myopathy causing pharyngeal dysphagia: a new entity. *Ann Otol Rhinol Laryngol.* (1996) 105:331–5. doi: 10.1177/000348949610500501
10. Williams RB, Grehan MJ, Hersch M, Andre J, Cook IJ. Biomechanics, diagnosis, and treatment outcome in inflammatory myopathy presenting as oropharyngeal dysphagia. *Gut.* (2003) 52:471–8. doi: 10.1136/gut.52.4.471
11. Lundberg IE, Tjarnlund A, Bottai M, Werth VP, Pilkington C, Visser M, et al. 2017 European League Against Rheumatism/American College of Rheumatology classification criteria for adult and juvenile idiopathic inflammatory myopathies and their major subgroups. *Ann Rheumat Dis.* (2017) 76:1955–64. doi: 10.1136/annrheumdis-2017-211468
12. Mariampillai K, Granger B, Amelin D, Guiguet M, Hachulla E, Maurier F, et al. Development of a new classification system for idiopathic inflammatory myopathies based on clinical manifestations and myositis-specific autoantibodies. *JAMA Neurol.* (2018) 75:1528–37. doi: 10.1001/jamaneurol.2018.2598
13. Neubauer PD, Rademaker AW, Leder SB. The yale pharyngeal residue severity rating scale: an anatomically defined and image-based tool. *Dysphagia.* (2015) 30:521–8. doi: 10.1007/s00455-015-9631-4
14. Warnecke T, Teismann I, Zimmermann J, Oelenberg S, Ringelstein EB, Dziewas R. Fiberoptic endoscopic evaluation of swallowing with simultaneous Tensilon application in diagnosis and therapy of myasthenia gravis. *J Neurol.* (2008) 255:224–30. doi: 10.1007/s00415-008-0664-6
15. Im S, Suntrup-Krueger S, Colbow S, Sauer S, Claus I, Meuth SG, et al. Reliability and main findings of the flexible endoscopic evaluation of swallowing-Tensilon test in patients with myasthenia gravis and dysphagia. *Eur J Neurol.* (2018) 25:1235–42. doi: 10.1111/ene.13688
16. Hey C, Pluschinski P, Zaretsky Y, Almahameed A, Hirth D, Vaerst B, et al. Penetration-Aspiration Scale according to Rosenbek. Validation of the German version for endoscopic dysphagia diagnostics. *HNO.* (2014) 62:276–81. doi: 10.1007/s00106-013-2815-z
17. Rosenbek JC, Robbins JA, Roecker EB, Coyle JL, Wood JL. A penetration-aspiration scale. *Dysphagia.* (1996) 11:93–8.
18. Crary MA, Mann GDC, Groher ME. Initial psychometric assessment of a functional oral intake scale for dysphagia in stroke patients. *Arch Phys Med Rehabil.* (2005) 86:1516–20. doi: 10.1016/j.apmr.2004.11.049
19. Zampieri S, Ghirardello A, Iaccarino L, Tarricone E, Gambari PF, Doria A. Anti-Jo-1 antibodies. *Autoimmunity.* (2005) 38:73–8. doi: 10.1080/08916930400022640
20. Casal-Dominguez M, Pinal-Fernandez I, Mego M, Accarino A, Jubany L, Azpiroz F, et al. High-resolution manometry in patients with idiopathic inflammatory myopathy: elevated prevalence of esophageal involvement and differences according to autoantibody status and clinical subset. *Muscle Nerve.* (2017) 56:386–92. doi: 10.1002/mus.25507
21. Murata K-Y, Kouda K, Tajima F, Kondo T. A dysphagia study in patients with sporadic inclusion body myositis (s-IBM). *Neurol Sci.* (2012) 33:765–70. doi: 10.1007/s10072-011-0814-y
22. Riminton DS, Chambers ST, Parkin PJ, Pollock M, Donaldson IM. Inclusion body myositis presenting solely as dysphagia. *Neurology.* (1993) 43:1241–3.

8

Association Between *Aldehyde dehydrogenase-2* Polymorphisms and Risk of Alzheimer's Disease and Parkinson's Disease

Jun Chen[1†], Wei Huang[1†], Chao-Hui Cheng[1], Lan Zhou[1], Guang-Bin Jiang[2]* and Yuan-Yuan Hu[3]*

[1] Department of Neurology, Taihe Hospital, Hubei University of Medicine, Shiyan, China, [2] Department of Radiology, Suizhou Central Hospital, Suizhou, China, [3] Department of Stomatology, Taihe Hospital, Hubei University of Medicine, Shiyan, China

***Correspondence:**
Lan Zhou
1902764052@qq.com
Guang-Bin Jiang
jgb126@126.com

† These authors have contributed equally to this work

Objective: A number of studies have reported that aldehyde dehydrogenase-2 (*ALDH2*) polymorphisms maybe associated with the risk of Alzheimer's disease (AD) and Parkinson's disease (PD). However, the results of such studies are inconsistent. We therefore conducted a meta-analysis to clarify the association between *ALDH2* polymorphisms and the risk of AD and PD.

Methods: Five online databases were searched and the relevant studies were reviewed from inception through May 10, 2018. Odds ratios (ORs) and corresponding 95% confidence intervals (CIs) were calculated in each genetic model of the general population and various subgroups. Furthermore, we simultaneously performed heterogeneity, cumulative, sensitivity, and publication bias analyses.

Results: Overall, nine case-control studies involving 5,315 subjects were included in this meta-analysis. Potential associations were found between the *ALDH2* rs671 G>A polymorphism and the risk of AD (A vs. G: OR = 1.46, 95%CI = 1.01–2.11, $P = 0.05$, $I^2 = 84.2\%$; AA vs. GG: OR = 2.22, 95%CI = 1.03–4.77, $P = 0.04$, $I^2 = 79.2\%$; AA vs. GG+GA: OR = 1.94, 95%CI = 1.03–3.64, $P = 0.04$, $I^2 = 71.1\%$). In addition, some similar results were observed in other subgroups. Moreover, no significant association between *ALDH2* polymorphisms and PD risk.

Conclusions: In conclusion, our meta-analysis indicated that the *ALDH2* rs671 G>A polymorphism plays an important role in AD development.

Keywords: ***Aldehyde dehydrogenase 2*****, neurodegenerative disorders, Alzheimer's disease, Parkinson's disease, polymorphiom**

INTRODUCTION

Neurodegenerative disorders are a family of heterogeneous disorders, in which progressive degeneration occurs in the structure and function of the central or peripheral nervous system (1). Neurodegenerative disorders would lead to progressive cognitive and motor disabilities, such as senile dementia, balance disorder, movement dyskinesia, and muscular tension abnormalities (2).

Alzheimer's disease (AD) and Parkinson's disease (PD) are the most common neurodegenerative disorders (3).Currently, there are more than 5 million patients with AD and this number is projected to increase to 7.1 million by 2025 (4). Indeed, the World Health Organization has predicted that AD and other causes of dementia, as well as such as PD and amyotrophic lateral sclerosis will overtake cancer to become the second leading cause of death following cardiovascular disease (5). Further, as the population ages, AD and PD will increasingly place substantial burdens on not only the families of individuals with these conditions, but also on society as a whole.

AD and PD are closely related to aging, can have multiple causative factors, such as oxidative damage, abnormal protein deposition, and neuroinflammation (6). Other factors, including atherosclerosis (7), diabetes (8), neuroinflammation (9), and various environmental effects (10), have also been proposed as interactive factors for AD and PD (11). Moreover, increasing evidence suggests that genetic abnormities, including genetic mutations, play important roles in the development of AD and PD (12, 13).

One such gene that is thought to be involved in AD and PD is the aldehyde dehydrogenase-2 (*ALDH2*) gene. This gene is located on chromosome 12q24.12, comprises 13 exons and 12 introns, and encodes an important biologically active enzyme, ALDH2. This enzyme participates in the metabolism and detoxification of aldehyde, and it can metabolize short-chain aliphatic aldehydes and converted acetaldehyde into acetate. Moreover, ALDH2 is involved in the metabolism of other biogenic aldehydes, such as 4-hydroxynonenal, 3,4-dihydroxyphenylacetaldehyde, and 3,4-dihydroxyphenylglycoaldehyde (14). Recent studies have indicated that ALDH2 exerts protective effects on the cardio-cerebral vascular system and central nervous system. Single nucleotide polymorphisms (SNPs) of the *ALDH2* gene have been reported to be associated with the risks for several diseases, such as coronary artery disease, ischemic stroke, digestive system cancer and allergic asthma. The A allele (*ALDH2*2*) of rs671, inherent in mainly the East Asian population, deregulates the ALDH2 activity intrinsically, and induces the accumulation of acetaldehyde. In 2000, Kamino et al. conducted the first case-control study in the Japanese population and found that the A allele and GA/AA genotypes are associated with an increased risk of AD (15). Subsequently, studies focusing on the association between *ALDH2* polymorphisms and the risk of AD and PD have been continually published, but the results are inconsistent. Therefore, we conducted a meta-analysis of all available studies to investigate the precise association between the *ALDH2* polymorphisms and the risk of AD and PD.

MATERIALS AND METHODS

This meta-analysis of observational studies was conducted according to the Preferred Reporting Items for Systematic Reviews and Meta-Analyses guidelines (16). All included data were collected from published studies, and no ethical issues were involved.

Search Strategy

Five online databases (PubMed, Embase, Web of Science, Chinese national knowledge infrastructure and Wanfang) were used to search for related studies on the association between *ALDH2* polymorphisms and the risk of AD and PD from inception through May 10, 2018. Only the studies published in English and Chinese were included. The bibliographies of the collected studies and relevant reviews were also checked to identify potential additional articles. The following search terms and strategy was adopted (e.g., in PubMed):

#1 *Aldehyde dehydrogenase 2*
#2 *Aldehyde Dehydrogenase-2*
#3 *ALDH2*
#4 rs671
#5 rs4767944
#6 rs441
#7 #1 OR #2 OR #3 OR #4 OR #5 OR #6
#8 polymorphism
#9 variant
#10 mutation
#11 #8 OR #9 OR #10
#12 neurodegenerative disorders
#13 Alzheimer's disease
#14 Parkinson's disease
#15#12 OR #13 OR #14 OR #15
#16 #7 AND #11 AND #15.

Eligibility Criteria

The following were our inclusion criteria: (1) observation studies focusing on the association between *ALDH2* polymorphisms and the risk of AD and PD; (2) studies containing sufficient data on the genotype in the control groups to evaluate crude odds ratios (ORs) and 95% confidence intervals (CIs); (3) studies published in English or Chinese, and (4) if overlapping or duplicate data were found on the same theme, only the largest or most recent sample data were included. The exclusion criteria included: (1) case report or review articles; (2) molecular biology research; (3) studies without efficient data; and (4) studies with duplicated or overlapping data.

Data Extraction and Quality Evaluation

Two authors (Chen and Huang) independently reviewed the included studies, and the following information was extracted and recorded for analysis: the first authors' name, publication date, study country, control design, genotyping method, sample sizes of the cases and controls, frequency data for the genotype distribution, assessment of Hardy-Weinberg equilibrium (HWE) in control, minor allele frequency, and disease type. The modified Newcastle-Ottawa scale (NOS) was used to evaluate the quality of all included studies (17). The scores ranged from 0 points (worst) to 11 points (best) (**Supplementary Table 1**). Studies with a score of 8 points or higher were classified as high quality.

Statistical Analysis

We calculated the crude ORs and 95% CIs to assess the statistical power of the association between *ALDH2* polymorphisms and the risk of AD and PD. For example, the following five genetic

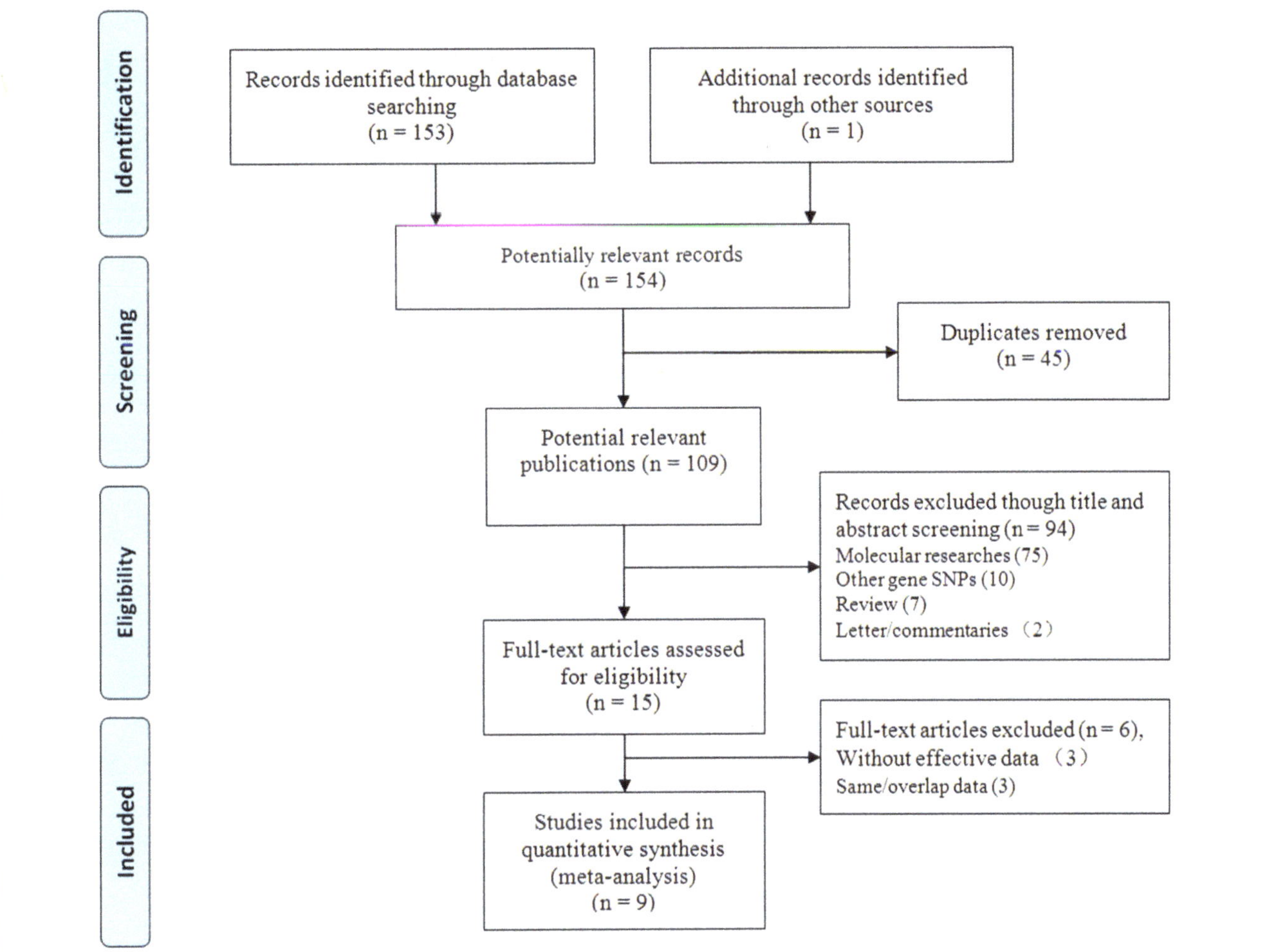

FIGURE 1 | Flow diagram of the study selection process.

models of the rs671 G>A locus were used: allele contrast (A vs. G), co-dominant models (GA vs. GG and AA vs. GG), dominant model (GA+AA vs. GG), and recessive model (AA vs. GG+GA). Heterogeneity among the included studies was examined using Cochran's Q tests and I^2-tests (18). A fixed-effects model was adopted when I^2 was $\leq$40%, but a random-effects model was adopted when I^2 was > 40%(19, 20). Subgroup analyses were performed according to the HWE status, study country, disease type, control design (population-based and hospital-based), subject number, NOS evaluation and gender diversity. Meta-regression was conducted to identify which factors contributed to the existing heterogeneity. A cumulative meta-analysis was performed to assess the statistical tendency of the results. Sensitivity analysis was used to examine the stability of the results by sequentially removing each study individually. Potential publication biases were assessed with Egger's linear regression test and Begg's funnel plots (21, 22). All statistical analyses were performed using STATA version 14.0 (Stata Corporation, College Station, TX, USA). Statistical significance was set at <0.05 (two-sided).

RESULTS

Study Characteristics

We initially identified 154 relevant articles through our systematic literature search. The selection process is shown in **Figure 1**. According to the eligibility criteria, 45 studies were excluded following duplicate screening, 94 studies were removed after the subsequent title and abstract reviews, and 9 studies were eliminated because of deficient data, and/or similar/overlapping data. Finally, nine publications (11 independent studies) involving 2,283 patients and 3,032 controls were included (15, 23–30). Three common SNPs were reported; eight studies focused on the rs671 G>A polymorphism (15, 23–29), two studies focused on the rs4767944 C>T polymorphism (27, 30), and one study focused on the rs441 T>C polymorphism (27). In all included studies, most subjects were from East Asians countries including China, Japan, and Korea, except for one study that was performed in the Iranian population (30). The HWE assessment of control revealed that there were two studies that deviated from or lacked the HWE index in the rs671

TABLE 1 | Characteristics of case-control studies on ALDH2 polymorphisms and AD and PD risk.

References	Country	Control design	Genotype method	Case	Control	Genotype distribution						P for HWE	MAF	NOS evaluation	Disease type
						Case			Control						
Rs671						GG	GA	AA	GG	GA	AA				
Kamino et al. (15)	Japan	HB	PCR-RFLP	447	447	232	183	32	280	138	29	0.04	0.22	7	AD
Kim et al. (23)	Korea	PB	PCR-RFLP	80	610	60[a]	20[b]		435[a]	175[b]		NA	NA	7	AD
Wang et al. (24)	China	HB	PCR-RFLP	188	223	54	92	42	124	84	15	0.88	0.26	7	AD
Zhou et al., (25)	China	HB	PCR-RFLP	106	100	65	32	9	54	38	8	0.72	0.27	7	AD
Komatsu et al. (26)	Japan	PB	TaqMan	158	130	81	62	15	67	54	9	0.67	0.28	8	AD
Ma et al., (29)	China	HB	PCR-RFLP	115	236	72	30	13	177	52	7	0.20	0.14	7	AD
Zhang et al. (27)	China	HB	PCR-RFLP	584	582	321	236	27	339	208	35	0.68	0.24	9	PD
Zhao et al. (28)	China	HB	PCR-RFLP	115	214	71	32	12	157	52	5	0.78	0.14	7	PD
Rs4767944						CC	CT	TT	CC	CT	TT				
Zhang et al. (27)	China	HB	PCR-RFLP	584	582	92	316	176	62	301	219	0.01	0.63	8	PD
Madadi et al. (30)	Iran	HB	PCR-RFLP	490	490	339	143	9	344	133	13	0.97	0.16	8	PD
Rs441						TT	TC	CC	TT	TC	TT				
Zhang et al. (27)	China	HB	PCR-RFLP	584	582	281	278	25	293	256	33	0.02	0.28	8	PD

HWE in control.
NA, Not available.
[a]*Data of the GG genotype;* [b]*Data of the GA/AA genotypes.*
HB, Hospital or healthy based; PB, Population based.
AD, Alzheimer's disease; PD, Parkinson's disease.

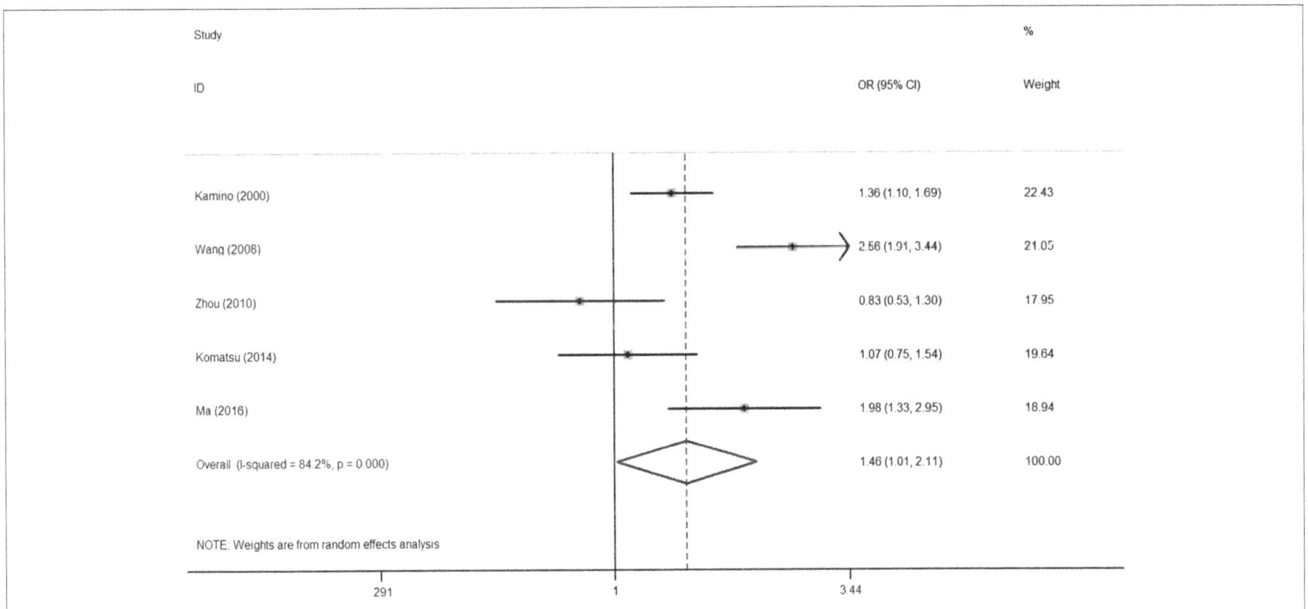

FIGURE 2 | OR and 95% CIs of the associations between ALDH2 rs671 G>A polymorphism and AD risk in A vs. G model.

G>A polymorphism (15, 23), and one study each that deviated from the HWE in the s4767944 C>T polymorphism (27) and rs441T>C polymorphism (27). The characteristics of all included studies are presented in **Table 1**.

Quantitative and Subgroup Analyses

Association between the rs671 polymorphism and the risk of AD and PD. There were six case-control studies involving 2,840 subjects focused on the association between the rs671 polymorphism and AD risk. The aggregated results indicated an increased risk of the rs671 G>A polymorphism in patients with AD (A vs. G: OR = 1.46, 95%CI = 1.01–2.11, P = 0.05, I^2 = 84.2% (**Figure 2**); AA vs. GG: OR = 2.22, 95%CI = 1.03–4.77, P =0.04, I^2 = 79.2%; AA vs. GG+GA: OR = 1.94, 95%CI = 1.03–3.64, P =0.04, I^2 = 71.1%). Subgroup analyses also revealed an increased AD risks in Chinese (AA vs. GG: OR = 3.15, 95%CI = 1.03–9.65, P =0.04, I^2 = 79.6%; AA vs. GG+GA: OR = 2.75, 95%CI = 1.23–6.14, P =0.02, I^2 = 63.0%) and Japanese (A vs. G: OR = 1.54, 95%CI = 1.00–2.36, P =0.05, I^2 = 17.1%) on the basis of country difference. The subsequent analysis based on the HWE status and other subgroup revealed the similar increased associations (**Table 2, Supplementary Figure S1** for other models) Heterogeneity was observed in all five genetic models; the meta-regression analysis was conducted with the above-mentioned stratified factors and did not identify any factor that contributed to the existing heterogeneity (e.g., A vs. G model: P =0.89 for HWE status, P =0.53 for study country, P =0.53 for control design, P =0.89 for subject number, and P =0.53 for NOS evaluation).

The accumulative analysis presented fluctuating findings and the results tending to show a potential association by Ma et al. (29) (**Figure 3** for A vs. G model, **Supplementary Figure S2** for other models). A sensitivity analysis was conducted by removing each included study, and fluctuating results were observed after several studies were removed (**Figure 4** for A vs. G model, **Supplementary Figure S3** for other models).

Publication biases were investigated, and the results did not show any obvious asymmetry in the five funnel plots (**Figure 5** for A vs. G model, **Supplementary Figure S4** for other models). All results were confirmed with Egger's linear regression test (A vs. G, P =0.76; GA vs. GG: P =0.40; AA vs. GG, P =0.94; GA+AA vs. GG, P =0. 42; AA vs. GG+GA, P =0.77).

Two case-control studies involving 1,495 subjects focused on the association between the rs671 polymorphism and PD risk and presented a negative relationship (**Table 2**).

Association between the rs4767944 and rs441 polymorphisms and the risk of PD. Two studies with 2,146 subjects focused on the association between the rs4767944 polymorphism and the risk of PD. The results of our aggregated analysis showed that the rs4767944 C>T polymorphism increased the PD risk in the homozygous model, but not in other genetic models. Only one study focused on the association between the rs441 polymorphisms and the risk of PD. The related information about the rs441 polymorphism is presented in **Table 1** (Quantitative calculation was not conducted).

DISCUSSION

AD and PD are the most important neurodegenerative disorders. The most intensively studied neurodegenerative disease is AD, which is known to be an established cause of aging-associated dementia, accounting for 60–70% of all neurodegenerative cases (31). Autopsy reports have demonstrated that the brain tissues of individuals with AD exhibit atrophied neurons, intraneuronal neurofibrillary tangles, and amyloid plaques. The

TABLE 2 | Summary ORs and 95% CI of ALDH2 polymorphisms and AD and PD risk.

	N*	OR	95% CI	*P*	I^2(%)	OR	95% CI	*P*	I^2(%)	OR	95% CI	*P*	I^2(%)	OR	95% CI	*P*	I^2(%)	OR	95% CI	*P*	I^2(%)
rs671			**A vs. G**				**GA vs. GG**				**AA vs. GG**				**GA+AA vs. GG**				**AA vs. GG+GA**		
AD Total	6	1.46	1.01–2.11	0.05	84.2	1.35	0.91–1.99	0.13	73.9	2.22	1.03–4.77	0.04	79.2	1.36	0.90–2.03	0.14	81.0	1.94	1.03–3.64	0.04	71.1
HWE–yes	4	1.48	0.88–2.49	0.14	87.4	1.26	0.72–2.21	0.41	79.4	2.57	1.01–6.53	0.05	78.1	1.45	0.77–2.73	0.25	86.0	2.23	1.18–4.60	0.01	61.4
HWE–no	2	1.36	1.10–1.69	0.01	NA	1.60	1.21–2.12	0.001	NA	1.33	0.78–2.27	0.29	NA	1.19	0.64–2.18	0.58	76.4	1.11	0.66–1.87	0.69	NA
COUNTRY																					
China	3	1.64	0.87–3.10	0.12	88.3	1.39	0.67–2.85	0.38	83.0	3.15	1.03–9.65	0.04	79.6	1.63	0.74–3.62	0.23	87.9	2.75	1.23–6.14	0.02	63.0
Japan	2	1.54	1.00–2.36	0.05	17.1	1.28	0.77–2.13	0.33	69.7	1.34	0.85–2.12	0.20	0	1.31	0.87–1.98	0.20	59.6	1.18	0.76–1.85	0.46	0
CONTROL DESIGN																					
HB	4	1.57	1.02–2.42	0.04	86.0	1.47	0.95–2.27	0.09	74.6	2.48	0.98–6.30	0.06	83.4	1.63	0.99–2.67	0.05	82.7	2.10	0.96–357	0.06	77.6
PB	2	1.07	0.75–1.54	0.71	NA	0.95	0.58–1.55	0.84	NA	1.38	0.57–3.35	0.48	NA	0.93	0.65–1.32	0.68	0	1.41	0.60–3.34	0.43	NA
SUBJECTS																					
>500	2	1.36	1.10–1.69	0.01	NA	1.60	1.21–2.12	0.001	NA	1.33	0.78–2.27	0.29	NA	1.19	0.64–2.18	0.58	76.4	1.11	0.66–1.87	0.69	NA
<500	4	1.48	0.88–2.49	0.14	87.4	1.26	0.72–2.21	0.41	79.4	2.57	1.01–6.53	0.05	78.1	1.45	0.77–2.73	0.25	86.0	2.23	1.18–4.60	0.01	61.4
NOS EVALUATION																					
NOS < 8	5	1.57	1.02–2.42	0.04	86.0	1.47	0.95–2.27	0.09	74.6	2.48	0.98–6.30	0.06	83.4	1.43	0.90–2.28 .92–2.18	0.13	82.9	2.10	0.96–357	0.06	77.6
NOS ≥8	1	1.07	0.75–1.54	0.71	NA	0.95	0.58–1.55	0.84	NA	1.38	0.57–3.35	0.748	NA	1.01	0.64–1.61	0.96	NA	1.41	0.60–3.34	0.43	NA
GENDER																					
Male	2	1.52	1.06–2.16	0.02	0	1.70	1.07–2.70	0.03	14.3	1.81	0.73–4.46	0.20	0	1.72	1.10–2.67	0.02	0	1.47	0.60–3.58	0.40	0
Female	2	0.90	0.40–2.10	0.79	83.4	0.94	0.35–2.57	0.891	81.5	0.93	0.37–2.32	0.88	43.8	0.91	0.33–1.2.49	0.86	84.3	0.98	0.57–1.69	0.95	0
PD Total	2	1.38	0.77–2.45	0.28	85.2	1.23	0.98–1.52	0.07	0	1.95	0.31–12.23	0.47	89.3	1.30	0.90–1.92	0.15	53.6	1.18	0.29–11.16	0.52	89.4
Rs4767944			T vs. C				CT vs. CC				TT vs. CC				CT+TT vs. CC				TT vs. CC+CT		
PD Total	2	0.87	0.67–1.14	0.31	70.9	0.89	0.58–1.36	0.60	71.3	0.57	0.40–0.80	<0.01	0	0.83	0.51–1.36	0.46	80.3	0.71	0.56–0.90	0.01	0

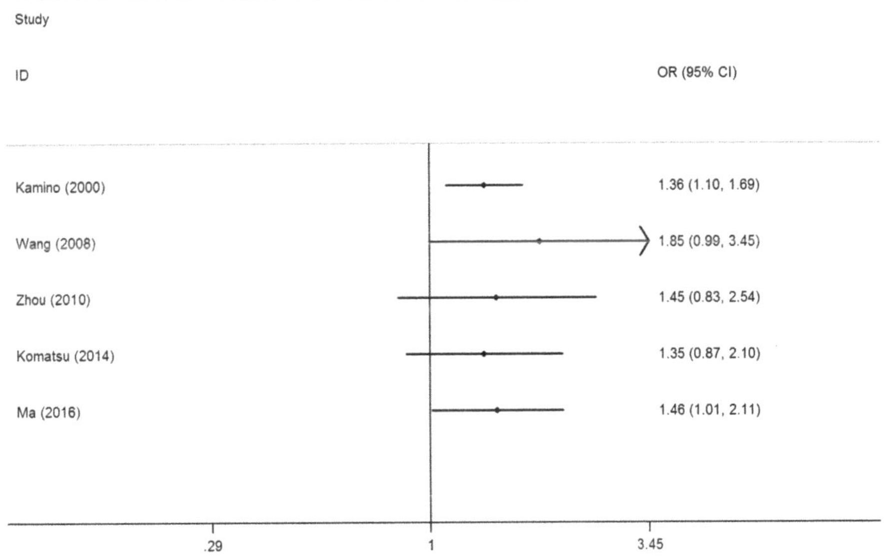

FIGURE 3 | Cumulative meta-analyses according to publication year in A vs. G model of ALDH2 rs671 G>A polymorphism and AD risk.

amyloid beta accumulation promotes oxidative stress and leads to mitochondrial dysfunction. As for PD, it is a chronic neurodegenerative disease without a clear etiology and is characterized by the classic triad of tremors, bradykinesia, and rigidity (32). Research has shown that >50% of patients with PD will develop dementia within 10 years after the initial diagnosis (33). The prominent pathological changes that occur in patients with PD are the degeneration of dopamine neurons in the mesencephalon, which causes a decrease of the dopamine content in the striatum.

Alcohol consumption is one of the most common habits of human beings. Alcohol is characterized by a high affinity for water and can be quickly distributed throughout the body after rapid absorption into the blood from the gastrointestinal tract. The majority of ethanol metabolism occurs in the liver and ALDH2 has a strong effect on acetaldehyde metabolism and accumulation (34). Current evidence suggests that alcohol intake can have two opposing effects on health. Specifically, consuming small doses of alcohol is believed to confer protection and decrease the risk of cardiovascular system dysfunction (35), while consuming large doses of ethanol can increase the alcohol content in the serum and seriously threaten human health, leading to cardiovascular disease and various oncological diseases. Most studies suggest that long-term and excessive alcohol consumption may damage the central nervous system cells and impair cognitive function (36).

Several important SNP loci have been identified and studied in the *ALDH2* gene. These SNPs change the nucleotide bases of the human genome, thus altering the protein expression levels and biological activity. The rs671 polymorphism is caused by a single-nucleotide mutation from G to A, which encodes an amino acid change from glutamate to lysine. Rs671is the most well-known dysfunctional SNP, and both the GA and AA genotypes severely reduce the activity of the ALDH2 enzyme

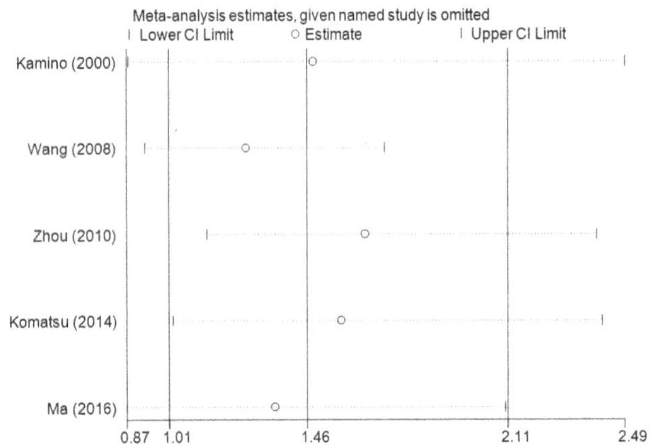

FIGURE 4 | Sensitivity analysis through deleting each study to reflect the influence of the individual dataset to the pooled ORs in A vs. G model of ALDH2 rs671 G>A polymorphism and AD risk.

and impair ethanol metabolism (37). The mutant genotypes and allele frequencies of rs671 are markedly different among different populations and are particularly more prevalent in East Asian populations (Chinese, Japanese and Korean individuals) than in other populations (38, 39). Many studies have demonstrated that the *ALDH2* rs671 G>A polymorphism maybe associated with the development of various diseases, such as digestive system cancer (40), diabetes (41), coronary heart disease (42), and ischemic stroke (43), especially in East Asians.

Since 2000, an increasing number of studies have focused on the relationship between *ALDH2* polymorphisms and the risk of AD. Kamino et al. conducted the first case-control study and found that the rs671 A allele would increase the risk for AD in the Japanese population (OR = 1.6, 95% CI = 1.19–2.03), and this

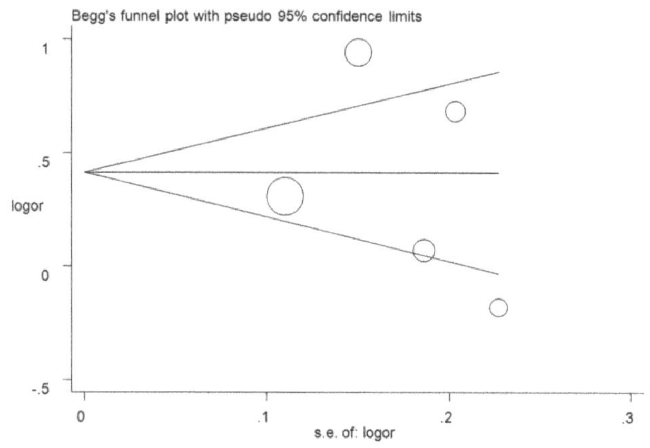

FIGURE 5 | Funnel plot analysis to detect publication bias for A vs. G model of ALDH2 rs671 G>A polymorphism and AD risk. Circles represent the weight of the studies.

trend was observed in both males and females. Wang et al. found an apparently increased AD risk in Chinese individuals with the rs671 A-allele (OR = 3.11, 95%CI = 2.06–4.69). Similarly, Zhao et al. and Ma et al. reported the similar elevated risk for PD (28) and AD with the rs671G>A mutation (29). However, Zhou et al., Komatsu et al., and Zhang et al. did not find any potential relationship between the rs671 G>A polymorphism and the risk of AD. Therefore, the discrepancies in these result promoted us to conduct this meta-analysis to investigate the precise association based on published studies.

To our knowledge, this is the first meta-analysis on the association between the *ALDH2* rs671 G>A polymorphism and the risk of AD and PD. All results suggest that the polymorphism locus of *ALDH2* rs671 G>A may be a potential risk factor for AD but not for PD in the East Asians. The current evidence indicated that the carriers with AA genotype were more dangerous compared with the GG genotype, which was also coincides with the decrease of ALDH2 protein activity that caused by allele A mutation. Moreover, the elevated risks we identified were also observed in some subgroups, such as in male groups. Among East Asians, males account for the majority of people who consume alcohol. The interactive effects of alcohol consumption and the deficient ALDH2 enzymatic activity caused by the rs671 mutation may contribute to AD development in males. Two of the studies we evaluated focused on the rs4767944 polymorphism, and the results revealed a slightly protective effect of this polymorphism against PD. In addition, no positive association was identified between rs441 polymorphism and the risk of PD with only one study. However, given the limited number of studies and included participants for this polymorphism, the results might not reflect the real relationship. Therefore, additional studies examining the association between the rs4767944 and rs441 polymorphisms and the risk of PD are necessary.

Given the inherent deficiencies in meta-analyses, this study has some limitations that should be considered when interpreting our findings. First, all subjects in the included studies were from East Asian countries. As such, the pooled results of this meta-analysis only reflect the East Asian population and thus are not generalizable to other ethnicities. Second, a slightly large sample size was only available for the *ALDH2* rs671 G>A polymorphism, but not for the rs4767944 and rs441 polymorphisms. The investigations of the associations of each of the three polymorphisms with the risk of AD and PD were conducted independently without adjusting for gene-gene interactions, such as through a haplotype analysis. Third, the interactions with some factors, such as body mass index, blood pressure, and unhealthy living habits, were not examined because of the lack of accurate individual information in the included studies. Finally, heterogeneity was observed in some of the genetic models in all included studies, and the meta-regression failed to identify any factors that contributed to the heterogeneity. Future studies that address these limitations will be required before any concrete conclusions about the relationships between these polymorphisms and AD and PD can be made.

In conclusion, the present results indicate that the *ALDH2* rs671 G>A polymorphism may be a potential risk factor for AD. Additional case-control studies are needed to investigate the underlying mechanism of the potential risk.

AUTHOR CONTRIBUTIONS

JC, WH, and LZ conceived the study and wrote the draft of the paper. JC, WH, and Y-YH searched the databases and extracted the data. C-HC and G-BJ analyzed the data and reviewed the manuscript. All the authors approved the final manuscript.

FUNDING

This study was supported by the Foundations of the Science and Technology Department of Hubei Province (No. 2016CFB567, 2014CFB364), and the Hubei Province health and family planning scientific research project (No. WJ2017F069, WJ2015Q041) and Taihe Hospital (2016BSQD02). The funders had no roles in study design, data collection and analysis, decision to publish, or preparation of the manuscript.

REFERENCES

1. Seeley WW, Crawford RK, Zhou J, Miller BL, Greicius MD. Neurodegenerative diseases target large-scale human brain networks. *Neuron.* (2009) 62:42–52. doi: 10.1016/j.neuron.2009.03.024
2. Matilla-Duenas A, Corral-Juan M, Rodriguez-Palmero Seuma A, Vilas D, Ispierto L, Morais S, et al. Rare neurodegenerative diseases: clinical and genetic update. *Adv Exp Med Biol.* (2017) 1031:443–96. doi: 10.1007/978-3-319-67144-4_25

3. Ridolfi B, Abdel-Haq H. Neurodegenerative disorders treatment: the MicroRNA role. *Curr Gene Ther.* (2017) 17:327–63. doi: 10.2174/1566523218666180119120726
4. Hebert LE, Weuve J, Scherr PA, Evans DA. Alzheimer disease in the United States (2010-2050) estimated using the 2010 census. *Neurology.* (2013) 80:1778–83. doi: 10.1212/WNL.0b013e31828726f5
5. Gammon K. Neurodegenerative disease: brain windfall. *Nature.* (2014) 515:299–300. doi: 10.1038/nj7526-299a
6. Maiti P, Dunbar GL. Use of curcumin, a natural polyphenol for targeting molecular pathways in treating age-related neurodegenerative diseases. *Int J Mol Sci.* (2018) 19:E1637. doi: 10.3390/ijms19061637
7. Bangen KJ, Nation DA, Delano-Wood L, Weissberger GH, Hansen LA, Galasko DR, et al. Aggregate effects of vascular risk factors on cerebrovascular changes in autopsy-confirmed Alzheimer's disease. *Alzheim Dement.* (2015) 11:394–403 e391. doi: 10.1016/j.jalz.2013.12.025
8. Yang Y, Song W. Molecular links between Alzheimer's disease and diabetes mellitus. *Neuroscience.* (2013) 250:140–50. doi: 10.1016/j.neuroscience.2013.07.009
9. Gelders G, Baekelandt V, Van der Perren A. Linking neuroinflammation and neurodegeneration in Parkinson's disease. *J Immunol Res.* (2018) 2018:4784268. doi: 10.1155/2018/4784268
10. Chen H, Kwong JC, Copes R, Tu K, Villeneuve PJ, van Donkelaar A, et al. Living near major roads and the incidence of dementia, Parkinson's disease, and multiple sclerosis: a population-based cohort study. *Lancet.* (2017) 389:718–26. doi: 10.1016/S0140-6736(16)32399-6
11. Xu W, Tan L, Wang HF, Jiang T, Tan MS, Zhao QF, et al. Meta-analysis of modifiable risk factors for Alzheimer's disease. *J Neurol Neurosurg Psychiatry.* (2015) 86:1299–306. doi: 10.1136/jnnp-2015-310548
12. Li Z, Del-Aguila JL, Dube U, Budde J, Martinez R, Black K, et al. Genetic variants associated with Alzheimer's disease confer different cerebral cortex cell-type population structure. *Genome Med.* (2018) 10:43. doi: 10.1186/s13073-018-0551-4
13. Freudenberg-Hua Y, Li W, Davies P. The role of genetics in advancing precision medicine for alzheimer's disease-a narrative review. *Front Med.* (2018) 5:108. doi: 10.3389/fmed.2018.00108
14. Chen CH, Joshi AU, Mochly-Rosen D. The role of mitochondrial aldehyde dehydrogenase 2 (ALDH2) in neuropathology and neurodegeneration. *Acta Neurol Taiwan.* (2016) 25:111–23.
15. Kamino K, Nagasaka K, Imagawa M, Yamamoto H, Yoneda H, Ueki A, et al. Deficiency in mitochondrial aldehyde dehydrogenase increases the risk for late-onset Alzheimer's disease in the Japanese population. *Biochem Biophys Res Commun.* (2000) 273:192–6. doi: 10.1006/bbrc.2000.2923
16. Moher D, Liberati A, Tetzlaff J, Altman DG. Preferred reporting items for systematic reviews and meta-analyses: the PRISMA statement. *BMJ.* (2009) 339:b2535. doi: 10.1136/bmj.b2535
17. Niu YM, Weng H, Zhang C, Yuan RX, Yan JZ, Meng XY, et al. Systematic review by multivariate meta-analyses on the possible role of tumor necrosis factor-alpha gene polymorphisms in association with ischemic stroke. *Neuromolecular Med.* (2015) 17:373–84. doi: 10.1007/s12017-015-8365-7
18. Huedo-Medina TB, Sanchez-Meca J, Marin-Martinez F, Botella J. Assessing heterogeneity in meta-analysis: Q statistic or I2 index? *Psychol Methods.* (2006) 11:193–206. doi: 10.1037/1082-989X.11.2.193
19. Mantel N, Haenszel W. Statistical aspects of the analysis of data from retrospective studies of disease. *J Natl Cancer Inst.* (1959) 22:719–48.
20. DerSimonian R. Meta-analysis in the design and monitoring of clinical trials. *Stat Med.* (1996) 15:1237–1248; discussion 1249–1252. doi: 10.1002/(SICI)1097-0258(19960630)15:12<1253::AID-SIM303>3.0.CO;2-R
21. Begg CB, Mazumdar M. Operating characteristics of a rank correlation test for publication bias. *Biometrics.* (1994) 50:1088–101. doi: 10.2307/2533446
22. Egger M, Davey Smith G, Schneider M, Minder C. Bias in meta-analysis detected by a simple, graphical test. *BMJ.* (1997) 315:629–34. doi: 10.1136/bmj.315.7109.629
23. Kim JM, Stewart R, Shin IS, Jung JS, Yoon JS. Assessment of association between mitochondrial aldehyde dehydrogenase polymorphism and Alzheimer's disease in an older Korean population. *Neurobiol Aging.* (2004) 25:295–301. doi: 10.1016/S0197-4580(03)00114-3
24. Wang B, Wang J, Zhou S, Tan S, He X, Yang Z, et al. The association of mitochondrial aldehyde dehydrogenase gene (ALDH2) polymorphism with susceptibility to late-onset Alzheimer's disease in Chinese. *J Neurol Sci.* (2008) 268:172–5. doi: 10.1016/j.jns.2007.12.006
25. Zhou S, Huriletemuer, Wang J, Zhang C, Zhao S, Wang de S, et al. Absence of association on *aldehyde dehydrogenase 2 (ALDH2)* polymorphism with Mongolian Alzheimer patients. *Neurosci Lett.* (2010) 468:312–5. doi: 10.1016/j.neulet.2009.11.022
26. Komatsu M, Shibata N, Ohnuma T, Kuerban B, Tomson K, Toda A, et al. Polymorphisms in the aldehyde dehydrogenase 2 and dopamine beta hydroxylase genes are not associated with Alzheimer's disease. *J Neural Transm.* (2014) 121:427–32. doi: 10.1007/s00702-013-1112-z
27. Zhang X, Ye YL, Wang YN, Liu FF, Liu XX, Hu BL, et al. Aldehyde dehydrogenase 2 genetic variations may increase susceptibility to Parkinson's disease in Han Chinese population. *Neurobiol Aging.* (2015) 36:2660 e2669–13. doi: 10.1016/j.neurobiolaging.2015.06.001
28. Zhao CC, Cai HB, Wang H, Pan SY. Role of ADH2 and ALDH2 gene polymorphisms in the development of Parkinson's disease in a Chinese population. *Genet Mol Res.* (2016) 15. doi: 10.4238/gmr.15038606
29. Ma L, Lu ZN. Role of ADH1B rs1229984 and ALDH2 rs671 gene polymorphisms in the development of Alzheimer's disease. *Genet Mol Res.* (2016) 15. doi: 10.4238/gmr.15048740
30. Madadi F, Khaniani MS, Shandiz EE, Ayromlou H, Najmi S, Emamalizadeh B, et al. Genetic analysis of the ZNF512B, SLC41A1, and ALDH2 polymorphisms in Parkinson's disease in the iranian population. *Genet Test Mol Biomarkers.* (2016) 20:629–32. doi: 10.1089/gtmb.2016.0133
31. Blennow K, de Leon MJ, Zetterberg H. Alzheimer's disease. *Lancet.* (2006) 368:387–403. doi: 10.1016/S0140-6736(06)69113-7
32. Assadeck H, Daouda MT, Djibo FH, Maiga DD, Omar EA. Clinical profile of Parkinson's disease: experience of niger. *J Neurosci Rural Pract.* (2018) 9:214–8. doi: 10.4103/jnrp.jnrp_337_17
33. Korczyn AD. Mild cognitive impairment in Parkinson's disease. *J Neural Transm.* (2013) 120:517–21. doi: 10.1007/s00702-013-1006-0
34. Heit C, Dong H, Chen Y, Thompson DC, Deitrich RA, Vasiliou VK. The role of CYP2E1 in alcohol metabolism and sensitivity in the central nervous system. *Subcell Biochem.* (2013) 67:235–47. doi: 10.1007/978-94-007-5881-0_8
35. de Gaetano G, Costanzo S, Di Castelnuovo A, Badimon L, Bejko D, Alkerwi A, et al. Effects of moderate beer consumption on health and disease: a consensus document. *Nutr Metab Cardiovasc Dis.* (2016) 26:443–67. doi: 10.1016/j.numecd.2016.03.007
36. Hassing LB. Light alcohol consumption does not protect cognitive function: a longitudinal prospective study. *Front Aging Neurosci.* (2018) 10:81. doi: 10.3389/fnagi.2018.00081
37. Peng GS, Yin SJ. Effect of the allelic variants of aldehyde dehydrogenase ALDH2*2 and alcohol dehydrogenase ADH1B*2 on blood acetaldehyde concentrations. *Hum Genomics.* (2009) 3:121–7. doi: 10.1186/1479-7364-3-2-121
38. Sakiyama M, Matsuo H, Nakaoka H, Yamamoto K, Nakayama A, Nakamura T, et al. Identification of rs671, a common variant of ALDH2, as a gout susceptibility locus. *Sci Rep.* (2016) 6:25360. doi: 10.1038/srep25360
39. Goedde HW, Agarwal DP, Fritze G, Meier-Tackmann D, Singh S, Beckmann G, et al. Distribution of ADH2 and ALDH2 genotypes in different populations. *Hum Genet.* (1992) 88:344–6. doi: 10.1007/BF00197271
40. Hidaka A, Sasazuki S, Matsuo K, Ito H, Sawada N, Shimazu T, et al. Genetic polymorphisms of ADH1B, ADH1C and ALDH2, alcohol consumption, and the risk of gastric cancer: the Japan Public Health Center-based prospective study. *Carcinogenesis.* (2015) 36:223–31. doi: 10.1093/carcin/bgu244

41. Li GY, Li ZB, Li F, Dong LP, Tang L, Xiang J, et al. Meta-analysis on the association of ALDH2 polymorphisms and type 2 diabetic mellitus, diabetic retinopathy. *Int J Environ Res Public Health.* (2017) 14:165. doi: 10.3390/ijerph14020165
42. Li YY, Wang H, Wu JJ, Kim HJ, Yang XX, Geng HY, et al. ALDH2 gene G487A polymorphism and coronary artery disease: a meta-analysis including 5644 participants. *J Cell Mol Med.* (2018) 22:1666–74. doi: 10.1111/jcmm.13443
43. Sung YF, Lu CC, Lee JT, Hung YJ, Hu CJ, Jeng JS, et al. Homozygous ALDH2*2 is an independent risk factor for ischemic stroke in taiwanese men. *Stroke.* (2016) 47:2174–9. doi: 10.1161/STROKEAHA.116.013204

9

Substance P Saliva Reduction Predicts Pharyngeal Dysphagia in Parkinson's Disease

Jens Burchard Schröder, Thomas Marian, Inga Claus, Paul Muhle, Matthias Pawlowski, Heinz Wiendl, Sonja Suntrup-Krueger, Sven G. Meuth, Rainer Dziewas, Tobias Ruck and Tobias Warnecke*

Department of Neurology, University Hospital Münster, Münster, Germany

***Correspondence:**
Jens Burchard Schröder
jensburchard.schroeder@ukmuenster.de

Introduction: Although patients with Parkinson's disease (PD) often suffer from oropharyngeal dysphagia, knowledge about the underlying pathophysiological mechanisms is limited. Substance P (SP) is a localization-independent neurotransmitter of the entire nervous system. Reduced levels of SP were found in saliva of patients with impaired cough reflex and in advanced stages of PD. The aim of the study was to investigate SP in PD patients in order to gain further insights into the underlying pathophysiology of PD-related dysphagia and to evaluate the potential of SP as a biomarker for early dysphagia.

Methods: Flexible endoscopic evaluation of swallowing (FEES) was used to objectively assess pharyngeal swallowing function. From a cohort of 105 consecutive PD patients 20 subjects were recruited: in 10 of them pharyngeal dysphagia was excluded by FEES, the other 10 subjects showed signs of early pharyngeal dysphagia defined as hypopharyngeal sensory deficit with mild to moderate vallecular residues after swallowing solid consistencies. Analysis of the Substance P level in saliva of the 20 included PD patients was performed in the clinical on state condition by ELISA-type immunoassay. Significant differences were calculated by using the Mann-Whitney test.

Results: Twenty PD patients with a mean age of 69.5 $\pm$ 12.5 years (8 female) were included in the study. No significant differences were found regarding gender, age, UPDRS III, Hoehn and Yahr stage, disease duration, and Levodopa equivalent dose between the non-dysphagic and dysphagic subjects. Dysphagia was mainly characterized by unrecognized residues in the valleculae without any aspiration risk for all of the tested consistencies in FEES and was thereby scored as mild in all cases. Saliva SP concentrations were significantly lower in PD patients with pharyngeal dysphagia compared to those with a normal pharyngeal swallowing function (9,644 vs. 17,591 pg/mL; $p = 0.001$).

Conclusion: Reduced saliva SP concentrations may predict early pharyngeal swallowing dysfunction in PD patients. This finding supports the hypothesis that an impaired SP mediated neurotransmission has a significant impact for the development of dysphagia in PD patients. Larger studies are needed to confirm SP as a clinical useful biomarker for early detection of PD-related dysphagia.

Keywords: Parkinson's disease, substance P, dysphagia, biomarker, neurodegeneration

INTRODUCTION

Following Alzheimer's disease, Parkinson's disease (PD) is the second most common neurodegenerative disorder (1, 2). Oropharyngeal dysphagia is a clinically relevant symptom in affected patients as the majority of PD patients will suffer from neurogenic dysphagia during the course of their disease (3–6). In addition to consecutive malnutrition, dehydration and insufficient medication intake, neurogenic dysphagia leads to loss of quality of life for affected patients and aspiration pneumonia, which is the leading cause of death in Parkinson's patients (4, 7–9).

However, clinical diagnosis of dysphagia in PD remains challenging. Particularly in early disease stages affected patients are usually unaware of their swallowing dysfunction and therefore do not report spontaneously about swallowing problems (10, 11). Furthermore, pharyngeal swallowing function cannot be assessed sufficiently by clinical neurological examination resulting in a significant delay of uncovering dysphagia in these patients (11–13). When more elaborate instrumental tools for swallowing evaluation like flexible endoscopic evaluation of swallowing (FEES) or videofluoroscopic swallowing study (VFSS) are systematically applied, dysphagia was found to be present in more than 50% of subjectively asymptomatic PD patients (14). However, access to FEES and VFSS is limited in many institutions.

Furthermore, the underlying pathophysiology of dysphagia in PD and particularly the role of substance P (SP) is still barely understood (15). SP is an ubiquitary neuropeptide in the nervous system (16). It mediates the response to local stimuli in the pharyngeal mucosa and thereby enhances the swallow and cough reflex (17–19). In a cohort of elderly patients with aspiration pneumonia, sputum levels of SP were found to be reduced (20). Probably due to a reduced concentration of SP in the saliva of patients in advanced stages of PD, protective reflexes with consecutive silent aspiration were observed (21, 22). However, it is so far unknown if substance P reduction is already present in PD patients with early pharyngeal dysphagia not showing any risk of aspiration.

The purpose of the present study was to investigate Substance P as a potential biomarker for early detection of pharyngeal dysphagia in PD and thereby gain further insights into pathophysiology.

MATERIAL AND METHODS

Protocol Approval, Registration, and Patient Consent

All patients were prospectively recruited from the movement disorder unit at the Department of Neurology, University Hospital Münster, Germany. Written informed consent was obtained from each subject after the nature of the study was explained in accordance to the principles of the declaration of Helsinki. The local ethics committee of the medical faculty at the University of Muenster approved the protocol of the study (2014-624-f-S).

Participants

From a cohort of 105 consecutive PD patients, who did not have subjective swallowing impairment and were evaluated for dysphagia with FEES, as part of the baseline dysphagia assessment in our clinic, 20 subjects were recruited between January 2017 and March 2018. Participants had to be on stable medication regimen and all examinations were done in the clinical "ON" phase. Exclusion criteria for this study were concomitant diseases that may cause neurogenic dysphagia, autoimmune diseases, anti-inflammatory co-medication (e.g., cytotoxic agents, steroids, non-steroid analgesia), sedatives, or evidence of an acute systemic inflammatory process at the time of Substance P measurement (elevated erythrocyte sedimentation rate above 25 mm/h, C-reactive protein above 0.5 mg/dL, or leukocytes above 11 × 103/μL). Patient characteristics are described in detail in **Table 1**.

Dysphagia Assessment

In all participants, Dysphagia was examined with fiberoptic endoscopic evaluation of swallowing in the on-state condition. FEES was performed in accordance with the standard protocol proposed by Langmore et al. as described in detail elsewhere (23).

Equipment consisted of a 3.1 mm-diameter flexible fiberoptic rhinolaryngoscope (11101RP2, Karl Storz, Tuttlingen, Germany), a light source and camera (rpCam-X, rpSzene®, Rehder/Partner, Hamburg, Germany), a color monitor (WMP-226, Wincomm, Taiwan) and a video recorder (AUCC2WV3F, Computar, CBC Group, Japan).

All PD patients were given nine test boluses in a standardized order. First, they received 8 ml of pudding (green jelly), second 5 ml blue-dyed liquid and finally three trials of white bread with the size of approximately 3 × 3 × 0.5 cm. During all swallowing tasks, the following parameters of swallowing function were assessed: premature spillage, material that enters the hypopharynx unintentionally from the oral cavity before the pharyngeal swallow was initiated, penetration-aspiration events or residues. When residues in FEES were observed, patients were asked explicitly if they perceived any foreign body sensation in their throat.

Swallowing dysfunction was classified with a FEES-based 4-grade dysphagia severity scale that has previously been developed and published: 0 = no relevant dysphagia, 1 = mild dysphagia (premature spillage and/or residues, but no penetration/aspiration events), 2 = moderate dysphagia (penetration/aspiration events with one consistency), 3 = severe dysphagia (penetration/aspiration events with two or more consistencies) (24–26). Substance P was collected from patients with either no signs of pharyngeal dysphagia (group 1), or endoscopic signs of early pharyngeal dysphagia (group 2). Dysphagia was defined as mild to moderate vallecular residues being present after swallowing solid consistencies (27). Patients showing an increased aspiration risk for any of the tested consistencies were excluded.

Sample Collection and Analysis:

Between 09 and 11 a.m., about 2 h after the intake of their regular dopaminergic medication, sputum was collected. Two

TABLE 1 | Subject characteristics and clinical features.

	All	Dysphagia +	Dysphagia −	*p*-value
Number of patients (M/F)	20 (12/8)	10 (8/2)	10 (4/6)	0.068
Mean age (year)	69.5 ± 12.5	71.7 ± 11.8	67.2 ± 13.3	0.172
Disease duration (year)	8.35 ± 5.8	10.9 ± 6.5	5.8 ± 3.7	0.403
Hoehn and Yahr stage[a]	2.4 ± 0.8	2.8 ± 0.6	2.0 ± 0.7	0.698
UPDRS III, points[a]	16.5 ± 4.7	18.2 ± 4.8	14.8 ± 4.1	0.120
L-Dopa-Dose-Equivalent, mg	768.8 ± 276.4	849.2 ± 264.7	688.3 ± 277.1	0.199
Saliva quantity, microliters	792.9 ± 122.5	752.1 ± 108.1	833.8 ± 127.5	0.287
PPI intake (*n*)	7	4	3	0.180

UPDRS, Unified Parkinson Disease Rating Scale.
[a]At clinical "On"-stage.

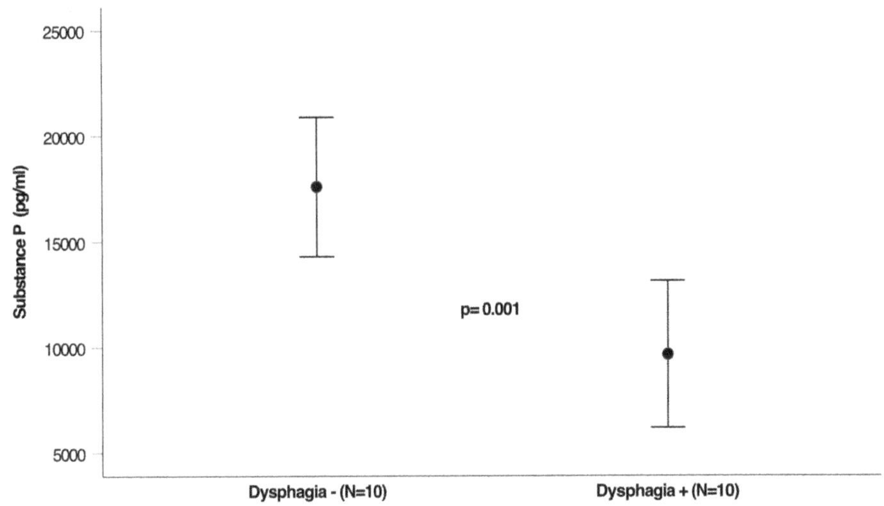

FIGURE 1 | Levels of Substance P in saliva of dysphagic and not dysphagic PD patients.

salivettes were placed into the patient's oral cavity for 1–3 min. Directly after collecting the saliva, the salivettes were centrifuged at 4,110 g for 5 min. Supernatants were stored in a deep freezer at −20°C until further analysis. Substance P levels were assessed by a commercially available competitive ELISA-type immunoassay according to the manufacturer's instructions (SP Immnunoassay, catalog no. KGE007; R&D Systems, Minneapolis, MN, USA).

Statistics

Statistical analysis was performed using SPSS Version 25.0. All data are reported as mean ± standard deviation, and the pre-chosen significance level for all confirmatory tests was $p < 0.05$. Substance P-Level was analyzed by using the Mann-Whitney test, presuming a non-Gaussian distribution.

RESULTS

FEES was successfully performed in all 20 subjects (12 male, 8 female, mean age 68.6 ± 12.5 years), presenting with either no ($n = 10$) or early pharyngeal dysphagia ($n = 10$). No adverse events occurred during the FEES examinations. **Table 1** summarizes patient's characteristics and clinical features of included patients. Gender and age were equally distributed in both study groups. In addition, no statistically significant differences were found regarding disease duration, L-Dopa equivalent doses, UPDRS III, and Hoehn & Yahr stages. PPI-intake was equally distributed between both groups.

Unnoticed pharyngeal residues were present in 10 patients (Group 2). They were located in the vallecular space in all subjects and, to a lesser extent in the pyriform sinuses (30%). Premature spillage and penetration/aspiration events were not observed for any consistency, i.e., liquid, semisolids, solids.

Figure 1 shows the concentration of SP in sputum among the 2 groups. Sputum SP concentrations were significantly lower in patients with dysphagia compared to those in control subjects (9,644 vs. 17,591 pg/mL; $p = 0.001$; see **Figure 1**).

DISCUSSION

This prospective study analyzed the saliva concentrations of SP in PD patients with early pharyngeal dysphagia compared to PD patients without any pharyngeal swallowing impairment.

The study's main finding is that early pharyngeal dysphagia in PD patients is associated with reduced levels of Substance P in patient's saliva.

PD-related dysphagia affects the oral, pharyngeal and the esophageal phase of swallowing and occurs in all stages of the disease (11, 28). Former studies have demonstrated a selective loss of vagal SP neurons in PD, potentially contributing to the emergence of esophageal motility disorders (29). In our study, also in patients with early pharyngeal dysphagia, as indicated by unnoticed significant pharyngeal residues, was associated with reduced SP concentrations. This finding broadens the results of a previous study, where significantly reduced levels of Substance P were found in PD patients with an impaired cough reflex sensitivity in a much more advanced stage of PD-related dysphagia. In early disease stages with by trend slightly lower Substance P levels cough sensitivity was not found to be impaired in this study (21). SP-immunoreactive fibers have been detected in the epithelium and basal membrane of pharyngeal mucosa, especially on the surface of the epiglottis (30). In this context, our findings could be another indication, that in early stages, loss of SP containing neurons in the pharyngeal mucosa may lead to pharyngeal hyposensitivity and merely incipient pharyngeal dysphagia.

Current diagnostic workup of suspected PD related dysphagia usually consists of questionnaires, swallowing assessment by speech language therapists and, in unclear cases, by using instrumental tools such as FEES or videofluoroscopic swallowing study (VFSS). Still, reliable screening methods are lacking 3, 27). FEES and VFSS are both considered to be the gold standard, but availability of instrumental assessment, especially in the outpatient setting, is often limited. In this context, the measurement of SP in saliva may have the potential to serve as a biomarker for the presence of clinically unrecognized pharyngeal dysphagia in early disease stages and thereby lead to earlier comprehensive dysphagia diagnosis and treatment.

Our study has several limitations that need to be addressed. First of all, PD patients were only assessed in one specific stage of their disease. Therefore, the results cannot be generalized over the entire PD population. For a possible use of substance P as a biomarker, in particular the establishment of reference values is necessary, which do not exist today. Furthermore, no follow-up of included patients was performed and, keeping in mind the basic experimental approach in the here presented pilot study, the sample size was rather low and no healthy controls were investigated. Any concomitant medication not excluded might have interfered with SP concentration. Impairment of motor function might as well have contributed to the emergence of dysphagia in our cohort. Furthermore, PD-related dysphagia is a complex symptom probably resulting from several central and peripheral mechanisms and thereby not being linked to one neurotransmitter system alone, and the exact localization of neurodegeneration, that leads to reduced SP release, cannot be identified in the clinical setting here (31).

In conclusion, this study showed for the first time, that reduced levels of SP occur in PD patients with signs of early pharyngeal dysphagia. Future studies should confirm this finding in larger cohorts. Moreover, agents like capsaicin, known to stimulate SP-release, should be investigated to assess their therapeutic potential by targeting the afferent sensory system within the swallowing network (32).

AUTHOR CONTRIBUTIONS

JS conceived, organized, executed the research project, and wrote the manuscript. TM reviewed the manuscript. PM reviewed the manuscript. IC reviewed the manuscript. MP reviewed the manuscript. HW helped to conceive the study and reviewed the manuscript. SS-K reviewed the manuscript. SM helped to conceive the study and reviewed the manuscript. RD reviewed the manuscript. TR conceived the research project, performed data analysis, and reviewed the manuscript. TW conceived and supervised the research project and reviewed the manuscript.

REFERENCES

1. Kalia LV, Lang AE. Evolving basic, pathological and clinical concepts in PD: Parkinson disease in 2015. *Nat Rev Neurol.* (2016) 12:65–6. doi: 10.1038/nrneurol.2015.249
2. de Lau LM, Breteler MM. Epidemiology of Parkinson's disease. *Lancet Neurol.* (2006) 5:525–35. doi: 10.1016/S1474-4422(06)70471-9
3. Kalf JG, de Swart BJM, Bloem BR, Munneke M. Prevalence of oropharyngeal dysphagia in Parkinson's disease: a meta-analysis. *Parkinsonism Relat Disord.* (2012) 18:311–5. doi: 10.1016/j.parkreldis.2011.11.006
4. Miller N, Allcock L, Hildreth AJ, Jones D, Noble E, Burn DJ. Swallowing problems in Parkinson disease: frequency and clinical correlates. *J Neurol Neurosurg Psychiatry.* (2009) 80:1047–9. doi: 10.1136/jnnp.2008.157701
5. Sapir S, Ramig L, Fox C. Speech and swallowing disorders in Parkinson disease. *Curr Opin Otolaryngol Head Neck Surg.* (2008) 16:205–10. doi: 10.1097/MOO.0b013e3282febd3a
6. Edwards L, Quigley EMM, Hofman R, Pfeiffer RF. Gastrointestinal symptoms in Parkinson disease: 18-month follow-up study. *Mov Disord.* (1993) 8:83–6. doi: 10.1002/mds.870080115
7. Plowman-Prine EK, Sapienza CM, Okun MS, Pollock SL, Jacobson C, Wu SS, et al. The relationship between quality of life and swallowing in Parkinson's disease. *Mov Disord Off J Mov Disord Soc.* (2009) 24:1352–8. doi: 10.1002/mds.22617
8. Morgante L, Salemi G, Meneghini F, Di Rosa AE, Epifanio A, Grigoletto F, et al. Parkinson disease survival: a population-based study. *Arch Neurol.* (2000) 57:507. doi: 10.1001/archneur.57.4.507
9. Lin J-H, Tu K-H, Chang C-H, Chen Y-C, Tian Y-C, Yu C-C, et al. Prognostic factors and complication rates for double-filtration plasmapheresis in patients with Guillain-Barré syndrome. *Transfus Apher Sci.* (2015) 52:78–83. doi: 10.1016/j.transci.2014.12.005
10. Coelho M, Marti MJ, Tolosa E, Ferreira JJ, Valldeoriola F, Rosa M, et al. Late-stage Parkinson's disease: the Barcelona and Lisbon cohort. *J Neurol.* (2010) 257:1524–32. doi: 10.1007/s00415-010-5566-8
11. Pflug C, Bihler M, Emich K, Niessen A, Nienstedt JC, Flügel T, et al. Critical dysphagia is common in Parkinson disease and occurs even in early stages: a prospective cohort study. *Dysphagia.* (2018) 33:41–50. doi: 10.1007/s00455-017-9831-1

12. Bird MR, Woodward MC, Gibson EM, Phyland DJ, Fonda D. Asymptomatic swallowing disorders in elderly patients with Parkinson's disease: a description of findings on clinical examination and videofluoroscopy in sixteen patients. *Age Ageing.* (1994) 23:251–4.
13. Bushmann M, Dobmeyer SM, Leeker L, Perlmutter JS. Swallowing abnormalities and their response to treatment in Parkinson's disease. *Neurology.* (1989) 39:1309–14.
14. Fuh J-L, Lee R-C, Wang S-J, Lin C-H, Wang P-N, Chiang J-H, et al. Swallowing difficulty in Parkinson's disease. *Clin Neurol Neurosurg.* (1997) 99:106–12.
15. Michou E, Hamdy S. Dysphagia in Parkinson's disease: a therapeutic challenge? *Expert Rev Neurother.* (2010) 10:875–8. doi: 10.1586/ern.10.60
16. Niel JP. Role of substance P in the nervous system control of digestive motility. *Arch Int Physiol Biochim Biophys.* (1991) 99:A65–76.
17. Renner B, Ahne G, Grosan E, Kettenmann B, Kobal G, Shephard A. Tonic stimulation of the pharyngeal mucosa causes pain and a reversible increase of inflammatory mediators. *Inflamm Res.* (2013) 62:1045–51. doi: 10.1007/s00011-013-0663-7
18. Imoto Y, Kojima A, Osawa Y, Sunaga H, Fujieda S. Cough reflex induced by capsaicin inhalation in patients with dysphagia. *Acta Otolaryngol.* (2011) 131:96–100. doi: 10.3109/00016489.2010.516013
19. Jin Y, Sekizawa K, Fukushima T, Morikawa M, Nakazawa H, Sasaki H. Capsaicin desensitization inhibits swallowing reflex in guinea pigs. *Am J Respir Crit Care Med.* (1994) 149:261–3.
20. Nakagawa T, Ohrui T, Sekizawa K, Sasaki H. Sputum substance P in aspiration pneumonia. *Lancet.* (1995) 345:1447. doi: 10.1016/S0140-6736(95)92638-0
21. Ebihara S, Saito H, Kanda A, Nakajoh M, Takahashi H, Arai H, et al. Impaired efficacy of cough in patients with Parkinson disease. *Chest.* (2003) 124:1009–15. doi: 10.1378/chest.124.3.1009
22. Troche MS, Brandimore AE, Okun MS, Davenport PW, Hegland KW. Decreased cough sensitivity and aspiration in Parkinson disease. *Chest.* (2014) 146:1294–9. doi: 10.1378/chest.14-0066
23. Langmore SE. Scoring a FEES examination. *Endosc Eval Treat Swallowing Disord N Y Thieme.* (2001) 101–43.
24. Warnecke T, Oelenberg S, Teismann I, Hamacher C, Lohmann H, Ringelstein EB, et al. Endoscopic characteristics and levodopa responsiveness of swallowing function in progressive supranuclear palsy. *Mov Disord Off J Mov Disord Soc.* (2010) 25:1239–45. doi: 10.1002/mds.23060
25. Warnecke T, Dziewas R. Chapter 106—swallowing in progressive supranuclear palsy and implications for nutrition. In: Martin CR, Preedy VR, editors. *Diet and Nutrition in Dementia and Cognitive Decline.* San Diego, CA: Academic Press. (2014) p. 1135–41.
26. Warnecke T, Suttrup I, Schroder JB, Osada N, Oelenberg S, Hamacher C, et al. Levodopa responsiveness of dysphagia in advanced Parkinson's disease and reliability testing of the FEES-Levodopa-test. *Parkinsonism Relat Disord.* (2016) 28:100–6. doi: 10.1016/j.parkreldis.2016.04.034
27. Suttrup I, Warnecke T. Dysphagia in Parkinson's Disease. *Dysphagia.* (2016) 31:24–32. doi: 10.1007/s00455-015-9671-9
28. Suttrup I, Suttrup J, Suntrup-Krueger S, Siemer M-L, Bauer J, Hamacher C, et al. Esophageal dysfunction in different stages of Parkinson's disease. *Neurogastroenterol Motil.* (2017) 29:e12915. doi: 10.1111/nmo.12915
29. Halliday GM, Li YW, Blumbergs PC, Joh TH, Cotton RG, Howe PR, et al. Neuropathology of immunohistochemically identified brainstem neurons in Parkinson's disease. *Ann Neurol.* (1990) 27:373–85.
30. Yoshida Y, Tanaka Y, Hirano M, Nakashima T. Sensory innervation of the pharynx and larynx. *Am J Med.* (2000) 108:51–61. doi: 10.1016/S0002-9343(99)00342-3
31. Mu L, Sobotka S, Chen J, Su H, Sanders I, Adler CH, et al. Altered pharyngeal muscles in Parkinson disease. *J Neuropathol Exp Neurol.* (2012) 71:520–30. doi: 10.1097/NEN.0b013e318258381b
32. Gamse R, Molnar A, Lembeck F. Substance P release from spinal cord slices by capsaicin. *Life Sci.* (1979) 25:629–36. doi: 10.1016/0024-3205(79)90558-7

10

Beyond Dopamine: GABA, Glutamate and the Axial Symptoms of Parkinson Disease

Ruth L. O'Gorman Tuura [1], Christian R. Baumann [2] and Heide Baumann-Vogel [2]*

[1] Center for MR Research, University Children's Hospital Zurich, Zurich, Switzerland, [2] Department of Neurology, University Hospital Zurich, Zurich, Switzerland

Correspondence:
Ruth L. O'Gorman Tuura
Ruth.tuura@kispi.uzh.ch

Introduction: The axial symptoms of Parkinson disease (PD) include difficulties with balance, posture, speech, swallowing, and locomotion with freezing of gait, as well as axial rigidity. These axial symptoms impact negatively on quality of life for many patients, yet remain poorly understood. Dopaminergic treatments typically have little effect on the axial symptoms of PD, suggesting that disruptions in other neurotransmitter systems beyond the dopamine system may underlie these symptoms. The purpose of the present study was to examine the relationship between the axial symptoms of PD and GABA and glutamate levels quantified with magnetic resonance spectroscopy.

Methods: The participant group included 20 patients with PD and 17 healthy control participants. Water-scaled GABA and Glx (glutamate + glutamine) concentrations were derived from GABA-edited MEGA-PRESS spectra acquired from the left basal ganglia and prefrontal cortex, and additional water-scaled Glx concentrations were acquired from standard PRESS spectra acquired from the pons. Spectra were analyzed with LCModel. The axial symptoms of PD were evaluated from subscales of the Unified Parkinson's Disease rating scale (MDS-UPDRS).

Results: PD patients demonstrated significantly higher GABA levels in the basal ganglia, which correlated with the degree of gait disturbance. Basal ganglia Glx levels and prefrontal GABA and Glx levels did not differ significantly between patient and control groups, but within the PD group prefrontal Glx levels correlated negatively with difficulties turning in bed. Results from an exploratory subgroup analysis indicate that the associations between GABA, Glx, and axial symptoms scores are typically more prominent in akinetic-rigid patients than in tremor-dominant patients.

Conclusion: Alterations in GABAergic and glutamatergic neurotransmission may contribute to some of the axial symptoms of PD.

Keywords: Parkinson disease, magnetic resonance spectroscopy, GABA, glutamate, basal ganglia, prefrontal cortex, gait, axial symptoms

INTRODUCTION

Parkinson disease (PD) is a progressive neurodegenerative disorder thought to affect over 4 million patients worldwide (1). The core motor symptoms of PD include akinesia, rigidity, resting tremor, and postural and balance difficulties, but patients can also suffer from a broad spectrum of non-motor symptoms (2). While some of the motor symptoms can be improved by dopaminergic (e.g., levodopa) therapy, the non-motor symptoms and the "axial" motor symptoms, including difficulties with gait, posture, speech, swallowing, and postural stability, typically do not respond well to dopaminergic therapy (3). These axial symptoms have a severe, long-lasting negative impact on quality of life and have been identified as a top research priority by patients, family members, and carers affected by PD, second only to the overarching aim to find an effective cure (2).

The neural origin of the axial symptoms of PD is not well-understood, and treatment options are limited. However, converging evidence indicates that disruptions in other neurotransmitter systems beyond the dopamine system are present in PD and may underlie some of the non-motor and axial symptoms (4–6).

Two of the other major neurotransmitter systems implicated in basal ganglia regulation and in PD, namely the glutamate and γ-amino butyric acid (GABA) systems, can be probed non-invasively using magnetic resonance spectroscopy (MRS) (7). Previous MRS studies in PD have reported increased GABA in the pons, basal ganglia, and thalamus (8–10), decreased cortical glutamate (11), and an increased GABA/glutamate ratio in the substantia nigra (12). In other neurodegenerative disorders, altered GABA and glutamate levels have been linked to symptoms which are also present in PD, including cognitive impairment (13, 14) and depression (15). In mice, altered GABA and Glycine neurotransmission was observed to trigger the cardinal features of rapid eye movement sleep behavior disorder (RBD) (16), a premotor symptom of PD which may represent a biomarker for overall disease severity (17). However, few studies have examined altered GABA and glutamate levels in relation to PD symptomatology, and currently the link between alterations in the GABAergic and glutamatergic systems and the axial symptoms of PD remains unclear. The purpose of the present study was to examine the relationship between the axial symptoms of PD, GABA, and glutamate levels in the basal ganglia and prefrontal cortex, and glutamate levels in the pons. Based on previous reports, we hypothesized that patients with PD would show increased GABA levels in the basal ganglia and decreased glutamate in the prefrontal cortex and pons, and that more pronounced abnormalities in the GABA and glutamate levels would correlate positively with the severity of the axial symptoms of PD.

MATERIALS AND METHODS

Participants

The patient group consisted of 20 patients with PD (4 female, mean age 63 years, range 50–75) recruited from the Neurology Department of the University Hospital of Zürich, Switzerland (see **Table 1** for demographics). All 20 patients had bilateral impairment, and 9/20 patients were treated with levodopa without dopamine agonists, while 11/20 patients were treated with a combination of levodopa and dopamine agonists. Patients were enrolled consecutively. Seventeen healthy control participants (4 female, mean age 62 years, range 28–77) with no history of neurological or psychiatric illness were also recruited. All participants gave written and verbal informed consent to participate in the study, which was approved by the cantonal ethics committee of the Canton of Zürich, Switzerland.

MRI/MRS Acquisition and Analysis

Magnetic resonance imaging and spectroscopy data were acquired with a 3T GE MR750 scanner (GE Healthcare, Milwaukee, WI, USA), using an 8-channel receive-only head coil. On the day of the scan, patients were scanned at a time when their dopaminergic medication was wearing off, before their next dose could be taken. The MRI protocol included a 3D T1-weighted fast spoiled gradient echo (SPGR) scan (echo time (TE) = 3 ms, repetition time (TR) = 8 ms, inversion time (TI)=600 ms; voxel resolution = $1 \times 1 \times 1$ mm^3, flip angle=8°), used for localisation of the MRS voxels and correction of the GABA and glutamate levels for partial volume CSF contamination (18).

Single voxel PRESS spectra were acquired from a 3.4 mL (15 × 15 × 15 mm3) voxel in the pons, with TE = 35 ms, TR = 3000 ms, 128 spectral averages, and 16 unsuppressed water reference lines, resulting in a total scan time of 7 min, (see **Figure 1** for an illustration of the voxel positions and representative spectra).

Single-voxel GABA-edited spectra were acquired from a 30 mL voxel centered on the left basal ganglia using the MEGAPRESS method (19), with TE = 69 ms, TR = 1800 ms, 320 spectral averages (160 edit ON/OFF pairs), and an eight-step phase cycle. MEGA-editing was achieved with 16-ms Gaussian editing pulses applied at 1.9 and 7.5 ppm in alternate spectral lines. For each metabolite spectrum, 16 unsuppressed water reference lines were also acquired, resulting in a total acquisition time of 10 min. To achieve a consistent voxel position between participants, voxels were prescribed on an axial plane where the putamen was widest in the lateral (right-left) direction, such that the anterior and medial borders of the voxel were aligned with the anterior and medial margins of the head of the caudate nucleus.

Additional GABA-edited MEGAPRESS spectra were collected from a subset of $n = 31$ participants ($n = 16$ PD patients, $n = 15$ controls), using a 30 mL voxel in in the left prefrontal cortex, with TE = 69 ms, TR = 1800 ms, 320 spectral averages (160 edit ON/OFF pairs), and an eight-step phase cycle. MEGA-editing was achieved as described above for the basal ganglia. In order to achieve a consistent voxel position between participants, the voxel was localized according to a standard set of anatomical measurements. (20).

Spectra were analyzed with LCModel version 6.31-H (21). Edited MEGA-PRESS spectra were analyzed with a simulated basis set including basis spectra for GABA, N-acetyl aspartate (NAA), glutamate (Glu), Glutamine (Gln), glutathione, and N-acetyl aspartyl glutamate (NAAG), using the control parameter sptype=mega-press-3 to avoid mis-assignment of the spectral baseline to the GABA peak (22). Since no attempt was

TABLE 1 | Patient characteristics and MDS-UPDRS scores.

Patient	Disease duration (years)	PD Type	Most affected side	LED	MDS-UPDRS			
					I	II	III	IV
1	18	Akinetic rigid	Right	1500	22	14	31	8
2	14	Tremor-dominant	Right	1300	18	10	41	6
3	5	Tremor-dominant	Right	600	8	15	13	6
4	6	Tremor-dominant	Left	900	17	16	31	4
5	11	Akinetic rigid	Left	1550	15	14	46	9
6	11	Akinetic rigid	Right	1200	10	12	18	1
7	8	Tremor-dominant	Left	800	8	7	25	6
8	8	Akinetic rigid	Left	1500	11	10	27	10
9	16	Akinetic rigid	Right	950	12	14	26	10
10	9	Tremor-dominant	Left	800	13	17	21	8
11	5	Akinetic rigid	Left	750	11	17	26	8
12	11	Akinetic rigid	Left	1500	20	14	31	10
13	12	Akinetic rigid	Right	1550	7	17	33	6
14	8	Tremor-dominant	Left	450	12	14	20	10
15	3	Akinetic rigid	Left	650	23	11	32	0
16	10	Akinetic rigid	Right	850	14	10	21	9
17	12	Akinetic rigid	Right	900	3	5	17	5
18	12	Tremor-dominant	Left	1050	8	12	40	7
19	4	Tremor-dominant	Left	1600	13	15	31	7
20	2	Tremor-dominant	Left	775	15	5	29	6

made to quantify the co-edited macromolecule underlying the GABA peak in the edited MEGAPRESS spectra, the GABA concentrations should be considered to represent GABA+ rather than pure GABA.

PRESS spectra from the pons were analyzed using a standard GE basis set including basis spectra for Alanine, Aspartate, Creatine, GABA, Glucose, Gln, Glu, glycerophosphorylcholine, phosphorylcholine, lactate, myo-inositol, NAA, NAAG, Scyllo-inositol, and Taurine. For all pontine PRESS spectra the default LCModel baseline fit settings were used.

Metabolite concentrations were calculated in institutional units (I.U.) after referencing each metabolite signal to the unsuppressed water signal and correcting both the metabolite and water signals for partial volume CSF contamination within the voxel (18). Additional water and metabolite relaxation time corrections were not performed. Since our hypotheses focused on alterations in the GABA and glutamate systems, only the GABA and Glx (Glu+Gln) levels from the basal ganglia and prefrontal cortex, and the Glx levels from the pons were entered into the statistical analysis (see below for statistical methods).

Symptom Evaluation

Axial symptoms were evaluated from subscales of the Unified Parkinson's Disease rating scale (MDS-UPDRS) (23) including speech/dysarthria (2.1), swallowing (2.3), turning in bed (2.9), arising from a chair (3.9), freezing of gait (2.13, 3.11), gait (3.10), postural stability (3.12), and posture (3.13). Since several symptom scores pertain to gait disturbance, a summary score for the gait symptoms was derived by summing together the individual scores for items 2.13, 3.10, and 3.11, and an overall summary score of the axial symptoms was also derived by adding together the symptom scores from each of the axial subscales. The UPDRS scores were derived while the patients were in the ON medication state.

Statistical Analysis

GABA and Glx concentrations and symptom scores were tested for normality with a Shapiro-Wilk test. Group comparisons (PD vs. control) were assessed with a two-sided *t*-test for normally-distributed variables and a Mann-Whitney test for non-normally distributed variables. A non-parametric bivariate correlation (Spearman's rho) was used to investigate the association between GABA and Glx levels and axial symptom scores from the MDS-UPDRS. In the event of a significant group difference or correlation emerging for Glx, *post-hoc* tests were performed to ascertain if this difference or association was driven by Glu or Gln. Since the patient group included both tremor-dominant and akinetic-rigid PD patients who are known to demonstrate differences in the progression of axial motor symptoms, (24–26) the relationship between GABA and Glx levels and the overall axial summary score was evaluated in the tremor-dominant and akinetic-rigid subgroups separately, after dichotomising patients according to their motor signs at disease onset (27). In the event of a significant association between the axial summary score and neurotransmitter levels emerging in one or both of the

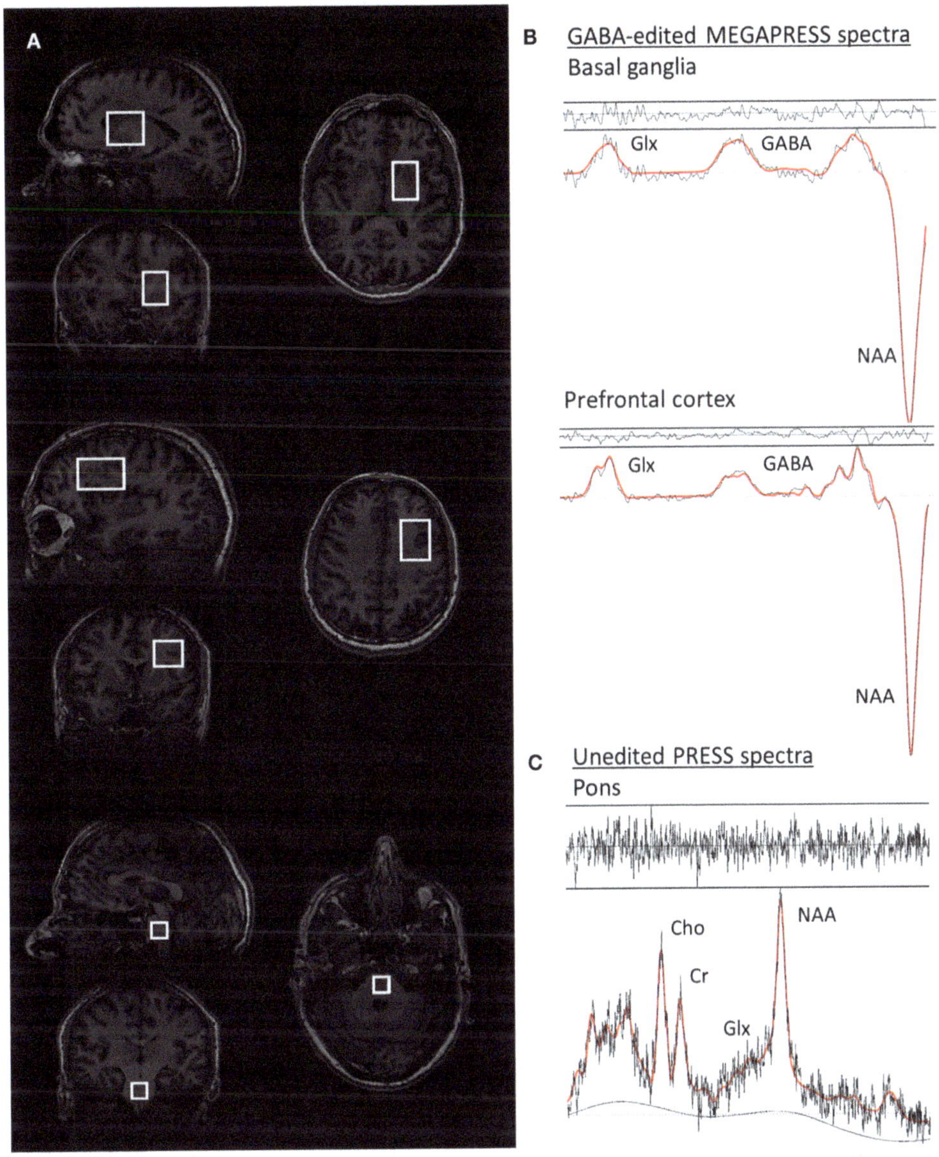

FIGURE 1 | Voxel positions and representative spectra from one PD patient. **(A)** voxel positions from the basal ganglia, prefrontal cortex, and pons voxels, respectively. **(B)** GABA-edited MEGAPRESS spectra from the basal ganglia (top) and prefrontal cortex (middle). The spectral data are plotted in black and the LCModel fit for each spectrum is overlaid in red. **(C)** PRESS spectrum from the pons, with the LCModel fit overlaid in red. For all spectra, the residuals of the fit are plotted above each spectrum.

subgroups, additional *post-hoc* correlations with the individual symptom scores were performed in the relevant subgroup(s) in order to ascertain which symptoms were likely to underly the observed association with neurotransmitter levels. In order to investigate the influence of medication on the association between neurotransmitter levels and symptom scores, additional *post-hoc* correlations were also performed for all significant associations between GABA, Glx, and symptom scores after controlling for the levodopa equivalent dose. All statistical analyses were performed with SPSS version 22, with a two-tailed significance threshold of $p < 0.05$. No correction was made for multiple comparisons.

RESULTS

Representative spectra from the pons, basal ganglia, and prefrontal cortex in one PD participant are shown in **Figure 1**, together with images depicting the voxel positions.

GABA-edited MEGAPRESS data was not collected from one patient with a lesion in the basal ganglia, and the basal ganglia Glx levels were excluded for one patient in whom an artifact was visible over the Glx doublet in the MEGA-PRESS subtraction spectrum.

Glx levels in the pons and GABA levels in the basal ganglia followed a normal distribution, but GABA and Glx levels in the

TABLE 2 | Demographic data and neurotransmitter levels for the PD and control groups.

	PD	Controls	PD vs. Control
Age (Median ± IQR)	62.9 ± 11.5	66.2 ± 12.4	$p = 0.563$
(Mean ± SD)	63.6 ± 6.8	62.5 ± 12.8	
Gender	16 M, 4 F	13 M, 4 F	$p = 0.798$
Left Basal Ganglia GABA[§]	4.61 ± 0.57	3.93 ± 0.75	$p = 0.005$*
Left Basal Ganglia Glx	8.27 ± 3.5	6.66 ± 2.0	$p = 0.069$
Left Prefrontal GABA	3.48 ± 0.90	2.96 ± 0.96	$p = 0.114$
Left Prefrontal Glx	8.19 ± 0.98	7.98 ± 0.84	$p = 0.114$
Pons Glx[§]	13.6 ± 4.02	14.2 ± 3.16	$p = 0.58$

[§]Indicates a normally distributed variable, described by Mean ± SD.
Data are summarized as median ± inter-quartile range and tested with a Mann-Whitney U test unless indicated otherwise. [MRS levels are given in institutional units (I.U.)].

prefrontal cortex and Glx levels in the basal ganglia were not normally distributed ($p < 0.05$, Shapiro–Wilk test). The axial symptom scores and the corresponding summary score were also not normally distributed ($p < 0.05$, Shapiro–Wilk test).

PD and control groups did not differ in terms of age or gender ($p > 0.5$, Mann–Whitney test, see **Table 2**). PD patients demonstrated increased GABA in the basal ganglia ($t = 2.874$, $p = 0.007$, 2-tailed t-test). After removal of one outlier in the PD group with a GABA level 6 standard deviations away from the mean, GABA levels in the basal ganglia remained significantly higher in the PD group ($t = 3.009$, $p = 0.005$, 2-tailed t-test). The corresponding Glx data for this outlier was also removed from further statistical analyses. No significant differences were observed between GABA and Glx levels in the prefrontal cortex or Glx levels in the basal ganglia and pons between the PD and control groups.

Significant associations between GABA and Glx concentrations and axial symptom scores are plotted in **Figure 2**. GABA levels in the left basal ganglia correlated positively with the gait summary score (Spearman's rho = 0.491, $p = 0.038$), as well as the individual gait (MDS 3.10) subscore (Spearman's rho = 0.495, $p = 0.037$) of the motor part of the MDS-UPDRS. Both correlations were present at trend level in the subgroup of akinetic-rigid patients (Gait summary score: Spearman's rho = 0.580, $p = 0.079$, MDS 3.10: Spearman's rho = 0.604, $p = 0.064$), but not in the tremor-dominant subgroup. For the summary score incorporating all the axial symptoms from the UPDRS, basal ganglia GABA levels showed a trend-level association in the full patient group (Spearman's rho = 0.441, $p = 0.067$), which was significant in the subgroup of akinetic rigid patients (Spearman's rho = 0.671, $p = 0.034$), but not in the subgroup of tremor-dominant patients (Spearman's rho = 0.345, $p = 0.403$). In the subgroup of akinetic-rigid patients, basal ganglia GABA levels were significantly correlated with difficulties arising from a chair (MDS 3.9, Spearman's rho = 0.838, p = 0.002 and with posture (MDS 3.13, Spearman's rho = 0.838, $p = 0.002$).

No significant correlations were observed between basal ganglia or pontine Glx levels and the axial symptom scores, but prefrontal Glx levels were negatively correlated with the turning in bed (MDS 2.9) subscore, both in the full patient group (Spearman's rho= −0.546, $p = 0.029$), and in the subgroup of akinetic-rigid patients (Spearman's rho = −0.686, $p = 0.041$). Prefrontal GABA levels were negatively correlated with the postural stability score (MDS 3.12, Spearman's rho = - 0.842, $p = 0.004$), in the akinetic-rigid subgroup only.

The correlations between basal ganglia GABA and the gait subscore and summary score became non-significant after controlling for the levodopa equivalent dose (Spearman's rho=0.324/0.341, $p = 0.224/0.196$ for the gait summary score and subscore, respectively), as did the correlation between basal ganglia GABA levels and the axial symptom summary score in the akinetic-rigid subgroup (Spearman's rho =0.403, $p = 0.322$) However, correlations between basal ganglia GABA levels and difficulties arising from a chair (MDS 3.9) remained significant in the akinetic-rigid subgroup after controlling for levodopa equivalent dose (Spearman's rho = 0.845, $p = 0.008$), as did the correlation between basal ganglia GABA and problems with posture (MDS 3.13, Spearman's rho = 0.845, $p = 0.008$). The correlation between prefrontal Glx and turning in bed diminished to trend level after controlling for levodopa equivalent dose (Spearman's rho = −0.491, $p = 0.074$), but the correlation between prefrontal GABA and difficulties with postural stability (MDS 3.12) in the akinetic-rigid subgroup remained significant after controlling for the levodopa equivalent dose (Spearman's rho = −0.76, $p = 0.047$).

DISCUSSION

Gait and locomotion, turning in bed, arising from a chair, and postural stability all depend on efficient sensorimotor integration (28, 29), which is affected in PD (30–32). The basal ganglia act as an important hub for sensorimotor integration (33, 34) and descending basal ganglia projections to the midbrain have been reported to play an important role in gait and postural control (35, 36). One of the ways in which the basal ganglia are thought to influence sensorimotor integration is by gating or controlling the access of sensory information to motor neurons, via a balance of neurotransmitter activity (30, 37, 38). In PD, the motor systems can become hypo-excitable following an increased inhibition of sensory inputs to the basal ganglia, leading to a diminished motor response to certain sensory stimuli (30). This diminished responsiveness to sensory stimuli is thought to underly the observed difficulties experienced by PD patients in regulating the amplitude of movements in the absence of external visual or auditory cues, when they are dependent on sensory feedback for accurate motor control, (31, 32, 38) and may also contribute to the axial symptoms.

In the present study, the observed link between increased GABA levels in the left basal ganglia in PD patients and the degree of gait disturbance (**Figure 2**) may be associated with an over-inhibition of the processing of sensory inputs necessary for maintaining posture and initiating locomotion. This observation is consistent with the reported role of GABAergic outputs from the basal ganglia in the control of posture and locomotion (35, 39, 40). However, since locomotion can be initiated by stimulation

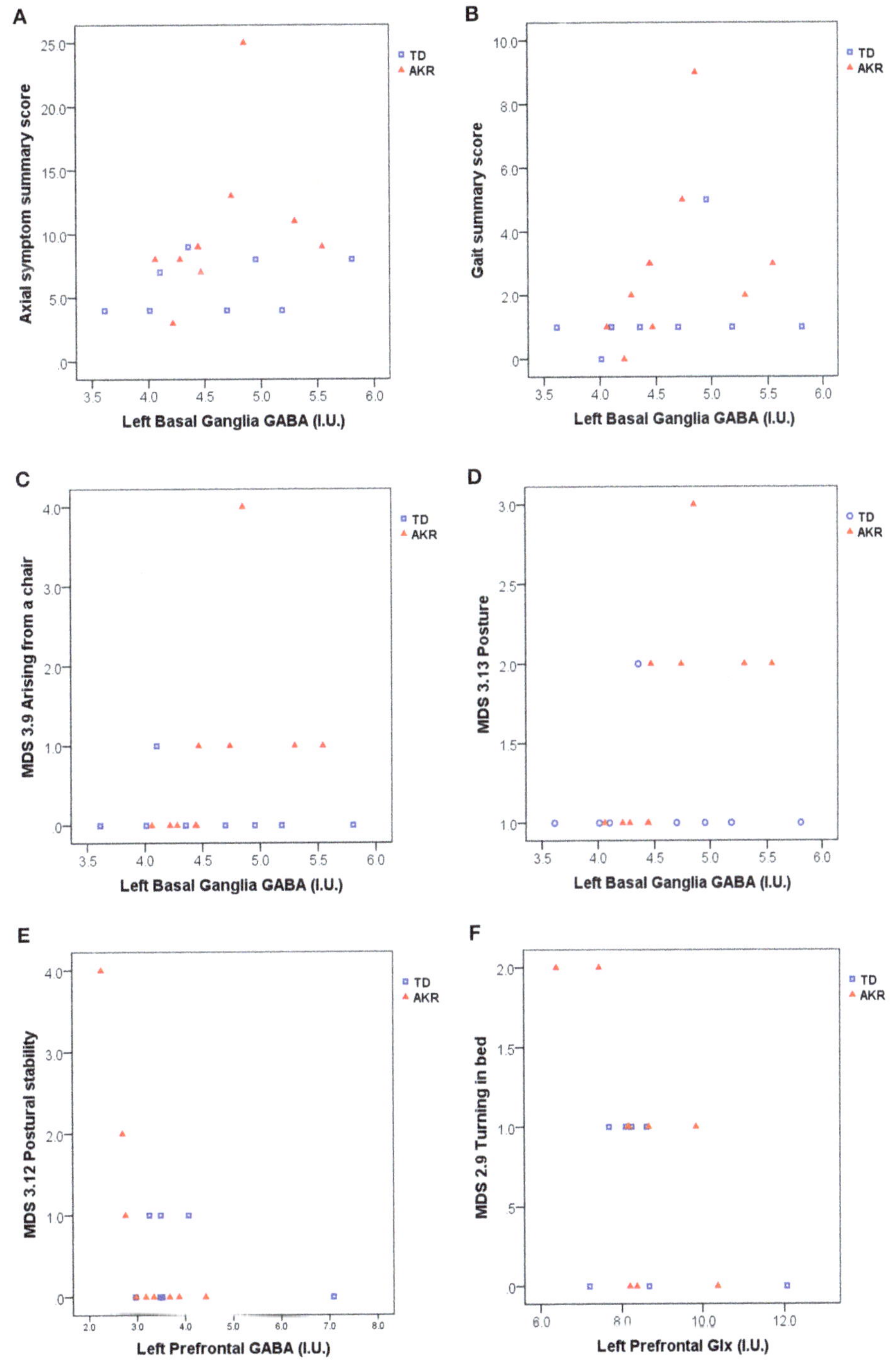

FIGURE 2 | Basal ganglia GABA, prefrontal GABA and prefrontal Glx appear to be associated with axial symptom scores including gait and postural difficulties assessed with the MDS-UPDRS. **(A)** left basal ganglia GABA levels were significantly associated with higher axial symptom summary scores in akinetic-rigid (AKR) patients ($p = 0.034$), but not in tremor-dominant (TD) patients ($p = 0.403$), while the full patient group showed a trend-level association between basal ganglia GABA and axial summary scores ($p = 0.067$). **(B)** Elevated GABA levels were also associated higher gait summary scores ($p = 0.038$, full group). In the AKR subgroup, increased GABA levels were significantly positively associated with difficulties arising from a chair (**C**, $p = 0.002$) and difficulties with posture (**D**, $p = 0.002$). Left prefrontal GABA levels were negatively associated with postural stability in the AKR subgroup ($p = 0.004$, **E**), while left prefrontal Glx levels were negatively associated difficulties turning in bed, both in the full group ($p = 0.029$, **F**), and in the AKR subgroup ($p = 0.041$, **F**).

of the midbrain locomotor region, (36) one would expect corresponding neurotransmitter abnormalities to be observed in the pons, related to problems with gait. In the present study, we were not able to measure GABA in the pons due to the large voxel size required for GABA measurement with MEGA-PRESS, but we did not observe any apparent relationship between the pontine Glx concentrations (from standard PRESS) and problems with gait. However, since the PRESS voxel volume (3.4 mL) is large in comparison to the size of the midbrain locomotor region or the peduculopontine nucleus of the pons, two of the pontine regions implicated in gait control and muscle tone regulation, the lack of an apparent relationship between pontine Glx and posture or gait symptoms may be due to a lack of regional specificity of the pontine MRS measurement. Future studies at higher field strengths (e.g., 7T), where smaller voxel volumes can be used and where GABA can be quantified without the need for spectral editing, may be able to extend the present findings to clarify the link between gait difficulties and pontine neurotransmitter levels.

In the subgroup analysis, the observed link between basal ganglia GABA levels and the gait and axial summary scores seemed to be mostly driven by GABA and symptom changes in the akinetic-rigid subgroup of patients rather than the tremor-dominant patients. Longitudinal studies have shown that the akinetic-rigid subtype of PD presents a risk factor for greater progression of the motor symptoms, including freezing of gait and other axial symptoms. (24–26) Akinetic-rigid PD patients have also been shown to demonstrate differences in structural and functional connectivity in comparison to tremor-dominant patients, (41–43) and differences in iron deposition between the subtypes indicates that different pathological mechanisms may underly the observed differences in symptom progression (44). In light of the small group sizes, the subgroup analysis in the present study should be considered exploratory, and we hope these results can be replicated in a larger sample. Given the evidence for differences in brain structure and function as well as symptom progression in different subtypes of PD, it would be interesting to examine differences in the metabolite profile, including neurotransmitter changes, between akinetic-rigid and tremor-dominant PD patients in more detail in a larger cohort.

While basal ganglia GABA levels appeared to be related to gait difficulties, prefrontal Glx levels correlated negatively with difficulties turning in bed (**Figure 2**), and prefrontal GABA levels correlated negatively with postural stability, in the akinetic-rigid subgroup. The negative correlation between prefrontal Glx and symptom scores would be consistent with previous reports of decreased cortical Glx in PD, (11) under the assumption that patients more severely affected by axial symptoms like turning in bed would have lower prefrontal Glx levels. However, since in the present study no significant differences in prefrontal Glx were observed at the group level, the apparent correlation between frontal Glx and symptom scores seen in the present study cannot be interpreted in the context of abnormal Glx levels in the patient group. The link between prefrontal GABA and posture is also consistent with the putative role of prefrontal and parietal cortical regions in maintaining postural equilibrium, (45) but should also be interpreted with caution in light of the lack of a significant difference in prefrontal GABA between the patient and control groups. It is possible that these associations with individual symptom scores may be affected by outliers, given the small group sizes and the limited distribution of symptoms in some domains. These results should therefore be considered with caution until they can be replicated in a larger sample.

Since the symptom scores were assessed while patients were in the ON medication state, while the MRS was performed just before the next dose was due and thus rather in an OFF state, medication effects could potentially confound the comparison between GABA and Glx levels and the axial symptom scores. While most of the axial symptoms do not typically respond well to levodopa, dopamine replacement therapy has been reported to reduce freezing of gait in patients with PD, (46) and in the present sample the levodopa equivalent dose showed a trend-level association with basal ganglia GABA ($p = 0.09$, Spearman's rho). The effect of levodopa on freezing of gait may explain why the correlations between basal ganglia GABA levels and the gait and axial symptom summary scores diminished in significance after controlling for the levodopa equivalent dose, particularly in akinetic-rigid patients. In contrast, the association between neurotransmitter levels and other symptom scores such as rising from a chair, turning in bed, posture, and postural stability, seemed relatively independent of levodopa effects, but in addition to levodopa 11 patients were additionally medicated with dopamine agonists. Previous studies in children with attention deficit hyperactivity disorder (ADHD) have reported that treatment with dopamine agonists like methylphenidate can reduce striatal Glx levels (47), although methylphenidate did not appear to influence frontal Glx levels, (47) and another study of medication-naïve and medicated adults with ADHD failed to find differences in Glx related to medication status (48). However, since treatment with dopamine agonists or other medications may introduce additional variability into the Glx and GABA signals measured MRS, it would be instructive to clarify the effects of dopaminergic and other medications on the GABA and Glx levels in a future study, where the cohort of PD patients is sufficiently large to enable separation into subgroups according to medication status.

CONCLUSION

MRS offers a unique opportunity to study the complex interplay between excitatory and inhibitory neurotransmitter activity both within and outside the motor network. The present pilot study provides evidence of a link between alterations in GABA and glutamate levels and the axial symptoms of Parkinson's disease, lending important insight into the neural origin of these symptoms, and opening up potential avenues for treatment.

AUTHOR CONTRIBUTIONS

RO: conception, organization, and execution of research project, design and execution of data analysis, and writing of the first draft of the manuscript. CB: conception of Research Project, design and review and critique of data analysis, and review and critique of the manuscript. HB-V: conception, organization, and execution of research project, design and review and critique of data analysis, and review and critique of the manuscript.

REFERENCES

1. Dorsey ER, Constantinescu R, Thompson JP, Biglan KM, Holloway RG, Kieburtz F. Projected number of people with Parkinson disease in the most populous nations, 2005 through 2030. *Neurology* (2007) 68:384–6. doi: 10.1212/01.wnl.0000247740.47667.03
2. Deane KH, Flaherty H, Daley DJ, Pascoe R, Penhale B, Clarke CE. et al. Priority setting partnership to identify the top 10 research priorities for the management of Parkinson's disease. *BMJ Open* (2014) 4:e006434. doi: 10.1136/bmjopen-2014-006434
3. Jankovic J, and Aguilar LG. Current approaches to the treatment of Parkinson's disease. *Neuropsychiatr Dis Treat* (2008) 4:743–57. doi: 10.2147/NDT.S2006
4. Bonnet AM. Involvement of non-dopaminergic pathways in Parkinson's disease. *CNS Drugs* (2000) 13:351–64. doi: 10.2165/00023210-200013050-00005
5. Barone P. Neurotransmission in Parkinson's disease: beyond dopamine. *Eur J Neurol.* (2010) 17:364–376. doi: 10.1111/j.1468-1331.2009.02900.x
6. Karachi C, Grabli D, Bernard FA, Tande D, Wattiez N, Belaid H. et al. Cholinergic mesencephalic neurons are involved in gait and postural disorders in Parkinson disease. *J Clin Invest.* (2010) 120:2745–54. doi: 10.1172/JCI42642
7. Rae CD. A guide to the metabolic pathways and function of metabolites observed in human brain 1H magnetic resonance spectra. *Neurochem Res.* (2014) 39:1–36. doi: 10.1007/s11064-013-1199-5
8. Emir UE, Tuite PJ, Oz G. Elevated pontine and putamenal GABA levels in mild-moderate Parkinson disease detected by 7 tesla proton MRS. *PLoS ONE* (2012) 7:e30918. doi: 10.1371/journal.pone.0030918
9. Dharmadhikari S, Ma R, Yeh CL, Stock AK, Snyder S, Zauber SE, et al. Striatal and thalamic GABA level concentrations play differential roles for the modulation of response selection processes by proprioceptive information. *Neuroimage* (2015) 120:36–42. doi: 10.1016/j.neuroimage.2015.06.066
10. O'Gorman Tuura RL, Baumann CR, Baumann-Vogel H. Neurotransmitter activity is linked to outcome following subthalamic deep brain stimulation in Parkinson's disease. *Parkins Relat Disord.* (2018) 50:54–60. doi: 10.1016/j.parkreldis.2018.02.014
11. Griffith, HR, Okonkwo OC, O'Brien T, Hollander JA. Reduced brain glutamate in patients with Parkinson's disease. *NMR Biomed.* (2008) 21:381–7. doi: 10.1002/nbm.1203
12. Oz G, Terpstra M, Tkac I, Aia P, Lowary J, Gruetter PJ. Proton MRS of the unilateral substantia nigra in the human brain at 4 tesla: detection of high GABA concentrations. *Magn Reson Med.* (2006) 55:296–301. doi: 10.1002/mrm.20761
13. Foy CM, Daly EM, Glover A, O'Gorman R, Simmons A, Murphy DG. et al. Hippocampal proton MR spectroscopy in early Alzheimer's disease and mild cognitive impairment. *Brain Topogr.* (2011) 24:316–22. doi: 10.1007/s10548-011-0170-5
14. Riese F, Gietl A, Zolch N, Henning A, O'Gorman R, Kalin AM, et al. Posterior cingulate gamma-aminobutyric acid and glutamate/glutamine are reduced in amnestic mild cognitive impairment and are unrelated to amyloid deposition and apolipoprotein E genotype. *Neurobiol Aging* (2015) 36:53–9. doi: 10.1016/j.neurobiolaging.2014.07.030
15. Kalueff AV, Nutt DJ. Role of GABA in anxiety and depression. *Depress Anxiety* (2007) 24:495–517. doi: 10.1002/da.20262
16. Brooks PL, Peever JH. Impaired GABA and glycine transmission triggers cardinal features of rapid eye movement sleep behavior disorder in mice. *J Neurosci.* (2011)31:7111–21. doi: 10.1523/JNEUROSCI.0347-11.2011
17. Chahine LM, Kauta SR Daley JT, Cantor CR, Dahodwala N. Surface EMG activity during REM sleep in Parkinson's disease correlates with disease severity. *Parkins Relat Disord.* (2014) 20:766–71. doi: 10.1016/j.parkreldis.2014.04.011
18. Chowdhury FA, O'Gorman RL, Nashef L, Elwes RD, Edden RA, Murdoch JB. et al. Investigation of glutamine and GABA levels in patients with idiopathic generalized epilepsy using megapress. *J Magn Reson Imaging* (2015) 41:694–99. doi: 10.1002/jmri.24611
19. Mescher M, Merkle H, Kirsch J, Garwood M, Gruetter R. Simultaneous *in vivo* spectral editing and water suppression. *NMR Biomed.* (1998) 11:266–72. doi: 10.1002/(SICI)1099-1492(199810)11:6<266::AID-NBM530>3.0.CO;2-J
20. Michels L, Martin E, Klaver P, Edden R, Zelaya F, LythgoeDJ. et al. Frontal GABA levels change during working memory. *PLoS ONE* (2012) 7:e31933. doi: 10.1371/journal.pone.0031933
21. Provencher SW. Estimation of metabolite concentrations from localized *in vivo* proton NMR spectra. *Magn Reson Med.* (1993) 30:672–9. doi: 10.1002/mrm.1910300604
22. Mullins PG, McGonigle DJ, O'Gorman RL, Puts NA, Vidyasagar R, Evans CJ, et al. Current practice in the use of MEGA-PRESS spectroscopy for the detection of GABA. *Neuroimage* (2014) 86:43–52. doi: 10.1016/j.neuroimage.2012.12.004
23. Goetz CG, Tilley BC, Shaftman SR, Stebbins GT, Fahn S, Martinez-Martin P. et al. Movement disorder society-sponsored revision of the unified parkinson's disease rating scale (MDS-UPDRS): scale presentation and clinimetric testing results. *Mov Disord.* (2008) 23:2129–70. doi: 10.1002/mds.22340
24. Post B, Merkus MP, de Haan RJ, Speelman JD. Prognostic factors for the progression of Parkinson's disease: a systematic review. *Mov Disord.* (2007) 22:1839–51; quiz 1988. doi: 10.1002/mds.21537
25. Reinoso G, Allen JC, Au WL, Seah SH, Tay KY, Tan LC. Clinical evolution of Parkinson's disease and prognostic factors affecting motor progression: 9-year follow-up study. *Eur J Neurol.* (2015) 22:457–63. doi: 10.1111/ene.12476
26. Zhang H, Yin X, Ouyang Z, Chen J, Zhou S, Zhang C. et al. A prospective study of freezing of gait with early Parkinson disease in Chinese patients. *Medicine (Baltimore)* (2016) 95:e4056. doi: 10.1097/MD.0000000000004056
27. Baumann CR, Held U, Valko PO, Wienecke M, Waldvogel D. Body side and predominant motor features at the onset of Parkinson's disease are linked to motor and nonmotor progression. *Mov Disord.* (2014) 29:207–13. doi: 10.1002/mds.25650
28. Peterka RJ. Sensorimotor integration in human postural control. *J Neurophysiol.* (2002) 88:1097–118. doi: 10.1152/jn.2002.88.3.1097
29. Hickok G, Houde J, Rong F. Sensorimotor integration in speech processing: computational basis and neural organization. *Neuron* (2011) 69:407–22. doi: 10.1016/j.neuron.2011.01.019
30. Schneider JS, Diamond SG, Markham CH. Deficits in orofacial sensorimotor function in Parkinson's disease. *Ann Neurol.* (1986) 19:275–82. doi: 10.1002/ana.410190309
31. Lewis GN, Byblow WD. Altered sensorimotor integration in Parkinson's disease. *Brain* (2002) 125(Pt. 9):2089–99. doi: 10.1093/brain/awf200
32. Abbruzzese G, Berardelli A. Sensorimotor integration in movement disorders. *Mov Disord.* (2003) 18:231–40. doi: 10.1002/mds.10327
33. De Long MR, Alexander GE. *The Basal Ganglia and Sensorimotor Integration.* Berlin: Springer Berlin Heidelberg (1987).
34. Albin RL, Young AB, Penney JB. The functional anatomy of basal ganglia disorders. *Trends Neurosci.* (1989) 12:366–75. doi: 10.1016/0166-2236(89)90074-X
35. Takakusaki K, Habaguchi T, Ohtinata-Sugimoto J, Saitoh K, Sakamoto T. Basal ganglia efferents to the brainstem centers controlling postural muscle tone and locomotion: a new concept for understanding motor disorders in basal ganglia dysfunction. *Neuroscience* (2003) 119:293–308. doi: 10.1016/S0306-4522(03)00095-2
36. Hikosaka O. GABAergic output of the basal ganglia. *Prog Brain Res.* (2007) 160:209–26. doi: 10.1016/S0079-6123(06)60012-5
37. Schneider JS, Denaro FJ, Lidsky TI. Basal ganglia: motor influences mediated by sensory interactions. *Exp Neurol.* (1982) 77:534–43. doi: 10.1016/0014-4886(82)90226-6
38. Adamovich SV, Berkinblit MB, Hening W, Sage J, Poizner H. The interaction of visual and proprioceptive inputs in pointing to actual and remembered targets in Parkinson's disease. *Neuroscience* (2001) 104:1027–1041. doi: 10.1016/S0306-4522(01)00099-9
39. Garcia-Rill E. The basal ganglia and the locomotor regions. *Brain Res.* (1986) 396:47–63. doi: 10.1016/0165-0173(86)90009-3
40. Takakusaki K, Saitoh K, Harada H, Kashiwayanagi M. Role of basal ganglia-brainstem pathways in the control of motor behaviors. *Neurosci Res.* (2004) 50:137–51. doi: 10.1016/j.neures.2004.06.015
41. Lewis MM, Du G, Sen S, Kawaguchi A, Truong Y, Lee S, et al. Differential involvement of striato- and cerebello-thalamo-cortical pathways in tremor- and akinetic/rigid-predominant Parkinson's disease. *Neuroscience* (2011) 177:230–9. doi: 10.1016/j.neuroscience.2010.12.060

42. Guan X, Xuan M, Gu Q, Xu X, Huang P, Wang N, et al. Influence of regional iron on the motor impairments of Parkinson's disease: a quantitative susceptibility mapping study. *J Magn Reson Imaging* (2017) 45:1335–42. doi: 10.1002/jmri.25434
43. Luo C, Song W, Chen Q, Yang J, Gong Q, Shang HF. White matter microstructure damage in tremor-dominant Parkinson's disease patients. *Neuroradiology* (2017) 59:691–8. doi: 10.1007/s00234-017-1846-7
44. Jin L, Wang J, Jin H, Fei G, Zhang Y, Chen W, et al. Nigral iron deposition occurs across motor phenotypes of Parkinson's disease. *Eur J Neurol.* (2012) 19:969–76. doi: 10.1111/j.1468-1331.2011.03658.x
45. Jacobs, J. V and Horak, F. B. Cortical control of postural responses. *J Neural Transm (Vienna)* (2007) 114:1339–48. doi: 10.1007/s00702-007-0657-0
46. Schaafsma JD, Balash Y, Gurevich T, Bartels AL, Hausdorff JM, Giladi N. Characterization of freezing of gait subtypes and the response of each to levodopa in Parkinson's disease. *Eur J Neurol.* (2003) 10:391–98. doi: 10.1046/j.1468-1331.2003.00611.x
47. Carrey N, MacMaster FP, Sparkes SJ, Khan SC, Kusumakar V. Glutamatergic changes with treatment in attention deficit hyperactivity disorder: a preliminary case series. *J Child Adolesc Psychopharmacol.* (2002) 12:331–36. doi: 10.1089/104454602762599871
48. Maltezos S, Horder J, Coghlan S, Skirrow C, O'Gorman R, Lavender, T. J. et al. Glutamate/glutamine and neuronal integrity in adults with ADHD: a proton MRS study. *Transl Psychiatry* (2014) 4:e373. doi: 10.1038/tp.2014.11

11

Identification of Cellular Pathogenicity Markers for SIL1 Mutations Linked to Marinesco-Sjögren Syndrome

*Christian Gatz[1], Denisa Hathazi[2,3], Ute Münchberg[2], Stephan Buchkremer[1], Thomas Labisch[1], Ben Munro[3], Rita Horvath[3], Ana Töpf[4], Joachim Weis[1] and Andreas Roos[1,2,5]**

[1] *Institute of Neuropathology, RWTH Aachen University Hospital, Aachen, Germany,* [2] *Leibniz-Institut für Analytische Wissenschaften—ISAS—e.V., Dortmund, Germany,* [3] *Department of Clinical Neuroscience, University of Cambridge, Cambridge, United Kingdom,* [4] *International Centre for Life, Institute of Genetic Medicine, Newcastle upon Tyne, United Kingdom,* [5] *Pediatric Neurology, Faculty of Medicine, University Childrens Hospital, University of Duisburg-Essen, Essen, Germany*

***Correspondence:**
Andreas Roos
andreas.roos@uk-essen.de;
andreas.roos@isas.de

Background and objective: Recessive mutations in the *SIL1* gene cause Marinesco-Sjögren syndrome (MSS), a rare neuropediatric disorder. MSS-patients typically present with congenital cataracts, intellectual disability, cerebellar ataxia and progressive vacuolar myopathy. However, atypical clinical presentations associated with *SIL1* mutations have been described over the last years; compound heterozygosity of SIL1 missense mutations even resulted in a phenotype not fulfilling the clinical diagnostic criteria of MSS. Thus, a read-out system to evaluate reliably the pathogenicity of amino acid changes in *SIL1* is needed. Here, we aim to provide suitable cellular biomarkers enabling the robust evaluation of pathogenicity of SIL1 mutations.

Methods: Five *SIL1* variants including one polymorphism (p.K132Q), three known pathogenic mutations (p.V231_I232del, p.G312R, and p.L457P) and one ambiguous missense variant (p.R92W) were studied along with the wild-type proteins in Hek293 *in vitro* models by cell biological assays, immunoprecipitation, immunoblotting, and immunofluorescence as well as electron microscopy. Moreover, the SIL1-interactomes were interrogated by tandem-affinity-purification and subsequent mass spectrometry.

Results: Our combined studies confirmed the pathogenicity of p.V231_I232del, p.G312R, and p.L457P by showing instability of the proteins as well as tendency to form aggregates. This observation is in line with altered structure of the ER-Golgi system and vacuole formation upon expression of these pathogenic SIL1-mutants as well as the presence of oxidative or ER-stress. Reduced cellular fitness along with abnormal mitochondrial architecture could also be observed. Notably, both the polymorphic p.K132Q and the ambiguous p.R92W variants did not elicit such alterations. Study of the SIL1-interactome identified POC1A as a novel binding partner of wild-type SIL1; the interaction is disrupted upon the presence of pathogenic mutants but not influenced by the presence of benign variants. Disrupted SIL1-POC1A interaction is associated with centrosome disintegration.

Conclusions: We developed a combination of cellular outcome measures to evaluate the pathogenicity of *SIL1* variants in suitable *in vitro* models and demonstrated that the p. R92W missense variant is a polymorphism rather than a pathogenic mutation leading to MSS.

Keywords: SIL1-interactome, Marinesco-Sjögren syndrome biomarkers, SIL1 missense mutation, POC1A, FAM134B, centrosome

INTRODUCTION

Marinesco-Sjögren syndrome (MSS) was established as an entity by the Romanian neurologist Georges Marinesco in 1931 based on the description of four individuals from a single family presenting with ataxia, cataracts, intellectual disability, and myopathy. This was followed by Torsten Sjögren who further defined the original four cases as well as 10 additional patients. Afterwards, cerebellar atrophy was described as part of the phenotypic spectrum (1). In 2005, two groups independently reported recessive mutations in the *SIL1* gene as the major genetic cause for MSS (2, 3). *SIL1* encodes a co-chaperone for the major Endoplasmic Reticulum (ER)-resident chaperone BiP and thus controls a variety of BiP-dependent functions such as protein folding (4). Hereby, SIL1 acts as a N-linked glycoprotein equipped with an N-terminal ER targeting sequence and a C-terminal ER retention signal. SIL1 dimerises at the N-terminus into a clamp-like configuration that interacts with the BiP ATPase domain and causes substrate release of BiP via the release of ADP (5).

The "clinical triad" of MSS is defined by presence of bilateral cataracts, ataxia, and myopathy whereas intellectual disability can manifest with very varying degree or can even be absent (6). So far, a clear genotype-phenotype correlation does not exist, and the phenotypical presentation becomes even more complex by the description of additional features: pectus carinatum and bilateral clinodactyly in a patient with a homozygous large indel in the $5'$UTR (7), Dandy-Walker malformations in a Chinese family with a non-stop mutation (8) and associated motor neuronopathy with a bradykinetic movement disorder in a 5-year-old child, suggesting an intriguing continuum between neurodevelopmental and neurodegenerative multisystem disorders intricately linked in the same cellular pathways (9). Moreover, the phenotypical variation has become even more complex by the first report of compound heterozygous *SIL1* missense mutations causing a neurological phenotype without signs of myopathy or cataracts but including spastic paraplegia, thus not fulfilling the clinical diagnostic criteria for MSS (10). Interestingly, the number of detected *SIL1* variants ($n = 488$; ExAC http://exac.broadinstitute.org/) as of 11/2018 includes 147 missense and 7 non-sense variants with various effects on the phenotype. Notably, these missense mutations also include the p.R92W variant of SIL1, described as segregating with the phenotype in a consanguineous family from Pakistan (11) but reported in ExAC with an allele frequency of nearly 4% in south Asian countries suggesting a polymorphic character. Given that *(i)* the MSS phenotype can present with prominent additional clinical features or characteristic features of the "clinical triad" can be absent, *(ii)* missense mutations may have a detrimental effect (10) and *(iii)* the detection of new *SIL1* sequence variants ever increasing in number, the need to classify the pathogenicity is indicated. Here we introduce an *in vitro* system designed to examine the consequences of *SIL1* mutations at the protein level, focussing on the stability of the variant SIL1 proteins, the morphology of cellular organelles, the build-up of aggregated proteins, the activation of proteolysis and on the SIL1-interactome. This procedure has allowed to differentiate between benign and pathogenic variants (mostly due to amino acid changes).

MATERIALS AND METHODS

Generation of SIL1-TAP and SIL1-HA Expression Constructs

Using the SIL1-TAP expression construct (pcDNA5/FRT/TO vector) (12) missense variants (listed below) as well as one deletion variant of recombinant human *SIL1* were generated by site-directed mutagenesis. To this end, the QuikChange Site-Directed Mutagenesis kit (Stratagene) was used according to the manufacturer's instructions. Primer sequences are available on request. All constructs were verified by sequencing the entire coding region of the inserts.

The ORF of the human *SIL1* cDNA was cloned in-frame into the carboxy-terminal hemagglutinin (HA) tag containing pRC/CMV expression vector. The same missense changes as for the pcDNA5/FRT/TO vector systems were introduced by site-directed mutagenesis using the QuikChange Site-Directed Mutagenesis kit (Stratagene). Primer sequences are available on request. All constructs were verified by sequencing the entire coding region of the inserts.

The following *SIL1* variants were selected and generated as expression systems based on the following reasons:

p.R92W

A missense variant of ambiguous pathogenic character: reported to cause MSS in a consanguineous Pakistani family (11) but present in ExAC with an allele frequency of nearly 4% and hereby also found to be homozygous in south Asian populations. Evaluation of its pathogenicity was one aim of the present study to address the suitability of our introduced *in vitro* system along with different tests.

p.K132Q

A missense variant of benign character (polymorphism) serving as a control. which should give the same results as the wild-type form of the SIL1 protein.

p.V231_I232del

A deletion variant with well-known pathogenicity based on stability of the protein as described previously by immunoblot and proteomics-based studies of MSS-patient-derived immortalized lymphoblastoid cells (6, 13).

p.G312R

A missense variant of well-known pathogenicity based on stability of the protein as described previously by immunoblot- and proteomics-based studies of MSS-patient derived immortalized lymphoblastoid cells (6, 13).

p.L457P

A missense variant with well-known pathogenicity *in vitro* tested in COS7 cells and associated with clinical presentation of MSS (14).

Cell Culture and Treatments:

Using the six pcDNA/FRT/TO-based expression constructs for SIL1-TAP (wild-type and five variants), stable inducible Hek293-TRex cell lines were generated as described previously (12). Cells were cultured in Dulbecco's Modified Eagle's medium (DMEM; Sigma-D5546) supplemented with 10 fetal calf serum (FCS; Sigma- F2442). Transient transfection of pRC/CMV-based constructs for SIL1-HA wildtype and variants was performed utilizing Lipofectamine 2000 (Thermo Fisher Scientific) according to the manufacturer's instructions.

Immunoprecipitation of the SIL1 Variants:

As SIL1 can act as a dimer (5), the ability to form protein dimers was addressed for the five protein variants of SIL1. Dimerization of the wildtype-protein was examined as a positive control to demonstrate functionality of the assay. The generated stable inducible Hek293-TRex cell lines (grown on 10 cm dishes) were additionally transfected with pRC/CMV-based constructs for SIL1-HA wildtype and variants and were collected 8 h post-transfection. Afterwards, cells were lysed in 500 μl of a buffer containing 1 mM EDTA (Sigma-Aldrich), 10% (v/v) glycerol (Roth), 20 mm HEPES (pH 7.5; Sigma-Aldrich), 150 mM NaCl (Sigma-Aldrich) and 0.8% (v/v) NP-40 (Roth) as well as 1 × Complete Protease Inhibitor Cocktail (Roche) for 1 h on ice. Next, centrifugation (1.500 rpm) of the lysates was performed at 4°C for 10 min to separate the protein extracts from cell debris. Protein concentrations were determined using the Pierce BCA protein assay kit (Thermo Fisher) according to manufacturer's instructions. Immunoprecipitation of the different HA-tagged forms of the SIL1 proteins via the TAP-tagged forms was carried out as described previously (12) using 100 μg of total protein extract.

For each experiment, cells overexpressing the solely the C-terminal TAP-Tag were included to exclude unspecific binding of the HA-Tagged versions of the SIL1 protein to the TAP-tag. All co-immunoprecipitation experiments were carried out three times.

Tandem-Affinity Purification of SIL1-Interactome and LC-MS/MS-Based Identification of Binding Partners

Interaction screening [tandem-affinity-purification (15) and subsequent mass spectrometry] of SIL1 wildtype protein as well as the five variant forms was carried out as described previously (6, 12) For each experiment, three independent biological replicates were analyzed.

Investigation of Cellular Fitness

Cellular fitness of Hek293-TRex cell lines overexpressing the wildtype SIL1 protein as well as of cells overexpressing the five variants was addressed by utilizing the WST-1 assay (Roche), according to the manufacturer's instructions. Cells treated with H_2O_2 were included as a positive control of decreased cellular fitness to demonstrate functionality of the assay. Moreover, cells overexpressing the TAP-Tag only were included to demonstrate that the presence/expression of the TAP-tag has no effect on cellular fitness. The relative absorption in cells overexpressing the SIL1 wildtype protein was considered as 100% of cellular fitness.

Native-PAGE, SDS-PAGE and Western Blotting:

Native-PAGE was carried out as described in a protocol available online (http://www.assay-protocol.com/molecular-biology/electrophoresis/native-page) and the immunoblot studies were performed as described previously (16). The following antibodies were used:

Immunofluorescence:

Distribution of SIL1 wildtype protein as well as of the five different variants was addressed in the stable inducible Hek293-TRex cell lines: the respective cell lines (2×10^5 cells) were plated onto 24-well plates on coverslips 12 h prior to induction of expression with doxycycline as described before (12). Beforehand, coverslips were coated with poly-L-lysine (Sigma-Aldrich) for 1 h at room and afterwards washed twice with ultra-pure water. Cells were fixed with 4% paraformaldehyde in PBS pH 7.4 for 20 min at room temperature. Afterwards, cells were washed 3 times with ice-cold PBS. For permeabilization, coverslips were incubated for 10 min in PBS containing 0.25% Triton X-100 (Roth). In the following step, cells were washed in PBS 3 times for 5 min. For blocking and immunostaining, coverslips were incubated in 1% BSA (in PBS+ 0.1% Tween 20) for 45 min and afterwards exposed to the anti-TAP antibody (Sigma-Aldrich) 1:100 diluted in 1% BSA in PBST in a humidified chamber overnight at 4°C. Afterwards, coverslips were washed 3 times in PBS (5 min each washing step) and then incubated with the secondary antibody (goat anti-rabbit Alexa Fluor® 568, Abcam) diluted 1:5,000 in 1% BSA-PBS for 1 h at room temperature in the dark. Next, three washing steps times in PBS (5 min each washing step) were carried out. Finally, cells were mounted with a drop of mounting medium (Thermo Fisher) and coverslips were sealed with nail polish to prevent drying and movement under microscope. For analysis of immunoreactivity, the Axiovert 200 M microscope from Zeiss (240525) was used. For each SIL1 variant as well as for the wildtype proteins 50 different cells were analyzed with more than 70% of cells giving similar results, respectively.

For co-localization studies of SIL1, Hek293 cells were permeabilized by incubation with 200 μL PBS buffer containing 0.1% Triton X-100 for 10 min and subsequently washed with PBS buffer. For blocking cells were incubated with 200 μL of PBS containing 0.1% TWEEN20 and 1% BSA for 30 min. Afterwards, cells were covered with 200 μL of blocking solution containing the respective combinations of both primary antibodies [α-CASQ1 (Sigma: C0618-200UL), α-FAM134B (Genetex: GTX46621), α-POC1A (Thermo Fisher Scientific: PA5-49028), α-SIL1 (Abcam: ab5639) dilution 1:300 each], incubated for 90 min and then washed with PBS. Secondary antibodies were diluted in 1% BSA (dilution 1:500 for Alexa488 probe, 1:300 for Alexa555 probe). Cells were covered with 200 μl of this antibody-solutions and incubated for 1 h in the dark. Next, antibody solution was removed, and samples were washed with BSA before the coverslips were directly mounted with fluorescent mounting medium ("Prolong Gold antifade reagent with DAPI" Invitrogen) and allowed to dry overnight (at 6°C). Fluorescence measurements were carried out with a modified Leica TCS SP8 CARS laser scanning Microscope using either a 20x objective (HC PL APO CS2 20x/0.75 DRY) or a 63x objective (HC PL APO CS2 63x/1.20 WATER). Images were acquired with a resolution of 2048 × 2048 pixel with a step size of 286 nm for 20x magnification and of 91 nm for 63x magnification. Fluorescence measurements on each position were performed sequentially using laser excitation at 488 nm and detection at 500–540 nm with a hybrid detector (LeicaHyD), excitation at 561 nm and detection at 566–620 nm with a HyD and excitation at 405 nm with detection at 425–500 nm using a PMT. All data processing was carried out using Matlab R2015a. Due to variations in fluorescence intensity between the samples as well as between the different dyes data were preprocessed for better comparability. To reduce background, noise data points having $<$ 2% of intensity were set to this lower threshold value. To account for cosmic spikes, the upper threshold was set so that a maximum of 0.1% of all data points above background showed fluorescence intensity above this limit. Intensities above the upper threshold were set to this value. Images were then rescaled to full range (8bit). For calculation of co-localization values in each channel, all data points exceeding an intensity value of 20% were determined. Data points that are above this value in both channels were considered to be co-localizing. The ratio of co-localization is calculated from the number of co-localizing points divided.

Electron Microscopy

Preparation of Hek293-TRex cell lines and subsequent transmission electron microscopic studies were carried out as described previously (12, 16). For each SIL1 variant as well as for the wildtype protein, at least 50 cells were analyzed showing similar (patho)morphology of subcellular organelles/structures.

RESULTS

Literature and *in silico*-Based Evaluation of the Pathogenicity of Selected SIL1-Variants

We chose one known polymorphism (p.K132Q), three notoriously pathogenic mutations (p.V231_I232del, p.G312R, and p.L457P) and p.R92W, a variant that was previously described as a pathogenic missense mutation (11). Notably, the two missense variants pR92W and p.K132Q are present in the control population with minor allele frequencies (MAF) of 0.5 and 0.7%, respectively, and in 29 and 72 healthy individuals in homozygous state. On the other hand, p.G312R is absent from a control population of $>$125,000 individuals (ExaC, http://exac.broadinstitute.org) and p.L457P is found in one allele count (MAF: 0.0004%) (http://gnomad.broadinstitute.org). The sites of the different variants/ mutations are depicted in **Figure 1A**. By affecting α-helix A8 of the SIL1-protein, the p.V231_I232del mutation directly impacts on the physiological SIL1-BiP interaction lobe IIb of the BiP-ATPase domain (major interaction site). Although the polymorphic variant p.K132Q and the reported pathogenic missense mutant p.G312R are also localized within the SIL1-BiP-binding domain, they do not directly affect α-helices mediating the physical interaction with BiP. The ambiguous missense variant, p.R92W, localizes within the N-terminal domain of the 461 amino acid SIL1 protein and p.L457P, another known pathogenic missense mutant of SIL1 affects one amino acid localized before the known ER-retention motif KDEL/KELR (17) (**Figure 1A**). Interestingly, *in silico* testing of pathogenicity with different platforms revealed controversial results including a probably damaging effect for all amino acid substitutions addressed in this study (**Figure 1B**). This result is in contrast with the observed allele frequencies in the control population and by the same token emphasizes the need to define biomarkers that can be used to evaluate the pathogenicity of *SIL1* mutations—in particular of amino acid substitutions.

Molecular Characteristics of Selected SIL1-Variants in a Non-reducing PAGE

First, molecular characteristics of the selected SIL1-variants were addressed in a non-reducing PAGE (and concomitant blotting to a PVDF-membrane) utilizing whole protein extracts. Detection of the different variant forms of the recombinant SIL1-protein utilizing an anti-SIL1 antibody (see **Table 1**) revealed no major differences in the detected molecular weight of wildtype SIL1-TAP in comparison to the ambiguous p.R92W and the benign p.K132Q variants of SIL1. In contrast, no band was detectable for p.V231_I232del-mutant SIL1 (16 h of induced overexpression) suggesting instability of the aberrant protein, a finding which is in line with our previous studies on patient derived cells (6, 12). However, absence of this mutant form of the protein might also arise from a changed antigenicity of this variant product. Immunoblots of the two well-known pathogenic mutant forms, p.G312R and p.L457P, did not only show protein bands of the predicted size of the recombinant fusion-protein (SIL1-TAP) but also additional bands corresponding to a higher molecular weight

A

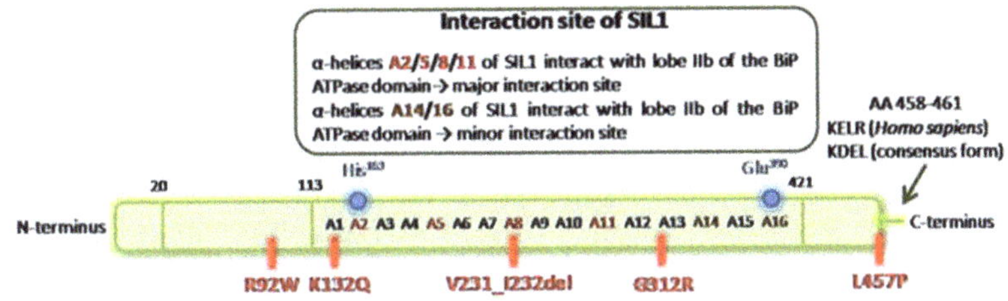

B

Nucleotide change	Location	Predicted aminoacid change	Family/ origin	ClinVar	In silico prediction	CADD score	Population frequency (homozygos)	Reference
c.274C>T	Exon 4	p.R92W	60078/ Pakistan	Likely benign	D;D;D;B	27,6	0,5% (14)	Riazuddin et al., 2009
c.394A>C	Exon 5	p.K132Q	n/a n/a	Likely benign/ benign	D;D;D;B	25,7	0,7% (29)	n/a
c.691_696del GTGATC	Exon 7	p.V231_ 232del	MSS24.1 Turkey	-	n/a	n/a	absent	Krieger et al., 2013
c.934G>A	Exon 9	p.G312R	MSS32.1 USA	-	D;D;D;B	27,8	absent	Krieger et al., 2013
c.1370T>C	Exon 10	p.L457P	M21 Japan	Patho-genic	D;P;D;P	24,2	absent	Anttonen et al., 2008

FIGURE 1 | Overview of investigated amino acid changes of SIL1. **(A)** Localization of SIL1 amino acid changes in the entire SIL1 protein. Schematic figure is modified from Yan et al. (5). **(B)** Table summarizing the *SIL1* variants by providing information regarding the corresponding nucleotide change/ deletion in different exons within the *SIL1* gene as well as origin of the respective MSS-patient and results of *in silico*-based testing of pathogenicity by "CADD score" and "ClinVar" as well as by "SIFT", "PluPhen2", "MutationTaster" and "FATHMM" (summarized as in silico prediction). D, damagingl; P, pathogenic; B, benign; T, tolerated.

which appear to be more pronounced for p.G312R (**Figure 2A**). The experiment was performed 6 times with similar results.

Influence of Amino Acid Substitutions/Deletions on SIL1-SIL1-Interactions:

Given that SIL1 can act as a dimer (6), we addressed the effect of the various amino acid changes and of the deletion of two amino acids (p.V231_I232del) on the formation of SIL1-protein homomers by immunoprecipitation and subsequent immunoblot analyses. As a proof-of-principle, the well-known homomerization of SIL1 wild-type proteins was confirmed (**Figure 2B**). Both, the ambiguous p.R92W and the benign p.K132Q variants showed a homomerization similar to the one observed for the wild-type SIL1-TAP-SIL1-HA complex (**Figures 2C,D**). Analyses of the well-known pathogenic p.V231_I232del mutation revealed no interaction of the resulting degradation products in terms of the formation of toxic (proteolytic) protein complexes (**Figure 2E**). Study of the two-known pathogenic SIL1-proteins, p.G312R and p.L457P, showed that they can form homomeric complexes along with their degradation products (**Figures 2F,G**). Immunoblot-based analyses of whole protein extracts/ straight lysates confirmed the expression of the respective recombinant SIL1-variants tagged with HA or TAP in each of the respective experiments. All immunoprecipitation and immunoblot experiments were performed three times with similar results.

Influence of Amino Acid Substitutions/ Deletions on the Fitness of the *in vitro* Models

Mitochondrial vulnerability has been repeatedly reported in MSS and woozy mouse tissues (13, 18–20), and in *in vitro* models of the disease (13, 16). As mitochondrial function is essential for cellular fitness, we examined metabolic activity of our *in vitro* models by focussing on processes related to mitochondrial activity as well as on mitochondrial morphology. The WST-1 assay (Roche) was used; in this assay the stable tetrazolium salt, WST-1, is cleaved to a soluble formazan. This conversion depends on the cellular availability of succinate-tetrazolium reductase system that belongs to the respiratory chain of the mitochondria (only active in metabolically intact cells). Thus, the amount of formazan dye formed directly correlates to the number of metabolically intact cells in the culture. Metabolic activity in WT-SIL1 cells was defined as 100% of cellular fitness. The WST-1 assay revealed no reduction in metabolic activity upon overexpression of the ambiguous p.R92W or of the benign p.K231Q variant of SIL1 (**Figure 3A**). Overexpression of the p.V231_I232del mutant form of the SIL1-protein (which displayed instability in our previous experiment, see above) resulted in a minor but significant decrease of the fitness (**Figure 3A**). In contrast, overexpression of the known pathogenic mutants p.G312R and p.L457P led to a 15–20% reduction in cellular viability compared to cells overexpressing the WT-SIL1 (or solely the TAP-Tag) suggesting an effect of

TABLE 1 | All immunoblot studies were carried out at least three times.

Antibody	Company	Dilution
α-Beclin	Novus Biologicals: NB110-87318	1:1000
α-CBP	Thermo Fisher Scientific: PA1-847	1:1000
α-CHOP	Novus Biologicals: NB600-1335SS	1:500
α-DJ-1	Santa Cruz: sc-55572	1:750
α-DNAJB6	Genetex: GTX33160	1:500
α-ERj3	Novus Biologicals: NBP1-68477	1:500
α-FAM134B	Genetex: GTX46621	1:500
α-GAPDH	Genetex: GTX627408	1:1000
α-GRP94	Genetex: GTX103203	1:1000
α-GRP170	Genetex: GTX102255	1:1000
α-HA	Sigma Aldrich: H3663-100UL	1:500
α-IRE1	Genetex: GTX130387	1:500
α-pEif2α (Ser52)	Thermo Fisher Scientific: 44-728G	1:1000
α-PERK	Abcam: ab65142	1:500
α-POC1A	Thermo Fisher Scientific: PA5-49028	1:500
α-SIL1	Abcam: ab5639	1:100
α-SOD1	Genetex: GTX100554	1:1000
α-VCP	Genetex: GTX101089	1:1000

List of antibodies used in the study.

their pathogenicity on cellular metabolism (**Figure 3A**). H_2O_2-treated Hek293 cells were included as a positive control for perturbed mitochondrial function based on massive oxidative stress burden (**Figure 3A**). The assay was carried out 4 times with similar results. Given that mitochondrial vulnerability might be connected to oxidative stress, a well-known epiphenomenon of ER-stress, levels of DJ1 and SOD1 (two proteins known to be modulated by oxidative stress burden) were studied by immunoblotting. Hek293 cells overexpressing the pathogenic missense variants of SIL1, p.G312R, and p.L457P, showed an increase in DJ1 (lower band), with a more pronounced effect in cells overexpressing p.G312R mutant SIL1. Cells overexpressing p.G312R mutant SIL1 showed a considerable increase in SOD1 protein, whereas there was no difference between the cells overexpressing the wildtype protein and those overexpressing the pathogenic p.L457P variant (**Figure 3B**). However, the increase of SOD1 in Hek293 cells overexpressing p.V231_I232del mutant form was comparable to the SOD1 increase in cells overexpressing the benign p.K132Q variant (**Figure 3B**. Notably, a parallel "trend" of abundances of DJ1 and SOD1 expression changes modulated by SIL1 variants can be observed. Prompted by the results of the WST-1 assay and by the immunoblot studies, mitochondrial-morphology was examined by electron microscopy. EM revealed normal ultrastructure of Hek293 cells overexpressing wild-type SIL1 as well as p.R92W- and p.K132Q variant forms of the SIL1 protein (**Figure 3C**). In contrast, Hek293 cells overexpressing the known pathogenic SIL1-missense mutations, p.G312R and p.L457P, presented with perturbed mitochondrial architecture including break-down of cristae and accumulation of electron-dense membranous material in the mitochondrial matrix most likely indicative of incipient mitophagy/ mitoptosis (21) (**Figure 3C**). Overexpression of the pathogenic but instable p.V231_I232del mutant form did not result in such a profound mitochondrial pathology. This might actually be due to the higher stability of the pathogenic missense mutant forms of SIL1 resulting in persistent mitochondrial stress. Pathomorphological mitochondria could be detected in 41 of 50 cells (82%) expressing the p.L457P and in 38 of 50 cells (76%) expressing the p.G312R mutant form whereas in cells expressing wildtype SIL1 or the variants p.R92W and p.K132Q, pathomorphological mitochondria were found in 10%, 18% and 14%, respectively (50 cells were analyzed for each *in vitro* model). Only 12% of Hek293 cells overexpressing the pathogenic but instable p.V231_I232del mutant displayed morphological aberrant mitochondria.

Pattern of Cellular SIL1 Staining—Polymorphic vs. Pathogenic Forms of the Protein:

Immunofluorescence studies of our Hek293 *in vitro* models overexpressing the different forms of the SIL1 protein in an inducible fashion were performed to address the question if the pattern of SIL1-TAP-immunoreactivity allows to differentiate between polymorphic variants and pathogenic mutations. Indeed, cells overexpressing WT-SIL1 in comparison to those overexpressing the two known pathogenic missense forms (p.G312R and p.L457P) showed significant differences regarding the pattern of immunoreactivity. WT-SIL1 was distributed in a reticular network in accordance with a regular ER-localization, whereas p.G312R- and p.L457P mutant SIL1 showed an altered non-reticular immunoreactivity pattern (**Figure 4A**). In contrast, p.V231_I232del mutant SIL1 (after 6 h of induced overexpression) showed a reticular distribution comparable to WT-SIL1 and the polymorphic p.K132Q form but with some focal accumulations (**Figure 4A**). Notably, immunoreactivity of p.R92W variant SIL1 does not show the same subcellular distribution as the p.G312R and p.L457P mutants and rather presents as a reticular network as observed for WT-SIL1 and p.K132Q but with some minor focal accumulations.

Influence of Amino Acid Substitutions/Deletions on ER-Morphology and Function in our *in vitro* Models

To follow up on the immunofluorescence studies described above, EM was performed. ER in Hek293 cells overexpressing WT-, p.R92W and p.K132Q versions of SIL1 showed a regular tubular structure. In cells overexpressing p.G312R and p.L457P mutant SIL1, the ER showed focal widening, occasionally associated with accumulation of electron dense material most likely corresponding to protein aggregates within the widened ER (black arrows in **Figure 4B**). In addition, cells overexpressing these two known-pathogenic mutants exhibited autophagic vacuoles that were often filled with membranous and granular osmophilic material (**Figure 4B**). Deposits of osmophilic material (mostly localized to autophagic vacuoles) were also detected in Hek293 cells with short-term (6 h) overexpression of p.V231_I232del mutant SIL1 (**Figure 4B**).

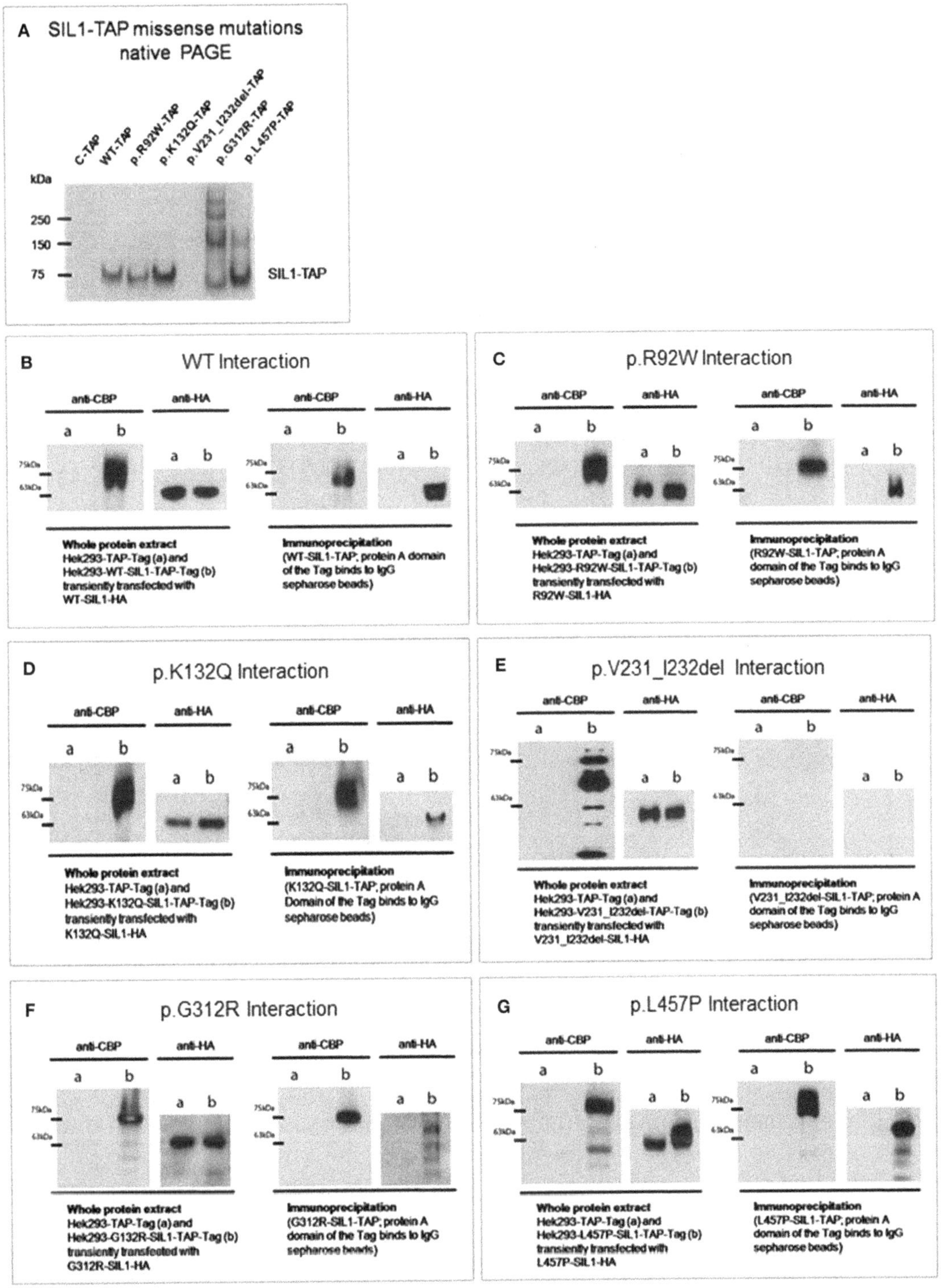

FIGURE 2 | Impact of amino acid substitutions and deletions on the molecular characteristics of SIL1. **(A)** Native-PAGE of SIL1 variants reveals absence of p.V231_I232del mutant SIL1 (16 h of induced overexpression) but no differences in the migration pattern of the different missense variants of SIL1. The two known pathogenic variants p.G312R- and p.L457P present additional bands of a higher molecular weight. **(B–G)** Immunoprecipitation and subsequent immunoblot analysis toward the study of SIL1-homomerization confirmed the known SIL1-SIL1 interaction of the wildtype form of the protein **(B)** and showed no effect of the p.R92W- or p.K132Q-amino acid substitutions on this interaction **(C,D)**. Study of p.V231_I232del mutant SIL1 (6 h of induced overexpression) did not show a physical interaction of the degradation products of this known pathogenic and instable form of SIL1 **(E)**. Analysis of the two known missense mutants p.G312R- and p.L457P revealed in both cases a homomerization of the full-length mutant proteins but also an interaction of the mutant full-length protein with the respective degradation products **(F,G)**.

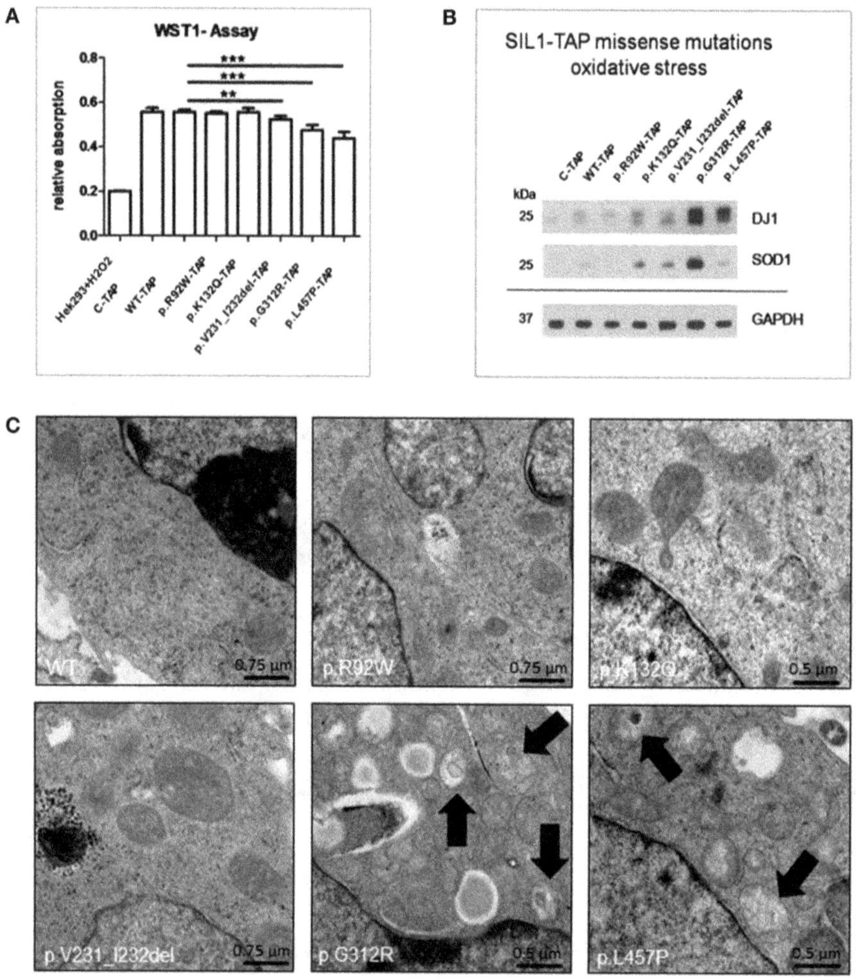

FIGURE 3 | Study of fitness of Hek293 cells overexpressing SIL1 or its variant forms in the context of mitochondrial vulnerability. **(A)** ELISA-based WST-1 assay showed a statistically significant reduction in the fitness of cells overexpressing the known pathogenic variants p.V231_I232del (6 h of induced overexpression), p.G312R and p.L457P, respectively. In accordance with the instability of p.V231_I232del mutant SIL1, the fitness is more reduced in Hek293 cells overexpressing p.G312R and p.L457P mutant forms of SIL1. Hek293 cells treated with H_2O_2 were included as positive control showing the functionality of the assay. **(B)** Immunoblot-based studies of DJ1 (lower band) and SOD1 as two representative marker proteins for oxidative stress (related to mitochondria) showed a considerable increase of DJ1 in cells overexpressing p.G312R or p.L457P mutant SIL1. Surprisingly, SOD1 was only markedly increased in cells overexpressing p.G312R mutant SIL1, but not in cells overexpressing p.L457P mutant SIL1. GAPDH was used to demonstrate equal protein loading. **(C)** EM revealed normal mitochondrial architecture in Hek293 cells overexpressing WT-SIL1, p.R92W and p.K132Q variant SIL1 as well as p.V231_I232del mutant SIL1 but disintegration of cristae and presence of membranous electron-dense material within the mitochondrial matrix (black arrows) in cells overexpressing the two known pathogenic missense variants p.G312R and p.L457P. **Statistically very significant; ***Statistically extremely significant.

Prompted by our ultra-structural findings, we next investigated the presence of ER-stress upon overexpression of wildtype SIL1 as well as the 5 different variants at the molecular level by immunoblotting by focussing on the abundances of 10 proteins modulating the unfolded protein response (UPR) and the ER-associated degradation pathway (ERAD). In accordance with our previous published data (12), overexpression of wildtype SIL1 results in the increased expression of these factors compared to cells overexpressing solely the TAP-Tag (**Figure 4C**). This in turn also explains the altered expression of these factors in Hek293 cells with long-term overexpression of the instable p.V231_I232del mutant form. However, overexpression of neither the polymorphic p.K132Q nor of the ambiguous p.R92W variant led to a sustained increase of the UPR-/ ERAD-related proteins compared to cells overexpressing the wildtype form of SIL1 (**Figure 4C**). Overexpression of p.G312R resulted in an increased expression of GRP170 and Beclin-1 as well as forced phosphorylation of eIF2α compared to cells overexpressing the TAP-tag only, the wildtype variant of SIL1 or the p.R29W and p.K132Q variants, respectively (**Figure 4C**). The overexpression of p.L457P mutant SIL1 even resulted in elevated abundance of all investigated UPR-/ ERAD-proteins except HSP40/ ERj3 (**Figure 4C**).

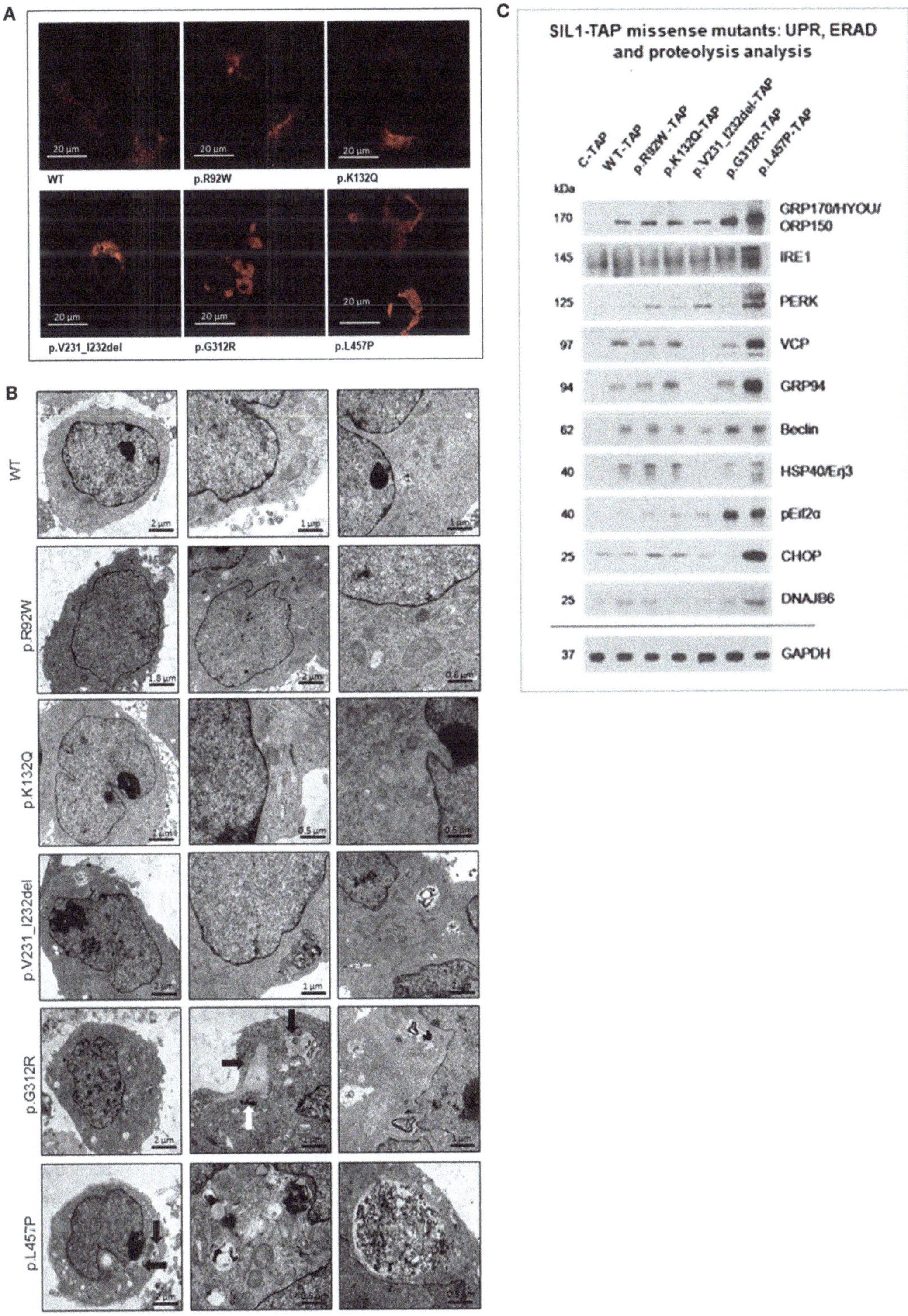

FIGURE 4 | Study of cellular SIL1 immunoreactivity and presence of ER-stress in Hek293 cells overexpressing SIL1 or its variant forms. **(A)** Immunofluorescence-based investigation of the SIL1-immunoreactivity pattern in Hek293 cell revealed a reticular distribution for WT-SIL1, p.R92W and p.K132Q variant forms of SIL1 but a non-reticular rather "clumpy" immunoreactivity for p.G312R and p.L457P mutant forms of SIL1. For p.V231_I232del mutant SIL1, a reticular distribution with focal accumulations was observed. **(B)** EM revealed widened and proliferated ER in cells overexpressing the mutant forms p.G312R and p.L457P, but not in cells overexpressing WT-SIL1, p.R92W, p.K132Q, and p.V231_I232del (6 h of induced overexpression) forms of the proteins. In addition, accumulation of electron dense material could occasionally be seen in cells overexpressing p.G312R and p.L457P muatnt SIL1 (black arrows). Along this line,

(Continued)

FIGURE 4 | overexpression of these two known missense mutants of SIL1 resulted in the build-up of electron dense material (most likely corresponding to aggregated protein) in the cytoplasm as well as in (autophagic) vacuoles. The white arrow highlights an abnormal centrosome in a Hek293 cell overexpressing p.G312R mutant SIL1. **(C)** Immunoblot-based studies aimed to investigate the presence of ER-Stress by focussing on marker proteins for activation of the unfolded protein response (GRP170, IRE1, PERK, GRP94, ERj3 & pEif2α), the ER-associated degradation pathway (VCP, DNAJB6) and proteolysis (Beclin). Results revealed a considerable presence of ER-stress in Hek293 cells overexpressing p.L457P mutant SIL1 than in cells overexpressing p.G312R mutant SIL1 where solely pEif2α and Beclin are increased compared to cells overexpressing WT-SIL1. p.R92W, p.K132Q variant SIL1, and p.V231_I232del mutant SIL1 (6 h of induced overexpression) do not show remarkable changes in abundances of the stress markers compared to cells overexpressing WT-SIL1. GAPDH was investigated to demonstrate equal protein loading. The differences in expression of these markers between C-TAP and WT-SIL1 overexpressing Hek293 cells have been described previously (12).

Influence of Amino Acid Substitutions/Deletions on SIL1-Protein-Binding and Subsequent Morphological Effects in our *in vitro* Models

To define another read-out measure enabling the robust evaluation of the pathogenicity of amino acid changes and deletions in *SIL1*, tandem-affinity-purification followed by mass spectrometric analysis of the different TAP-tagged variants of the SIL1 protein was performed. Overexpression of p.V231_I232del mutant SIL1 was induced by doxycycline treatment for 6 h to study binding partners prior degradation of this instable pathogenic SIL1 protein. Results of this screening approach are presented in **Figure 5A** and show that all variants of the SIL1-protein bind to BiP, Mortalin and the small subunit of Calpain-1. Moreover, our protein-interaction studies revealed a precipitation of ERj3 along with the two pathogenic mutants of SIL1, p.G312R, and p.L457P, but not with the two variants p.R92W and p.K132Q or the wildtype form of SIL1. Remarkably, our unbiased studies focusing on interaction of different forms of SIL1 to other proteins revealed that the wildtype protein as well as the p.R92W and p.K132Q variants are precipitating with POC1A whereas immunoprecipitation of p.G312R and p.L457P mutant SIL1 along with their interactors and subsequent mass spectrometry studies did not result in the identification of POC1A as a binding partner. Given that mutations in *POC1A* are causative for SOFT (short stature, onychodysplasia, facial dysmorphism, and hypotrichosis) syndrome (22) and short stature is also a clinical finding in MSS patients, a regulatory effect of abundances of the SIL1-wildtype protein on level of POC1A was confirmed by immunoblot studies. Our findings highlight an effect of cellular SIL1 level on POC1A protein abundance (**Figure 5B**, left). *POC1A* encodes for a protein linking centrosomes to Golgi assembly and function, and recessive mutations affecting this gene result in perturbed Golgi structures and cytosolic vesicle accumulations, in addition to abnormal multipolar spindles *in vitro* (22, 23). This known POC1A function along the mentioned pathological findings resulting from mutations in the corresponding gene prompted us to also study the level of FAM134B, a newly identified cis-Golgi protein with a pivotal role in neuronal function and survival (24) in relation to the expression of SIL1 wildtype protein as well as the morphology of Golgi and centrosomes. Indeed, immunoblot studies of FAM134B showed a beneficial effect of SIL1 expression on the abundance of this Golgi-protein (**Figure 5B**, left). Results of expression studies in Hek293 cells expressing different mutant forms of the protein show a clear influence of the pathogenicity of SIL1-mutations on the abundance of the FAM134B and POC1A proteins (**Figure 5B**, right).

Prompted by our SIL1-protein interaction findings suggestive for a localization of SIL1 also to the Golgi-apparatus, further immunofluorescence studies have been performed and revealed an expected co-localization of SIL1 with calsequestrin (CASQ1; a known ER-marker protein) and additionally co-localizations with golgin-97 (a known marker protein of the Golgi apparatus) as well as with FAM134B and POC1A. Quantification of these co-localizations revealed that the excessive proportion of the SIL1 protein localizes to the ER but almost equal co-localization with golgin-97, FAM134B and POC1A indicates a minor localization of SIL1 also within the Golgi apparatus (**Figure 5C**).

Results of further ultra-morphological studies focussing on the integrity of Golgi and centrosomes revealed proliferated and dispersed Golgi cisternae in Hek293 cells overexpressing p.G312R or p.L457P but not in cells overexpressing the wildtype form of the protein (**Figure 5D**). Whereas, neither the polymorphic p.K132Q nor the ambiguous p.R92W variant of SIL1 presented with changes in Golgi architecture compared to cells overexpressing WT-SIL1 (data not shown), Hek293 cells with short-term overexpression of p.V231_I232del showed only a very mild widening of Golgi cisternae (**Figure 5D**). Interestingly, altered Golgi structures could frequently be detected adjacent to abnormal centrosomes as exemplified for p.V231_I232del and p.G312R in **Figure 5D** (black arrows). Along this line, overexpression of the pathogenic forms of the SIL1 protein in Hek293 cells repeatedly resulted in disintegration of centrosome architecture including centriole-multiplications and -proliferations as well as mis-localization of centrioles to lysosomes and vacuoles (**Figure 5E**).

DISCUSSION

On a general note, the need of suitable *in vitro* systems allowing a reliable testing of ambiguous gene mutations potentially affecting stability and localization of the corresponding protein is crucial in the cases that patient-derived tissue is not available to perform verification studies. Here, using MSS as a paradigmatic rare neurogenetic disease, we demonstrate that Hek293 cells overexpressing different mutant forms of the SIL1 protein are suitable to evaluate the pathogenicity of SIL1 mutations such as missense variants and in-frame-amino acid deletions. MSS has been selected for our studies as:

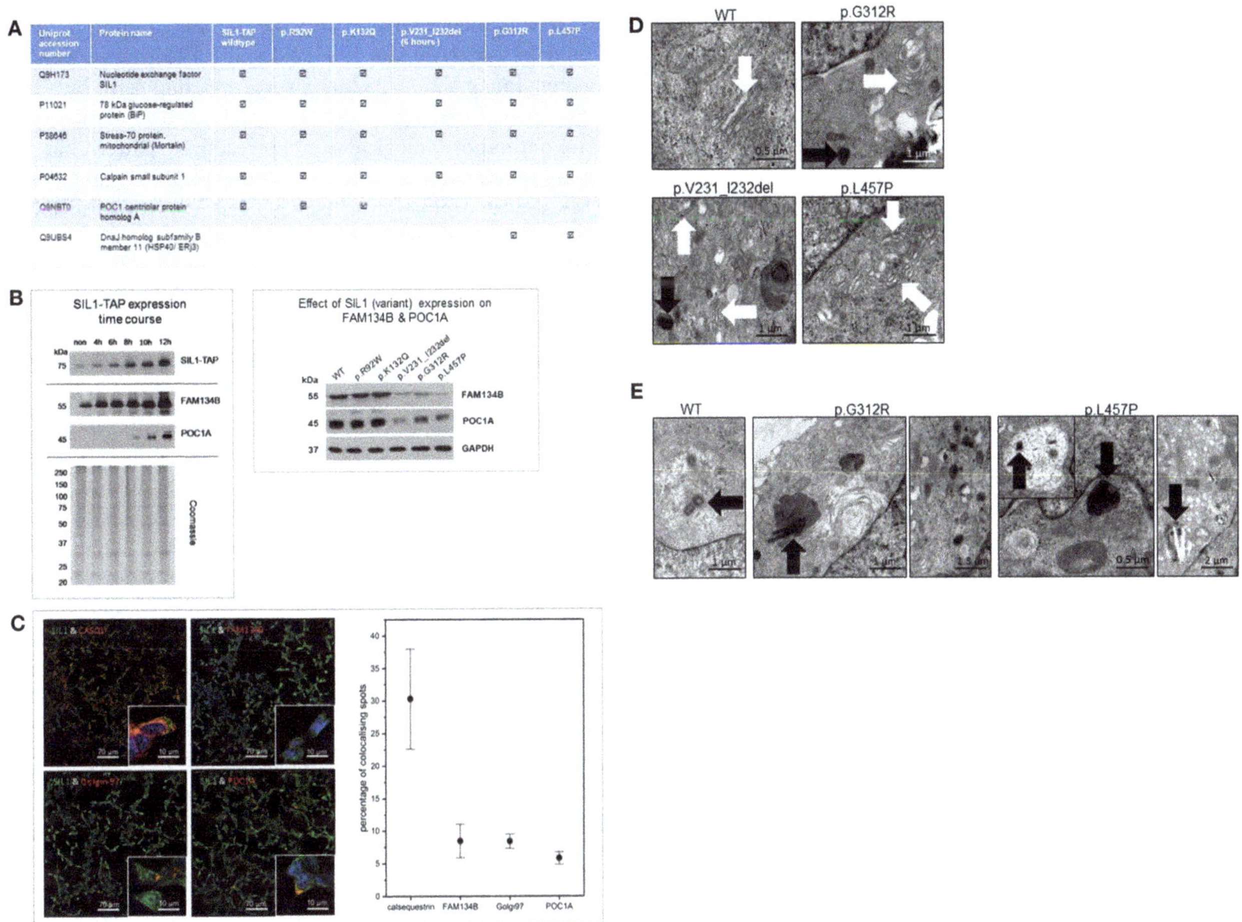

Figure 5_1

FIGURE 5 | Study of SIL1-interactome and impact of interaction on subcellular morphologies. **(A)** Table presenting SIL1-protein interactions identified by tandem-affinity-purification and subsequent mass spectrometry in an unbiased fashion: whereas WT-SIL1 and its (polymorphic and pathogenic) variants interact with BiP, Mortalin and the small subunit of Calpain-1, solely WT-SIL1, p.R92W and p.K132Q variant forms of SIL1 precipitated POC1A. In contrast, solely p.G312R and p.L457P mutant SIL1 precipitated ERj3, a known BiP-binding protein controlled by ER-stress. the detection of SIL1—as shown in the table presented—refers to the identification/ detection of tryptic peptides unique for the SIL1 protein in the mass spectrometric analysis. The peptides identified for the respective SIL1-variant arise from the overexpression of same ones and show the reliability of the combined IP-LC-MS/MS data. **(B)** Immunoblot-based study of FAM134B and POC1A revealed increased expression of both proteins upon elevation of the cellular SIL1 level. Coomassie-staining was carried out to demonstrate equal protein loading (left panel). Results of expression studies in Hek293 cells expressing different mutant forms of the protein show a clear influence of the pathogenicity of SIL1-mutations on the abundance of the FAM134B and POC1A proteins (right panel). **(C)** Results of our co-immunofluorescence studies focussing on SIL1 localizations revealed co-localizations of SIL1 with CASQ1 (calsequestrin), golgin-97, FAM134B, and POC1A. Representative overviews of cells are shown for each respective co-localization study which have also been used for the quantifications of co-localizations (right diagram). **(D)** EM of Golgi morphology revealed a regular architecture in Hek293 cells overexpressing WT-SIL1, but proliferated and dispersed Golgi with widened terminal cisternae (white arrows) and vesicle accumulations in cells overexpressing p.G312R or p.L457P mutant SIL1. In cells overexpressing p.V231_I232del mutant SIL1, solely a mild pathology of the Golgi apparatus (widened cisternae indicated by white arrows) could be observed. **(E)** EM of centrosome morphology revealed a regular architecture in Hek293 cells overexpressing WT-SIL1, but proliferated, multiplicated and dispersed centrosomes in cells overexpressing the pathogenic missense mutant pG312R or p.L457P (black arrows). Remarkably, in cells overexpressing these two known pathogenic forms of SIL1, a mis-localization of abnormal centrosomes to lysosomes (black arrows in pictures 2 and 4) or to vacuoles (black arrow in the inset of picture for as well as in picture 5) was observed.

- The phenotype can present with prominent additional clinical features or characteristic features of the "clinical triad" can be absent thus complicating the evaluation of detected variants in terms of phenotype-causative mutations
- Missense mutations may have a detrimental effect on the clinical presentation (10)
- Detection of new *SIL1* sequence variants is ever increasing in number thus indicating the need to classify their pathogenicity.

Indeed, the combination of different biochemical, morphological and functional studies utilizing Hek293 cells overexpressing different variants of SIL1 of known and ambiguous pathogenicity allowed to introduce a system enabling the *in vitro*-based evaluation of *SIL1* variants leading to amino acid substitutions or deletions: results of our SIL1-protein studies in a non-reducing PAGE suggest that although the pathogenic variants do not cause essential changes in the behavior of the main SIL1 band, bands of higher molecular weight occur which most likely correspond to aberrant SIL1 protein complexes. The absence of these bands under reducing conditions (data not shown) indicates that these aberrant complexes are soluble. Hence, the presence of additional (higher molecular weight) SIL1 bands in a non-reducing PAGE might serve as a read-out measure to evaluate the pathogenicity of amino acid substitutions in SIL1. The absence of these bands in immunoblots of WT-SIL1, p.K132Q and p.R92W variants of SIL1 suggest that p.R92W is a benign variant rather than a pathogenic mutation.

In addition, studies focussing on the influence of amino acid substitutions/ deletions on SIL1-SIL1-interactions provided a new outcome measure toward the evaluation of the pathogenicity of SIL1 variants: given that degradation products of the p.V231_I232del, the p.G312R and the p.L457P mutant forms of SIL1 can be identified utilizing the straight protein lysates of the SIL1-SIL1 interaction experiment and anti-HA/TAP antibodies (detecting the respective Tags at the C-terminus of the recombinant proteins) a N-terminal initiated degradation of these mutant forms of the protein is suggested. The presence of degradation products for p.G312R and p.L457P mutant SIL1 (**Figures 2F,G**) in combination with the detected higher molecular weight bands for these forms as presented in **Figure 2A** suggests formation of protein aggregates and breakdown. A comparison of the degradation of the variant forms of SIL1 with known pathogenic character suggests a much higher instability of SIL1 exhibiting deletion of two amino acids compared to the two forms with C-terminal substitutions. Taken together, this assay shows that precipitation of degradation products might be indicative for a pathogenic character of amino acid changes in SIL1.

Given that mitochondria display a considerable vulnerability in the etiology of MSS (13, 18–20), WST-1 assay has been performed to investigate mitochondrial activity in our MSS *in vitro* models and results suggest a benign character of the p.R92W and p.K132Q amino acid changes in SIL1 whereas the pathogenic character of the p.G312R and p.L457P missense mutants could be confirmed. The mild reduction of the cellular fitness in cells overexpressing the instable p.V231_I232del mutant form of SIL1 (while cells still also express the endogenous SIL1 protein) might arise from impairment of cellular processes until degradation of the mutant recombinant protein is fully achieved. Findings of this assay suggest a reduced metabolic activity as a cellular biomarker or read-out measure of pathogenicity of *SIL1* mutations. As the expression of pathogenic SIL1 variants also impacts on morphological integrity of mitochondria, presence of oxidative stress and perturbed mitochondrial architecture might represent further useful read-out measures for the *in vitro* evaluation of pathogenicity of overexpressed *SIL1* mutations that are associated with a loss of function rather than a loss of protein. However, the less pronounced oxidative stress burden in the case of overexpression of p.L457P mutant SIL1 (**Figure 3B**) suggests that analysis of oxidative stress should not serve as a mere measure to evaluate the pathogenic character of SIL1 missense variants.

To address cellular SIL1 immunoreactivity and distribution as a further measure to evaluate pathogenicity of SIL1 amino acid substitutions and deletions immunofluorescence studies have been carried out and -in comparison to the Hek293 cells over expressing the SIL1 wildtype protein—altered immunoreactivity could be observed for p.G312R and p.L457P and to a minor degree for p.V231_I232del overexpressing cells but not for cells overexpressing p.R92W or p.K132Q variants of SIL1. As a pathomorphological immunoreactivity-pattern has already been demonstrated for p.L457P mutant SIL1 in COS7 cells (14), the recapitulation in Hek293 cells confirms the suitability of these cells to investigate pathogenicity of *SIL1* mutations. Moreover, a similar pattern of immunoreactivity has been shown *in vitro* upon overexpression of a pathogenic form of *SIL1* caused by a deletion of thymidine at base-pair position 1366 of the corresponding gene (17). Consequently, our immunofluorescence findings confirm the pathogenicity of p.G312R mutant SIL1. One might speculate that the small focal accumulations of the p.V231_I232del mutant form of SIL1 represent early stages of degradation of the mutant protein, an assumption that is in line with the detection of degradation bands upon short-term overexpression (**Figure 2B**) and the absence of the protein upon long-term overexpression (**Figure 2A**). As immunofluorescence studies of p.R29W did not reveal pathological changes compared to the cells overexpressing the wildtype or the p.K132Q variant form of SIL1, the combined results support the notion that p.R92W is a polymorphic variant rather than a pathogenic mutation and also indicate that the pattern of SIL1 immunoreactivity might serve as another cellular biomarker or read-out measure allowing the evaluation of pathogenicity of SIL1 amino acid substitutions.

The altered distribution and aggregation of p.G312R and p.L457P mutant forms of SIL1 prompted us to focus on subcellular ultrastructural alterations suggestive for protein aggregation and proteolysis. Indeed, electron microscopic studies revealed the presence of vacuoles in Hek293 cells overexpressing these two pathogenic missense variants of SIL1. One might assume that these vacuoles result from impaired ER-function and thus protein processing resulting in accumulation of osmophilic material which could also be observed in the cytoplasm (not localized within vacuoles; white arrows in **Figure 4B**). As the p.V231_I232del pathogenic mutation is instable, protein aggregates and vacuoles identified by electron microscopy might correlate to the degradation of the mutant SIL1 protein. Importantly, build-up of electron-dense aggregates and altered ER morphology have also been described in immortalized lymphoblastoid cells from patients [including heterozygosity for p.V231_I232del and p.G312R, (6, 13)] as well as in Hek293 cells with depleted SIL1 expression (16) but also in MSS-patient derived fibroblasts (25). This in turn confirms the suitability of our generated *in vitro* overexpression models to evaluate the pathogenicity of SIL1 mutations on the ultra-structural level. However, results of our immunoblot-studies focussing on ER-stress and activation of proteolysis suggested a more profound ER-vulnerability and proteolytic activation in Hek293 cells overexpressing the p.L457P-mutant form of SIL1 and furthermore again suggest that the p.R92W is in fact a polymorphic missense variant of SIL1. Based on the relatively low effect of the overexpression of p.G312R (showing a detrimental effect on oxidative homeostasis; see above) on ER-homeostasis and proteolysis compared to overexpression of p.L457P, the necessity of parallel investigations of different read-out measures to draw a meaningful conclusion regarding the pathogenicity of *SIL1* variants is indicated.

SIL1-interactome has been addressed as a potential further measure to evaluate the pathogenicity of amino acid changes in SIL1 and results showed that all variants of the SIL1-protein investigated in this study bind to BiP, Mortalin and the small subunit of Calpain-1. In this context it is important to note that an ER localization of Mortalin which shows a high homology to BiP has already been described (26). Given that Calpain-1 acts as a non-lysosomal thiol-protease catalyzing proteolytic cleavage of substrate proteins, its binding to all five variants of SIL1 as well as to WT-SIL1 might result from protein overexpression and serves toward the elimination of excessive level, an assumption supported by our previous findings in Hek293 cells with WT-SIL1 overexpression (12). As BiP represents a well-known binding partner of SIL1 but also acts as a major chaperone in the UPR facilitating the re-folding of misshaped proteins, it is difficult to evaluate whether the interaction of BiP with the different variants of SIL1 is physiological or a result of an attempt to warrant a native folding of the protein in case of the binding to the pathogenic forms of SIL1. Notably, localization of p.V231_I232del- and p.G312R-amino acid changes in the BiP-binding domain of SIL1 (**Figure 1A**) are suggestive for a binding of BiP to these SIL1-forms (or degradation products) toward re-folding and antagonization of build-up of (toxic) protein aggregates. This hypothesis is further supported by the fact that DNAJB11/ERj3 serves as another BiP co-chaperone (stimulating ATPase activity) by direct binding to both unfolded ERAD-substrates and nascent unfolded peptides, but dissociates from the BiP-unfolded protein complex before folding is completed (27) and our molecular observation of ERj3 binding to p.G312R and p.L457P mutant SIL1 but not to WT-SIL1, and the p.R92W and p.K132Q variants. Thus, it seems plausible that the functional ERj3-BiP complex is recruited to the pathogenic missense variants based on pathophysiological circumstances. On a general note, this finding moreover suggests that ERj3 binding to SIL1 or rather the SIL1-BiP complex might serve as a molecular measure/ biomarker to evaluate the pathogenicity of stable SIL1 missense variants. However, results of our immunoblot studies of ER-stress related proteins did not show elevated ERj3 level in Hek293 cells overexpressing p.G312R and p.L457P mutant SIL1 compared cells overexpressing the wildtype SIL1 protein (**Figure 4C**) indicating that cellular available ERj3 pools are re-located to the two pathogenic mutant forms of SIL1. Mass spectrometry-based analysis of SIL1-interacotme moreover revealed that the wildtype protein as well as the p.R92W and p.K132Q variants bind to POC1A. Interestingly, immunoprecipitation of the p.G312R and p.L457P forms of SIL1 along with their interactors did not result in the identification of the binding to POC1A. This finding defines the interaction of POC1A with SIL1 variants as further read-out measure to evaluate the pathogenicity of amino acid substitutions and deletions in *SIL1* and by the same token underlines our previous findings suggesting that the p.R92W variant form of SIL1 is in fact a polymorphic variant rather than a pathogenic mutant of the BiP co-chaperone. On a more general note, our immunoprecipitation data support the previous description of an interaction of POC1A with the SIL1-BiP machinery as identified by BioPlex 2.0 [Biophysical Interactions of ORFEOME-derived complexes; (28)].

TABLE 2 | Overview of cellular markers and respective analytical approaches toward evaluation of pathogenicity of SIL1-mutants.

Test	Cellular marker of pathogenicity
Native and reducing PAGE with subsequent Western-Blot of SIL1 protein	Higher and lower molecular weight bands as signs of protein aggregates (in native PAGE) and degradation products
WST-1 viability assay	Reduced viability
Immunofluorescence of SIL1-protein	Non-reticular pattern of immunoreactivity
Electron microscopy	Abnormal mitochondria, vacuoles & protein aggregates, dispersed Golgi, disintegrated centrosomes
SIL1-interactome	Loss of interaction with POC1A and binding to DNAJB11/ ERj3
Immunoblot analysis of cellular stress markers	Oxidative- and/ or ER-stress burden
SIL1-SIL1 homomerization	Occurrence of degradation products of pathogenic mutant SIL1-protein which do not present rapid degradation

Prompted by the fact POC1A mutations are causative for a phenotype defined by short stature, onychodysplasia, facial dysmorphism, and hypotrichosis (SOFT syndrome; 22) and short stature is also a recurrent clinical finding in MSS patients, effect of SIL1 expression (wildtype and variant forms) has been studied and highlighted an increasing effect of elevated SIL1 protein level on POC1A protein abundance (**Figure 5B**). Same effect could be observed for p.R92W and p.K132Q but not p.G312R, p.L457P or p.V231_I232del mutant forms of SIL1. This effect indicates that the molecular interaction between the two proteins might also be of relevance for the clinical manifestation of MSS upon loss of (functional) SIL1. Given that POC1A links centrosomes to Golgi assembly and function we further studied level of FAM134B, a newly identified cis-Golgi protein with a pivotal role in neuronal function and survival (24) in relation to the expression of SIL1 wildtype protein. Here same results as for POC1 could be obtained (**Figure 5B**) suggesting an impact of SIL1 expression on the Golgi apparatus, an assumption which accords with the newly identified SIL1-POC1A interaction and the results of our further immunofluorescence studies not only showing a co-localization of SIL1 with POC1A and FAM134B but also with golgin-97, a known Golgi-marker protein (**Figure 5C**). Results of these immunofluorescence-based localization studies in combination with our immunoprecipitation findings also suggest that SIL1 localizes (although to a minor degree) to subcellular compartments beyond the ER. However, to follow the hypothesis that pathogenic SIL1 variant significantly impact on function and structure of centrosome and the Golgi apparatus, ultra-structural studies focussing on their integrity have been carried out and revealed proliferated and dispersed Golgi cisternae as well as centriole-multiplications and -proliferations in Hek293 cells overexpressing the known pathogenic forms of SIL1 but not in cells overexpressing the wildtype or the p.R92W or p.K132Q forms of the protein (**Figures 5D,E**). These pathomorphological findings in turn further support the concept of an impact of SIL1 on Golgi and centrosome function and integrity and by the same token define changes in Golgi and centrosome structures as further read-out measures enabling the evaluation of the pathogenicity of *SIL1* mutations. In this context, it is important to note that depletion of SIL1 expression in Hek293 cells could be linked to vulnerability of the Golgi apparatus on both the structural and the biochemical level (16).

CONCLUSIONS

Generation and subsequent functional, biochemical and morphological phenotyping of our *in vitro* models overexpressing different (benign and pathogenic) forms of the SIL1 protein allowed to define cellular markers to evaluate the pathogenicity of SIL1-mutations, an aspect of significant importance for genetic counseling and genotype-phenotype correlations. Suitable assays and respective read-out measures (in terms of cellular biomarkers for pathogenicity of changes in SIL1 amino acid composition) are summarized in **Table 2.**

AUTHOR CONTRIBUTIONS

AR and JW conceptualized and designed the study, corrected the manuscript and supervised the experimental work. SB generated the different expression constructs used in this study. TL assisted CG in the generation of the stable-inducible cell Hek293 cell lines. DH performed the mass spectrometric analysis of the SIL1-interactome. AT performed the *in silico*-based analysis of pathogenicity of selected variants. UM performed the immunofluorescence-based co-localization studies of SIL1. CG performed all other experiments and drafted the first version of the manuscript. RH and BM gave expert opinion regarding the mitochondrial findings.

FUNDING

This work was supported by a grant from the French Muscular Dystrophy Association (AFM-Téléthon; #21644; grant to AR). Financial support was moreover obtained from the Ministerium für Kultur und Wissenschaft des Landes Nordrhein-Westfalen and the Bundesministerium für Bildung und Forschung (031A360E) as well as from the Senatsverwaltung für Wirtschaft, Technologie und Forschung des Landes Berlin.

REFERENCES

1. Georgy BA, Snow RD, Brogdon BG, Wertelecki W. Neuroradiologic findings in Marinesco-Sjogren syndrome. *AJNR Am J Neuroradiol.* (1998) 19:281–3.
2. Senderek J, Krieger M, Stendel C, Bergmann C, Moser M, Breitbach-Faller N, et al. Mutations in SIL1 cause Marinesco-Sjogren syndrome, a cerebellar ataxia with cataract and myopathy. *Nat Genet.* (2005) 37:1312–4. doi: 10.1038/ng1678
3. Zhao L, Longo-Guess C, Harris BS, Lee JW, Ackerman SL. Protein accumulation and neurodegeneration in the woozy mutant mouse is caused by disruption of SIL1, a cochaperone of BiP. *Nat Genet.* (2005) 37:974–9. doi: 10.1038/ng1620
4. Dudek J, Benedix J, Cappel S, Greiner M, Jalal C, Muller L, et al. Functions and pathologies of BiP and its interaction partners. *Cell Mol Life Sci.* (2009) 66:1556–69. doi: 10.1007/s00018-009-8745-y
5. Yan M, Li J, Sha B. Structural analysis of the Sil1-Bip complex reveals the mechanism for SIL1 to function as a nucleotide-exchange factor. *Biochem J.* (2011) 438:447–55. doi: 10.1042/BJ20110500
6. Krieger M, Roos A, Stendel C, Claeys KG, Sonmez FM, Baudis M, et al. SIL1 mutations and clinical spectrum in patients with Marinesco-Sjogren syndrome. *Brain.* (2013) 136:3634–44. doi: 10.1093/brain/awt283
7. Nair P, Hamzeh AR, Mohamed M, Tawfiq N, Al-Ali MT, Bastaki F. Marinesco-Sjogren syndrome in an emirati child with a novel mutation in SIL1 affecting the 5' untranslated region. *Med Princ Pract.* (2016) 25:580–2. doi: 10.1159/000449225
8. Gai N, Jiang C, Zou YY, Zheng Y, Liang DS, Wu LQ. Novel SIL1 nonstop mutation in a Chinese consanguineous family with Marinesco-Sjogren syndrome and Dandy-Walker syndrome. *Clin Chim Acta.* (2016) 458:1–4. doi: 10.1016/j.cca.2016.04.018
9. Byrne S, Dlamini N, Lumsden D, Pitt M, Zaharieva I, Muntoni F, et al. SIL1-related Marinesco-Sjoegren syndrome (MSS) with associated motor neuronopathy and bradykinetic movement disorder. *Neuromuscul Disord.* (2015) 25:585–8. doi: 10.1016/j.nmd.2015.04.003
10. Noreau A, La Piana R, Marcoux C, Canada F, Dion PA, Brais B, et al. Novel SIL1 mutations cause cerebellar ataxia and atrophy in a French-Canadian family. *Neurogenetics.* (2015) 16:315–8. doi: 10.1007/s10048-015-0455-z
11. Riazuddin SA, Amiri-Kordestani L, Kaul H, Butt T, Jiao X, Riazuddin S, et al. Novel SIL1 mutations in consanguineous Pakistani families mapping to chromosomes 5q31. *Mol Vis.* (2009) 15:1050–6.
12. Labisch T, Buchkremer S, Phan V, Kollipara L, Gatz C, Lentz C, et al. Tracking effects of SIL1 increase: taking a closer look beyond the consequences of elevated expression level. *Mol Neurobiol.* (2018) 55:2524–46. doi: 10.1007/s12035-017-0494-6
13. Kollipara L, Buchkremer S, Coraspe JAG, Hathazi D, Senderek J, Weis J, et al. (2017). In-depth phenotyping of lymphoblastoid cells suggests selective cellular vulnerability in Marinesco-Sjogren syndrome. *Oncotarget.* 8, 68493–68516. doi: 10.18632/oncotarget.19663
14. Anttonen AK, Siintola E, Tranebjaerg L, Iwata NK, Bijlsma EK, Meguro H, et al. Novel SIL1 mutations and exclusion of functional candidate genes in Marinesco-Sjogren syndrome. *Eur J Hum Genet.* (2008) 16:961–9. doi: 10.1038/ejhg.2008.22
15. Puig O, Caspary F, Rigaut G, Rutz B, Bouveret E, Bragado-Nilsson E, et al. The tandem affinity purification (TAP) method: a general procedure of protein complex purification. *Methods.* (2001) 24:218–29. doi: 10.1006/meth.2001.1183
16. Roos A, Kollipara L, Buchkremer S, Labisch T, Brauers E, Gatz C, et al. Cellular signature of SIL1 depletion: disease pathogenesis due to alterations in protein composition beyond the ER machinery. *Mol Neurobiol.* (2016) 53:5527–41. doi: 10.1007/s12035-015-9456-z
17. Howes J, Shimizu Y, Feige MJ, Hendershot LM. C-terminal mutations destabilize SIL1/BAP and can cause Marinesco-Sjogren syndrome. *J Biol Chem.* (2012) 287:8552–60. doi: 10.1074/jbc.M111.333286
18. Sewry CA, Voit T, Dubowitz V. Myopathy with unique ultrastructural feature in Marinesco-Sjogren syndrome. *Ann Neurol.* (1988) 24:576–80. doi: 10.1002/ana.410240416
19. Roos A, Buchkremer S, Kollipara L, Labisch T, Gatz C, Zitzelsberger M, et al. Myopathy in Marinesco-Sjogren syndrome links endoplasmic reticulum

chaperone dysfunction to nuclear envelope pathology. *Acta Neuropathol.* (2014) 127:761–77. doi: 10.1007/s00401-013-1224-4

20. Buchkremer S, Gonzalez Coraspe JA, Weis J, Roos A. Sil1-mutant mice elucidate chaperone function in neurological disorders. *J Neuromuscul Dis.* (2016) 3:169–81. doi: 10.3233/JND-160152
21. Mijaljica D, Prescott M, Devenish RJ. Mitophagy and mitoptosis in disease processes. *Methods Mol Biol.* (2010) 648:93–106. doi: 10.1007/978-1-60761-756-3_6
22. Sarig O, Nahum S, Rapaport D, Ishida-Yamamoto A, Fuchs-Telem D, Qiaoli L, et al. Short stature, onychodysplasia, facial dysmorphism, and hypotrichosis syndrome is caused by a POC1A mutation. *Am J Hum Genet.* (2012) 91:337–42. doi: 10.1016/j.ajhg.2012.06.003
23. Shaheen R, Faqeih E, Shamseldin HE, Noche RR, Sunker A, Alshammari MJ, et al. POC1A truncation mutation causes a ciliopathy in humans characterized by primordial dwarfism. *Am J Hum Genet.* (2012) 91:330–6. doi: 10.1016/j.ajhg.2012.05.025
24. Kurth I, Pamminger T, Hennings JC, Soehendra D, Huebner AK, Rotthier A, et al. Mutations in FAM134B, encoding a newly identified Golgi protein, cause severe sensory and autonomic neuropathy. *Nat Genet.* (2009) 41:1179–81. doi: 10.1038/ng.464
25. Ezgu F, Krejci P, Li S, De Sousa C, Graham JM Jr, Hansmann I, et al. Phenotype-genotype correlations in patients with Marinesco-Sjogren syndrome. *Clin Genet.* (2014) 86:74–84. doi: 10.1111/cge.12230
26. Ran Q, Wadhwa R, Kawai R, Kaul SC, Sifers RN, Bick RJ, et al. Extramitochondrial localization of mortalin/mthsp70/PBP74/GRP75. *Biochem Biophys Res Commun.* (2000) 275:174–9. doi: 10.1006/bbrc.2000.3237
27. Shen Y, Hendershot LM. ERdj3, a stress-inducible endoplasmic reticulum DnaJ homologue, serves as a cofactor for BiP's interactions with unfolded substrates. *Mol Biol Cell.* (2005) 16:40–50. doi: 10.1091/mbc.e04-05-0434
28. Huttlin EL, Bruckner RJ, Paulo JA, Cannon JR, Ting L, Baltier K, et al. Architecture of the human interactome defines protein communities and disease networks. *Nature.* (2017) 545:505–9. doi: 10.1038/nature 22366

12

Longitudinal Associations Between Serum Cytokine Levels and Dementia

*Ju-Wan Kim[1], Robert Stewart[2], Hee-Ju Kang[1], Kyung-Yeol Bae[1], Sung-Wan Kim[1], Il-Seon Shin[1], Jin-Sang Yoon[1] and Jae-Min Kim[1]**

[1] Department of Psychiatry, and Depression Clinical Research Centre, Chonnam National University Medical School, Gwangju, South Korea, [2] Institute of Psychiatry, King's College London, London, United Kingdom

***Correspondence:**
Jae-Min Kim
jmkim@chonnam.ac.kr

Background: The purpose of this study was to investigate whether long-term inflammation is related to the incidence of dementia in a prospective observational study.

Methods: In total, 732 Korean community-dwelling elderly people >65 years were evaluated at baseline. Of the 625 without dementia, 518 (83%) were followed over a 2.4-years period, and the incidence of dementia was determined. Cytokine [interleukin (IL)-1α, IL-1β, IL-6, IL-8, and tumor necrosis factor (TNF)-α] levels were measured at baseline and follow-up. The individual and combined effects of cytokine levels on dementia were evaluated after adjusting for potential covariates (lifestyle factors, demographics, disability, cognitive function, and presence of the APOE e4 allele) and a Bonferroni correction.

Results: Incident dementia was associated with increased serum cytokine levels after 2 years; the association remained significant for TNF-α, IL1-α, and IL-1β concentrations even after applying a Bonferroni correction. The analysis of the combined effects of the five cytokines showed independent associations between increases in the summed number of higher cytokine levels, between baseline and follow-up. However, incident dementia was not expected based on higher baseline pro-inflammatory cytokine levels.

Conclusion: Our results suggest that dementia may precede changes in serum cytokine levels and inflammatory processes, rather than resulting from elevated pro-inflammatory cytokines.

Keywords: cytokines, dementia, geriatric psychiatry, inflammation, longitudinal studies

INTRODUCTION

Dementia is a group of symptoms involving impairments in attention, memory, language, executive function, perception, and social cognition (1). As dementia has a high prevalence and a progressive, irreversible course in older adults (2, 3), it has become a global challenge for public health (4, 5). Understanding the etiology of dementia is essential for early diagnosis and treatment. Dementia has complex and heterogeneous etiologies, including amyloid plaques, tau-pathy, and cerebrovascular disease (6–8). Recently, the inflammatory process has received attention in the pathogenesis of dementia (9, 10).

Cytokines play a pivotal role in regulating the inflammatory response. The involvement of cytokines in dementia is supported by studies (11–13) showing that the levels of pro-inflammatory cytokines [e.g., tumor necrosis factor alpha (TNF-α), interleukin (IL)-1α, IL-1β, IL-6, and IL-8] are altered. A recent meta-analysis study reported significantly higher levels of the proinflammatory cytokines TNF-α, IL-6, IL-1β, IL-2, and IL-18 in peripheral blood samples of patients with Alzheimer's disease (AD) compared with a control group (14). However, causal relationships cannot be confirmed from case-control and cross-sectional investigations because increases in pro-inflammatory processes could be caused by disease pathophysiology (15, 16). Therefore, longitudinal studies are needed for clarification, although such studies have been scarce and have reported inconsistent findings. Some previous longitudinal studies have reported that the incidence of dementia is associated with TNF-α, IL-6, and C-reactive protein (CRP) concentrations (10, 17, 18), whereas other studies have found no relationship between baseline inflammation and future risk of dementia after adjusting for confounding factors (19, 20). These studies of inflammation-related dementia risk were conducted at a single time point, providing only the temporality of disease progression. Therefore, whether increased cytokine levels at a baseline evaluation can predict dementia risk remains unknown. To address these limitations, we analyzed data from a 2.4-years longitudinal cohort study to investigate prospectively the associations between five serum cytokine levels estimated at baseline and at follow-up with the incidence of dementia.

METHODS

Study Overview and Participants

This prospective cohort study was carried out from 2001 to 2003 in Kwangju, South Korea. Details of the study design have been described previously (21). Briefly, 732 community dwelling subjects aged >65 years from Kwangju, South Korea, were recruited from national resident registration lists. Of the 732 participants, 625 did not receive a dementia diagnosis at the baseline evaluation. Among these, 518 (83%) finished all assessments at follow-up. A secondary analysis was carried out with these 518 participants. The study was performed in accordance with the Declaration of Helsinki. Written informed consent was obtained for the study, and this study was approved by the Chonnam National University Hospital Institutional Review Board.

Baseline Sampling and Assessments

Examinations included a fully structured diagnostic interview for AD and vascular dementia, peripheral blood sampling for five serum pro-inflammatory cytokines, and a formal evaluation of covariate factors.

Dementia Evaluation

Dementia assessments were performed at the baseline and follow-up. Examinations included the Mini-Mental State Examination (MMSE) (22), the Instrumental Activities of Daily Living Scale (23), the Clinical Dementia Rating scale (24), history, and a neurological examination. Clinical researchers assigned consensus diagnoses using standard criteria for dementia (1), AD (25), and vascular dementia (26). If AD and vascular dementia pathologies were mixed, they were diagnosed as either, using the criteria. In this study, we divided the participants into two different groups of incident dementia and no incident dementia.

Biochemical Analyses

Blood samples were collected from the participants in a fasting state and were taken in the morning when possible. The blood samples were collected in EDTA tubes, centrifuged, separated into plasma aliquots, and frozen at −70°C within 2 h of collection. Biochemical assays were conducted for five serum cytokines: IL-1α, IL-1β, IL-6, IL-8, and TNF-α. Serum cytokine levels were analyzed using a solid-phase sandwich enzyme-linked immunosorbent assay (ELISA) kit (Invitrogen, Camarillo, CA, USA) according to the manufacturer's instructions. To reduce assay variation, all specimens were analyzed on the same day, in duplicate, in random order, by a technician blinded to the participant's status. The inter-assay coefficients of variation were 4–8% for IL-1α, 5–9% for IL-1β, 6–9% for IL-6, 3–6% for IL-8, and 5–7% for TNF-α. The intra-assay coefficients of variation were 4–6% for IL-1α, 4–7% for IL-1β, 4–5% for IL-6, 2–4% for IL-8, and 3–6% for TNF-α.

Covariates

Several potential factors that may be associated with serum cytokine levels were investigated based on previous studies (6–8). Age, gender, and education were recorded. Depression was evaluated by the community version of the Geriatric Mental State schedule (GMS) (27). Functional disability was measured by the Korean version of the World Health Organization Disability Assessment Schedule II (WHODAS II) (28). Smoking status was investigated and participants were categorized into current smokers or not current (ex- and never) smokers. History of alcohol use was ascertained from the participants, and verified by family members. Low risk alcohol drinking was defined, based on consuming more than 14 drinks per week during the previous 3 months for men or more than 7 drinks per week for women, following the guidelines from the National Institute of Alcohol Abuse and Alcoholism (29). Physical activity was checked at baseline by asking about work and leisure activities on a 4-point scale (not at all active, not very active, fairly active, and very active) according to the standard protocol (30). A summary vascular risk score was calculated by summing self-reported disorders (stroke, heart disease, hypertension, and diabetes), hypercholesterolemia (fasting cholesterol >200 mg/dl), and obesity (body mass index >25 kg/m^2). The apolipoprotein E (APOE) genotype was reflected as a covariate in analyses of the relationship with AD.

Follow-Up Assessments

The follow-up was carried out in 2003 (31). Attempts were made to follow up 2 years after the baseline appointment (mean interval [standard deviation (SD)], 2.4 (0.3) years). Blood samples were collected to determine five serum pro-inflammatory cytokines, centrifuged within the hour, and stored at −70°C. The same biomedical assays were carried out using the ELISA method described above. Clinical researchers

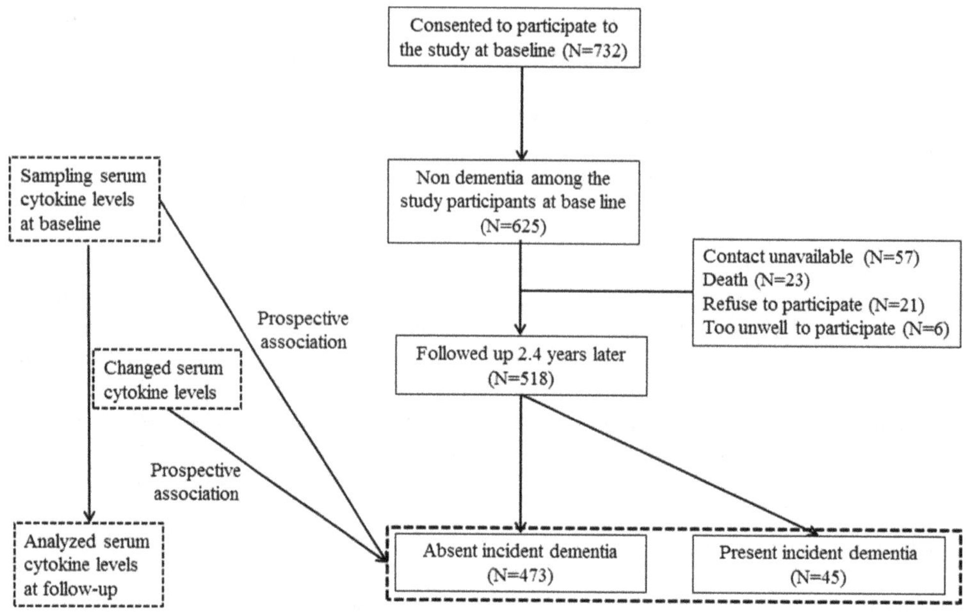

FIGURE 1 | Flow chart of the study.

assigned consensus diagnoses using standard criteria (1, 25, 26).

Statistical Analysis

The study design is outlined in **Figure 1**. Associations between baseline characteristics, demographics, assessment scales (MMSE, WHODAS II, and GMS depression) (27, 28, 32), smoking, alcohol, physical activity, and vascular risk score with incident dementia were analyzed using t- or χ^2-tests as appropriate. Results with significant associations (p-value < 0.05) were reflected in subsequent multivariate analyses. Unadjusted associations between the incidence of dementia and baseline serum cytokine concentrations and changes (from baseline to follow-up) were investigated using the Mann–Whitney U-test. The baseline levels and changes in levels were recorded as binary values of "lower" or "higher" (i.e., below or above the median value). Odds ratios and 95% confidence intervals were calculated for the associations between the baseline cytokine values and increases in cytokine levels during the follow-up in subjects with dementia. These associations were analyzed before and after adjusting for significant baseline covariates using logistic regression models. Because cytokines have demonstrated additive and synergistic effects on AD (21), the combined effects of the pro-inflammatory cytokines were calculated by summing the number of cytokines with higher levels at baseline and the number of cytokines with higher levels at the follow-up, and then assigning ordinal values (0, 1, 2, 3, 4, 5) to each. Associations between baseline values and the summed number of higher cytokine levels with the incidence of dementia were assessed initially by the χ^2-test for a linear trend (i.e., 1 df), and then with the same logistic regression models to adjust for covariates. The Bonferroni correction was applied to maintain an overall type I error rate of 0.05 against the multiple comparisons. All statistical analyses were performed with SPSS software (ver. 21.0; SPSS Inc., Chicago, IL, USA).

RESULTS

Participant Characteristics

The recruitment procedure for the baseline and follow-up aspects of the study and distribution of dementia diagnoses are shown in **Figure 1**. Among the 625 subjects without dementia at the baseline evaluation, 518 (83%) completed all evaluations. At follow-up, incident dementia [mean interval (SD), 2.4 (0.3) years] was diagnosed in 45 participants (8.7%): 34 (6.6%) had AD, seven (1.4%) had vascular dementia, and four had "other" dementia (0.8%). Median [interquartile range (IQR)] IL-1α, IL-1β, IL-6, IL-8, and TNF-α levels were 40.3 (32.3–48.3), 12.0 (11.1–12.9), 9.5 (8.9–10.5), 20.1 (18.7–23.1), and 40.7 (37.5–43.9) pg/ml, respectively. Baseline characteristics are compared by the dementia diagnosis in **Supplementary Table 1**. Incident dementia was associated with older age, lower education, lower MMSE score, higher WHODAS II score, lower physical activity, and presence of the APOE e4 allele. The median (IQR) changes from baseline to follow-up for IL-1α, IL-1β, IL-6, IL-8, and TNF-α levels were +0.3 (0.3–1.9), +0.6 (0.4–0.8), +0.6 (0.6–4.0), +0.3 (0.1–1.8), and +1.2 (1.0–3.9), pg/ml, respectively. Baseline levels of and follow-up changes in serum cytokine concentrations according to the dementia diagnosis are shown in **Supplementary Table 2**.

Baseline and Follow-Up Concentrations of Serum Cytokines by Dementia Incidence

Unadjusted associations between serial serum cytokine levels and incident dementia are summarized in **Table 1**. Incident dementia was associated with increases in all five serum

TABLE 1 | Baseline levels of and follow-up changes in serum cytokine concentrations by incident dementia status.

	No incident dementia (*N* = 473)	Incident dementia (*N* = 45)	*P*-value*
BASELINE VALUES			
Tumor necrosis factor-α	40.3 (32.5–48.5)	40.7 (31.7–50.4)	0.921
Interleukin-1α	12.1 (11.1–12.9)	11.9 (11.2–14.1)	0.505
Interleukin-1β	9.5 (8.9–10.5)	9.3 (8.8–10.5)	0.981
Interleukin-6	20.0 (18.0–22.3)	21.0 (17.7–25.0)	0.146
Interleukin-8	40.4 (37.3–43.5)	43.0 (40.5–50.3)	**<0.001**
FOLLOW-UP VALUES			
Tumor necrosis factor-α	42.1 (36.5–47.7)	42.1 (37.1–47.1)	0.469
Interleukin-1α	13.2 (12.2–14.2)	13.9 (13.2–14.6)	**0.001**
Interleukin-1β	10.1 (9.5–11.1)	11.2 (10.0–12.6)	**<0.001**
Interleukin-6	22.1 (19.5–24.7)	24.6 (22.6–28.1)	**<0.001**
Interleukin-8	41.1 (38.4–44.6)	45.0 (38.5–53.5)	**0.002**
CHANGED VALUES			
Tumor necrosis factor-α	+1.2 (1.0–1.4)	+4.5 (−0.3–6.0)	**0.002**
Interleukin-1α	+0.3 (0.3–1.9)	+1.8 (1.1–2.0)	**0.001**
Interleukin-1β	+0.6 (0.6–0.7)	+2.2 (0.0–2.6)	**<0.001**
Interleukin-6	+0.6 (0.6–3.3)	+4.8 (0.8–6.0)	0.005
Interleukin-8	+0.3 (0.0–0.6)	+3.6 (−3.9–7.6)	0.100

**Mann Whitney test, Bold character denotes statistical significance after Bonferroni correction.*
Data are median (IQR).

TABLE 2 | Associations of incident dementia with (binary) higher baseline cytokine levels and (binary) more pronounced increase in levels over follow-up.

	Unadjusted	Adjusted[a]
BASELINE HIGHER LEVELS		
Tumor necrosis factor-α	1.05 (0.57–1.93)	0.83 (0.43–1.60)
Interleukin-1α	0.97 (0.47–1.59)	1.29 (0.65–2.56)
Interleukin-1β	0.78 (0.42–1.45)	1.09 (0.56–2.14)
Interleukin-6	1.16 (0.63–2.14)	1.22 (0.63–2.36)
Interleukin-8	2.67 (1.37–5.21)†	2.56 (1.25–5.23)*
MORE PRONOUNCED INCREASE IN LEVELS		
Tumor necrosis factor-α	**7.83 (3.92–15.63)‡**	**8.44 (4.02–17.70)‡**
Interleukin-1α	**7.26 (3.31–15.95)‡**	**8.20 (3.58–18.82)‡**
Interleukin-1β	**7.16 (3.64–14.09)‡**	**7.19 (3.47–14.94)‡**
Interleukin-6	**5.23 (2.63–10.40)‡**	**5.01 (2.43–10.32)‡**
Interleukin-8	**3.80 (2.02–7.16)‡**	**3.73 (1.90–7.32)‡**

[a]Adjusted for age, education, scores on Mini-Mental State Examination and World Health Organization Disability Assessment Scale II, APOE and physical activity.
**p-value < 0.05; †p-value < 0.01; ‡p-value < 0.001.*
Bold character denotes statistical significance after Bonferroni correction.
Data are displayed as odds ratios (95% confidence intervals).

cytokines during the follow-up, and the strength of the significance remained for TNF-α, IL1-α, and IL-1β after applying the Bonferroni correction. Incident dementia was associated with a higher IL-8 level at baseline, and the strength of the significance remained after applying the Bonferroni correction. The same analyses were repeated by dementia diagnosis and are presented in **Supplementary Table 2**. Incident AD was significantly associated with increases in IL1-α, IL-1β, and IL-6 levels but not with baseline cytokine levels after applying Bonferroni corrections. Incident vascular dementia was not associated any cytokine value.

Binary Higher Baseline Levels and Increasing Follow-up Level Categories of Serum Cytokines by Incident Dementia Status

The logistic regression results show a positive relationship between baseline and follow-up cytokine levels with the incidence of dementia (**Table 2**). Incident dementia was associated with IL-8 levels at baseline in unadjusted analyses. However, the association was not significant after adjusting for covariates. Incident dementia was significantly associated with higher levels of all five cytokines before and after adjustment, even after applying the Bonferroni correction. Incident dementia was not associated with higher pro-inflammatory cytokine level category at baseline before or after adjusting for covariates.

Sums of Higher Baseline Cytokine Levels and Increases in Cytokine Levels by Dementia Incidence

Figure 2 shows the combined effects of baseline and follow-up cytokine levels on dementia incidence. Incident dementia was associated with increases in the number of changes to higher cytokine levels during follow-up in unadjusted analyses ($\chi^2 = 50.91$; p-value < 0.001). However, no association was found between the incidence of dementia and increases in the summed number of higher cytokine levels at baseline ($\chi^2 = 0.604$; $p = 0.438$). After adjusting for older age, lower education, lower MMSE score, higher WHODAS II score, lower physical activity, and presence of the APOE e4 allele, the incidence of dementia increased significantly with increases in the summed number of changes to higher cytokine levels at follow-up. No association was found between incident dementia and increases in the summed number of higher cytokine levels at baseline.

DISCUSSION

The principal findings of this study were that the incidence of dementia was significantly associated with increases in all five serum cytokines, considered as both continuous and dichotomized variables, at follow-up, and the strength of these associations remained significant after applying the Bonferroni correction and relevant adjustments. The analysis of the combined effects of the five cytokines showed independent associations between increases in the summed number of higher cytokine levels between baseline and follow-up before and after adjustment. The incidence of dementia was only predicted by higher IL-8 levels at baseline, but this association was no longer significant in a multivariate analysis after applying the Bonferroni correction.

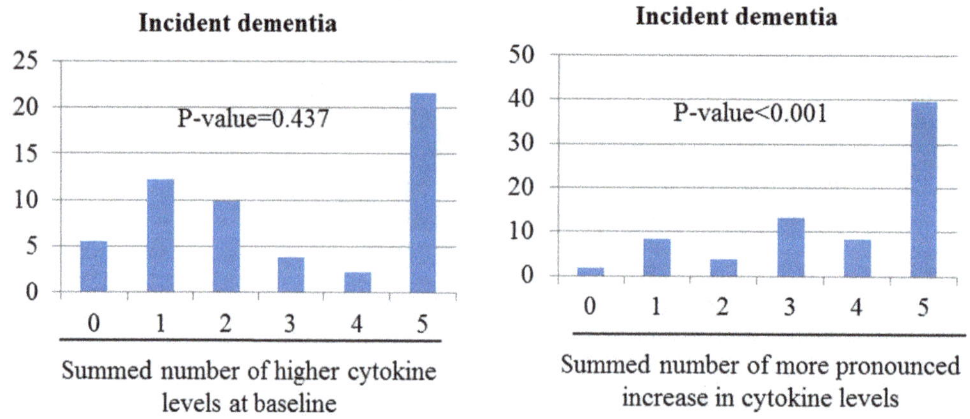

FIGURE 2 | Associations of incident dementia with number of cytokine levels categorize as high at baseline or as showing more pronounced increase over the follow-up period. Odds ratios (95% confidence intervals) for the association between incident depression and increased summed number of higher cytokine levels at baseline was 1.08 (0.88–1.33), p-value = 0.437; and between incident dementia and increased summed number of changed higher cytokine levels was 1.91 (1.55–2.34), p-value < 0.001 after adjustment for sex, cognitive function, disability, physical activity, and presence of the APOE e4 allele.

Inflammation may be an important mechanism underlying dementia (33, 34); however, it is unclear whether the inflammatory response is associated with the onset of dementia or is an outcome of dementia. To understand how inflammatory cytokines change, and possibly exert negative effects in dementia, a prospective cohort study with numerous inflammatory markers is needed. Very few studies have incorporated data from multiple time points in a clinical sample (35–37). Among them, only one study reported no association between AD and longitudinal inflammation (35), and two studies described an association between increases in inflammatory markers from baseline to follow-up and subsequent AD (36, 37). In this study, incident dementia was significantly associated with increases in cytokine levels during the study period. Several potential mechanisms might explain these findings. First, the level of inflammation may serve as a marker of active pathological processes. Hyperphosphorylation of the tau protein forming neurofibrillary tangles and amyloid beta (Aβ) accumulation in plaques are trademarks of AD progression (38). The abnormal Aβ clearance process results from the distortion of astrocytes or microglia to a pro-inflammatory state. This process is represented by elevated levels of pro-inflammatory cytokines and dysregulation of clear Aβ, and it leads to Aβ accumulation and worsened immune activation (39). In this study, 41 of 45 (91.1%) participants with dementia had AD and vascular dementia. Although the etiologies of AD and vascular dementia may be different, and thus lead to different disease outcomes, they may begin as a similar cascade of cytokine production in response to neuronal injury (8, 38, 39). Increased cytokine levels were significantly associated with incident AD but not with vascular dementia. However, due to the small sample size, there is a possibility of a type II error in the non-significant associations with vascular dementia. Second, it is also possible that cytokines increased due to causes other than dementia during the follow-up period. For example, normal aging can cause an increase in peripheral cytokines (33, 40). Our longitudinal observations support this hypothesis. Five cytokines increased during the follow-up period in both the dementia and control groups. The term sensitization is often used to describe induction of an immune response. Here, the incidence of dementia was associated with an increase in cytokine levels, but not with the absolute concentrations of baseline cytokine levels. Therefore, when conditions other than aging occur that can accelerate inflammation, such as amyloid plaques and neurofibrillary tangles (9), depression (9), genetic conditions (41), infections (42), trauma, and vascular events (8), immune sensitization can occur, which can accelerate cognitive impairment.

Previous studies of cross-sectional cytokine levels as predictors of the incidence of dementia have resulted in heterogeneous findings (35, 43–45). Those studies were limited by differences in study design, such as participant characteristics. In our study, baseline IL-8 level was associated with incident dementia in unadjusted analyses, but was not significant in the multivariate analysis after applying the Bonferroni correction. Furthermore, the impacts of cytokines have been revealed to be synergistic and, given the inconsistent outcome of a single cytokine level, the combined effect of multiple cytokines represents a more practical approach (21, 46). No associations were detected when high cytokine levels were summed. Together, these data do not support the hypothesis that cytokines result in dementia-related dysfunction but, instead, suggest that cytokine levels are elevated by dementia-related processes.

This study has several strengths. Cytokine levels were assessed serially, which could help to clarify causal relationships. In addition, the follow-up rate was reasonable and a number of potential covariates were considered in the analyses. This study also has several limitations. First, due to limited resources, we only measured five cytokines, and other important anti-inflammatory (e.g., IL-4 and IL-10) and pro-inflammatory (e.g., IL-13 and IL-18) cytokines were not evaluated (47). It is important to determine the exact function of various cytokines and disease progression. Overproduction of several cytokines could result in damage to neurons, and these cytokines may play a role in the progression of dementia, but their protective effects have also been considered (47). Second, we collected blood samples from the periphery to measure inflammation in the central nervous system. Several studies have been conducted using imaging technology, including positron emission tomography, to measure neuroinflammation directly in subjects with dementia (48, 49). More studies are required to demonstrate the relationships between these cytokines and dementia. Third, due to protein degradation, it is recommended that blood samples be examined immediately. In this instance, due to technical difficulties, they were centrifuged at 3,000 rpm for 10 min, and sera were stored at −70°C until we finished specimen collection. However, most studies follow this procedure (20, 50). Fourth, the small set of covariate-adjusted analyses leaves the possibility of confounding bias. For example, we adjusted for age, education, MMSE, WHODAS, and physical activity but not for alcohol, smoking, or body mass index, which did affect the associations between cytokine levels and dementia, although these factors were not significantly associated with incident dementia at the follow-up (**Supplementary Table 1**). In particular, we could not provide an accurate diagnosis for smoking and alcohol use. Varying the cutoff points may lead to a different interpretation of the results of a trial. Thus, our adjustment might have been suboptimal. Fifth, conclusions regarding dementia that fully reflect the complex disease status are improbable, as stated above. In this study, due to a limitation in the study design, the probability that increases in cytokines may arise transiently, as in acute infectious disease, or continuously because of chronic inflammatory disease, may have influenced the heterogeneity, and both diseases may contribute to incident dementia. In addition, it was difficult to diagnose mixed dementia due to a lack of brain imaging data. However, this limitation is common in most epidemiological studies. Finally, because this study did not specify the timing of the dementia diagnosis, it was not possible to state clearly that dementia preceded inflammation. Furthermore, only 2 years of follow-up visits were carried out. Because dementia progresses over decades, having a longer follow-up is crucial to identifying the developmental trajectory of the disease. Additional follow-up studies will be needed to address these limitations.

Our findings suggest that incident dementia may lead changes in serum cytokine levels and inflammation, rather than resulting from elevated pro-inflammatory cytokines. It has been reported that patients with dementia, particularly those at more advanced stages, are at a higher risk for developing stroke and depression (51, 52), which could, theoretically, be mediated by inflammation. As mentioned above, our findings must be replicated in future studies with more cytokines. Furthermore, interactions between cytokine levels and genes need further assessment, as there is sufficient evidence that the transcriptional activity of specific polymorphisms influences cytokine production (53).

AUTHOR CONTRIBUTIONS

J-WK conducted the data analysis and drafted the article. RS and H-JK helped to analyze the data and to draft the article. K-YB, S-WK, I-SS, and J-SY helped to recruit the participant and perform dementia assessment and management. All authors approved the final version of manuscript to be published. J-MK had full access to all of the data in the study and take responsibility for the integrity of the data and the accuracy of the data analysis.

FUNDING

This study was supported by a grant (BCRI 18018) Chonnam National University Hospital Biomedical Research Institute to J-MK.

REFERENCES

1. American Psychiatric Association. *Diagnostic and Statistical Manual of Mental Disorder*. 5th ed. Washington, DC: American Psychiatric Press (2013).
2. Tai SY, Huang SW, Hsu CL, Yang CH, Chou MC, Yang YH. Screening dementia in the outpatient department: patients at risk for dementia. *ScientificWorldJournal* (2014) 2014:138786. doi: 10.1155/2014/138786
3. Thies W, Bleiler L. Alzheimer's disease facts and figures. *Alzheimers Dement.* (2011) 7:208–44. doi: 10.1016/j.jalz.2011.02.004
4. Martin P, Matthew P, Maëlenn G. *World Alzheimer Report 2013: Journey of Caring a Analysis of Long-Term Care for Dementia* (2013). Available online at: http://www.alz.co.uk/research/WorldAlzheimerReport2013.pdf?m
5. Schneider J, Murray J, Banerjee S, Mann A. EUROCARE: a cross-national study of co-resident spouse carers for people with Alzheimer's disease: I–factors associated with career burden. *Int J Geriatr Psychiatry* (1999) 14: 651–61.
6. Carlson MC, Helms MJ, Steffens DC, Burke JR, Potter GG, Plassman BL: Midlife activity predicts risk of dementia in older male twin pairs. *Alzheimers Dement.* (2008) 4: 324–31. doi: 10.1016/j.jalz.2008.07.002
7. van den Biggelaar AH, Gussekloo J, de Craen AJ, Frolich M, Stek ML, van der Mast RC, et al. Inflammation and interleukin-1 signaling network contribute to depressive symptoms but not cognitive decline in old age. *Exp Gerontol.* (2007) 42: 693–701. doi: 10.1016/j.exger.2007.01.011
8. Tarkowski E, Rosengren L, Blomstrand C, Wikkelso C, Jensen C, Ekholm S, et al. Intrathecal release of proand anti-inflammatory cytokines during stroke. *Clin Exp Immunol.* (1997) 110:492–9. doi: 10.1046/j.1365-2249.1997.4621483.x
9. Akiyama H, Barger S, Barnum S, Bradt B, Bauer J, Cole GM, et al. Inflammation and Alzheimer's disease. *Neurobiol Aging* (2000) 21:383–421. doi: 10.1016/S0197-4580(00)00124-X
10. Tan ZS, Beiser AS, Vasan RS, Roubenoff R, Dinarello CA, Harris TB, et al. Inflammatory markers and the risk of Alzheimer disease: the Framingham Study. *Neurology* (2007) 68:1902–8. doi: 10.1212/01.wnl.0000263217.36439.da
11. Tarkowski E, Liljeroth AM, Minthon L, Tarkowski A, Wallin A, Blennow K. Cerebral pattern of pro- and anti-inflammatory cytokines

in dementias. *Brain Res Bull.* (2003) 61:255–60. doi: 10.1016/S0361-9230(03)00088-1
12. Dursun E, Gezen-Ak D, Hanagasi H, Bilgiç B, Lohmann E, Ertan S, et al. The interleukin 1 alpha, interleukin 1 beta, interleukin 6 and alpha-2-macroglobulin serum levels in patients with early or late onset Alzheimer's disease, mild cognitive impairment or Parkinson's disease. *J Neuroimmunol.* (2015) 283:50–7. doi: 10.1016/j.jneuroim.2015.04.014
13. Swardfager W, Lanctôt K, Rothenburg L, Wong A, Cappell J, Herrmann N. A meta-analysis of cytokines in Alzheimer's disease. *Biol Psychiatry* (2010) 68:930–41. doi: 10.1016/j.biopsych.2010.06.012
14. Lai KSP, Liu CS, Rau A, Lanctot KL, Kohler CA, Pakosh M, et al. Peripheral inflammatory markers in Alzheimer's disease: a systematic review and meta-analysis of 175 studies. *J Neurol Neurosurg Psychiatry* (2017) 88:876–82. doi: 10.1136/jnnp-2017-316201
15. Metti AL, Cauley JA. How predictive of dementia are peripheral inflammatory markers in the elderly? *Neurodegener Dis Manag.* (2012) 2:609–22. doi: 10.2217/nmt.12.68
16. Wyss-Coray T. Inflammation in Alzheimer disease: driving force, bystander or beneficial response? *Nat Med.* (2006) 12:1005–15. doi: 10.1038/nm1484
17. Engelhart MJ, Geerlings MI, Meijer J, Kiliaan A, Ruitenberg A, van Swieten JC, et al. Inflammatory proteins in plasma and the risk of dementia: the Rotterdam study. *Arch Neurol.* (2004) 61:668–72. doi: 10.1001/archneur.61.5.668
18. Schmidt R, Schmidt H, Curb JD, Masaki K, White LR, Launer LJ. Early inflammation and dementia: a 25-year follow-up of the Honolulu-Asia Aging Study. *Ann Neurol.* (2002) 52:168–74. doi: 10.1002/ana.10265
19. Eriksson UK, Pedersen NL, Reynolds CA, Hong MG, Prince JA, Gatz M, et al. Associations of gene sequence variation and serum levels of C-reactive protein and interleukin-6 with Alzheimer's disease and dementia. *J Alzheimers Dis.* (2011) 23:361–9. doi: 10.3233/JAD-2010-101671
20. Ravaglia G, Forti P, Maioli F, Chiappelli F, Tumini E, Mariani E, et al. Blood inflammatory markers and risk of dementia: The Conselice Study of Brain Aging. *Neurobiol Aging* (2007) 28:1810–20. doi: 10.1016/j.neurobiolaging.2006.08.012
21. Kang HJ, Kim JM, Kim SW, Shin IS, Park SW, Kim YH, et al. Associations of cytokine genes with Alzheimer's disease and depression in an elderly Korean population. *J Neurol Neurosurg Psychiatry* (2015) 86:1002–7. doi: 10.1136/jnnp-2014-308469
22. Park JH, Kwon YC. Modification of the mini-mental state examination for use in the elderly in a non-western society: Part I. Development of Korean version of Mini-Mental State Examination. *Int J Geriatr Psychiatry* (1990) 5:381–7. doi: 10.1002/gps.930050606
23. Lawton MP, Brody EM. Assessment of older people: self-maintaining and instrumental activities of daily living. *Gerontologist* (1969) 9:179–186. doi: 10.1093/geront/9.3_Part_1.179
24. Hughes CP, Berg L, Danziger WL, Coben LA, Martin RL. A new clinical scale for the staging of dementia. *Br J Psychiatry* (1982) 140:566–72. doi: 10.1192/bjp.140.6.566
25. McKhann G, Drachman D, Folstein M, Katzman R, Price D, Stadlan EM. Clinical diagnosis of Alzheimer's disease: report of the NINCDS-ADRDA Work Group under the auspices of Department of Health and Human Services Task Force on Alzheimer's Disease. *Neurology* (1984) 34:939–44. doi: 10.1212/WNL.34.7.939
26. Román GC, Goldstein M. Facts, myths, and controversies in vascular dementia. *N Engl J Med.* (1993) 329:63.
27. Copeland JR, Dewey ME, Griffiths-Jones HM. A computerized psychiatric diagnostic system and case nomenclature for elderly subjects: GMS and AGECAT. *Psychol Med.* (1986) 16:89–99. doi: 10.1017/S0033291700057779
28. Kim JM, Stewart R, Glozier N, Prince M, Kim SW, Yang SJ, et al. Physical health, depression and cognitive function as correlates of disability in an older Korean population. *Int J Geriatr Psychiatry* (2005) 20:160–7. doi: 10.1002/gps.1266
29. National Institute of Alcohol Abuse and Alcoholism. *The Physicians' Guide to Helping Patients With Alcohol Problems.* Bethesda, MD: National Institutes of Health Publication (1995). p. 95–3769.
30. Prince M. 10/66 Dementia Research Group. Care arrangements for people with dementia in developing countries. *Int J Geriatr Psychiatry* (2004) 19:170–7. doi: 10.1002/gps.1046
31. Kim JM, Stewart R, Kim SW, Yang SJ, Shin IS, Yoon JS. Predictive value of folate, vitamin B12 and homocysteine levels in late-life depression. *Br J Psychiatry* (2008) 192:268–74. doi: 10.1192/bjp.bp.107.039511
32. Folstein MF, Fostein SE, McHugh PR. "Mini-Mental State": a practical method for grading the cognitive state of patients for the clinician. *J Psychiatr Res.* (1975) 12:189–98. doi: 10.1016/0022-3956(75)90026-6
33. Brüünsgaard H, Pedersen BK. Age-related inflammatory cytokines and disease. *Immunol Allergy Clin North Am.* (2003) 23:15–39. doi: 10.1016/S0889-8561(02)00056-5
34. Launer LJ. Nonsteroidal anti-inflammatory drugs and Alzheimer disease. What's next? *JAMA* (2003) 289:2865–7. doi: 10.1001/jama.289.21.2865
35. Lanzrein AS, Johnston CM, Perry VH, Jobst KA, King Em, Smith AD. Longitudinal study of inflammatory factors in serum, cerebrospinal fluid, and brain tissue in Alzheimer's disease: interleukin-1b, interleukin-6, interleukin-1 receptor antagonist, tumornecrosis factor-a, the soluble tumor necrosis factor receptors I and II, and a-1-antichymotrypsin. *Alzheimer Dis Assoc Disord.* (1998) 12:215–27.
36. Leung R, Proitsi P, Simmons A, Lunnon K, Guntert A, Kronenberg D, et al. Inflammatory proteins in plasma are associated with severity of Alzheimer's disease. *PLoS ONE* (2013) 8:e64971. doi: 10.1371/journal.pone.0064971
37. Sundelöf J, Kilander L, Helmersson J, Larsson A, Ronnemaa E, Degerman-Gunnarsson M, et al. Systemic inflammation and the risk of Alzheimer's disease and dementia: a prospective population-based study. *J Alzheimers Dis.* (2009) 18:79–87. doi: 10.3233/JAD-2009-1126
38. Kumar A, Singh A, Ekavali. A review on Alzheimer's disease pathophysiology and its management: an update. *Pharmacol Rep.* (2015) 67:195–203. doi: 10.1016/j.pharep.2014.09.004
39. Zheng C, Zhou XW, Wang JZ. The dual roles of cytokines in Alzheimer's disease: update on interleukins, TNF-α, TGF-β and IFN-γ. *Transl Neurodegener.* (2016) 5:1–15. doi: 10.1186/s40035-016-0054-4
40. Lee DH, Kim M, Kim M, LeeYJ, Yoo HJ, Lee SH, et al. Age-dependent alterations in serum cytokines, peripheral blood mononuclear cell cytokine production, natural killer cell activity, and prostaglandin F2α. *Immunol Res.* (2017) 65:1009–16. doi: 10.1007/s12026-017-8940-0
41. Cribbs DH, Berchtold NC, Perreau V, Coleman PD, Rogers J, Tenner AJ, et al. Extensive innate immune gene activation accompanies brain aging, increasing vulnerability to cognitive decline and neurodegeneration: a microarray study. *J Neuroinflammation* (2012) 9:1–18. doi: 10.1186/1742-2094-9-179
42. Perry VH, Cunningham C, Holmes C. Systemic infections and inflammation affect chronic neurodegeneration. *Nat Rev Immun.* (2007) 7:161–7. doi: 10.1038/nri2015
43. Miwa K, Okazaki S, Sakaguchi M, Mochizuki H, Kitagawa K. Interleukin-6, interleukin-6 receptor gene variant, small-vessel disease and incident dementia. *Eur J Neurol.* (2016) 23:656–63. doi: 10.1111/ene.12921
44. Franciosi S, Choi HB, Kim SU, McLarnon JG. IL-8 enhancement of amyloid-beta (Abeta 1-42)-induced expression and production of pro-inflammatory cytokines and COX-2 in cultured human microglia. *J Neuroimmunol.* (2005) 159:66–74. doi: 10.1016/j.jneuroim.2004.10.006
45. Richartz E, Stransky E, Batra A, Simon P, Lewczuk P, Buchkremer G, et al. Decline of immune responsiveness: a pathogenic factor in Alzheimer's disease? *J Psychiatr Res.* (2005) 39:535–43. doi: 10.1016/j.jpsychires.2004.12.005
46. Schiepers OJ, Wichers MC, Maes M. Cytokines and major depression. *Prog Neuropsychopharmacol Biol Psychiatry* (2005) 29:201–17. doi: 10.1016/j.pnpbp.2004.11.003
47. Zhang F, Jiang L. Neuroinflammation in Alzheimer's disease. *Neuropsychiatr Dis Treat.* (2015) 11:243–56. doi: 10.2147/NDT.S75546
48. Herholz K, Carter SF, Jones M. Positron emission tomography imaging in dementia. *Br J Radiol.* (2007) 80:S160–7. doi: 10.1259/bjr/97295129
49. Nordberg A, Rinne JO, Kadir A, Långström B. The use of PET in Alzheimer disease. *Nat Rev Neurol.* (2010) 6:78–87. doi: 10.1038/nrneurol.2009.217
50. Baune BT, Ponath G, Golledge J, Varga G, Arolt V, Rothermundt M, et al. Association between IL-8 cytokine and cognitive performance in an elderly

general population–the MEMO-Study. *Neurobiol Aging* (2008) 29:937–44. doi: 10.1016/j.neurobiolaging.2006.12.003

51. Bunn F, Burn AM, Goodman C, Rait G, Norton S, Robinson L, et al. Comorbidity and dementia: a scoping review of the literature. *BMC Med.* (2014) 12:192. doi: 10.1186/s12916-014-0192-4
52. Kitching D. Depression in dementia. *Aust Prescr.* (2015) 38:209–11. doi: 10.18773/austprescr.2015.071
53. de Craen AJ, Posthuma D, Remarque EJ. Heritability estimates of innate immunity: an extended twin study. *Genes Immun.* (2005) 6:167–70. doi: 10.1038/sj.gene.6364162

13

Proteomic Profiling Unravels a Key Role of Specific Macrophage Subtypes in Sporadic Inclusion Body Myositis

Andreas Roos[1,2†], *Corinna Preusse*[3†], *Denisa Hathazi*[2], *Hans-Hilmar Goebel*[3] *and Werner Stenzel*[3,4*]

[1] *Department of Neuropediatrics, Developmental Neurology and Social Pediatrics, Centre for Neuromuscular Disorders in Children, University Children's Hospital Essen, University of Duisburg-Essen, Essen, Germany,* [2] *Leibniz-Institut für Analytische Wissenschaften -ISAS- e.V., Dortmund, Germany,* [3] *Department of Neuropathology, Charité -Universitätsmedizin Berlin, Corporate Member of Freie Universität Berlin, Humboldt-Universität zu Berlin, and Berlin Institute of Health, Berlin, Germany,* [4] *Leibniz Science Campus Chronic Inflammation, Berlin, Germany*

Correspondence:
Werner Stenzel
werner.stenzel@charite.de

† *These authors share first authorship*

Unbiased proteomic profiling was performed toward the identification of biological parameters relevant in sIBM, thus giving hints about the pathophysiological processes and the existence of new reliable markers. For that purpose, skeletal muscle biopsies from 13 sIBM and 7 non-diseased control patients were analyzed with various methods, including liquid chromatography coupled to tandem mass spectrometry (four patients). Subsequent data analysis identified key molecules further studied in a larger cohort by *q*PCR, immunostaining, and immunofluorescence *in situ*. Proteomic signature of muscle biopsies derived from sIBM patients revealed the chaperone and cell surface marker CD74, the macrophage scavenger molecule CD163 and the transcription activator STAT1 to be among the highly and relevantly expressed proteins suggesting a significant contribution of immune cells among the myofibers expressing these markers. Moreover, *in silico* studies showed that 39% of upregulated proteins were involved in type I or mixed type I and type II interferon immunity. Indeed, further studies via immunohistochemistry clearly confirmed the prominent involvement of the key type I interferon signature-related molecules, ISG15 as well as IRF8 with MHC class II^{+} myofibers. Siglec1 colocalized with CD163^{+} macrophages and MHC class II molecules also co-localized with CD74 on macrophages. STAT1 co-localized with Siglec1^{+} macrophages in active myofibre myophagocytosis while STAT6 colocalized with endomysial macrophages. These combined results show involvement of CD74, CD163, and STAT1 as key molecules of macrophage activation being crucially involved in mixed and specific type I interferon, and interferon gamma associated-pathways in sIBM. On a more general note, these results also highlight the type of immune-interaction between macrophages and myofibers in the etiopathology of sIBM.

Keywords: CD74, SIGLEC1, CD163, STAT1, STAT6, type I interferon (IFN), muscle proteomics

INTRODUCTION

Inclusion body myositis is a chronic muscle-specific disease of adulthood leading to progressive and very characteristic hip flexor and quadriceps paresis, long finger flexor paresis, and swallowing difficulties (1–4). Muscle biopsy reveals a severe myopathic/dystrophic process with the characteristic complex inflammatory infiltrate composed of different types of T cells, macrophages and other mononuclear cells. Additional degenerative changes with the presence of amyloidogenic protein deposits, disturbed autophagy, and mitochondrial abnormalities are present. Clinical and muscle biopsy characteristics are the basis of a precise diagnosis of sIBM (1, 3, 5, 6). The autoantibody cN1A can be used as a marker of severity in sIBM, however, its role in the pathogenicity of this disease has not been fully elucidated (7–9). Despite the characteristic clinical picture and well-known biopsy findings, the pathogenesis of sIBM is still elusive and not fully understood. So far, therapeutic approaches have not been broadly successful, questioning the (auto)-immune pathogenesis. Moreover, these therapeutic interventions present attempts to address the degenerative autophagic dysfunction (10).

Proteomics and subsequent specific data analysis of diseased tissue such as skeletal muscle can help to identify key pathogenic molecules or groups of molecules involved in certain processes, which may be of relevance in inflammatory or genetic diseases affecting muscle fiber integrity [exemplified in (11)].

In this study, we applied unbiased proteomic profiling and identified CD74, CD163, and STAT1 among the highly expressed proteins in muscle biopsies of sIBM patients. Notably, these proteins were found to localize to macrophages and partially to the sarcolemma of myofibers. Further analyses were performed in the larger context of associated immune responses in skeletal muscle tissue. These approaches revealed a specific and key role of the cellular interaction of specifically activated macrophages with myofibers.

MATERIALS AND METHODS

Patients

Clinical data of all IBM patients enrolled in this study are listed in **Table 1**. We included patients with clinical, and morphological signs and symptoms consistent with sIBM, according to present criteria (12), as well as sex- and age-matched patients defined as non-diseased controls (NDCs). We chose as controls subjects who had undergone a muscle biopsy, but who were found not to have any inflammatory muscle disease. They had suffered from non-specific complaints like myalgia, but objective muscle weakness and morphological abnormalities on skeletal muscle biopsy were absent. CK levels were normal and no signs of systemic inflammation and no myositis-specific antibodies (MSA) or myositis-associated antibodies (MAA) were detectable. sIBM patients had moderate illness (still ambulatory) and homogeneous muscle biopsy findings (not severely atrophic muscle bulk). Informed consent was obtained from all patients and the Charité ethics committee (EA2/163/17), had granted ethical approval.

Skeletal Muscle Specimens

In this study, we analyzed skeletal muscle biopsies derived from sIBM patients (clinically and morphologically definite sIBM) (12). Skeletal muscle biopsies from sIBM patients were used to produce proteomic results (four biopsies) and qualitative morphological characteristics *in situ* (whole cohort). In addition, four control muscle biopsies were included for the proteomic profiling and additional nine biopsies for subsequent immunohistochemical and *q*PCR studies. All skeletal muscle specimens were cryopreserved at −80°C prior to analysis.

Morphological Analysis

All stains were performed on 7 µm cryomicrotome sections, according to standard procedures. Immunohistochemical and double immunofluorescence reactions were carried out as described previously (13). The following antibodies were used for staining procedures:

Mouse anti-human CD163, 1:50, St. John's Lab/polyclonal; rabbit anti-human CD74, 1:100 St. John's Lab/polyclonal; mouse anti-human CD68, 1:100 Dako/EBM1; rabbit anti-human iNOS, ready-to-use, Genetex/polyclonal; rabbit anti-human ISG15, 1:100, abcam/polyclonal; MHCI, 1:1.000, Dako/W6/32; mouse anti-human MHC class II, 1:100, DAKO/ CR3/43; rat anti-human STAT1, 1:50, R&D Systems/246523; mouse anti-human STAT6, 1:50, R&D Systems/253906; mouse anti-human Siglec1, 1:100, Novus Biologicals/HSn7D2; IRF8, 1:100 Abcam/polyclonal.

Proteomics

Proteomic profiling of four sIBM-patient derived and four control quadriceps muscles was carried out as described previously (14).

In Silico Studies

Further *in silico* studies included "Proteomaps" (www.proteomaps.net), "Interferome" (www.interferome.org), "Cytoscape" (www.cytoscape.org) and "STRING" (www.string-db.org) and have been carried out to unravel functional connections and interdependences between the proteins vulnerable in sIBM with a special focus on such involved in the interferon-mediated immune response. All regulated proteins (24 down, 119 up-regulated) were used for the analyses.

"Proteomaps" enables us to obtain a picture of the quantitative composition of vulnerable pathways and cellular processes with a focus on individual protein functions controlling these pathways and processes. The visualization of affected pathways (and responsible proteins) is built automatically from the computerized proteome data and based on the "KEGG Pathways" gene classification. Hereby, individual proteins are shown as polygons and to emphasize the fold of regulation, polygon-sizes reflect fold of changes abundances. Functionally related proteins are arranged in proximity. This *in silico* tool has been applied

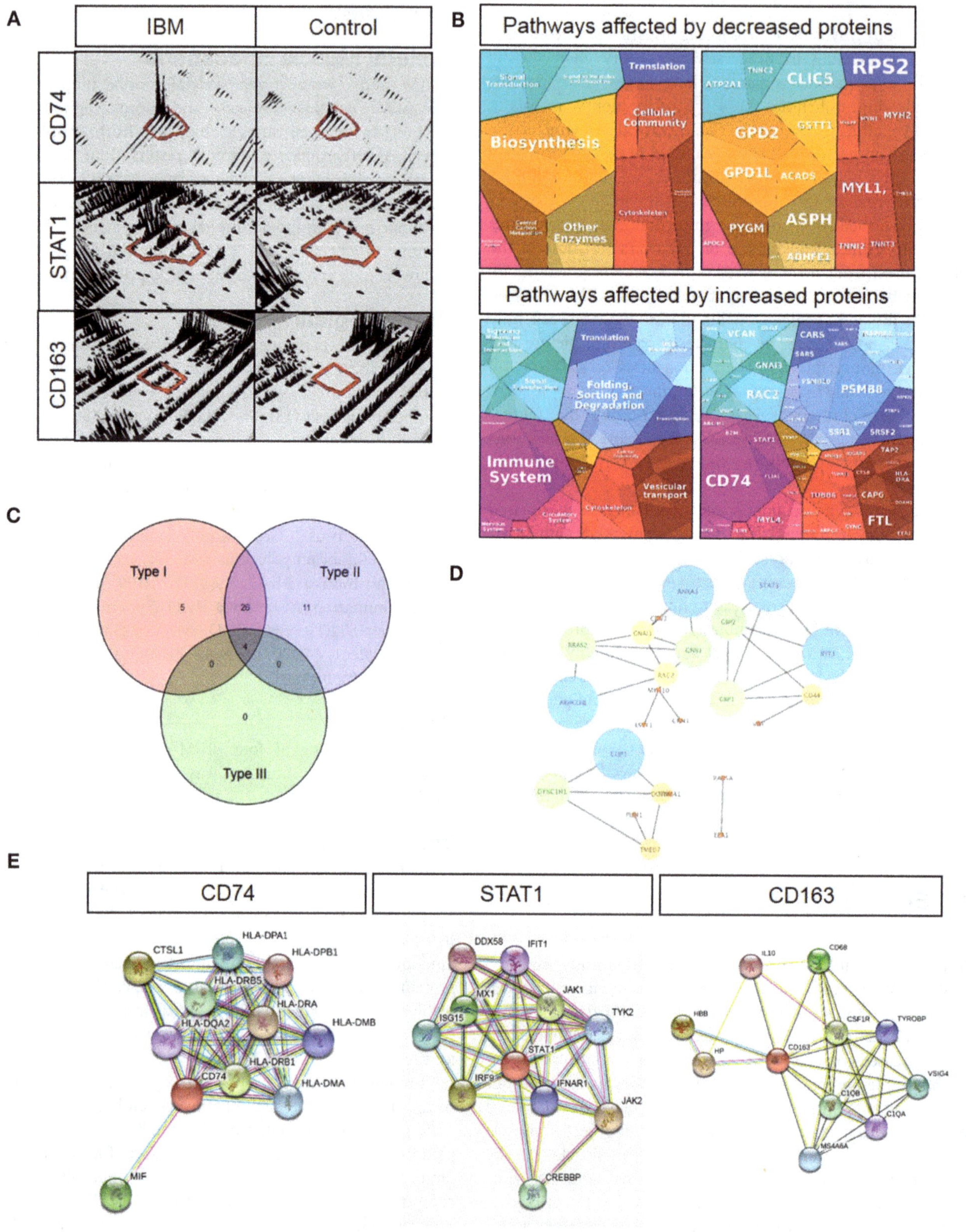

FIGURE 1 | Key proteomic findings and subsequent *in silico* analyses. **(A)** 3-D montages of representative tryptic peptides highlighting the increased abundance of the corresponding proteins, CD47, STAT1, and CD163. **(B)** Proteomaps-based analysis of cellular processes addressed by up- and down-regulated proteins in sIBM-patient-derived muscle (left figures) as well as of proteins predominating the respective cellular processes by taking their relative abundance/fold of regulation

(Continued)

FIGURE 1 | into consideration (right figures). **(C)** Venn diagram-based categorization of proteins increased in sIBM-patient-derived muscle and modulated by the three different interferon types (detailed list of increased proteins controlled by interferons is provided in **Table 2**). **(D)** Cytoscape-based visualization of functional networks of upregulated proteins controlled by interferons. **(E)** STRING-based analysis of functional protein networks of CD74 (left figure), STAT1 (figure in the middle) and CD163 (right figure) toward the identification of further interferon-modulated and macrophage-expressed proteins with pathophysiological significance in sIBM.

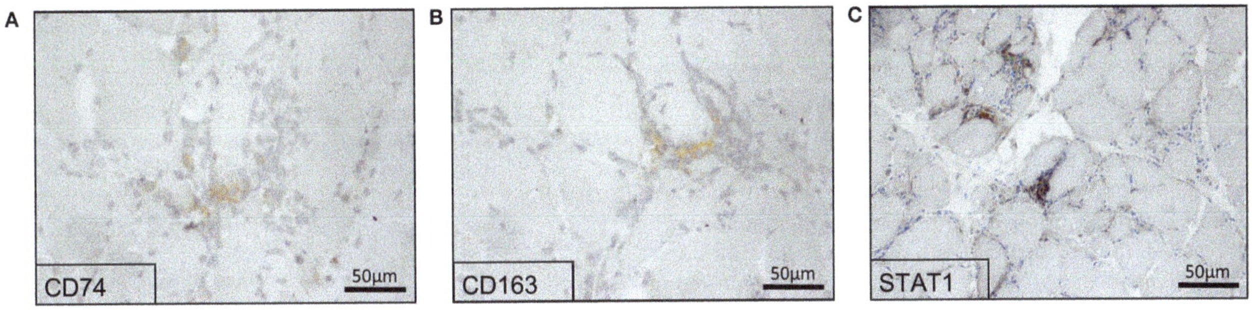

FIGURE 2 | Immunohistochemical reactions of potential key players in the skeletal muscle biopsies from sIBM patients. Proteomics-based identified key players showed a positive staining in sIBM patients' skeletal muscle biopsies, where CD74 **(A)**, as well as CD163 **(B)** highlighted macrophages. STAT1 **(C)** was expressed in macrophages in active myophagocytosis, while it was not present at the sarcolemma of myofibers.

to proteins showing a statistically significant altered abundance and thus vulnerability in sIBM-diseased muscle. "Interferome" enables the reliable identification of individual interferon-regulated genes or respective molecular signatures. Here, "Ensembl IDs" have been utilized to filter for interferon-regulated genes (or rather corresponding proteins) based on our proteomic findings. "Cytoscape" as an additional open source *in silico* tool enabling the visualization of molecular and functional protein-protein interaction networks. Here, we applied "Cytoscape" to proteins modulated by the interferon-response (based on the results of our "Interferome"-based data analysis). "STRING" (Search Tool for the Retrieval of Interacting Genes/Proteins) represents an *in silico* tool enabling the delineation of (direct and functionally related) protein-protein interactions and thus allows to identify functional interdependences of proteins with altered abundances in diseased tissues such as sIBM muscle. Here, we applied "STRING" to decipher proteins interacting with CD74, STAT1, and CD63.

Quantitative Reverse Transcription PCR (*q*RT-PCR)

Total RNA was extracted from muscle specimens using the technique described previously (13). Briefly, cDNA was synthesized using the High-Capacity cDNA Archive Kit (Applied Biosystems, Foster City, CA). For qPCR reactions, 2 ng of cDNA were used and for subsequent analysis, the 7900HT Fast Real-Time PCR System (Applied Biosystems, Foster City, CA) was utilized with the following, running conditions: 95°C 0:20, 95°C 0:01, 60°C 0:20, 45 cycles (values above 40 cycles were defined as not expressed). All targeted transcripts were run as triplicates. For each of these runs, the reference gene *PGK1* has been included as internal control to normalize the relative expression of the targeted transcripts. The qPCR assay identification numbers, TaqMan® Gene Exp Assay from Life Technologies/ThermoFisher are listed as follows: STAT1 Hs01013989_m1, STAT6 Hs00598625_m1, PGK1 Hs99999906_m1. The ΔCT of non-diseased controls was subtracted from the ΔCT of sIBM patients muscles to determine the differences (ΔΔCT) and fold change (2^ − ΔΔCT) of gene expression. Gene expression was illustrated by the log10 of fold change values compared to NDCs.

Statistical Analysis

Statistical analysis of proteomic data has been carried out as described previously (14). Kruskal-Wallis one-way ANOVA followed by Bonferroni-Dunn correction of the *post hoc* tests was used to analyze quantitative differences of mRNA transcripts. Data are presented as mean ± SEM. The level of significance was set at $P < 0.05$. GraphPad Prism 5.02 software (GraphPad Software, Inc., La Jolla, CA, USA) was used for statistical analysis.

RESULTS

Proteomic Signature: CD74, CD163, and STAT1 Are Highly Expressed in Skeletal Muscle Biopsies of sIBM Patients

Since the precise pathogenesis of IBM is still unclear, we aimed to analyze the proteomic signature via label-free profiling as an unbiased approach to gather new relevant molecules that might play decisive roles in the disease pathogenesis. The proteomic analysis unraveled that CD74 (6.7-fold; log_2-ratio), STAT1 (5-fold; log_2-ratio), and CD163 (4.8-fold; log_2-ratio) are among the highly expressed proteins in skeletal muscle specimens derived from sIBM patients (**Figure 1A**). *In silico* studies (proteomap: https://www.proteomaps.net/) of all proteins altered in abundance (out of 1375 quantified proteins, 24 are statistically significantly decreased and 119 are increased; vulnerability of 10.4% of the investigated proteome) in sIBM-patient derived skeletal muscles, revealed alteration of biosynthesis, cellular composition, cytoskeleton and altered protein processing (folding, sorting, and degradation) along with vesicular transport. Moreover, the activation of the immune response is a predominating mechanism mirrored by an increase in specific proteins (**Figure 1B**). Remarkably, proteomap-based linking of altered cellular processes to key proteins (taking their fold of regulation into consideration) revealed that CD74 and STAT1 hereby seem to be major molecular "determinators" of modulation of the immune response. Prompted by this finding and by the fact that CD74, STAT1, and CD163 are well-known modulators of interferon-mediated processes (15–21), all up-regulated proteins (total of 119 proteins) were additionally analyzed *in silico* using the "interferome" platform (http://www.interferome.org). This resulted in the identification of a total 46 transcripts corresponding to the proteins up-regulated in the muscle of sIBM patients which are controlled by interferon-modulated processes (**Figure 1C**). Hereby 26 out of the 46 up-regulated transcripts are controlled by both types I and II interferon and four proteins by types I, II, and III. Five transcripts are controlled either by type 1 interferons while eleven are by type 2 interferons (**Figure 1C**). An additional analysis of the interferon-pathway controlled proteins via the "cytoscape" platform (https://cytoscape.org/) confirmed a functional interdependence of these proteins (**Figure 1D**), thus suggesting a functional relevance in sIBM-pathogenesis.

A further STRING analysis (https://string-db.org) toward the identification of functional protein-protein networks confirmed the functional interplay of the proteins encoded by these transcripts (**Figure 1D**), suggesting a fundamental role of interferon-modulated processes in the etiopathology of sIBM. An individual STRING analysis of CD74, STAT1, and CD163 confirmed a functional link of these immune-response proteins to a variety of interferon-induced proteins (**Figure 1E**).

Based on the dense networks of predicted functional protein-protein interplays, we evaluated the potential reaction partners and hence decided to focus on some key players for further studies. The selected key players are MIF—Macrophage migration inhibitory factor, involved in the interferon type response and showing a functional interplay with CD74 (**Figure 1E**) as well as ISG15, which was not upregulated in our analyses, but represents a well-known partner (22) for e.g., STATs, JAKs and IL-6, which are all found in our STRING analysis (**Figure 1E**). Both of these molecules showed an increased immunoreactivity within macrophages in sIBM-patient derived muscle biopsy specimens, thus supporting the concept of the involvement of different types of interferon-mediated downstream intracellular activation programs in macrophages. The concept of a particular role of macrophage-mediated interferon response in sIBM is not only further supported by increased abundance of Macrophage-capping protein (CAPG; identified via proteomic profiling; **Table 2**), but also by the identification of increased immunoreactivity of additional key players such as Siglecl and CD68 within macrophages in sIBM muscle (see below), adding additional markers to the subsequent analyses.

TABLE 1 | Summarized clinical information of all IBM patients included in the study.

Patient No.	Age	Sex	Duration of disease (years)	Muscle symptoms
sIBM1	72	M	?	Symmetric LL prox. and distal paresis, CK 3-fold elevated
sIBM2	78	F	3	Prox. LL and paresis of finger flexors, CK 2-fold elevated
sIBM3	64	M	2	Prox. tetraparesis and paresis of distal forearms, CK 2-fold elevated
sIBM4	68	F	3	Chronic progressive tetraparesis, significant muscle atrophy
sIBM5	66	M	5	Prox. paresis LL, significant atrophy of vastus lateralis
sIBM6	75	F	?	Prox. paresis LL and distal paresis UL, CK 6-fold elevated
sIBM7	64	M	?	Prox. paresis and distal paresis of fingers
sIBM8	75	M	2	Prox. progressive paresis LL and exercise induced pain, CK 3-fold elevated
sIBM9	66	M	?	Dysphagia, distal and proximal tetraparesis, CK 1.5-fold elevated
sIBM10	79	F	11	Prox. tetraparesis, progressive muscle atrophy
sIBM11	76	M	>2	Muscle pain, proximal weakness, muscle atrophy, CK normal
sIBM12	72	F	7	Prox. tetraparesis, muscle atrophy
sIBM13	71	M	?	Prox. tetraparesis

Cellular Localization of CD74, CD163, and STAT1 in Skeletal Muscle Biopsies From sIBM Patients

To verify the *in silico* results and the respective increased expression of CD74, CD163, and STAT1 in sIBM muscle biopsies, we stained sections of muscle biopsy specimens in a larger cohort of sIBM patients ($n = 13$). In sIBM patients' skeletal muscle biopsies, CD74 mostly stained endomysial macrophages (**Figure 2A**). CD163 highlighted macrophages in the endomysium but was not positive on the sarcolemma of the myofibres (**Figure 2B**). STAT1 was expressed in macrophages in active myophagocytosis but not in the endo- and perimysium, independently of macrophages. STAT1 antibodies did not stain the sarcolemma of myofibers (**Figure 2C**). In summary and on a descriptive first approach, all three molecules are detectable on a variety of macrophages in the endomysium or in myophagocytosis.

Significance of CD74, CD163, and STAT1 to Immunological Processes in Skeletal Muscle of sIBM Patients

To expand these descriptive findings and to further implement functional association of the above-mentioned quantitatively and qualitatively highly relevant proteins, we analyzed additional proteins which are predicted to interact with those *in situ* and studied co-expression of several markers by immunofluorescence. CD74 stained some muscle fibers sarcolemmaly and co-localized with CD68^{+} macrophages (**Figure 3A**), as well as with sarcolemmal MHC class II immunoreactivity (**Figure 3B**). On the contrary, the macrophage migration inhibitory factor MIF did not co-stain with CD74 (**Figure 3C**). Furthermore, our immunostaining studies revealed that many CD163^{+} macrophages co-stained with Siglec1 (CD169) in the endomysium (**Figure 3D**).

In addition, Siglec1^{+} macrophages expressed the transcription factor STAT1 in active myophagocytic clusters (**Figure 4A**), while STAT6 was expressed endomysially (**Figure 4B**), demonstrating the involvement of different yet complementary immune mechanisms in the course of sIBM-associated muscle inflammation. Importantly, both markers were also significantly elevated on the transcript level in skeletal muscle biopsies of sIBM patients as compared to NDCs (**Figure 4E**), with gene expression of *STAT1* being elevated around 15-fold, and of *STAT6* around 4,5-fold. Of note, activated MHC class II^{+} macrophages strongly co-stained with key proteins of the type I interferon pathway such as IRG8 and ISG15 (**Figures 4C,D** and **Table 2**).

DISCUSSION

In the present study, data from unbiased proteomic analysis highlighted the presence of certain proteins playing decisive roles in immune response to be highly abundant in sIBM patients' skeletal muscle biopsies. *In silico* analyses and subsequent morphological studies in skeletal muscle revealed their key characteristics in pathways driving specific macrophage responses. Along this line, Siglec1^{+} CD163^{+} and Siglec1^{+} STAT1^{+} macrophages were identified. Furthermore, MHC class II^{+} macrophages co-expressed ISG15 and IRF8 in patient-derived muscles highlighting a tight bond between these activated macrophages and the type I and type II interferon responses. Additionally, MHC class II^{+} macrophages and the sarcoplasm of adjacent muscle fibers expressed CD74.

These findings have important implications for the current understanding of the role of specifically activated macrophages in the pathogenesis of sIBM. Several ways of addressing the activation of macrophages *in vivo* and *in vitro* by using targeted and unbiased approaches notoriously exist (13, 23–27). Flexible states of macrophage activation have been found to occur according to their vast duties in physiology and pathophysiology of different diseases, specifically in chronic inflammatory and fibrotic diseases (24, 28–31). In sIBM, the vast majority of studies focusing on the immune-system have addressed the adverse effects of systemic T cell function and dysfunction or T cell dysfunction within the muscle itself (1, 5, 32–38). In contrast, only few studies have had a broader approach in tackling additional aspects of the immune response (48, 49) or genetic factors influencing the pathogenesis such as the *SQSTM1* or *VCP* variants (39). Proteomic analysis has recently helped to decipher new and unexpected molecules involved in the pathophysiology of sIBM such as FYCO1 and its role in autophagy or the composition of protein aggregates in rimmed vacuoles (40). While the latter studies have focused on the elucidation of vacuole pathophysiology, in the present study we have used the whole protein extracts of skeletal muscle biopsies to obtain molecular information about the entire tissue, and thus, to gain a better and unbiased understanding of the etiology of the disease. This approach revealed that CD74, CD163 and STAT1, driving inflammatory responses, were at the forefront of the highly expressed proteins within the diseased skeletal muscle tissue. This finding accords with our hypothesis of a major role for molecules driving macrophage polarization since sIBM biopsies feature very strong immunity-related aspects over all with macrophages being by far the most abundant cell type in the lesion. Hence, we were able to characterize the immunity of these macrophages in more detail and found molecules identified by proteomic analysis and subsequently verified by immunohistochemistry in biopsies which are strongly related to type I/II interferon responses, specifically IRF8, ISG15, GBP1, GBP1P1, HLA-DOB, IFIT3, STAT1, TAP2. Since macrophages can adopt a great variety of functional states (24, 31, 41, 42), it was not surprising to identify a further important subgroup consisting of STAT1^{+}Siglec1^{+} macrophages in active myophagocytosis. This type of macrophages is implicated in acute clearance of necrotic muscle fibers, a process which, despite the explicitly chronic character of the disease (active over decades), is a constant muscle biopsy feature. Of note, we also identified STAT6^{+}Siglec1^{+} macrophages in the endomysium at distance of myophagocytic and necrotic fibers, highlighting that both downstream transcription factors may become activated in certain macrophages, which have then different duties and fates. A specific immune phenotype of Caucasian sIBM patients with HLA-A3 suggesting MHC class I activation has been described (43), MHC class II staining patterns were recently described for sIBM patients in comparison to dermatomyositis and anti-synthetase syndrome-associated myositis (44). This finding is in keeping with our proteomic identification of elevated CD74, as a protein regularly interacting with MHC class II molecules. Our findings also indicate that macrophages (which are mentioned as being the most abundant mononuclear inflammatory cells in skeletal muscle biopsies of sIBM patients) have been underestimated as cellular key players in the etiopathology of sIBM. The second relevant finding of this study, is the type I and type II interferon response identified both by proteomic profiling, subsequent *in silico* studies, and immunohistochemistry, expanding previous data where the interferon signature genes have been addressed by transcriptomics (45). Notably, the signatures of type I and type II Interferons, identified here, differ from the ones that have been described to be crucial in dermatomyositis (45–47). Herewith, the relevant role of macrophages as versatile multifunctional immune cells playing a decisive role in the etiopathology of sIBM was shown. These findings may define a molecular starting

TABLE 2 | List of proteins altered in abundance and controlled by interferon-mediated processes (based on "Interferome" database).

Acces-sion #	Peptide count/unique peptides	Anova (p)	Description	Gene Symbol	Ensembl ID	Fold of regu-lation [log2]
UPREGULATED PROTEINS						
Q99972	1/1	0.04	Myocilin	*MYOC*	ENSG00000034971	6.49
P15153	1/1	<0.0005	Ras-related C3 botulinum toxin substrate 2	*RAC2*	ENSG00000128340	5.21
P42224	9/9	0.01	Signal transducer and activator of transcription 1-alpha/beta	*STAT1*	ENSG00000115415	4.99
Q14764	8/8	<0.0005	Major vault protein	*MVP*	ENSG00000013364	4.66
Q9UJU6	1/1	<0.0005	Drebrin-like protein	*DBNL*	ENSG00000136279	4.60
P08754	1/1	0.01	Guanine nucleotide-binding protein G(k) subunit alpha	*GNAI3*	ENSG00000065135	4.44
P33241	1/1	0.02	Lymphocyte-specific protein 1	*LSP1*	ENSG00000130592	4.29
Q03519	1/1	0.01	Antigen peptide transporter 2	*TAP2*	ENSG00000204267 ENSG00000250264	3.95
O95865	2/2	<0.0005	N(G),N(G)-dimethylarginine dimethylaminohydro-lase 2	*DDAH2*	ENSG00000213722	3.89
P32455	4/3	0.03	Interferon-induced guanylate-binding protein 1	*GBP1*	ENSG00000117228 ENSG00000225492	3.72
Q9UKY7	1/1	<0.0005	Protein CDV3 homolog	*CDV3*	ENSG00000091527	3.65
O14879	1/1	0.03	Interferon-induced protein with tetratricopeptide repeats 3	*IFIT3*	ENSG00000119917	3.58
Q9UHD8	4/3	<0.0005	Septin-9	*SEPT9*	ENSG00000184640 ENSG00000261843	3.58
Q14203	3/3	<0.0005	Dynactin subunit 1	*DCTN1*	ENSG00000204843	3.46
P49756	1/1	<0.0005	RNA-binding protein 25	*RBM25*	ENSG00000119707	3.32
Q9Y3B3	1/1	0.01	Transmembrane emp24 domain-containing protein 7	*TMED7*	ENSG00000134970	3.19
P78559	1/1	0.02	Microtubule-associated protein 1A	*MAP1A*	ENSG00000166963	3.16
Q14980	1/1	0.02	Nuclear mitotic apparatus protein 1	*NUMA1*	ENSG00000137497	3.12
P35580	9/4	0.04	Myosin-10	*MYH10*	ENSG00000133026	2.91
P23142	3/3	0.02	Fibulin-1	*FBLN1*	ENSG00000077942	2.87
Q13033	1/1	0.01	Striatin-3	*STRN3*	ENSG00000196792	2.79
O75534	1/1	0.03	Cold shock domain-containing protein E1	*CSDE1*	ENSG00000009307	2.77
Q99536	4/4	<0.0005	Synaptic vesicle membrane protein VAT-1 homolog	*VAT1*	ENSG00000108828	2.77
Q9BSJ8	6/6	<0.0005	Extended synaptotagmin-1	*ESYT1*	ENSG00000139641	2.76
P62070	1/1	<0.0005	Ras-related protein R-Ras2	*RRAS2*	ENSG00000133818	2.75
Q07065	2/2	0.01	Cytoskeleton-associated protein 4	*CKAP4*	ENSG00000136026	2.75
Q9Y696	4/4	0.01	Chloride intracellular channel protein 4	*CLIC4*	ENSG00000169504	2.75
O60240	9/8	0.05	Perilipin-1	*PLIN1*	ENSG00000166819	2.73
P32456	3/2	0.01	Interferon-induced guanylate-binding protein 2	*GBP2*	ENSG00000162645	2.72
Q15075	4/3	0.02	Early endosome antigen 1	*EEA1*	ENSG00000102189	2.72
P04275	5/5	<0.0005	von Willebrand factor	*VWF*	ENSG00000110799	2.71
P04083	9/8	<0.0005	Annexin A1	*ANXA1*	ENSG00000135046	2.70
P51911	2/2	0.01	Calponin-1	*CNN1*	ENSG00000130176	2.66
Q9Y4L1	2/2	0.04	Hypoxia up-regulated protein 1	*HYOU1*	ENSG00000149428	2.61
P09936	5/4	0.02	Ubiquitin carboxyl-terminal hydrolase isozyme L1	*UCHL1*	ENSG00000154277	2.57
P16070	1/1	<0.0005	CD44 antigen	*CD44*	ENSG00000026508	2.52

(Continued)

TABLE 2 | Continued

Acces-sion #	Peptide count/unique peptides	Anova (p)	Description	Gene Symbol	Ensembl ID	Fold of regu-lation [log2]
DOWNREGULATED PROTEINS						
P02585	9/9	0.01	Troponin C, skeletal muscle	*TNNC2*	ENSG00000101470	−2.25
P48788	12/12	0.01	Troponin I, fast skeletal muscle	*TNNI2*	ENSG00000130598	−2.21
P45378	21/20	0.01	Troponin T, fast skeletal muscle	*TNNT3*	ENSG00000130595	−2.19
P16219	5/5	0.02	Short-chain specific acyl-CoA dehydrogenase, mitochondrial	*ACADS*	ENSG00000122971	−1.83
P30711	3/2	0.01	Glutathione S-transferase theta-1	*GSTT1*	ENSG00000184674	−1.37
Q12797	1/1	0.01	Aspartyl/asparaginyl beta-hydroxylase	*ASPH*	ENSG00000198363	−1.11
P11217	55/42	0.01	Glycogen phosphorylase, muscle form	*PYGM*	ENSG00000068976	−1.10
Q8N335	8/7	0.01	Glycerol-3-phosphate dehydrogenase 1-like protein	*GPD1L*	ENSG00000152642	−1.10

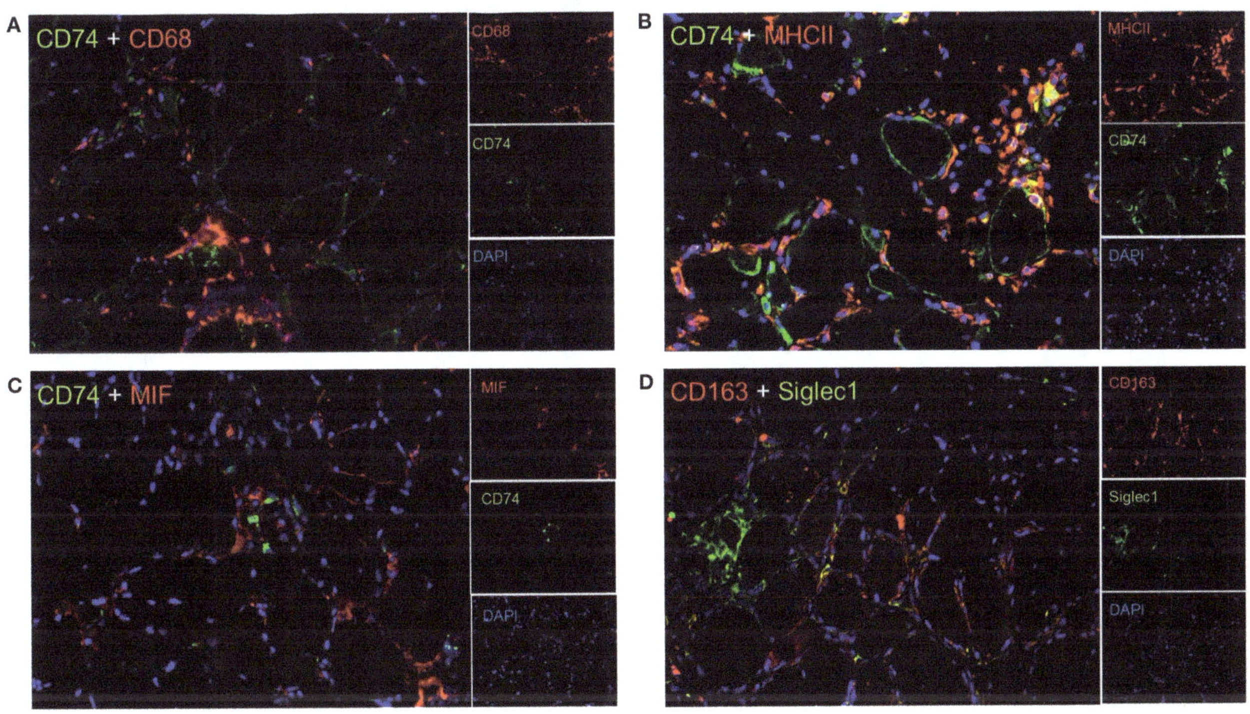

FIGURE 3 | Double immunflorescent staining reveal functional interactions in sIBM patients' muscle tissue. Co-staining of various proteins revealed that CD74 co-labels with CD68+ macrophages **(A)**, and MHC class II **(B)**, but not with the macrophage migration inhibitory factor MIF **(C)**. In addition, CD163^{+} macrophages partially co-express Siglec1 **(D)**.

point for future therapeutic approaches in sIBM utilizing JAK-STAT inhibitors.

SUMMARY

In summary, we demonstrate that unbiased proteomic profiling of skeletal muscle biopsies provides important insights into the molecular etiology of a disease and more precisely in the context of sIBM revealed proteins prominently involved in immunity and characterizing a pattern of macrophage activation. Application of immunohistochemical verification and analysis of these cells in the context of the type I and type II interferon signature *in situ* allowed the attribution of these proteins to specific functional states of

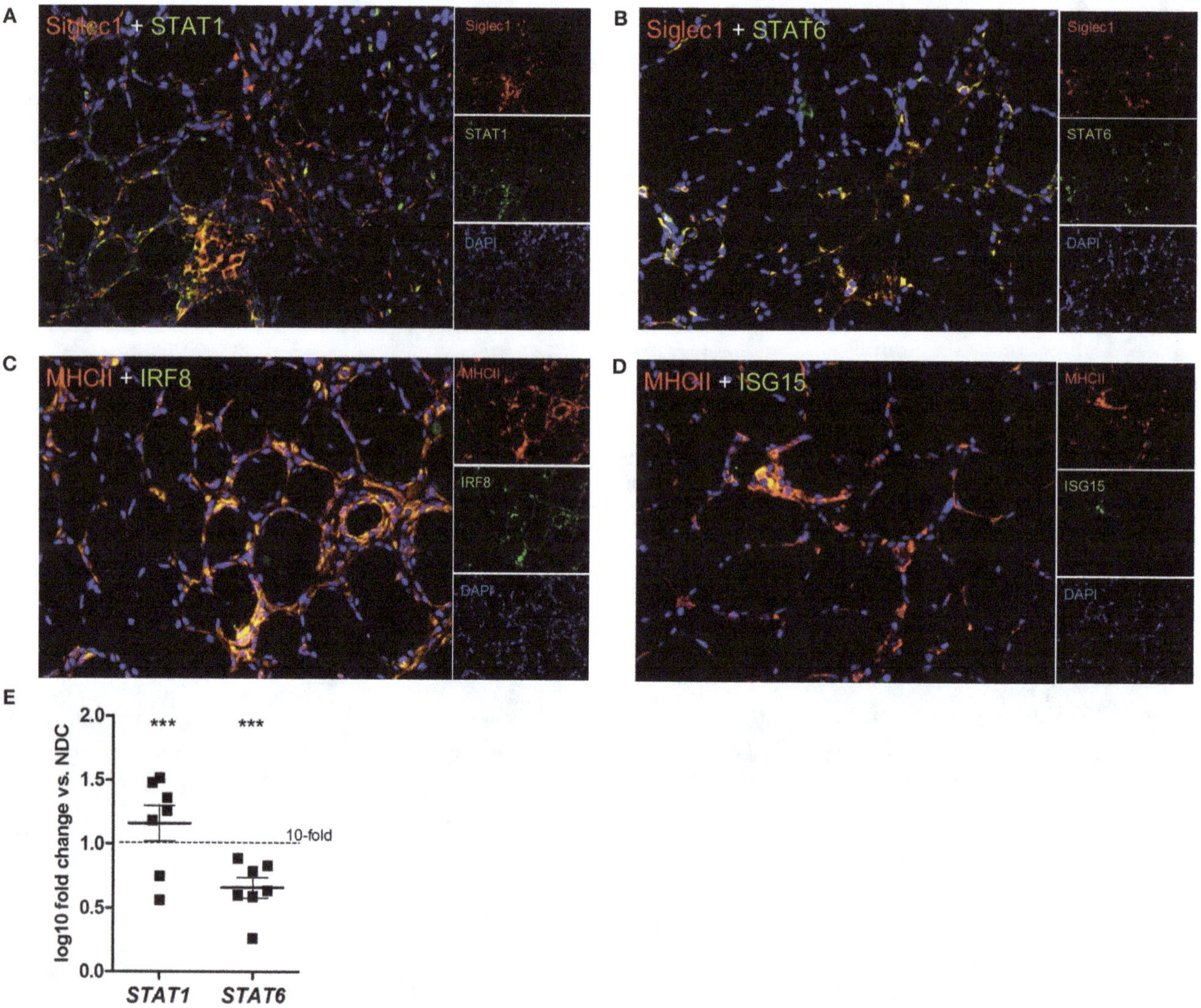

FIGURE 4 | different subforms of macrophages, as well as type I interferon pathways are found in sIBM. We could demonstrate Siglec1+ macrophages, which express STAT1 **(A)**, or STAT6 **(B)**, hinting at involvement of different macrophage subtypes in sIBM muscle inflammation. The activation of STAT1 and STAT6 could also be demonstrated by significantly elevated gene expression levels **(E)**, $p < 0.01$. MHC class II+ macrophages also clearly co-stained with key proteins of the type I interferon pathway like IRF8 **(C)** and ISG15 **(D)**.

macrophage activation. Hence, we show that several different types of macrophages are actively affecting the immune response in sIBM, via a prominent type I interferon signature among others.

AUTHOR CONTRIBUTIONS

AR and CP: design of the study, acquisition, analysis and interpretation of data, as well as drafting the manuscript. DH: acquisition and analysis of data, as well as revising the manuscript. H-HG: design of the study and revising the manuscript. WS: design of the study, interpretation of data, as well as drafting the manuscript.

ACKNOWLEDGMENTS

The authors thank Petra Matylewski for technical assistance. This work was supported by a grant from the Deutsche Gesellschaft für Muskelkranke (to AR). Moreover, financial support by the French Muscular Dystrophy Association (AFM-Téléthon; grant 21466 to AR) and the Ministerium für Innovation, Wissenschaft und Forschung des Landes Nordrhein-Westfalen, the Senatsverwaltung für Wirtschaft, Technologie und Forschung des Landes Berlin and the Bundesministerium für Bildung und Forschung is gratefully acknowledged.

REFERENCES

1. Benveniste O, Stenzel W, Hilton-Jones D, Sandri M, Boyer O, Van Engelen BGM. Amyloid deposits and inflammatory infiltrates in sporadic inclusion body myositis: the inflammatory egg comes before the degenerative chicken. *Acta Neuropathol.* (2015) 611–24. doi: 10.1007/s00401-015-1384-5
2. De Bleecker JL, Lundberg IE, De Visser M. 193rd ENMC international workshop pathology diagnosis of idiopathic inflammatory myopathies 30 November - 2 December 2012, Naarden, The Netherlands. *Neuromusc Dis.* (2013) 23:945–51. doi: 10.1016/j.nmd.2013.07.007
3. Brady S, Squier W, Hilton-Jones D. Clinical assessment determines the diagnosis of inclusion body myositis independently of pathological features. *J Neurol Neurosurg Psychiatry.* (2013) 84:1240–6. doi: 10.1136/jnnp-2013-305690
4. Dimachkie MM. Idiopathic inflammatory myopathies. *J Neuroimmunol.* (2011) 231:32–42. doi: 10.1016/j.jneuroim.2010.10.013
5. Benveniste O, Guiguet M, Freebody J, Dubourg O, Squier W, Maisonobe T, et al. Long-term observational study of sporadic inclusion body myositis. *Brain.* (2011) 134:3176–84. doi: 10.1093/brain/awr213
6. Lloyd TE, Mammen AL, Amato AA, Weiss MD, Needham M, Greenberg SA. Evaluation and construction of diagnostic criteria for inclusion body myositis. *Neurology.* (2014) 83:426–33. doi: 10.1212/WNL.0000000000000642
7. Larman HB, Salajegheh M, Nazareno R, Lam T, Sauld J, Steen H, et al. Cytosolic 5′-nucleotidase 1A autoimmunity in sporadic inclusion body myositis. *Ann Neurol.* (2013) 73:408–18. doi: 10.1002/ana.23840
8. Pluk H, van Hoeve BJ, van Dooren SH, Stammen-Vogelzangs J, van der Heijden A, Schelhaas HJ, et al. Autoantibodies to cytosolic 5′-nucleotidase 1A in inclusion body myositis. *Ann Neurol.* (2013) 73:397–407. doi: 10.1002/ana.23822
9. Goyal NA, Cash TM, Alam U, Enam S, Tierney P, Araujo N, et al. Seropositivity for NT5c1A antibody in sporadic inclusion body myositis predicts more severe motor, bulbar and respiratory involvement. *J Neurol Neurosurg Psychiatry.* (2016) 87:373–8. doi: 10.1136/jnnp-2014-310008
10. Benveniste O, Hogrel JY, Annoussamy M, Bachasson D, Rigolet A, Servais L, et al. Rapamycin vs. placebo for the treatment of inclusion body myositis: improvement of the 6 min walking distance, a functional scale, the FVC and muscle quantitative, M. R. I. *Arthr Rheumatol.* (2017) 58:375–6. doi: 10.1093/rheumatology/key043
11. González Coraspe JA, Weis J, Anderson ME, Münchberg U, Lorenz K, Buchkremer S, et al. Biochemical and pathological changes result from mutated caveolin-3 in muscle. *Skeletal Muscle.* (2018) 8:28. doi: 10.1186/s13395-018-0173-y
12. Rose MR, ENMC IBM Working Group. 188th ENMC international workshop: inclusion body myositis, 2-4 December 2011, Naarden, The Netherlands. *Neuromuscul Disord.* (2013) 23:1044–55. doi: 10.1016/j.nmd.2013.08.007
13. Preuße C, Allenbach Y, Hoffmann O, Goebel HH, Pehl D, Radke J, et al. Differential roles of hypoxia and innate immunity in juvenile and adult dermatomyositis. *Acta Neuropathol Commun.* (2016) 4:45. doi: 10.1186/s40478-016-0308-5
14. Ladislau L, Suárez-Calvet X, Toquet S, Landon-Cardinal O, Amelin D, Depp M, et al. JAK inhibitor improves type i interferon induced damage: proof of concept in dermatomyositis. *Brain.* (2018) 141:1609–21. doi: 10.1093/brain/awy105
15. Moeller JB, Nielsen MJ, Reichhardt MP, Schlosser A, Sorensen GL, Nielsen O, et al. CD163-L1 is an endocytic macrophage protein strongly regulated by mediators in the inflammatory response. *J Immunol.* (2012) 188:2399–409. doi: 10.4049/jimmunol.1103150
16. van de Garde MD, Martinez FO, Melgert BN, Hylkema MN, Jonkers RE, Hamann J. Chronic Exposure to glucocorticoids shapes gene expression and modulates innate and adaptive activation pathways in macrophages with distinct changes in leukocyte attraction. *J Immunol.* (2014) 192:1196–208. doi: 10.4049/jimmunol.1302138
17. Gutiérrez-González A, Martínez-Moreno M, Samaniego R, Arellano-Sánchez N, Salinas-Muñoz L, Relloso M, et al. Evaluation of the potential therapeutic benefits of macrophage reprogramming in multiple myeloma. *Blood.* (2016) 128:2241–52. doi: 10.1182/blood-2016-01-695395
18. Court M, Petre G, Atifi MEL, Millet A. Proteomic signature reveals modulation of human macrophage polarization and functions under differing environmental oxygen conditions. *Mol Cell Proteom.* (2017) 16:2153–68. doi: 10.1074/mcp.RA117.000082
19. Tanese K, Hashimoto Y, Berkova Z, Wang Y, Samaniego F, Lee JE, et al. Erratum: cell surface CD74-MIF interactions drive melanoma survival in response to interferon-γ. *J Invest Dermatol.* (2015) 135:2775–84. doi: 10.1038/jid.2015.204
20. Chmielewski S, Olejnik A, Sikorski K, Pelisek J, Błaszczyk K, Aoqui C, et al. STAT1 Dependent signal integration between IFNγ and TLR4 in vascular cells reflect pro-atherogenic responses in human atherosclerosis. *PLoS ONE.* (2014) 9:e113318. doi: 10.1371/journal.pone.0113318
21. Buechler C, Ritter M, Orsó E, Langmann T, Klucken J, Schmitz G. Regulation of scavenger receptor CD163 expression in human monocytes and macrophages by pro- and antiinflammatory stimuli. *J Leukocyte Biol.* (2000) 67:97–103. doi: 10.1002/jlb.67.1.97
22. Chairatvit K, Wongnoppavich A, Choonate, S. Up-regulation of interferon-stimulated gene15 and its conjugates by tumor necrosis factor-α via type I interferon-dependent and -independent pathways. *Mol Cell Biochem.* (2012) 368:195–201. doi: 10.1007/s11010-012-1360-5
23. Pesce JT, Ramalingam TR, Mentink-Kane MM, Wilson MS, El Kasmi KC, Smith AM, et al. Arginase-1-expressing macrophages suppress Th2 cytokine-driven inflammation and fibrosis. *PLoS Pathogens.* (2009) 5:e1000371. doi: 10.1371/journal.ppat.1000371
24. Ginhoux F, Schultze JL, Murray PJ, Ochando J, Biswas SK. New insights into the multidimensional concept of macrophage ontogeny, activation and function. *Nat Immunol.* (2015) 17:34–40. doi: 10.1038/ni.3324
25. Preuße C, Goebel HH, Held J, Wengert O, Scheibe F, Irlbacher K, et al. Immune-mediated necrotizing myopathy is characterized by a specific th1-m1 polarized immune profile. *Am J Pathol.* (2012) 181:2161–71. doi: 10.1016/j.ajpath.2012.08.033
26. Stenzel W, Preuße C, Allenbach Y, Pehl D, Junckerstorff R, Heppner FL, et al. Nuclear actin aggregation is a hallmark of anti-synthetase syndrome-induced dysimmune myopathy. *Neurology.* (2015) 84:1346–54. doi: 10.1212/WNL.0000000000001422
27. Schultze JL, Schmieder A, Goerdt S. Macrophage activation in human diseases. *Sem Immunol.* (2015) 27:249–56. doi: 10.1016/j.smim.2015.07.003
28. Villalta SA, Nguyen HX, Deng B, Gotoh T, Tidball JG. Shifts in macrophage phenotypes and macrophage competition for arginine metabolism affect the severity of muscle pathology in muscular dystrophy. *Hum Mol Genet.* (2009) 18:482–96. doi: 10.1093/hmg/ddn376
29. Tidball JG, Villalta SA. Regulatory interactions between muscle and the immune system during muscle regeneration. *Am J Physiol Regul Integr Comp Physiol.* (2010) 298:R1173–87. doi: 10.1152/ajpregu.00735.2009
30. Wynn TA. Fibrotic disease and the T(H)1/T(H)2 Paradigm. *Nat Rev Immunol.* (2004) 4:583–94. doi: 10.1038/nri1412
31. Murray PJ, Wynn TA. Obstacles and opportunities for understanding macrophage polarization. *J Leukocyte Biol.* (2011) 89:557–63. doi: 10.1189/jlb.0710409
32. Zajac AJ, Blattman JN, Murali-Krishna K, Sourdive DJ, Suresh M, Altman JD, et al. Viral immune evasion due to persistence of activated T cells without effector function. *J Exp Med.* (1998) 188:2205–13. doi: 10.1084/jem.188.12.2205
33. Crespo J, Sun H, Welling TH, Tian T, Zou W. T cell anergy, exhaustion, senescence and stemness in the tumor microenvironment. *Curr Opin Immunol.* (2013) 25:214–21. doi: 10.1016/j.dcn.2011.01.002
34. Wherry EJ. T cell exhaustion. *Nat Immunol.* (2017) 12:492–9. doi: 10.1038/ni.2035
35. Ivanidze J, Hoffmann R, Lochmüller H, Engel AG, Hohlfeld R, Dornmair K. inclusion body myositis: laser microdissection reveals differential up-regulation of IFN-γ signaling cascade in attacked versus nonattacked myofibers. *Am J Pathol.* (2011) 179:1347–59. doi: 10.1016/j.ajpath.2011.05.055
36. Allenbach Y, Solly S, Grégoire S, Dubourg O, Salomon B, Butler-Browne G, et al. Role of regulatory T cells in a new mouse model of experimental autoimmune myositis. *Am J Pathol.* (2009) 174:989–98. doi: 10.2353/ajpath.2009.080422

37. Dalakas MC. Polymyoisits, dermatomyositis, and inclusion-body-myositis. *N Engl J Med.* (1991) 325:1487–98.
38. Muth IE, Barthel K, Bähr M, Dalakas MC, Schmidt J. Proinflammatory cell stress in sporadic inclusion body myositis muscle: overexpression of alphab-crystallin is associated with amyloid precursor protein and accumulation of beta-amyloid. *J Neurol Neurosurg Psychiatry.* (2009) 80:1344–9. doi: 10.1136/jnnp.2009.174276
39. Gang Q, Bettencourt C, Machado PM, Brady S, Holton JL, Pittman AM, et al. Rare variants in SQSTM1 and VCP genes and risk of sporadic inclusion body myositis. *Neurobiol Aging.* (2016) 47:218.e1–218.e9. doi: 10.1016/j.neurobiolaging.2016.07.024
40. Güttsches AK, Brady S, Krause K, Maerkens A, Uszkoreit J, Eisenacher M, et al. Proteomics of rimmed vacuoles define new risk allele in inclusion body myositis. *Ann Neurol.* (2017) 81:227–39. doi: 10.1002/ana.24847.
41. Murray PJ, Wynn TA. Protective and pathogenic functions of macrophage subsets. *Nat Rev Immunol.* (2011) 11:723–37. doi: 10.1038/nri3073
42. Schultze JL, Freeman T, Hume DA, Latz E. A transcriptional perspective on human macrophage biology. *Sem Immunol.* (2015) 27:44–50. doi: 10.1016/j.smim.2015.02.001
43. Price P, Santoso L, Mastaglia F, Garlepp M, Kok CC, Allcock R, et al. Two major histocompatibility complex haplotypes influence susceptibility to sporadic inclusion body myositis: critical evaluation of an association with HLA-DR3. *Tissue Antigens.* (2014) 64:575–80. doi: 10.1111/j.1399-0039.2004.00310.x
44. Rigolet M, Hou C, Amer YB, Aouizerate J, Periou B, Gherardi RK, et al. Distinct interferon signatures stratify inflammatory and dysimmune myopathies. *RMD Open.* (2019) 5:10–4. doi: 10.1136/rmdopen-2018-000811
45. Greenberg SA. Dermatomyositis and type 1 interferons. *Curr Rheumatol Rep.* (2011) 12:198–203. doi: 10.1007/s11926-010-0101-6.Dermatomyositis
46. Suárez-Calvet X, Gallardo E, Nogales-Gadea G, Querol L, Navas M, Díaz-Manera J, et al. Altered RIG-I/DDX58-mediated innate immunity in dermatomyositis. *J Pathol.* (2014) 233:258–68. doi: 10.1002/path.4346
47. Greenberg SA, Pinkus JL, Pinkus GS, Burleson T, Sanoudou D, Tawil R, et al. Interferon-alpha/beta-mediated innate immune mechanisms in dermatomyositis. *Ann Neurol.* (2005) 57:664–78. doi: 10.1002/ana.20464
48. De Bleecker JL, De Paepe B, Aronica E, de Visser M, Amato A, Benveniste O, et al. 205th ENMC international workshop: pathology diagnosis of idiopathic inflammatory myopathies part II 28-30 March 2014, Naarden, The Netherlands. *Neuromuscul Disord.* (2015) 25:268–72. doi: 10.1016/j.nmd.2014.12.001
49. Paepe BD, Creus KK, De Bleecker JL. Role of cytokines and chemokines in idiopathic inflammatory myopathies. *Curr Opin Rheumatol.* (2009) 21:610–6. doi: 10.1097/BOR.0b013e3283317b31

14

Combinatory Biomarker Use of Cortical Thickness, MUNIX and ALSFRS-R at Baseline and in Longitudinal Courses of Individual Patients with Amyotrophic Lateral Sclerosis

Anna M. Wirth[1,2], Andrei Khomenko[1], Dobri Baldaranov[1], Ines Kobor[1], Ohnmar Hsam[1], Thomas Grimm[1], Siw Johannesen[1], Tim-Henrik Bruun[1], Wilhelm Schulte-Mattler[1], Mark W. Greenlee[2] and Ulrich Bogdahn[1†]*

[1] Department of Neurology, University Hospital of Regensburg, Regensburg, Germany, [2] Department of Experimental Psychology, University of Regensburg, Regensburg, Germany

***Correspondence:**
Ulrich Bogdahn
uli.bogdahn@ukr.de

†Senior authorship.

Objective: Amyotrophic lateral sclerosis (ALS) is a progressive neurodegenerative process affecting upper and lower motor neurons as well as non-motor systems. In this study, precentral and postcentral cortical thinning detected by structural magnetic resonance imaging (MRI) were combined with clinical (ALS-specific functional rating scale revised, ALSFRS-R) and neurophysiological (motor unit number index, MUNIX) biomarkers in both cross-sectional and longitudinal analyses.

Methods: The unicenter sample included 20 limb-onset classical ALS patients compared to 30 age-related healthy controls. ALS patients were treated with standard Riluzole and additional long-term G-CSF (Filgrastim) on a named patient basis after written informed consent. Combinatory biomarker use included cortical thickness of atlas-based dorsal and ventral subdivisions of the precentral and postcentral cortex, ALSFRS-R, and MUNIX for the musculus abductor digiti minimi (ADM) bilaterally. Individual cross-sectional analysis investigated individual cortical thinning in ALS patients compared to age-related healthy controls in the context of state of disease at initial MRI scan. Beyond correlation analysis of biomarkers at cross-sectional group level ($n = 20$), longitudinal monitoring in a subset of slow progressive ALS patients ($n = 4$) explored within-subject temporal dynamics of repeatedly assessed biomarkers in time courses over at least 18 months.

Results: Cross-sectional analysis demonstrated individually variable states of cortical thinning, which was most pronounced in the ventral section of the precentral cortex. Correlations of ALSFRS-R with cortical thickness and MUNIX were detected. Individual longitudinal biomarker monitoring in four slow progressive ALS patients revealed evident differences in individual disease courses and temporal dynamics of the biomarkers.

Conclusion: A combinatory use of structural MRI, neurophysiological and clinical biomarkers allows for an appropriate and detailed assessment of clinical state and course of disease of ALS.

Keywords: amyotrophic lateral sclerosis, magnetic resonance imaging, cortical thickness, MUNIX, ALSFRS-R

INTRODUCTION

Amyotrophic lateral sclerosis (ALS) is a rapidly progressive neurodegenerative disorder affecting upper and lower motor neurons as well as non-motor systems (1). The degeneration of motor neurons results in muscular fasciculation, progressive weakness, and eventual paralysis (2). Average survival in ALS is 3–5 years, but patients evidently vary in phenotype and disease progression (2, 3). The great clinical heterogeneity in ALS is reflected by different phenotypes with variability regarding the involvement of upper motor neuron (UMN) and lower motor neuron (LMN) signs, site of onset (bulbar, limb), rate of progression, and involvement of neurobehavioral deficits (2, 4). Therefore, clinical and biological biomarkers are helpful in describing disease severity and progression (3).

Magnetic resonance imaging (MRI) has produced potential biomarkers that clarify the role of brain structure and function in the progress of the disease (5, 6). In structural morphometric studies, cortical thickness compared to surface and volume was most sensitive to disease-related changes (7). A variety of studies investigating structural surface-based morphometry showed reduced cortical thickness primarily in the precentral cortex (8–16). Cortical thinning was not restricted to the primary motor cortex. Several studies reported cortical thinning to spread to non-motor cortex areas like the temporal, frontal, parietal, and postcentral cortex (8, 10, 15). However, not all published MRI studies detected alterations in the cortical thickness (17) or cortical volume (18, 19) of the precentral cortex of ALS patients. Essentially, precentral cortical thinning was reported to be focal, and dependent on the clinical phenotype, rate of progression, and age (8, 11, 13). Additionally, several longitudinal MRI studies revealed no further cortical thinning of the precentral cortex in the course of disease (9, 14–17).

In addition to MRI, clinical and electrophysiological biomarkers are among the most currently used and prominent biomarkers (20). The widely used ALS-specific functional rating scale revised (ALSFRS-R) and its subscales are correlated with survival (3). However, correlations between precentral cortical thickness and ALSFRS-R scores were rather weak (10, 21) or not detected in several neuroimaging studies so far (9, 12, 13, 16, 22). While MRI is considered a suitable biomarker for UMN function, neurophysiological motor unit number estimation (MUNE) and motor unit number index (MUNIX) are treated as biomarkers for the estimation of functional lower motor units (23, 24). MUNE is calculated from the division of maximal compound muscle action potential (CMAP) by the mean surface single motor unit action potential (SMUP) (25). In contrast, MUNIX is derived from a mathematical model based on CMAP and electromyographic surface interference patterns (SIP) (26). MUNE and MUNIX scores are inter-correlated in ALS patients (23). As the acquisition of MUNIX is easier and less time consuming than that of MUNE, MUNIX has become a promising biomarker of motor unit loss (27, 28). MUNIX scores were correlated with ALSFRS-R scores (26), but they declined faster than ALSFRS-R scores over time in ALS patients (29). Only few studies investigated the relationship between neurophysiological biomarkers and cortical thickness and failed to find a significant correlation with MUNE or other motor evoked potential indices (21, 30). To our knowledge, no published study investigated correlations between cortical thickness and MUNIX as a biomarker potentially affected by both lower and UMN function (23).

Aim of the study was to investigate individual states of cortical thinning of the precentral and postcentral cortex in a limb-onset ALS sample with respect to young-onset, and slow disease progression. It is the first study to analyze combinatory biomarker use of MRI cortical thickness, neurophysiological MUNIX, and routine ALSFRS-R in both cross-sectional group analysis of the whole sample, and in longitudinal monitoring exploring differences in temporal dynamics between biomarkers in a subgroup of slow progressive ALS patients.

MATERIALS AND METHODS

Participants

Cross-sectional group analysis included 20 limb-onset classical ALS patients (5 females, $M = 48$ years, $SD = 11$) compared to 30 age-related healthy controls (14 females, $M = 45$ years, $SD = 13$). Mean age of ALS patients was lower than that reported in other ALS studies, as the sample included several young-onset patients. Mean ALSFRS-R score across all 20 patients at the time point of first MRI scan was 36 score points ($SD = 8$; range: 23–48). The sample included both slow and fast progressive ALS patients indicated by disease progression rates ($M = 0.51$, $SD = 0.27$; range: 0.00–1.00). The presence of both UMN and LMN signs in all patients allowed no clear differentiation in UMN or LMN predominance of disease. Patients' characteristics are

Abbreviations: ADM, abductor digiti minimi; ALS, amyotrophic lateral sclerosis; ALSFRS-R, ALS-specific functional rating scale revised; CMAP, compound muscle action potential; G-CSF, granulocyte-colony stimulating factor; LMN, lower motor neuron; MNI, Montreal Neurological Institute; MPRAGE, magnetization prepared rapid gradient echo sequence; MRI, magnetic resonance imaging; MUNE, motor unit number estimation; MUNIX, motor unit number index; PoD, postcentral dorsal; PoV, postcentral ventral; PreD, precentral dorsal; PreV, precentral ventral; ROI, region of interest; SIP, surface interference pattern; SMN, sensorimotor network; SMUP, single motor unit potential; UMN, upper motor neuron.

TABLE 1 | Patients' characteristics at baseline.

#	Range of age	ALSFRS-R [0 48]	MUNIX left	MUNIX right	Time span since onset	Onset	Progression rate
1	21–25	30	6.63	10.43	49	Arm	0.37
2	26–30	35	8.20	29.21	28	Arm	0.46
3	31–35	24	6.94	2.83	28	Leg	0.86
4	41–45	24	*	*	28	Leg	0.86
5	41–45	41	54.12	38.00	19	Leg	0.37
6	41–45	28	4.85	0.70	38	Arm	0.53
7	41–45	46	*	*	16	Arm	0.13
8	46–50	39	138.10	41.88	56	Leg	0.16
9	46–50	48	170.10	187.30	19	Leg	0.00
10	46–50	24	48.37	18.51	24	Arm	1.00
11	46–50	46	213.60	193.00	3	Leg	0.67
12	46–50	40	114.50	97.18	21	Leg	0.38
13	46–50	38	*	*	25	Leg	0.40
14	51–55	42	27.25	21.62	7	Arm	0.86
15	51–55	35	*	*	33	Leg	0.39
16	56–60	38	123.90	101.60	29	Leg	0.34
17	56–60	44	126.90	0.00	13	Leg	0.31
18	61–65	42	83.10	119.00	10	Leg	0.60
19	61–65	24	12.34	9.66	33	Leg	0.73
20	66–70	21	6.94	2.83	36	Leg	0.75

*Summary of baseline characteristics of all 20 limb-onset ALS patients including age (in ranges of years), ALSFRS-R sum score upon initial MRI scan (48 in clinical non affected), neurophysiological MUNIX scores for left and right ADM upon initial MRI scan, the length of time span between symptom onset and initial MRI scan in months, onset of disease (arm, leg), and progression rate. In four out of 20 ALS patients (marked with *), neurophysiological assessment was still conducted using MUNE technique (patient 4: left MUNE = 2, right MUNE = 1; patient 7: left MUNE =3, MUNE right = 77; patient 13: left MUNE = 275, right MUNE = 85; patient 15: left MUNE = 240, right MUNE = 120). No MUNIX scores were obtained in these four patients. Progression rates were calculated by [48-ALSFRS-R sum score/months since symptom onset; see (8)]. Neuropsychological assessment using the Edinburgh Cognitive and Behavioral ALS Screen (ECAS) was conducted only in patient 3 (129/136 score points) and patient 9 (100/136 score points).*

summarized in **Table 1**. These included age (in ranges of years), ALSFRS-R sum scores and neurophysiological MUNIX scores for left and right ADM upon initial MRI scan, time interval between symptom onset and initial T1 MRI scan (in months), onset of disease (arm, leg), and progression rates [(48-ALSFRS-R)/months since symptom onset] (8). Genetic background of ALS was exhibited in one patient only (patient 8). All other patients were diagnosed as sporadic ALS.

All patients received standard Riluzole treatment and additional G-CSF (granulocyte-colony stimulating factor, Filgrastim) treatment on a named patient basis. Application modes and doses of G-CSF were individually adapted, treatment duration was up to 7 years. For safety and monitoring of progression, structural MRI and MUNIX were assessed every 3 months. ALSFRS-R scores were acquired monthly, but were integrated in the analysis only at the time points of MRI scanning. MRI cortical thickness was combined with ALSFRS-R sum scores, and MUNIX scores for left and right ADM in both cross-sectional analysis and longitudinal biomarker monitoring.

The unicenter project was carried out in accordance with the Declaration of Helsinki (31) and approved by the ethics committee at the University of Regensburg (ethics approval: 15-101-0106). Written informed consent was obtained prior to participation in all participants.

Data Acquisition

Structural MRI was conducted at a 1.5 Tesla clinical scanner (Aera, Siemens Medical, Erlangen, Germany). For each patient, a high-resolution T1-weighted structural scan was obtained by a magnetization prepared rapid gradient echo sequence (MPRAGE; time-to-repeat TR: 2220 ms, time-to-echo TE: 5.97 ms, flip angle FA: 15°, voxel size: $1 \times 1 \times 1$ mm^3, field of view FOV: 256×256 mm^2, 176 sagittal slices covering the whole brain).

MUNIX estimates the number of motor units in a muscle by a mathematical algorithm involving both the compound muscle action potentials (CMAP) and the continuous electromyographic surface interference pattern (SIP) of the muscles (23, 27). In contrast to original MUNIX, MUNIX recordings of this project implicated continuous SIP recordings during increasing muscle contraction. SIP data were modified by baseline correction, filter settings, rectifications, and SIP intervals. Artifacts were corrected by exclusion of SIP intervals below a specified baseline threshold. As MUNIX was introduced more recently as a neurophysiological biomarker, four out of 20 ALS patients received the assessment of MUNE only (see **Table 1**).

MRI Data Preprocessing

T1-weighted structural images were reconstructed by Freesurfer software version 5.3 (Martinos Center for Biomedical Imaging,

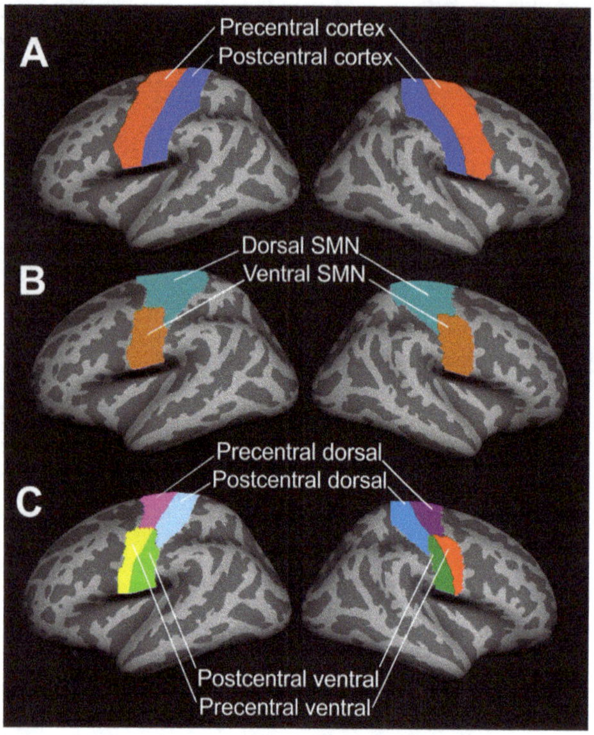

FIGURE 1 | Definition of regions of interest. **(A)** Precentral (red) and postcentral (blue) cortex were identified by the Desikan-Killiany parcellation atlas (34). **(B)** The resting-state-fMRI based atlas of Yeo et al. (35) was used to define dorsal (marine blue) and ventral (brown) segments of the sensorimotor network (SMN). **(C)** Final subdivision of the precentral and postcentral cortex into dorsal and ventral segments resulted in four ROIs (precentral dorsal, precentral ventral, postcentral dorsal, postcentral ventral) in both left and right hemisphere. ROIs were mapped upon the Freesurfer average brain surface.

Charlestown, MA). The reconstruction procedure included automatic segmentation of gray matter and subcortical white matter (32) and tessellation and registration of the cortical surface to a spherical atlas (33). For group analysis, T1-weighted images of the 20 individual patients' brains were registered to the Freesurfer average structural brain by using the Freesurfer linear and non-linear image registration tools (FLIRT, FNIRT).

ROI Definition

Cortical thickness analysis focused on precentral and postcentral regions of interest (ROI) as defined by the Desikan-Killiany parcellation atlas [(34); see **Figure 1A**]. Dorsal and ventral subdivisions of the sensorimotor network were defined by a resting-state-functional MRI (fMRI) data-based atlas (35) in volumetric MNI (Montreal Neurological Institute) space. These ROIs were subsequently registered to the Freesurfer volumetric space and then to the Freesurfer average brain surface (see **Figure 1B**). As all ROIs were mapped upon the Freesurfer average brain space, ROIs were identically sized in each patient and healthy control.

Computation of Cortical Thickness

Cortical thickness was computed according to a workflow recommended by Freesurfer software. Individual surface-based cortical thickness data were mapped upon the Freesurfer average brain surface. By the use of a segmentation statistical tool of Freesurfer software, cortical thickness in each of the four ROIs (PreD: precentral dorsal, PreV: precentral ventral, PoD: postcentral dorsal, PoV: postcentral ventral, see **Figure 1C**) was calculated and extracted as a mean value across vertices.

Cross-Sectional Group Analysis

Group-analysis of mean cortical thickness was conducted using a repeated measures ANOVA with the within-subject factors region (PreD, PreV, PoD, PoV) and hemisphere (left vs. right), and the between-subject factors group (ALS vs. controls), gender (male vs. female), and the covariate age. Differences in cortical thickness between regions were investigated by paired *t*-tests and differences between patients and controls were analyzed using independent-samples *t*-tests. *T*-tests were corrected by Bonferroni correction. Correlation analyses were conducted to investigate relations between cortical thickness, ALSFRS-R sum scores and subscores, and MUNIX by the Bravais-Pearson correlation coefficient. Significance level was set to $p < 0.05$. Multiple comparison errors were controlled by Bonferroni correction procedure in *post-hoc* analyses.

Individual Cortical Thickness Analysis

In addition to cross-sectional group analysis, this project focused on the interindividual variability of cortical thinning. For this purpose, we compared the cortical thickness of all 20 patients to age-related controls, resulting in individual *z*-transformed deviations of cortical thickness from healthy control level. As age effects on cortical thickness are well described (36), ALS patients were compared to one out of two possible age groups. Based on the mean age of ALS patients, the 30 healthy controls were differentiated into two comparably sized subgroups (1: age <48 years, $n = 17$; 2: age ≥ 48 years, $n = 13$). Furthermore, *z*-transformed deviations of cortical thickness from healthy controls as well as biomarkers MUNIX and ALSFRS-R were monitored in four individual slow progressive ALS patients over a time course of at least 18 months (patient 1, 2, 8, 9, see **Table 1**). All other patients exhibited MRI time courses of a maximum of 9 months only (3 scans: $n = 2$; 2 scans $n = 6$; 1 scan: $n = 8$) due to high disability and lack of T1 MRI data.

RESULTS

Cross-Sectional Group Analysis

As Mauchly's test indicated that the assumption of sphericity was violated [$\chi^2_{(5)} = 22.42$, $p < 0.001$], degrees of freedom were corrected using Greenhouse-Geisser estimates of sphericity ($\varepsilon = 0.79$). Cortical thickness was not significantly different between patients and healthy controls [$F_{(1, 45)} = 1.314$; $p = 0.258$] at cross-sectional group level. Cortical thickness significantly varied across cerebral regions [$F_{(3, 135)} = 23.351$, $p < 0.001$] and with respect to age [$F_{(1, 45)} = 21.776$, $p < 0.001$]. Cortical thickness was significantly higher in precentral than in

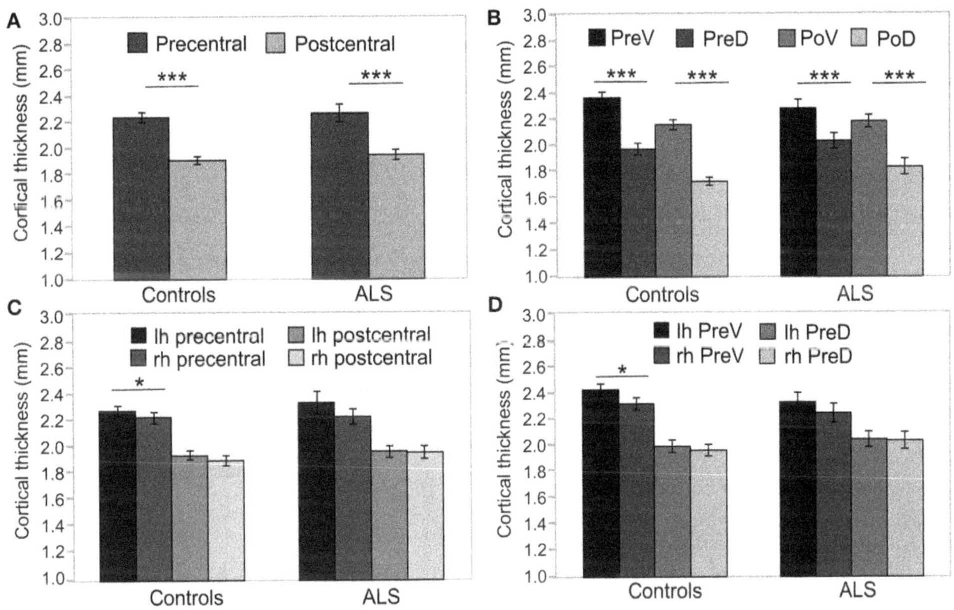

FIGURE 2 | Precentral and postcentral cortical thickness. Cross-sectional analyses of cortical thickness of ALS patients (n = 20) and healthy controls (n = 30). **(A)** Precentral cortical thickness averaged across left (lh) and right (rh) hemisphere was significantly higher than postcentral cortical thickness in both ALS patients and healthy controls. **(B)** Cortical thickness of ventral segments of both precentral (PreV) and postcentral (PoV) cortex were similarly higher than in dorsal segments (PreD, PoD) in both ALS patients and healthy controls. Hemispheric differences were detected only in the precentral **(C)** and precentral ventral cortex **(D)** of healthy controls. Significance level was set to $p < 0.05$. Bonferroni correction was used for multiple comparisons. Lh, left hemisphere; Rh, right hemisphere; PreV, precentral ventral; PreD, precentral dorsal; PoV, postcentral ventral; PoD, postcentral dorsal. Asterisks refer to the height of p-value: $^{*}p < 0.05$, $^{***}p < 0.001$.

postcentral regions in both ALS patients [$T_{(19)} = 8.584, p < 0.05$, corrected], and healthy controls [$T_{(29)} = 16.521$, $p < 0.05$, corrected] (**Figure 2A**). Ventral subdivisions of precentral and postcentral cortex showed greater cortical thickness than dorsal subdivisions in both ALS patients [$T_{(19)} = 9.906$, $p < 0.05$, corrected] and healthy controls [$T_{(29)} = 12.389$; $p < 0.05$, corrected] (**Figure 2B**). The ANOVA revealed no significant main effect of hemisphere, as significant hemispheric differences in cortical thickness were restricted to the precentral [$T_{(29)} = 3.445$, $p < 0.05$, corrected] (**Figure 2C**) and precentral ventral cortex [$T_{(29)} = 3.596$, $p < 0.05$, corrected] of healthy controls (**Figure 2D**). ALSFRS-R sum scores correlated with cortical thickness of the precentral ventral cortex ($r = 0.570, p = 0.009$) and the postcentral ventral region ($r = 0.481, p = 0.032$). Cortical thickness did not significantly correlate with MUNIX scores for left and right ADM in any ROI. MUNIX scores for the left ($r = 0.767, p < 0.05$, corrected) and right ($r = 0.791, p < 0.05$, corrected) ADM correlated with ALSFRS-R sum scores. Highest correlations of cortical thickness with ALSFRS-R subscores were found for turning (PreV: $r = 0.501$, $p = 0.024$; PoV: $r = 0.652$, $p = 0.002$), walking (PoV: $r = 0.603$, $p = 0.005$), and cutting (PreV: $r = 0.453$, $p = 0.045$). MUNIX scores predominantly correlated with ALSFRS-R subscores on handwriting (left ADM: $r = 0.637$, $p = 0.008$; right ADM: $r = 0.678$, $p = 0.005$), cutting (left ADM: $r = 0.840, p < 0.001$; right ADM: $r = 0.834$, $p < 0.001$), dressing (left ADM: $r = 0.793, p < 0.001$, right ADM: $r = 0.806$, $p < 0.001$), turning (left ADM: $r = 0.609$, $p = 0.012$; right ADM: $r = 0.663, p = 0.007$), and climbing stairs (left ADM: $r = 0.563$, $p = 0.023$; right ADM: $r = 0.611$, $p = 0.016$). ALS patients were separated *post-hoc* in arm-onset ($n = 7$) and leg-onset ($n = 13$) groups. Arm-onset patients showed significantly lower MUNIX scores for ADM (left: $M = 19$, $SD = 19$; right: $M = 16, SD = 11$) than leg-onset patients (left: $M = 95, SD = 69$; right: $M = 72$, $SD = 72$) [left ADM: $T_{(14)} = -3.399$, $p < 0.05$, corrected; right ADM: $T_{(14)} = -2.506$; $p = 0.029$]. Arm-onset and leg-onset patients did not significantly differ in disease progression, ALSFRS-R sum scores and subscores.

Variability of Cortical Thinning

Thirty healthy controls were differentiated into two groups of age (1. age <48 years, 2. age ≥48 years, see section Individual Cortical Thickness Analysis). In each of the two subgroups, means of cortical thickness of all precentral and postcentral ROIs (see **Table 2**) were calculated. These mean values were used as reference values for the calculation of z-transformed deviations of ROI-specific cortical thickness of individual ALS patients (for patient numbers see **Table 1**) from healthy control level.

Cortical thickness alterations below at least one deviation from healthy control level were detected in eleven out of twenty patients (patients 1, 2, 3, 4, 6, 10, 14, 16, 18, 19, 20) and marginally indicated in two patients (patients 5, 9). Cortical thinning was primarily observed in the precentral cortex, especially in the ventral segment (**Figure 3A**). Most pronounced cortical thinning in all precentral ROIs was detected in patient 10 and patient 19. Leg-onset patient 19 was characterized by older age (range: 61–65 years), low ALSFRS-R score (24 score points), low MUNIX

TABLE 2 | References values of cortical thickness.

		Lh PreV (mm)	Rh PreV (mm)	Lh PreD (mm)	Rh PreD (mm)	Lh PoV (mm)	Rh PoV (mm)	Lh PoD (mm)	Rh PoD (mm)
1	*M*	2.542	2.442	2.106	2.068	2.276	2.205	1.804	1.798
	SD	0.205	0.139	0.194	0.158	0.165	0.188	0.158	0.163
2	*M*	2.249	2.132	1.827	1.807	2.072	2.016	1.663	1.584
	SD	0.184	0.275	0.242	0.232	0.198	0.244	0.141	0.145

Cortical thickness (mm) of healthy control participants subdivided into two age groups (1: age <48 years, 2: age ≥48 years). Mean age of the two subgroups: Group 1: $M = 36$, $SD = 7$, $n = 17$; Group 2: $M = 52$, $SD = 15$, $n = 13$. Lh, left hemisphere; Rh, right hemisphere; PreV, precentral ventral; PreD, precentral dorsal; PoV, postcentral ventral; PoD, postcentral dorsal.

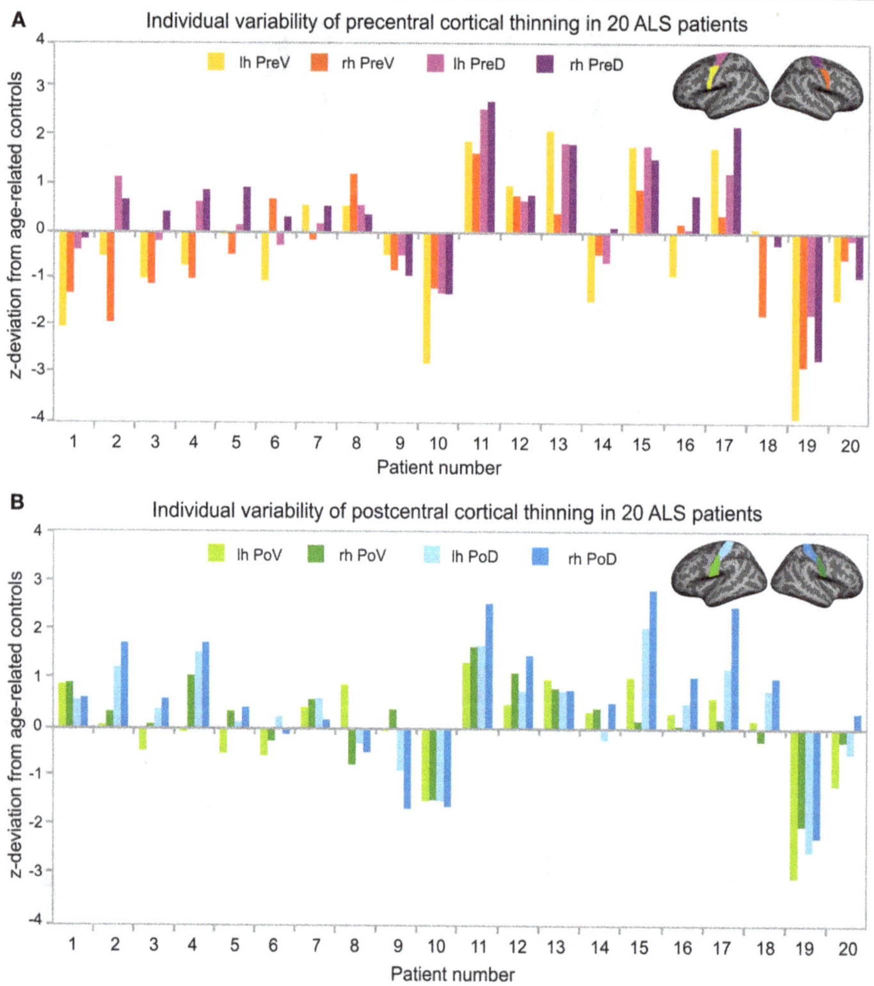

FIGURE 3 | Individual variability of cortical thinning in ALS patients. Z-transformed deviation of cortical thickness from age-related healthy controls (see **Table 2**) in all 20 individual ALS patients. Patient numbers refer to **Table 1**. Patients were sorted by age. *Z*-transformed deviations of cortical thickness were considered relevant at least one deviation from healthy controls. **(A)** Individual variability of cortical thickness of the left (lh, yellow) and right (rh, red) precentral ventral (PreV) and left (lh, pink) and right (rh, purple) precentral dorsal (PreD) ROIs. **(B)** Deviations of individual cortical thickness of the left (lh, light green) and right (rh, dark green) postcentral ventral (PoV) and the left (lh, bright blue) and right (rh, dark blue) postcentral dorsal (PoD) region in the same 20 individual patients. Precentral **(A)** and postcentral **(B)** ROIs were visualized upon the Freesurfer average brain surface. Lh, left hemisphere; Rh, right hemisphere; PreV, precentral ventral; PreD, precentral dorsal; PoV, postcentral ventral; PoD, postcentral dorsal.

scores of ADM, and high disease progression rate (0.73). Patient 10 was much younger (range: 46–50 years), but showed low ALSFRS-R score (24 score points), and the highest progression rate (1.00) of the entire patient sample (see **Table 1**). The two youngest ALS patients (patients 1–2, age ranges: 21–25 and 26–30 years) shared similar patterns of cortical thinning, similar mode of disease (arm-onset), low ALSFRS-R scores, low MUNIX scores for ADM, and similar disease progression rates (see **Table 1**, see **Figure 3A**). Cortical thinning in the postcentral cortex was detected in four patients (patients 9, 10, 19, 20; **Figure 3B**). Three out of these four patients also exhibited evident precentral cortical thinning. Leg-onset patient 9 stood out of the sample with the highest ALSFRS-R score, high MUNIX scores for ADM, lowest progression rate (0.00), and more pronounced cortical thinning of the postcentral cortex than of the precentral cortex. Increased levels of cortical thickness above healthy control level were more prominent in the postcentral cortex than in the precentral cortex. Seven patients exhibited unremarkable levels of cortical thickness (patients 7, 8, 11, 12, 13, 15, 17). Six (patients 7, 8, 12, 13, 15, 17) out of these seven patients exhibited disease progression rates less or equal to 0.40 (see **Table 1**).

Longitudinal Monitoring of Cortical Thickness, ALSFRS-R, and MUNIX

Repeated long-term follow-up T1 MRI data exceeding 18 months were available in two leg-onset patients (patients 8, 9) and two arm-onset patients (patients 1, 2). The four patients presented different initial levels and longitudinal courses of ALSFRS-R sum scores (**Figure 4A**), MUNIX scores (**Figure 4B**), and cortical thickness alterations (**Figures 4C–F**). Both patients 1 and 2 have in common young-onset (21–30 years), arm-onset diagnosis, low levels of ALSFRS-R scores (patient 1: 30 score points, patient 2: 35 score points) upon first MRI scan, low MUNIX scores for left and right ADM (see **Table 1**), and similar progression rates (patient 1: 0.37, patient 2: 0.46). In both patients, ALSFRS-R sum scores decreased over time (patient 1: blue; patient 2: green; **Figure 4A**). In contrast, MUNIX for left and right ADM stagnated at low level (patient 1: blue; patient 2: green;

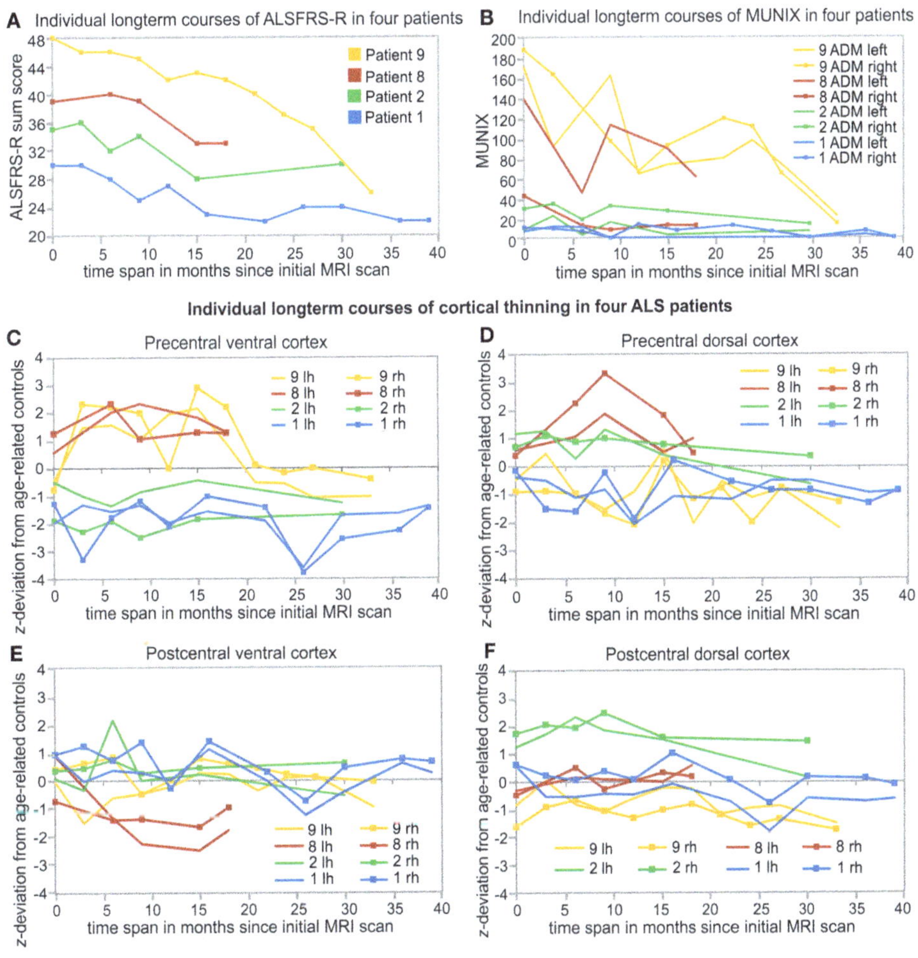

FIGURE 4 | Individual and long-term biomarker monitoring over at least 18 months. Arm-onset and young-onset patients (patient 1, 2) showed higher progression rates (see **Table 1**) than leg-onset similarly aged patients 8 and 9. Patient 9 (yellow), Patient 8 (red), Patient 2 (green), patient 1 (blue) are sorted based on the initial levels of ALSFRS-R sum scores. **(A)** Courses of ALSFRS-R sum scores of the four individual patients starting at different baseline values and developed differently over the measured time span. **(B)** Long-term courses of MUNIX scores for the left and right ADM of the same four patients. Individual long-term monitoring of cortical thickness of these four patients in the precentral ventral (PreV, **C)** and dorsal cortex (PreD, **D)** and postcentral ventral (PoV, **E)** and dorsal (PoD, **F)** cortex of both hemispheres. Individual cortical thickness is *z*-transformed to age-related healthy control level (see **Table 2**). Lh, left hemisphere; Rh, right hemisphere.

Figure 4B). Cortical thickness of the precentral ventral cortex persisted below healthy control level over time in both patients (patient 1: blue, patient 2: green; **Figure 4C**). Cortical thickness of the precentral dorsal cortex decreased below healthy control level in patient 1 in the longitudinal course (**Figure 4D**). No cortical thinning consistently below healthy control level was found for the postcentral ROIs in both patients 1 and 2 (**Figures 4E,F**). Patient 8 and 9 (both aged 46–50 years) were diagnosed with leg-onset disease and obtained high ALSFRS-R sum scores at time point of initial MRI scan (**Table 1**). Progression rates of patient 8 (0.16) and 9 (0.00) were much lower than for patients 1 and 2. In both patients, ALSFRS-R sum scores declined over time (patient 8: red, patient 9: yellow, **Figure 4A**). MUNIX scores of patient 9 similarly decreased for the left and right ADM (yellow, **Figure 4B**). In patient 8, MUNIX scores for the left ADM started at much higher level than for the right ADM and showed a more pronounced decline of scores over time (red, **Figure 4B**). Patient 8 exhibited progressive cortical thinning only in the postcentral ventral cortex (**Figure 4E**). In patient 9, cortical thinning of the right precentral dorsal cortex spread to the left hemisphere over the time course (yellow, **Figure 4D**). Cortical thickness of the postcentral dorsal cortex further decreased over time (yellow, **Figure 4F**). Despite fluctuations, ventral sections of precentral and postcentral cortex of patient 9 persisted at healthy control level (yellow, **Figures 4C,E**).

DISCUSSION

Cortical thinning was heterogenous and most pronounced in the precentral ventral cortex. ALSFRS-R sum score was associated with both cortical thickness and MUNIX scores. Individual longitudinal monitoring of clinical ALSFRS-R, neurophysiological MUNIX, and MRI cortical thickness indicated both interindividual differences among ALS patients as well as differences in temporal dynamics between biomarkers over the course of disease.

Cortical Thickness of the Precentral and Postcentral Cortex

Cortical thickness was highly age-dependent and significantly different between precentral and postcentral cortex as well as between ventral and dorsal subdivisions of precentral and postcentral cortex. Postmortem (37) and MRI (38, 39) studies showed approximately 1.5 times greater cortical thickness of the precentral compared to the postcentral cortex. The only study addressing gradients of postcentral cortical thickness in humans (40) reported greatest cortical thickness in the area defined as ventral segment in our study. Age effects on precentral and postcentral cortical thickness have been well described (36).

Variability of Cortical Thinning

Individual cross-sectional analysis revealed heterogenous individual states of cortical thinning, which was more pronounced in the precentral than in the postcentral cortex. Postcentral cortical thinning was only present in four patients. Three out of these four patients also showed pronounced cortical thinning of the precentral cortex. These observations are consistent with studies reporting postcentral atrophy was rather less prominent or not detectable (12, 41). Instead, postcentral atrophy was discussed to result from the spread of cortical degeneration in the course of disease (41, 42). With respect to the spread of disease, interestingly, individual longitudinal analysis revealed that patient 8 developed postcentral cortical thinning despite lack of precentral cortical thinning. Cortical thinning was most pronounced in the ventral segment of the precentral cortex. The precentral ventral cortex as defined here was also reported to exhibit alterations in ALS patients in other studies (14, 43, 44). Seven out of twenty patients exhibited no indications of cortical thinning. This finding is supported by a meta-analysis reporting cortical atrophy only in a percentage of ALS cases (45) and other MRI studies failing to find alterations in the precentral cortex of ALS patients (17–19). The lack of cortical thinning in ALS patients may be explained by low progression rates and young-onset. Cortical thinning was primarily observed in ALS patients with faster progression or advanced stage of disease (46). Six out of seven patients exhibiting no indications of cortical thinning were characterized with disease progression rates less or equal to 0.40. Moreover, the ALS sample of the current study was much younger than ALS patients involved in most MRI studies (8, 13, 17, 43, 47, 48). Individual cross-sectional analysis also revealed enhanced levels of cortical thickness predominantly in the postcentral cortex. Future studies may investigate if enhanced levels of cortical thickness may be associated with processes of neuroplasticity or treatment effects. Finally, heterogeneous alterations in cortical thickness (including increases and decreases) argue for the need of individual perspective on ALS patients beyond group averages (6).

Longitudinal Monitoring of Cortical Thickness, ALSFRS-R, and MUNIX

Longitudinal monitoring of cortical thickness in four patients revealed differences in temporal dynamics of clinical ALSFRS-R, neurophysiological MUNIX, and MRI cortical thickness in the same individual patients. The long-term biomarker monitoring was limited to the patients who survived for longer periods of time and who underwent more than three MRI scans. All other patients of the sample received three MRI scans or less due to short survival or lack of scan capability. Similar to Abhinav et al. (49), patients showed very different baseline levels and various progression types of ALSFRS-R sum scores over time. While the decline of high-level ALSFRS-R sum scores of patient 9 (ALSFRS-R baseline: 48) was evidently observable, changes in ALSFRS-R sum scores of progressed stage patient 1 (ALSFRS-R baseline: 30) were less evident. These observations are consistent with ALSFRS-R being considered to be less sensitive for short-term time windows and slow disease progression (3, 24, 50). ALSFRS-R is also regarded as a rather general severity summary scale without sensitivity for mode of disease (17, 29). The unspecific character of ALSFRS-R may also explain why correlations between ALSFRS-R and cortical thickness were weak or not detectable (9, 15, 21). In contrast to ALSFRS-R, MUNIX significantly differentiated between arm and leg-onset of disease. Corresponding to Grimaldi et al. (26), MUNIX scores significantly correlated with ALSFRS-R scores, but showed much faster longitudinal dynamics than ALSFRS-R scores as reported by Neuwirth et al. (29). Once at very low level MUNIX scores stagnated across time in arm-onset patients 1 and 2. The phenomenon of a floor effect of MUNIX measurements at low level in completely wasted muscles was described by Neuwirth et al (51). In contrast, higher level MUNIX scores for ADM in leg-onset patients 8 and 9 showed a fast decrease over time. Consistent with these observations, clinical markers are considered to be more sensitive to changes than MRI markers (17). Although MUNIX is considered a candidate biomarker like MUNE for LMN function (24), MUNIX scores may be influenced by both lower and UMN function (23). Existing studies investigating correlations of cortical thickness to MUNE or other neurophysiological techniques failed to find significant correlations (21, 30). As the first study combining MRI cortical thickness with MUNIX, we also found no significant correlations. Differences in both individual state of disease and within-subject temporal dynamics of various biomarkers may explain the difficulty to find significant correlations in multimodal biomarker use.

Methodological Limitations

Some methodological limitations need to be considered. First, the sample size was limited to 20 patients. As ALS MRI studies suffer from high costs and high drop-out rates due to increasing disability of patients (50), many published unicenter ALS MRI studies included samples smaller than 20 ALS patients (12, 41, 52, 53). Second, the MRI magnetic field strength was 1.5T. Although MRI magnetic field strength of 3T may have been beneficial, 1.5T still was sufficient for the detection of gray matter alterations in ALS MRI studies (11, 12, 22, 41, 54). Third, by the use of a more conservative ROI based approach than a vertex-based approach, the study may have failed to detect very focal cortical thinning inside of the ROIs. However, this approach did not only reduce the influence of false positive results but still successfully detected cortical thinning. Fourth, MUNIX scores were not assessed in leg muscles. However, this study is the first cross-sectional and longitudinal study combining cortical thickness analysis with both ALSFRS-R and MUNIX with respect to the individual patient. Fifth, longitudinal monitoring of biomarkers was limited to four patients of the sample due to high disability ($n = 6$), death ($n = 4$), lack of T1 data ($n = 6$). Still, our long-term biomarker monitoring analysis is unique, as to our knowledge, none of the published longitudinal MRI studies showed longitudinal courses of both MRI cortical thickness and MUNIX biomarkers using as many repeated measures in a time course longer than 18 months as presented in the current study. Moreover, most MRI studies focused on group analysis irrespective of the individual patient (9, 10, 14–17), although the individual perspective has been increasingly demanded in ALS neuroimaging research (6, 24, 55, 56).

CONCLUSIONS

The present study demonstrated that MRI is a potential biomarker for the differentiation of individual states of cortical thinning in an ALS sample including young-onset and slow progressive patients. Longitudinal monitoring of MRI, clinical, and neurophysiological biomarkers in the same patient reveal substantial differences in temporal dynamics. Combinatory biomarker use contributes a substantial gain of information about individual state of disease beyond group averages. Future studies may expand the idea of combining neuroimaging techniques with other clinical or molecular biomarkers to deepen our understanding of multisystem/multifactorial ALS disease progression.

AUTHOR CONTRIBUTIONS

AW: substantial contribution to the conception and the design of the study, acquisition, analysis, interpretation of the MRI data, and composition of the manuscript. AK and DB: substantial contribution to the conception of the study, data acquisition, interpretation of the data, and revision of the manuscript. IK, TG, SJ, WS-M, T-HB, and UB: substantial contribution to the conception of the study, acquisition, analysis, and interpretation of clinical and neurophysiological data, and revision of the manuscript. SJ, OH, AK, DB, WS-M, and UB: care for ALS patients in outpatient clinic, treatment concept. MG: substantial contribution to the conception of the study, supervision of MRI data analysis and data interpretation, and revision of the manuscript.

FUNDING

This work was supported by the German Federal Ministry of Education and Research (BMBF, Project GO-Bio, 031A386).

REFERENCES

1. Riva N, Agosta F, Lunetta C, Filippi M, Quattrini A. Recent advances in amyotrophic lateral sclerosis. *J Neurol.* (2016) 263:1241–54. doi: 10.1007/s00415-016-8091-6
2. Calvo AC, Manzano R, Mendonca DMF, Munoz MJ, Zaragoza P, Osta R. Amyotrophic lateral sclerosis: a focus on disease progresssion. *Biomed Res Int.* (2014) 2014:925101. doi: 10.1155/2014/925101
3. Rosenfeld J, Strong MJ. Challenges in the understanding and treatment of Amyotrophic Lateral Sclerosis/Motor Neuron disease. *Neurotherapeutics* (2015) 12:317–25. doi: 10.1007/s13311-014-0332-8
4. Chio A, Calvo A, Moglia C, Mazzini L, Mora G, PARALS study group, et al. Phenotypic heterogeneity of amyotrophic lateral sclerosis: a population based study. *J Neurol Neurosurg Psychiatry* (2011) 82:740–6. doi: 10.1136/jnnp.2010.235952
5. Agosta F, Chio A, Cosottini M, De Stefano N, Falini A, Mascalchi M, et al. The present and the future of neuroimaging in amyotrophic lateral sclerosis. *Am J Neuroradiol.* (2010) 31:1769–77. doi: 10.3174/ajnr.A2043

6. Simon NG, Turner MR, Vucic S, Al-Chalabi A, Shefner J, Lomen-Hoerth C, et al. Quantifying disease progression in amyotrophic lateral sclerosis. *Ann Neurol.* (2014) 76:643–57. doi: 10.1002/ana.24273
7. Turner MR, Verstraete E. What does imaging reveal about the pathology of amyotrophic lateral sclerosis. *Curr Neurol Neurosci Rep.* (2015) 15:45. doi: 10.1007/s11910-015-0569-6
8. Agosta F, Valsasina P, Riva N, Copetti M, Messina MJ, Prelle A, et al. The cortical signature of amyotrophic lateral sclerosis. *PLoS ONE* (2012) 7:e42816. doi: 10.1371/journal.pone.0042816
9. De Albuquerque M, Branco LMT, Rezende TJR, de Andrade HMT, Nucci A, Franca, M. C. F. Jr. Longitudinal evaluation of cerebral and spinal cord damage in Amyotrophic Lateral Sclerosis. *Neuroimage Clin.* (2017) 14:269–76. doi: 10.1016/j.nicl.2017.01.024
10. Kwan JY, Meoded A, Danielian LE, Wu T, Floeter MK. Structural imaging differences in longitudinal changes in primary lateral sclerosis and amyotrophic lateral sclerosis. *NeuroImage Clin.* (2013) 2:151–60. doi: 10.1016/j.nicl.2012.12.003
11. Mezzapesa DM, D'Errico E, Tortelli R, Distaso E, Cortese R, Tursi M, et al. (2013). Cortical Thinning and clinical heterogeneity in Amyotrophic Lateral Sclerosis. *PLoS ONE* 8:e80748. doi: 10.1371/journal.pone.0080748
12. Roccatagliata L, Bonzano L, Mancardi G, Canepa C, Caponnetto C. Detection of motor cortex thinning and corticospinal tract involvement by quantitative MRI in amyotrophic lateral sclerosis. *Amyotroph Lateral Scler.* (2009) 10:47–52. doi: 10.1080/17482960802267530
13. Schuster C, Kasper E, Matchts J, Bittner D, Kaufmann J, Benecke R, et al. Focal thinning of the motor cortex mirrors clinical features of amyotrophic lateral sclerosis and their phenotypes: a neuroimaging study. *J Neurol.* (2013) 260:2856–64. doi: 10.1007/s00415-013-7083-z
14. Schuster C, Kasper E, Machts J, Bittner D, Kaufmann J, Benecke R, et al. Longitudinal course of cortical thickness decline in amyotrophic lateral sclerosis. *J Neurol.* (2014) 261:1871–80. doi: 10.1007/s00415-014-7426-4
15. Verstraete E, Veldink JH, Hendrikse J, Schelhaas HJ, van den Heuvel MP, van den Berg LH. Structural MRI reveals cortical thinning in amyotrophic lateral sclerosis. *J Neurol Neurosurg Psychiatry* (2012) 83:383–8. doi: 10.1136/jnnp-2011-300909
16. Walhout R, Westeneng HJ, Verstraete E, Hendrikse J, Veldink JH, van den Heuvel MP, et al. Cortical thickness in ALS: towards a marker for upper motor neuron involvement. *J Neurol Neurosurg Psychiatry* (2015) 86:288–94. doi: 10.1136/jnnp-2013-306839
17. Cardenas-Blanco A, Machts J, Acosta-Cabronero J, Kaufman J, Abdulla S, Kollewe K, et al. Structural and diffusion imaging versus clinical assessment to monitor amyotrophic lateral sclerosis. *Neuroimage Clin.* (2016) 11:408–14. doi: 10.1016/j.nicl.2016.03.011
18. Ellis CM, Suckling J, Amaro, E. Jr., Bullmore ET, Simmons A, Williams SC, et al. Volumetric analysis reveals corticospinal tract degeneration and extramotor involvement in ALS. *Neurology* (2001) 57:1571–8. doi: 10.1212/WNL.57.9.1571
19. Mezzapesa DM, Ceccarelli A, Dicuonzo F, Carella A, De Caro MF, Lopez M, et al. Whole-brain and regional brain atrophy in amyotrophic laterals sclerosis. *Am. J. Neuroradiol.* (2007) 28:255–259.
20. Benatar M, Boylan K, Jeromin A, Rutkove SB, Berry J, Atassi N, et al. ALS Biomarkers for therapy development: State of the field and future directions. *Muscle Nerve* (2016) 53:169–82. doi: 10.1002/mus.24979
21. Cosottini M, Donatelli G, Costagli M, Caldarazzo Ienco E, Frosini D, Pesaresi I, et al. High-resolution 7T MR imaging of the motor cortex in amyotrophic lateral sclerosis. *Am J Neuroradiol.* (2016) 37:455–61. doi: 10.3174/ajnr.A4562
22. Thorns J, Jansma H, Peschel T, Grosskreutz J, Mohammadi B, Dengler R, et al. Extent of cortical involvement in amyotrophic lateral sclerosis – an analysis based on cortical thickness. *BMC Neurol.* (2013) 13:148. doi: 10.1186/1471-2377-13-148
23. Stein F, Kobor I, Bogdahn U, Schulte-Mattler W. Toward the validation of a new method (MUNIX) for motor unit number assessment. *J Electromyogr Kinesiol.* (2016) 27:73–7. doi: 10.1016/j.jelekin.2016.02.001
24. Van Es MS, Hardiman O, Chio A, Al-Calabi A, Pasterkamp RJ, Veldink JH, et al. Amyotrophic lateral sclerosis. *Lancet* (2017) 390:2084–98. doi: 10.1016/S0140-6736(17)31287-4
25. Gooch CL, Doherty TJ, Chan KM, Bromberg MB, Lewis RA, Stashuk DW, et al. Motor unit number estimation: a technology and literature review. *Muscle Nerve* (2014) 50:884–93. doi: 10.1002/mus.24442
26. Grimaldi S, Duprat L, Grapperon AM, Verschueren A, Delmont E, Attarian S. Global motor unit number index sum score for assessing the loss of lower motor neurons in amyotrophic lateral sclerosis. *Muscle Nerve* (2017) 56:202–6. doi: 10.1002/mus.25595
27. Grimm T, Schulte-Mattler W. Update – Neurophysiologische Methoden zur Bestimmung motorischer Einheiten in menschlichen Muskeln. *Klinische Neurophysiol.* (2017) 48:14–150. doi: 10.1055/s-0043-115149
28. Escorcio-Bezerra ML, Abrahao A, de Castro I, Chieia MAT, de Avezado LA, Pinheiro DS, et al. MUNIX: Reproducibility and clinical correlations in Amyotrophic Lateral Sclerosis. *Clin Neurophysiol.* (2016) 127:2979–84. doi: 10.1016/j.clinph.2016.06.011
29. Neuwirth C, Barkhaus PE, Burkhardt C, Castro J, Czell D, de Carvalho M, et al. Motor Unit Number Index (MUNIX) detects motor neuron loss in pre-symptomatic muscles in Amyotrophic Lateral Sclerosis. *Clin Neurophysiol.* (2017) 128:495–500. doi: 10.1016/j.clinph.2016.11.026
30. Mitsumoto H, Ulug AM, Pullman SL, Gooch CL, Chan S, Tang MX, et al. Quantitative objective markers for upper and lower motor neuron dysfunction in ALS. *Neurology* (2007) 68:1402–10. doi: 10.1212/01.wnl.0000260065.57832.87
31. World Medical Association. World medical association declaration of Helsinki: Ethical principles for medical research involving human subjects. *JAMA* (2013) 310:2191–4. doi: 10.1001/jama.2013.281053
32. Fischl B, Salat DH, Busa E, Albert M, Dieterich M, Haselgrove C, et al. Whole brain segmentation: automated labeling of neuroanatomical structures in the human brain. *Neuron* (2002) 33:341–355. doi: 10.1016/S0896-6273(02)00569-X
33. Fischl B, Sereno MI, Dale AM. Cortical surface-based analysis. II: inflation, flattening, and a surface-based coordinate system. *Neuroimage* (1999) 9:195–207. doi: 10.1006/nimg.1998.0396
34. Desikan RS, Ségonne F, Fischl B, Quinn BT, Dickerson BC, Blacker D, et al. An automated labeling system for subdividing the human cerebral cortex on MRI scans into gyral based regions of interest. *Neuroimage* (2006) 31:968–80. doi: 10.1016/j.neuroimage.2006.01.021
35. Yeo BTY, Krienen FM, Sepulcre J, Sabuncu MR, Lashkari D, Hollinshead M, et al. The organization of the human cerebral cortex estimated by intrinsic functional connectivity. *J Neurophysiol.* (2011) 106:1125–65. doi: 10.1152/jn.00338.2011
36. Salat DH, Buckner RL, Snyder AZ,Greve DN, Desikan RSR, Busa E, et al. Thinning of the cerebral cortex in aging. *Cereb Cortex* (2004) 14:721–30. doi: 10.1093/cercor/bhh032
37. Meyer JR, Roychowdhury S, Russell EJ, Callahan C, Gitelman D, Mesulam MM. Location of the central sulcus via cortical thickness of the precentral and postcentral gyri on MRI. *Am J Neuroradiol.* (1996) 17:1699–706.
38. Fischl B, Dale AM. Measuring the thickness of the human cerebral cortex from magnetic resonance images. *Proc Natl Acad Sci USA.* (2000) 97:11050–5. doi: 10.1073/pnas.200033797
39. Sahin N, Mohan S, Maralani PJ, Duddukuri S, O'Rourke DM, Melhem ER, et al. Assignment confidence in localization of the hand motor cortex: comparison of structural imaging with functional MRI. *Am J Roentgenl.* (2016) 207:1263–1270. doi: 10.2214/AJR.15.15119
40. Wagstyl K, Ronan L, Goodyer IM, Fletcher PC. Cortical thickness gradients in structural hierarchies. *Neuroimage* (2015) 111:241–50. doi: 10.1016/j.neuroimage.2015.02.036
41. Grosskreutz J, Kaufmann J, Fradrich J, Dengler R, Heinze HJ, Peschel T. Widespread sensorimotor and frontal cortical atrophy in Amyotrophic Lateral Sclerosis. *BMC Neurol.* (2006) 6:17. doi: 10.1186/1471-2377-6-17
42. Brettschneider J, Del Tredici K, Toledo JB, Robinson JL, Irwin DJ, Grossman M, et al. Stages of pTDP-3 pathology in amyotrophic lateral sclerosis. *Ann Neurol.* (2013) 74:20–38. doi: 10.1002/ana.23937
43. Lillo P, Mioshi E, Burrell JR, Kiernan MC, Hodges JR, Hornberger M. (2012). Grey and white matter changes across the amyotrophic lateral sclerosis-frontotemporal dementia continuum. *PLoS ONE* 7:e43993. doi: 10.1371/journal.pone.0043993.

44. Schuster C, Hardiman O, Bede P. Survival prediction in Amyotrophic lateral sclerosis based on MRI measures and clinical characteristics. *BMC Neurol.* (2017) 17:73. doi: 10.1186/s12883-017-0854-x
45. Chen Z, Ma L. Grey matter volume changes over the whole brain in amyotrophic lateral sclerosis: a voxel-wise meta-analysis of voxel based morphometry studies. *Amyotroph Lateral Scler.* (2010) 11:549–54. doi: 10.3109/17482968.2010.516265
46. Meadowcroft MD, Mutic NJ, Bigler DC, Wang JL, Simmons Z, Connor JR, et al. Histological-MRI correlation in the primary motor cortex of patients with amyotrophic lateral sclerosis. *J Magn Reson Imaging* (2015) 41:665–75. doi: 10.1002/jmri.24582
47. Agosta F, Ferraro PM, Riva N, Spinelli EG, Cio A, Canu E, et al. Structural brain correlates of cognitive and behavioral impairment in MND. *Hum Brain Mapping* (2016) 37:1614–26. doi: 10.1002/hbm.23124
48. Spinelli EG, Agosta F, Ferraro PM, Riva N, Lunetta C, Falzone YM, et al. Brain MR imaging in patients with lower motor neuron-predominant disease. *Radiology* (2016) 280:545–56. doi: 10.1148/radiol.2016151846
49. Abhinav K, Yeh FC, El-Doklar A, Ferrando LM, Chang YF, Lacomis D, et al. Use of diffusion spectrum imaging in preliminary longitudinal evaluation of amyotrophic lateral sclerosis: development of an imaging biomarker. *Front Neurosci.* (2014) 8:270. doi: 10.3389/fnhum.2014.00270
50. Rutkove SB. Clinical measures of disease progression in amyotrophic lateral sclerosis. *Neurotherapeutics* (2015) 12:338–93. doi: 10.1007/s13311-014-0331-9
51. Neuwirth C, Barkhaus PE, Burkhardt C, Castro J, Czell D, de Carvalo M, et al. Tracking motor neuron loss in a set of six muscles in amyotrophic lateral sclerosis using the Motor Unit Number Index (MUNIX): a 15-month longitudinal multicentre trial. *J Neurol Neurosurg Psychiatry* (2015) 86:1172–9. doi: 10.1136/jnnp-2015-310509
52. Cosottini M, Cecchi P, Piazza S, Pesaresi I, Fabbri S, Diciotti S, et al. Mapping cortical degeneration in ALS with magnetization transfer ratio and voxel-based morphometry. *PLoS ONE* (2013) 8:e68279. doi: 10.1371/journal.pone.0068279
53. Verstraete E, van den Heuvel MP, Veldink JH, Blanken N, Mandl RC, Hulshoff Pol HE, et al. (2010). Motor network degeneration in amyotrophic lateral sclerosis: a structural and functional connectivity study. *PLoS ONE* 5:e13664. doi: 10.1371/journal.pone.0013664
54. Tavazzi E, Lagana MM, Bergsland N, Tortorella P, Pinardi G, Luneta C, et al. Grey matter damage in progressive multiple sclerosis versus amyotrophic lateral sclerosis: a voxel-based morphometry MRI study. *Neurol Sci.* (2015) 36:371–7. doi: 10.1007/s10072-014-1954-7
55. Turner MR, Bowser R, Brujn L, Dupuis L, Ludolph A, McGrath M, et al. Mechanisms, models and biomarkers in amyotrophic lateral sclerosis.Amyotroph. *Lateral Scler Frontotemporal Degener.* (2013) 14:19–32. doi: 10.3109/21678421.2013.778554
56. Verstraete E, Foerster BR. Neuroimaging as a new diagnostic modality in amyotrophic lateral sclerosis. *Neurotherapeutics* (2015) 12:403–16. doi: 10.1007/s13311-015-0347-9

15

Lymphocyte Count and Body Mass Index as Biomarkers of Early Treatment Response in a Multiple Sclerosis Dimethyl Fumarate-Treated Cohort

*Alessia Manni[1], Antonio Iaffaldano[1], Giuseppe Lucisano[1,2], Mariangela D'Onghia[3], Domenico Maria Mezzapesa[1], Vincenzo Felica[1], Pietro Iaffaldano[1], Maria Trojano[1] and Damiano Paolicelli[1]**

[1] *Department of Basic Medical Sciences, Neurosciences and Sense Organs, University of Bari "Aldo Moro", Bari, Italy,* [2] *Center for Outcomes Research and Clinical Epidemiology, Pescara, Italy,* [3] *Operative Unit of Neurology, "Dimiccoli" General Hospital, Barletta, Italy*

Correspondence:
Damiano Paolicelli
damiano.paolicelli@uniba.it

Introduction: In relapsing Multiple Sclerosis (RMS) patients treated with disease modifying drugs (DMDs), few data are available regarding the biomarkers of treatment response. We aimed to assess the predictive value of lymphocyte count (LC) and Body Mass Index (BMI) for treatment response in a real life setting of dimethyl fumarate (DMF) treated patients.

Materials and Methods: We included in our observational analysis 338 patients who were prescribed DMF in an Italian MS Center. We collected clinical and demographic data at the beginning of DMF (T0), and assessed White Blood Cells (WBC) and LC at T0 and at 3 (T3), 6 (T6), 9 (T9), and 12 (T12) months. Gadolinium enhancing (Gd+), new T2 lesions and relapses within the first year of treatment (T12) were recorded in order to evaluate clinical activity at 12 months. Analysis of correlation was performed to correlate WBC, LC and BMI with clinical and radiological responses. We evaluated whether BMI or LC can predict treatment response by using multivariate logistic regression models at each follow-up.

Results: Our cohort was followed up for a mean period of 19.8 $\pm$ 6.8 months. The mean BMI at baseline was 24.19 $\pm$ 4.48. The multivariate models gave as predictive factors for Gd+ lesions at T12, LC at T3 (OR = 1.003, 95% CI = 1.00-1.07; $p = 0.046$) and baseline BMI (OR = 0.71, 95% CI = 0.52–0.98; $p = 0.037$). Predictive factors for new T2 lesions at T12 were LC at T3 (OR = 1.01 95%CI = 1.00–1.95; $p = 0.005$) and baseline BMI (OR = 0.99, 95% CI = 0.98–1.00; $p = 0.026$).

Conclusions: In our real life-experience, BMI and LC may be early biomarkers to predict treatment response during DMF.

Keywords: dimethyl fumarate, lymphocyte count, body mass index, biomarkers, treatment response

INTRODUCTION

Multiple Sclerosis (MS) is a chronic immune-mediated disease of the central nervous system mainly affecting young adults (1). The development of disease modifying drugs (DMDs) has made an important contribution to MS treatment, allowing a reduction in the frequency of relapses and delaying disease progression. In recent decades there has been a constant increase in the availability of DMDs with different mechanisms of action, routes of administration and safety profiles. Interferon-β (IFN-β) and glatiramer acetate (GA) are well-established MS therapies which have well-characterized safety profiles and have shown a reduction of relapse rate by approximately one third. However, these DMDs are administered through weekly or daily injections and patients may experience breakthrough disease activity and tolerability may be suboptimal (2, 3). These drawbacks have prompted the search for drugs that could reduce the burden of medication administration and be somehow more efficacious. All newer DMDs have the aim of regulating or suppressing the immune system through specific pathways, and in many cases this has resulted in foreseeable adverse effects (lymphopenia).

Dimethyl fumarate (DMF) is a DMD that was approved for the treatment of relapsing–remitting MS (RRMS) in 2013 in the USA and in 2014 in the European Union. Two Phase III studies and their ongoing long-term extensions have proved that DMF reduces Annualized Relapse Rate (ARR) by ~50% and also reduces the number of new or enlarging T2 hyperintense lesions, new T1 hypointense lesions, and gadolinium-enhancing (Gd+) lesions (4–6). Although its exact mechanism of action has not been fully explained, DMF has proven capable of reducing white blood cell (WBC) counts and absolute lymphocyte counts (LC) by ~30% from the baseline within the first year of treatment (7). Of the patients treated for at least 6 months, 2.2% experienced LC <500 mm^3 [grade 3 lymphopenia, according to Common Terminology Criteria for Adverse Events -CTCAE- vs. 4.0 (8)] persisting for at least 6 months (5). However, the clinical implications of DMF-induced leukopenia and lymphopenia on treatment response are not yet fully understood. Nevertheless, the need for a careful surveillance is strong given the cases of progressive multifocal leukoencephalopathy (PML) occurring in DMF treated patients with sustained lymphopenia (grade 3 lymphopenia for >6 months) (9).

In addition to acting via the immunomodulation of various cells, DMF also appears to act through neuroprotection since it induces the nuclear factor erythroid 2–related factor 2 (Nrf2) pathway (10). It has been demonstrated that Nrf2 activity is lessened in diabetes and that body weight could modify its activity (11). In recent years, several studies have investigated the role of the Body Mass Index (BMI) in the pathogenesis of autoimmune diseases, such as MS. It has been shown that obesity may worsen the disease course in several autoimmune diseases (12) and studies have reported a positive association between BMI and disability among MS patients (13). Although this evidence supports the role of obesity as a risk factor for MS and its progression, the potential effects of BMI on treatment response have not yet been fully understood. Our work attempted to assess the predictive value of LC and BMI for treatment response in a real-life cohort of DMF-treated relapsing Multiple Sclerosis (RMS) patients. For this purpose, we evaluated the temporal profile of WBC and LC during the first year of treatment and also correlated clinical and Magnetic Resonance Imaging (MRI) (T1 Gd+ lesions, new or enlarging T2 lesions) variables with BMI and with WBC and LC variation in order to identify potential biomarkers of treatment response.

METHODS

Study Design, Study Population, and Follow-Up

This is an observational, retrospectively acquired cohort study, approved by the Local Ethics Committee. At the beginning of DMF all patients provided their written informed consent to authorize the use of their clinical and MRI data. A total number of 456 patients started DMF-treatment at the Center for Multiple Sclerosis of the University of Bari between 2014 and 2016; we studied a cohort of 338 patients with RMS according to McDonald and Polman criteria (14, 15), who had reached at least 1-year follow up (**Figure 1**). Three patients (0.5%) had an unscheduled MRI before the sixth month of treatment (mean time of MRI acquisition = 2.8 ± 0.2 months), showing, according to their treating physician, a high MRI disease activity compared with the baseline MRI; therefore they interrupted the treatment before reaching the sixth month follow up, underwent a high-dose intravenous glucocorticoids, and were then switched to second line DMDs. Five patients (1.1%) experienced a disabling relapse within the third month of treatment and were therefore treated with high dose steroids. Three of these patients were also treated with plasma exchange. All five interrupted DMF treatment. These eight patients were not included in the study cohort.

At the beginning of the treatment (baseline), the following demographic, clinical and MRI data were collected from all patients using the electronic iMed database: age and gender, weight, height, BMI, disease duration, number of relapses, previous DMDs, presence/absence of new/enlarging T2 lesions, and presence/absence of Gd+ lesions. To avoid the slight weight gain (16), possibly caused by a steroid cycle, patients weight and BMI were recorded at least 30 days after the last day of steroids intake. Patients were assessed for neurological disability using the Expanded Disability Status Scale (EDSS) (17) at baseline and at 3-month intervals, and an additional neurological assessment was performed in the event of a relapse. Relapses were defined as episodes of neurological symptoms occurring at least 30 days after the onset of any previous episode, lasting at least 24 h, not attributable to any other causes, occurring in the absence of an infection or fever, and accompanied either by new clinical signs, i.e., changes in the neurological examination, or by an increased EDSS score (1). Peripheral blood (PB) samples were collected in order to monitor WBC and LC at baseline (T0), and then at 3-month intervals. To avoid any possible confounders due to the effect of steroid treatment in the case of relapses/MRI activity, PB samples were collected at least 30 days after the last day of corticosteroids intake. WBC count and LC were evaluated using

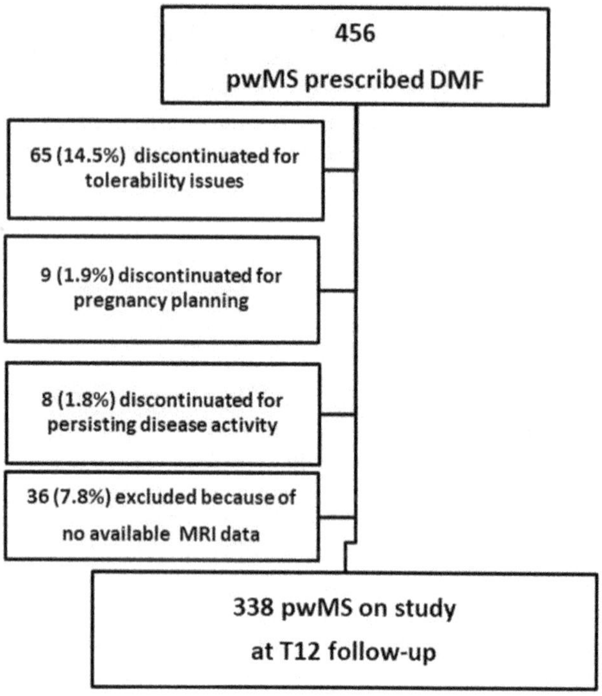

FIGURE 1 | Flow diagram of the study. pwMS, people with Multiple Sclerosis; DMF, dimethyl fumarate; MRI, Magnetic Resonance Imaging; T12, 1 year follow-up.

the quality reference of the same laboratory at the Center for Multiple Sclerosis of the University of Bari.

MRI scans were performed on a 1.5 T Achieva scanner (Philips Healthcare, Best, Netherlands) and 8-channel head coil. Dual-echo sequences (to obtain T2 weighted images; TR 2,800 ms, TE 21/120 ms, flip angle: 90°) and fluid attenuated inversion recovery (FLAIR; TR/TE/TI, 8,900/190/2,500 ms, flip angle: 90°) were acquired in axial orientation (50 slices, 3-mm thick, 1-mm gap, FOV 256 x 256, matrix 400 x 400). Before and after gadolinium administration, T1 weighted images (TR /TE 1,000/12.5 ms, flip angle: 69°) were acquired in axial orientation (22 slices, 5-mm thick, 1-mm gap, FOV 230 × 230, matrix 320 × 320). Spinal cord MRI protocol included T2-weighted (TR/TE 3,500/120 ms) and T1-weighted (before and after gadolinium administration; TR/TE 400/7.5 ms), acquired in sagittal orientation (13 slices, 3.5-mm thick, 0.35-mm gap, FOV 522 × 522, matrix 1,024 × 1,024). Baseline MRI scans were performed no more than 6 months before the start of DMF treatment (mean time of MRI acquisition = 3.8 ± 1.4 months), and then at 6-month intervals (±30 days). MRI outcomes were defined as follows: presence/absence of new/enlarging T2 lesions; presence/absence of Gd+ lesions. Trained neuro-radiologists performed the lesion count by visual analysis of two successive MRI images.

Clinical Variables

The quantitative variation in WBC and LC, considered both in terms of absolute value and of the "delta" (Δ = the difference between the absolute values of WBC and LC between two consecutive time-points), were analyzed. The baseline (T0) was compared with four different periods of treatment: T3 (3rd month ± 30 days), T6 (6th month ± 30 days), T9 (9th month ± 30 days), and T12 (12th month ± 30 days). Moreover, in order to investigate the impact of the DMF-induced lymphopenia (DIL) on the risk of clinical and MRI activity, the median of the absolute LC was calculated at each observation time, and patients were divided into two groups: those with a high DIL (DIHL, above the median) and those with a low DIL (DILL, below the median). We used this statistical (not clinical) classification to divide the study population into two equal-sized groups (50% of the LC distribution for each group).

Outcomes

- Presence/absence of new T2 lesions at the T12 MRI follow-up;
- Presence/absence of Gd+ lesions at the T12 MRI follow-up;
- Presence/absence of relapses within the first year of DMF treatment;
- Variation in WBC and LC over time.

Statistical Analysis

Baseline characteristics were reported for continuous variables as mean ± standard deviation (SD) and for categorical variables as percentages. Characteristics were compared in subjects with and without an event (presence/absence of Gd+ lesions, presence/absence of new T2 lesions, presence/absence of relapses) using the *T*-test for continuous variables and the chi-squared test for categorical variables. For the comparison over time, we used the Wilcoxon matched pair test, and analysis of Pearson correlation was performed to correlate WBC and BMI.

We used multivariate analysis testing the following covariates: sex, age at the start of DMF, presence/absence of T2 lesions at the baseline MRI, presence/absence of Gd+ lesions at the baseline MRI, presence/absence of relapses in the year before starting DMF, previous DMD exposure (naïve patients vs. patients treated with a first-line DMD vs. those treated with a second-line DMD), variation in WBC from T0 to T3, LC at T3, baseline BMI, DIHL at T3 and at T6. Multivariate logistic regression models always considered as covariates the baseline clinical and demographic characteristics of the cohort, and those covariates significant at the univariate analysis, and were used to evaluate whether BMI or LC can predict the outcome. We used a multivariate logistic regression approach for each follow-up because there were no exact dates for follow-up evaluation. Results were expressed as odds ratio (OR) and 95% confidence intervals (95% CI). A 2-sided $p<0.05$ was considered significant. All analyses were performed using the SPSS version 19.0 (SPSS Inc., Chicago, Illinois).

RESULTS

The mean ± standard deviation (SD) follow-up of our cohort was 19.8 ± 6.8 months. The baseline demographic and clinical characteristics of the study population are shown in **Table 1**. Our cohort consisted of 197 (58.3%) female patients and 141 (41.8%) male patients. The mean age at DMF initiation was

TABLE 1 | Baseline demographic, anthropometric, and clinical characteristics of the study population.

Number of patients	338
Sex: n (F/M)	197/141
Age at DMF beginning (years, mean± SD)	38 ± 10.7
Disease duration (years, mean± SD)	12.5±7.3
EDSS at DMF initiation (mean± SD)	3.0 ± 1.5
Patients with comorbidities (%)	118 (34.9%)
BMI at DMF beginning (kg/m^2, mean± SD)	24.19 ± 4.48
LC (cells/mm^3 mean± SD)	1,940 ± 667.60
WBC (cells/mm^3 mean± SD)	6380.8 ± 2051.93
Previous DMDs	
-Naïve: *n* (%)	50 (14.8%)
-Only first line treatments: *n* (%)	257 (76%)
-First and second line treatments; *n* (%)	31 (9.2%)

DMF, Dimethyl fumarate; SD, standard deviation; EDSS, Expanded Disability Status Scale; BMI, Body Mass Index; LC, lymphocyte count; WBC, white blood cells; DMDs, Disease modifying drugs.

38 ± 10.7 years, and the mean disease duration was 12.5 ± 7.3 years. The mean EDSS at DMF initiation was 3.0 ± 1.5 and the ARR in the previous year was 0.5. The mean BMI at baseline was 24.19 ± 4.48. Fifty patients were treatment-naïve (14.8%), while 257 switched to DMF from a first-line DMD, and 31 from second-line treatments. The latter 31 patients (2 with Mitoxantrone, 2 with Azathioprine, 21 patients with Fingolimod and 4 patients with Natalizumab), because of a possible overlap of immunosuppressive effects, observed a washout period sufficient to restore immune function and bring LC and WBC back within normal ranges. For patients switching from a first-line DMD, a wash-out period of at least 4 weeks was observed (longer if specifically reported by Summary of Product Characteristics or in accordance with treating-physicians' decisions).

Temporal Profile of WBC and LC

Figure 2 shows WBC and LC values at the beginning of DMF and at 3-month intervals during the first year of treatment. We compared the LC and WBC between T0 and T3, and we observed a reduction of 15.4% in LC (from 1,940 ± 667.60 to 1642.18 ± 184.75; $p < 0.0001$) and a reduction of 5.9% in WBC (from 6380.80 ± 2051.93 to 6010.29 ± 1601.30; $p = 0.124$). In T0–T6, a reduction of 33.2% was observed in LC (from 1,940 ± 667.60 to 1296.06 ± 584.03; $p < 0.001$) and a reduction of 14.9% in WBC (from 6380.80 ± 2051.93 to 5,436 ± 1585.63; $p < 0.001$). In T0–T9, a reduction of 39.1% was observed in LC (from 1,940 ± 667.60 to 1181.86 ± 480.80; $p < 0.001$), and a reduction of 19.9% in WBC (from 6380.80 ± 2051.93 to 5119.28 ± 1252.66; $p < 0.001$). Finally, in T0–T12, a reduction of 37.14% was observed in LC (from 1,940 ± 667.60 to 1213.01 ± 577.6; $p < 0.001$) and a reduction of 15.7% in WBC (from 6380.80 ± 2051.93 to 5383.33 ± 1313.82; $p < 0.001$). From T3, 29 patients presented GRADE I CTCAE lymphopenia (<LLN-800 u/mm^3), and 24 presented GRADE II lymphopenia (<800–500 u/mm^3). The nadir of reduction was observed at T9, both for WBC ($p < 0.0001$) and LC ($p < 0.0001$), with a reduction, respectively, of 19.8 and 39.1% from T0.

Correlation Between WBC and LC Variation and Disease Activity

During the first year of treatment, in our cohort, the ARR was significantly lower than ARR as recorded in our clinical database for the previous year (0.25 vs. 0.51, $p = 0.001$). We evaluated the correlation between WBC and LC variation and outcomes of disease activity during DMF-treatment (**Table 2**).

In the univariate analysis, patients who experienced relapses within the first year of treatment had a higher WBC count at T3 (6,031 ± 1,687/µl vs. 5,660 ± 1,110/µl, $p = 0.05$) as well as a lower variation in WBC between T0 and T3 (−59.53 ± 1006.33 vs. 167.79 ± 1660.78, $p = 0.05$) than patients who experienced no relapse (**Table 2**). However, multivariate analysis confirmed the reduction in WBC as a predictive factor for relapses occurring during the entire first year of treatment (OR = 1.054, 95% CI = 1.03–2.65; $p = 0.043$, **Table 3**).

We observed no differences in the absolute value or the delta of WBC between patients presenting new Gd+/T2 lesions and patients who did not. On the other hand, LC was higher at T3 in patients who experienced new Gd+ lesions at T6 (1,845 ± 455 vs. 1,486 ± 556, $p = 0.043$), in patients who experienced new T2 lesions at T12 (1,952 ± 317 vs. 1,495 ± 592; $p = 0.040$), and in patients experiencing a relapse during the first year of treatment (1,761 ± 465 vs. 1,386 ± 402; $p = 0.033$) (**Table 2**). Multivariate analysis showed that LC at T3 was a predictive factor for Gd+ lesions at T12 (OR = 1.003, 95% CI = 1.00–1.07; $p = 0.046$) (**Table 3**) and new T2 lesions at T12 (OR = 1.01; 95% CI = 1.00–1.95; $p = 0.005$) (**Table 3**).

In order to investigate the impact of the lymphocytes on the risk of relapses and on worsening MRI, the median values of LC at T3, T6 and T9 were calculated, and the population was divided into two groups:

- Patients with LC below the median calculated (with low number of DMF-induced lymphocytes -DILL-),
- Patients with LC above the median calculated (with high number of DMF-induced lymphocytes -DIHL-).

In the univariate analysis, during the first and second semesters of treatment, no differences were found between the clinical activity of patients with DIHL and patients with DILL (**Table 2**). However, considering MRI activity at T12, patients with DIHL at T3 (OR = 1.31, 95% CI = 1.12–5.34, $p = 0.043$) and at T6 (OR = 1.14, 95% CI = 1.13–6.33; $p = 0.05$) had a higher risk of Gd+ lesions (**Table 3**). Patients with DIHL at T3 (OR = 1.26, 95% CI = 1.07–1.96; $p = 0.04$) and at T6 (OR = 1.48, 95% CI = 1.15–2.59; $p = 0.035$) also had a higher risk of new T2 lesions at T12, compared to patients with DILL (**Table 3**).

Role of BMI

Patients experiencing a relapse during the first year of treatment presented a lower baseline BMI (20.9 ± 2.4 vs. 24.7 ± 4.4; $p = 0.001$) (**Table 2**). Multivariate analysis, confirmed baseline BMI as a predictive factor for GD+ lesions at T12 (OR = 0.71; CI = 0.52–0.98; $p = 0.037$) (**Table 3**) and also for new T2 lesions at T12

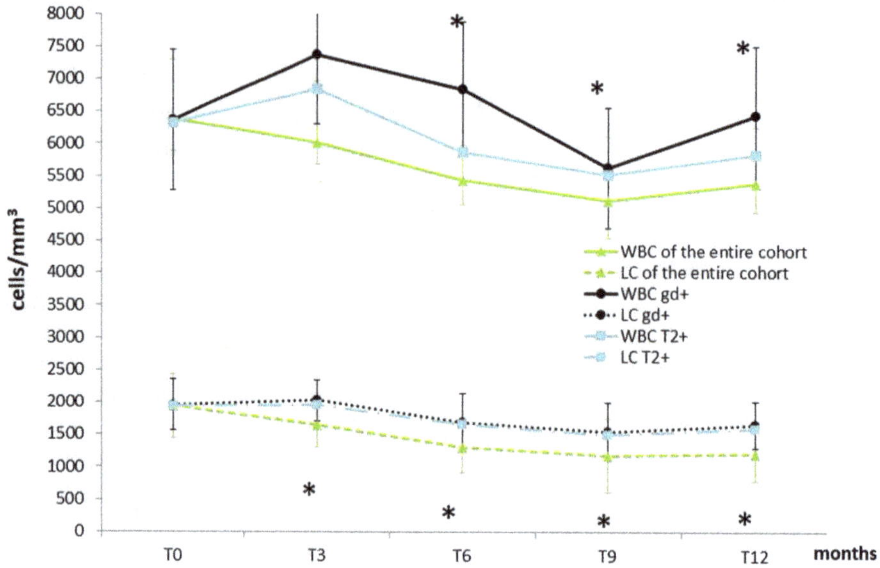

FIGURE 2 | Temporal profile of WBC and LC of the entire cohort compared with patients showing MRI activity at T12. Data are presented as mean ± SD. WBC, white blood cell; LC, lymphocyte count; MRI, Magnetic Resonance Imaging; Gd+, Gadolinium enhancing; T2+, new hyperintense lesions; T0, baseline; T3, 3 months follow up; T6, 6 months follow-up; T9, 9 months follow up; T12, one year follow-up.*Indicates Wilcoxon matched pair test $P < 0.05$ (vs. T0) in the entire sample size.

(OR = 0.99, 95% CI = 0.98–1.00; $p = 0.026$) (**Table 3**). **Figure 3** graphically represents the BMI in patients with and without new T2 lesions at T12.

At T0 we observed a direct correlation between the WBC count and BMI ($r = 0.42$; $p = 0.001$; **Figure 4**); we had also expected a correlation between BMI and LC, as often found in other diseases, but we did not observe this. No other correlations were found between baseline WBC and LC values and any clinical-demographic variable (baseline age and gender, disease duration, number of relapses within the previous year, previous DMDs, presence/absence of new/enlarging T2 lesions, and presence/absence of Gd+ lesions). We further investigated whether any comorbidities, presented by 34.9% of our population (118 patients), could influence BMI at baseline, but we found no difference between BMI in patients with and without comorbidities (24.7 ± 3.8 vs. 23.9 ± 5.4; $p = 0.117$). We also observed a direct correlation between BMI and WBC at T3 ($r = 0.23$; $p = 0.016$); no other correlations were found between baseline BMI and variations in WBC and LC values.

DISCUSSIONS AND CONCLUSIONS

Several DMDs used to treat MS can reduce the occurrence of relapses and slow the progression of neurological disability, thus improving patients' quality of life. However, variability in response to DMDs in patients with MS represents a significant clinical challenge. Potentially, treatment delays may occur in suboptimal responder patients, exposing them to adverse effects without significant benefit. Therefore, biomarkers of treatment response are urgently needed. In our cohort, after 1 year of therapy, DMF was effective in reducing both clinical and MRI disease activity, as shown by the multivariate models used that take into account the absence of exact date of both clinical and MRI relapses. We tried to identify some possible factors that could influence DMF effectiveness, avoiding potential confounders such as baseline disease activity and other patient specific characteristics that were considered in our analysis. Building our hypothesis we also considered the drug effects that involve immunomodulatory action as well as neuroprotection (10, 18). DMF, in fact, reduces cytokine production (19), down-regulates the migratory activity of immune cells at the blood–brain barrier (20) and activates the antioxidant nuclear factor NRF2 transcriptional pathway (10, 21). Considering that the Nrf2 pathway plays an important role in energy metabolism (11, 22) and that recent data demonstrate that DMF is a negative regulator of preadipocyte differentiation mediated by STAT3 inhibition (23), we tried to link patients' BMI with both clinical (relapses) and MRI outcomes. There have been studies indicating that overweight and obese patients have a lesser chance of obtaining complete remission and Non-Evidence of disease Activity (NEDA)-status during IFN-β-treatment, although it remains to be determined whether this is due to a suboptimal treatment response or to a generally more aggressive disease (24). Moreover, Krupp et al. have argued that a higher BMI in US adolescents could be a relevant explanation for their worse outcomes during IFN-ß therapy (25). Obesity, however, is known to effect serum inflammatory markers, promoting a chronic low-grade inflammatory state (26), also through the activation of the nuclear factor (NF) κB pathway (27), and DMF has been shown to prevent the induction of NFκB dependent transcription (28). In our cohort, a lower BMI was

TABLE 2 | LC and WBC of the patients stratified for Gd+ lesions, new T2 lesions and relapses.

	GD+ lesions at baseline MRI (YES) *N* = 95 (28%)	**GD+ lesions at baseline MRI (NO) *N* = 243 (72%)**	**Gd+ lesions at T6 (YES) *N* = 48 (14.2%)**	**Gd+ lesions at T6 (NO) *N* = 290 (85.8%)**	**Gd+ lesions at T12 (YES) *N* = 30 (8.9%)**	**Gd+ lesions at T12 (NO) *N* = 308 (91.1%)**
Baseline LC (cells/mm^3)	1,846 ± 554	1,986 ± 720	1,857 ± 584.4	2,102 ± 912.4	1,903 ± 503	1,967 ± 498
Baseline WBC (cells/mm^3)	6,300 ± 1,030	6,466 ± 2,222	6,630 ± 2,033	6,228 ± 1,995	6,630 ± 917	6,204 ± 1,649
LC at T3 (cells/mm^3)	1,925 ± 1,281	1,588 ± 583	*1,845 ± 455**	*1,486 ± 556**	2,024 ± 337	1,518 ± 581
WBC at T3 (cells/mm^3)	6,208 ± 1,326	6,006 ± 1680	5,875 ± 1,277	5,788 ± 1624	7,376 ± 1165	5,962 ± 1,575
	New T2 lesions at baseline MRI (YES) *N* = 125 (37%)	**New T2 lesions at baseline MRI (NO) *N* = 213 (63%)**	**New T2 lesions at T6 (YES) *N* = 91(26.9%)**	**New T2 lesions at T6 (NO) *N* = 247 (73.1%)**	**New T2 lesions at T12 (YES) *N* = 50 (14.8%)**	**New T2 lesions at T12 (NO) *N* = 288 (85.2%)**
Baseline LC (cells/mm^3)	2,069 ± 740	1,880 ± 642	1,855 ± 546.1	2021.63 ± 837.5	1903.8 ± 614	1,941 ± 393
Baseline WBC (cells/mm^3)	6,344 ± 2,244	6,478 ± 2,000	6,001 ± 2,024	6,419 ± 1,986	6,312 ± 1,090	6,234 ± 1,678
LC at T3 (cells/mm^3)	1,811 ± 1,826	1,518 ± 570	1,739 ± 571	1,461 ± 653	*1,952 ± 317**	*1,495 ± 592**
WBC at T3 (cells/mm^3)	6,247 ± 1,539	5,936 ± 1,357	5,969 ± 1,392	5,729 ± 1,641	6,840 ± 1,073	5,963 ± 1,940
	Relapse before DMF (YES) *N* = 152 (45%)	**Relapse before DMF (NO) *N* = 186 (55%)**	**Relapse within T6 (YES) *N* = 41 (12%)**	**Relapse within T6 (NO) *N* = 297 (88%)**	**Relapse within T12 (YES) *N* = 63 (18.6%)**	**Relapse within T12 (NO) *N* = 275 (81.4%)**
Baseline LC (cells/mm^3)	1,837 ± 622	2,027 ± 696	2054.18 ± 956	1,858.15 ± 561	1,702 ± 549	1,868 ± 858
Baseline WBC (cells/mm^3)	6,194 ± 2,073	6,553 ± 2,033	6,324 ± 2,126	6,216 ± 1,972	6,165 ± 1,045	5,600 ± 1,275
LC at T3 (cells/mm^3)	1,551 ± 574	1,725 ± 1,548	1,687 ± 353	1,597 ± 537	*1,761 ± 465**	*1,386 ± 402**
WBC at T3 (cells/mm^3)	6,193 ± 1,662	5,841 ± 1,537	6,243 ± 1,398	5,850 ± 1,688	*6,031 ± 1,687**	*5,660 ± 1,110**

Values expressed as mean (±SD).
*LC, lymphocyte count; WBC, white blood cells; T3, 3 months follow-up; T6, 6-months follow up; T12, 1 year follow up. * underlines $p < 0.05$.*

TABLE 3 | Predictors of relapses and MRI disease outcomes at T12: multivariate logistic regression analysis.

	OR (95% CI); *p*-value		
Variable	**Relapse within T12**	**New T2 lesions at T12**	**Gd+ lesions at T12**
Gender (F)	0.635 (0.09–4.13); 0.630	0.313 (0.06–15.14); 0.557	0.095 (0.001–5.23); 0.566
Age	0.851 (0.697–1.04); 0.060	0.63 (0.56–11.25); 0.991	0.411 (0.062–2.73); 0.358
Baseline Gd+ (YES)	0.045 (0.005–0.44); 0.080	0.032 (0.001–1.23); 0.994	0.011 (0.001–1.96); 0.088
Baseline T2 (YES)	1.99 (0.25–16.07); 0.510	1.22 (0.28–2.21); 0.198	0.31 (0.074–1.29); 0.109
Relapses pre-DMF (YES)	0.73 (0.61-1.60); 0.060	1.016 (0.175–14.5); 0.993	1.76 (0.175–15.32); 0.998
1st line DMD vs. naive	1.002 (0.045–3.47); 0.990	6.37 (0.19–7.52); 0.988	0.15 (0.001–69.9); 0.545
2nd line DMD vs. naive	0.236 (0.008–6.74); 0.380	2.25 (0.03–2.29); 0.862	0.31 (0.07–1.3); 0.109
Variation in WBC	*1.054 (1.03-2.65); 0.043*	–	–
LC at T3	1.08 (0.98–2.80), 0.090	*1.01 (1.00–1.95); 0.005*	*1.003 (1.00–1.07); 0.046*
Baseline BMI	0.828 (0.61–1.15); 0.213	*0.99 (0.98–1.00); 0.026*	*0.71 (0.52–0.98); 0.037*
DIHL at T3	2.5 (0.77–8.05); 0.125	*1.26(1.07–1.96); 0.040*	*1.31(1.12–5.34); 0.043*
DIHL at T6	0.62 (0.16–2.42); 0.493	*1.48 (1.15–2.59); 0.035*	*1.14 (1.133–6.33); 0.050*

*WBC, white blood cells; BMI, Body Mass Index; LC, lymphocyte count; DIHL, high number of DMF-induced lymphocytes; T3, 3 months follow-up; T6, 6-months follow up; T12, 1 year follow up. *Models always considered as covariates baseline clinical and demographic characteristics of the cohort, and those covariates significant at the univariate analysis. Underlined values are those statistically significant (p<0.05).*

a predictive factor for MRI activity at T12, and we tried to explain this finding with the differences in DMF action according to the amount of adipose tissue; we may hypothesize that the higher the amount of adipocytes, the greater the action that DMF can exert on the inflammatory aspect of the disease. Nowadays, in fact, adipocytes are attributed a metabolically active role in biochemical mechanisms that may contribute to a chronic low-grade inflammatory status (29), increasing ROS oxidative stress. Reactive oxygen and nitrogen species have been described to induce damage to biological macromolecules in MS lesions (30, 31). Moreover, in RR and also in progressive MS, active lesions are associated with inflammation (32), although not always present in the latter form of the disease.

We also found that LC at T3 was a predictive factor for clinical and MRI activity. DMF suppresses lymphocytes and induces T-cell apoptosis. DMF-induced lymphopenia could theoretically be linked to disease control. However, in DEFINE and CONFIRM, the reduction in ARR at 2 years in patients treated with DMF 240 mg bid vs. placebo was not substantially different in patients with lymphopenia (≥1LC < lower limit of normal) compared to those without lymphopenia (all LCs ≥lower limit of normal) (7). However, real-life data are sometimes discordant on this point; for example, data from a Dallas Multiple Sclerosis Center (33) have shown a greater risk of relapses in patients with higher LC at 3 months [$p < 0.001$, hazard ratio [HR]: 1.82], just as we found in our cohort. Moreover, the Dallas examiners stratified LC by tertile, and found a reduced risk in patients with lower LC values: 1,200 cells/mL compared with mid-tier (1,210–1,800 cells/mL) and the highest tertile (>1,810 cells/mL) ($p < 0.01$). We obtained comparable results by stratifying patients according to the LC median during the follow-up, and found that patients with DIHL at T3, T6, and T12 had a higher risk of MRI activity than those with DILL. Conversely, in another cohort from the MS Center of Washington (34), DMF-induced lymphopenia did not predict a good clinical response to therapy. In this Washington study, the authors examined predictive factors of lymphopenia including recent natalizumab exposure as risk factors of developing moderate to severe lymphopenia during treatment with DMF. In our cohort, the previous treatment was not associated with a different incidence in reduction of WBC or LC, and we found no significant correlation between the previous DMD and the disease activity. However, we observed a direct correlation between the WBC count and BMI ($r = 0.32$; $p = 0.001$) at T0; since fat tissue releases inflammatory cytokines, this may explain why in our cohort we found a direct correlation between WBC (which can be considered a non-specific marker of inflammation) and BMI. Moreover, while BMI and LC are independently linked to DMF effectiveness, the association test performed on these did not prove to be a statistically significant effect of either clinical or MRI activity. The reason for this may be that our cohort contained few underweight or obese patients. Another possible explanation could be that the two variables did not change to the same extent: BMI remained constant during the observation period, while there was a reduction (15.36%) in LC which was statistically significant from the third month and tended to stabilize around the ninth month. This finding differs from what has been observed in an integrated analysis of long-term extension studies on DMF (7), which demonstrated that LC decreased by 30% during the first year and then plateaued, remaining above the lower limit of normal (LLN).

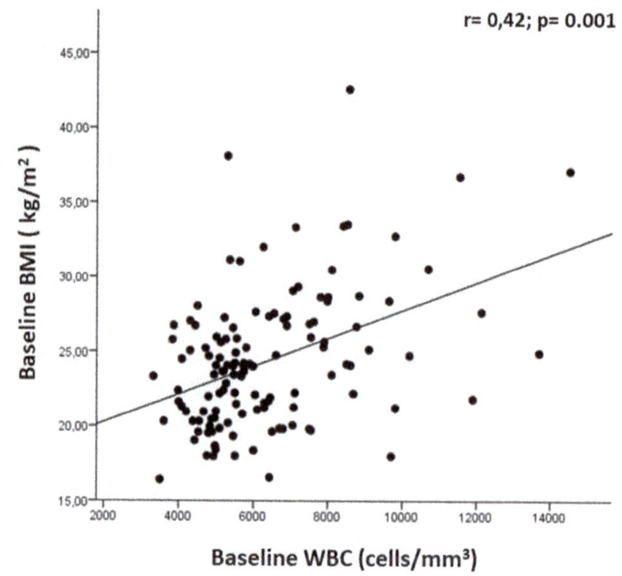

FIGURE 3 | Correlation between baseline BMI and WBC. WBC, white blood cell; BMI, Body Mass Index.

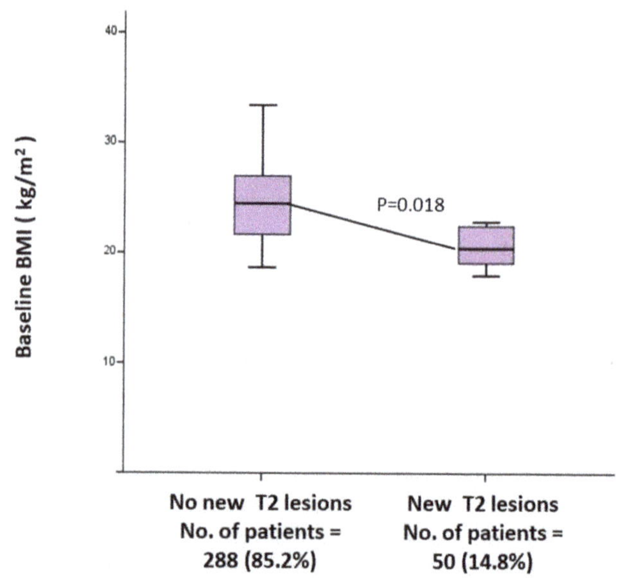

FIGURE 4 | Univariate between baseline BMI and MRI activity at T12. BMI, Body Mass Index; MRI, Magnetic Resonance Imaging; T12, 1 Year follow up.

Our analysis did not investigate the influence of different lymphocytes subsets (LS) on disease activity during DMF. A recent study demonstrated that patients under DMF therapy who remained stable (with no radiological or clinical evidence of disease activity) tended to exhibit greater reductions of CD3+, CD4+, CD8+, and CD19+ cells compared to active MS patients, and they also presented significantly higher CD4/CD8 ratios (35). However, since the monitoring of the immune system re-modulation in DMF relapsing MS patients is not required during the routine clinical practice, we did not perform, in this real life setting, analyses on specific LS variations and this is one of the limitations of our study. Other limitations may be the lack of a control group treated with a different DMD, as well as the lack of details regarding metabolic parameters of patients (blood glucose levels and urine tests), the metabolic state of immune cells, and patients' consumption behavior. Further studies will be performed that will include these details in order to have a more in-depth analysis of the role of BMI in predicting DMF effectiveness. Another limitation is that, given the oral administration of the drug, we did not check patients' adherence. Finally, the most important limitation may be the observational design of our study: our findings may only reflect a unique sample population and, thus, may not be generalized to other groups.

In conclusion, elucidating the significance of DMF-induced lymphopenia could be important for clinical decisions, including the frequency of monitoring and the possibility of predicting both clinical or MRI activity. This becomes an even more appealing prospect when it is considered that changes in LC can be detected from the third month of treatment, and might therefore offer the possibility of formulating an early prediction of a possible suboptimal response. Moreover, the use of an easily detectable baseline characteristic (BMI), could allow better profiling of patients for a tailored treatment. However, given the observational nature of our work, there is a need for further studies on larger cohorts in order to support the clinical importance of our results.

AUTHOR CONTRIBUTIONS

AM participated in the design of the study, collected the data, and drafted the manuscript. AI collected the data and revised the manuscript, helped to give final approval. GL participated in the design of study, performed statistical analysis and helped to given final approval. MD participated in the design of study and revised the manuscript. DM revised the manuscript and helped to give final approval. VF revised the manuscript. PI helped to draft the manuscript. MT revised the manuscript and helped to give final approval. DP conceived of the study, and participated in its design, revised the manuscript and helped to give final approval of the version to be published.

ACKNOWLEDGMENTS

Preliminary data regarding this topic were presented at the 4th Congress of the European Academy of Neurology - Lisbon 2018 (EPO3067 - Lymphocyte count and Body Mass Index as biomarkers of treatment response in a Multiple Sclerosis Dimethyl-Fumarate-treated cohort).

REFERENCES

1. Olsson T, Barcellos LF, Alfredsson L. Interactions between genetic, lifestyle and environmental risk factors for multiple sclerosis. *Nat Rev Neurol.* (2017) 13:25–36. doi: 10.1038/nrneurol.2016.187
2. Goodin DS. Disease-modifying therapy in MS: a critical review of the literature. Part II: assessing efficacy and dose-response. *J Neurol.* (2004) 251(Suppl. 5):v50–6. doi: 10.1007/s00415-004-1508-7
3. Rudick RA, Polman CH. Current approaches to the identification and management of breakthrough disease in patients with multiple sclerosis. *Lancet Neurol.* (2009) 8:545–59. doi: 10.1016/S1474-4422(09)70082-1
4. Gold R, Kappos L, Arnold DL, Bar-Or A, Giovannoni G, Selmaj K, et al. DEFINE Study Investigators. Placebo-controlled phase 3 study of oral BG-12 for relapsing multiple sclerosis. *N Engl J Med.* (2012) 367:1098–107. doi: 10.1056/NEJMoa1114287
5. Fox RJ, Miller DH, Phillips JT, Hutchinson M, Havrdova E, Kita M, et al. CONFIRM Study Investigators. Placebo-controlled phase 3 study of oral BG-12 or glatiramer in multiple sclerosis. *New Engl J Med.* (2012) 367:1087–97. doi: 10.1056/NEJMoa1206328
6. Gold R, Arnold DL, Bar-Or A, Hutchinson M, Kappos L, Havrdova E, et al. Long-term effects of delayed-release dimethyl fumarate in multiple sclerosis: interim analysis of ENDORSE, a randomized extension study. *Mult Scler.* (2017) 23:253–65. doi: 10.1177/1352458516649037
7. Fox RJ, Chan A, Gold R, Phillips JT, Selmaj K, Chang I, et al. Characterizing absolute lymphocyte count profiles in dimethyl fumarate-treated patients with MS: patient management considerations. *Neurol Clin Pract.* (2016) 6:220–9. doi: 10.1212/CPJ.0000000000000238
8. National Cancer Institute. *Common Terminology Criteria for Adverse Events v4.0, NCI, NIH, DHHS.* Bethesda, MD: NIH publication (2009).
9. European Medicines Agency. *Updated Recommendations to Minimise the Risk of the Rare Brain Infection PML With Tecfidera.* (2015). Available online at: https://www.ema.europa.eu/en/news/updated-recommendations-minimise-risk-rare-brain-infection-pml-tecfidera (accessed May 20, 2019).
10. Linker RA, Lee DH, Ryan S, van Dam AM, Conrad R, Bista P, et al. Fumaric acid esters exert neuroprotective effects in neuroinflammation via activation of the Nrf2 antioxidant pathway. *Brain.* (2011) 134(Pt 3):678–92. doi: 10.1093/brain/awq386
11. Pi J, Leung L, Xue P, Wang W, Hou Y, Liu D, et al. Deficiency in the nuclear factor E2-related factor-2 transcription factor results in impaired adipogenesis and protects against diet-induced obesity. *J Biol Chem.* (2010) 285:9292–300. doi: 10.1074/jbc.M109.093955
12. Versini M, Jeandel PY, Rosenthal E, Shoenfeld Y. Obesity in autoimmune diseases: not a passive bystander. *Autoimmun. Rev.* (2014) 13:981–1000. doi: 10.1016/j.autrev.2014.07.001
13. Oliveira SR, Simão AN, Kallaur AP, de Almeida ER, Morimoto HK, Lopes J, et al. Disability in patients with multiple sclerosis: influence of insulin resistance, adiposity, and oxidative stress. *Nutrition.* (2014) 30:268–73. doi: 10.1016/j.nut.2013.08.001
14. McDonald WI, Compston A, Edan G, Goodkin D, Hartung HP, Lublin FD, et al. Recommended diagnostic criteria for multiple sclerosis: guidelines from the International Panel on the diagnosis of multiple sclerosis. *Ann Neurol.* (2001) 50:121–7. doi: 10.1002/ana.1032
15. Polman CH, Reingold SC, Banwell B, Clanet M, Cohen JA, Filippi M, et al. Diagnostic criteria for multiple sclerosis: 2010 revisions to the "McDonald criteria". *Ann Neurol.* (2011) 69:292–302. doi: 10.1002/ana.22366
16. Durelli L, Cocito D, Riccio A, Barile C, Bergamasco B, Baggio GF, et al. High-dose intravenous methylprednisolone in the treatment of multiple sclerosis: clinical-immunologic correlations. *Neurology.* (1986) 36:238–43 doi: 10.1212/WNL.36.2.238
17. Kurtzke JF. Rating neurologic impairment in multiple sclerosis: an expanded disability status scale (EDSS). *Neurology.* (1983) 33:1444–52. doi: 10.1212/WNL.33.11.1444
18. Scannevin RH, Chollate S, Jung MY, Shackett M, Patel H, Bista P, et al. Fumarates promote cytoprotection of central nervous system cells against oxidative stress via the nuclear factor (Erythroid-Derived 2)-like 2 pathway. *J Pharmacol Exp Ther.* (2012) 341:274–84. doi: 10.1124/jpet.111.190132
19. McGuire VA, Ruiz-Zorrilla Diez T, Emmerich CH, Strickson S, Ritorto MS, Sutavani RV, et al. Dimethyl fumarate blocks pro-inflammatory cytokine production via inhibition of TLR induced M1 and K63 ubiquitin chain

formation. *Sci Rep.* (2016) 6:31159. doi: 10.1038/srep31159

20. Loewe R, Holnthoner W, Gröger M, Pillinger M, Gruber F, Mechtcheriakova D, et al. Dimethylfumarate Inhibits TNF-induced nuclear entry of NF-jB/p65 in human endothelial cells. *J Immunol.* (2002) 168:4781–7. doi: 10.4049/jimmunol.168.9.4781
21. Wang Q, Chuikov S, Taitano S, Wu Q, Rastogi A, Tuck SJ. et al. Dimethyl fumarate protects neural stem/progenitor cells and neurons from oxidative damage through Nrf2-ERK1/2 MAPK Pathway. *Int J Mol Sci.* (2015) 16:13885–907. doi: 10.3390/ijms160613885
22. Hou Y, Xue P, Bai Y, Liu D, Woods CG, Yarborough K, et al. Nuclear factor erythroid-derived factor 2-related factor 2 regulates transcription of CCAAT/enhancer-binding protein β during adipogenesis. *Free Radic Biol Med.* (2012) 52:462–72. doi: 10.1016/j.freeradbiomed.2011.10.453
23. Kang HJ, Seo HA, Go Y, Oh CJ, Jeoung NH, Park KG, et al. Dimethylfumarate suppresses adipogenic differentiation in 3T3-L1 preadipocytes through inhibition of STAT3 activity. *PLoS ONE.* (2013) 8:e61411. doi: 10.1371/journal.pone.0061411
24. Kvistad SS, Myhr KM, Holmøy T, Šaltytė Benth J, Wergeland S, Beiske AG, et al. Body mass index influence interferon-beta treatment response in multiple sclerosis. *J Neuroimmunol.* (2015) 288:92–7. doi: 10.1016/j.jneuroim.2015.09.008
25. Krupp LB, Pohl D, Ghezzi A, Boyko A, Tenembaum S, Chen L, et al. REPLAY Study Group, Subcutaneous interferon β-1a in pediatric patients with multiple sclerosis: regional differences in clinical features, disease management, and treatment outcomes in an international retrospective study, *J Neurol Sci.* (2016) 363:33–8 doi: 10.1016/j.jns.2016.01.023
26. Cao H. Adipocytokines in obesity and metabolic disease. *J Endocrinol.* (2014) 220:T47–59. doi: 10.1530/JOE-13-0339
27. Yuan M, Konstantopoulos N, Lee J, Hansen L, Li ZW, Karin M, et al. Reversal of obesity- and diet-induced insulin resistance with salicylates or targeted disruption of Ikkbeta. *Science.* (2001) 293:1673–7. doi: 10.1126/science.1061620
28. Loewe R, Pillinger M, de Martin R, Mrowietz U, Gröger M, Holnthoner W, et al. Dimethylfumarate inhibits tumor-necrosis-factor-induced CD62E expression in an NF-kappa B-dependent manner. *J Invest Dermatol.* (2001) 117:1363–8. doi: 10.1046/j.0022-202x.2001.01576.x
29. Palavra F, Almeida L, Ambrósio AF, Reis F. Obesity and brain inflammation: a focus on multiple sclerosis. *Obes Rev.* (2016) 17:211–24. doi: 10.1111/obr.12363
30. van Horssen J, Schreibelt G, Drexhage J, Hazes T, Dijkstra CD, van der Valk P, et al. Severe oxidative damage in multiple sclerosis lesions coincides with enhanced antioxidant enzyme expression. *Free Radic Biol Med.* (2008) 45:1729–37. doi: 10.1016/j.freeradbiomed.2008.09.023
31. Haider L, Fischer MT, Frischer JM, Bauer J, Höftberger R, Botond G, et al. Oxidative damage in multiple sclerosis lesions. *Brain.* (2011) 134(Pt 7):1914–24. doi: 10.1093/brain/awr128
32. Frischer JM, Bramow S, Dal-Bianco A, Lucchinetti CF, Rauschka H, Schmidbauer M, et al. The relation between inflammation and neurodegeneration in multiple sclerosis brains. *Brain.* (2009) 132(Pt 5):1175–89. doi: 10.1093/brain/awp070
33. Wright K, Winkler MD, Newton BD, Sormani MP, Okuda DT. Patient outcomes influenced by reduced lymphocyte counts after dimethyl fumarate initiation. *Neurol Neuroimmunol Neuroinflamm.* (2017) 4:e397 doi: 10.1212/NXI.0000000000000397
34. Longbrake EE, Naismith RT, Parks BJ, Wu GF, Cross AH. Dimethyl fumarate-associated lymphopenia: risk factors and clinical significance. *MSJ Exp Transl Clin.* (2015) 1:1–8. doi: 10.1177/2055217315596994
35. Fleischer V, Friedrich M, Rezk A, Bühler U, Witsch E, Uphaus T, et al. Treatment response to dimethyl fumarate is characterized by disproportionate CD8+ T cell reduction in MS. *Mult Scler.* (2018) 24:632–41. doi: 10.1177/1352458517703799

16

Inverse Phosphatidylcholine/Phosphatidylinositol Levels as Peripheral Biomarkers and Phosphatidylcholine/Lysophosphatidylethanolamine-Phosphatidylserine as Hippocampal Indicator of Postischemic Cognitive Impairment in Rats

*Angelica Maria Sabogal-Guáqueta[1], Javier Gustavo Villamil-Ortiz[1], Julian David Arias-Londoño[2] and Gloria Patricia Cardona-Gómez[1]**

[1] *Neuroscience Group of Antioquia, Cellular and Molecular Neurobiology Area – School of Medicine, Sede de Investigación Universitaria (SIU), University of Antioquia, Medellín, Colombia,* [2] *Department of Systems Engineering, University of Antioquia, Medellín, Colombia*

***Correspondence:**
Gloria Patricia Cardona-Gómez
patricia.cardonag@udea.edu.co;
patricia.cardona@neurociencias.udea.edu.co

Vascular dementia is a transversal phenomenon in different kinds of neurodegenerative diseases involving acute and chronic brain alterations. Specifically, the role of phospholipids in the pathogenesis of dementia remains unknown. In the present study, we explored phospholipid profiles a month postischemia in cognitively impaired rats. The two-vessel occlusion (2-VO) model was used to generate brain parenchyma ischemia in adult male rats confirmed by alterations in myelin, endothelium, astrocytes and inflammation mediator. A lipidomic analysis was performed via mass spectrometry in the hippocampus and serum a month postischemia. We found decreases in phospholipids (PLs) associated with neurotransmission, such as phosphatidylcholine (PC 32:0, PC 34:2, PC 36:3, PC 36:4, and PC 42:1), and increases in PLs implied in membrane structure and signaling, such as lysophosphatidylethanolamine (LPE 18:1, 20:3, and 22:6) and phosphatidylserine (PS 38:4, 36:2, and 40:4), in the hippocampus. Complementarily, PC (PC 34:2, PC 34:3, PC 38:5, and PC 36:5) and ether-PC (ePC 34:1, 34:2, 36:2, 38:2, and 38:3) decreased, while Lyso-PC (LPC 18:0, 18:1, 20:4, 20:5, and LPC 22:6) and phosphatidylinositol (PI 36:2, 38:4, 38:5, and 40:5), as neurovascular state sensors, increased in the serum. Taken together, these data suggest inverse PC/LPC-PI levels as peripheral biomarkers and inverse PC/LPE-PS as a central indicator of postischemic cognitive impairment in rats.

Keywords: global ischemia, cognitive impairment, phospholipid profile, biomarkers, serum, hippocampus

---

Abbreviations: ePC ether phosphatidylcholine; ePE, ether phosphatidylethanolamine; ePS, ether phosphatidylserine; LPC, lysophosphatidylcholine; LPE, lysophosphatidylethanolamine; PA, phosphatidic acid; PC, phosphatidylcholine; PCA, principal component analyses; PE, phosphatidylethanolamine; PG, phosphatidylglycerol; PI, phosphatidylinositol; PLS-DA, partial least squares analysis; PS, phosphatidylserine; SM, sphingomyelin.

INTRODUCTION

Cognitive impairment and dementia are common phenomena induced by acute and chronic brain injury, including Alzheimer's disease, stroke, and traumatic brain injury (TBI) (Nucera and Hachinski, 2018). Additionally, these conditions are predisposed to or worsened by poor lifestyles, including obesity, metabolic disorders, sedentary habits, smoking, and cardiocerebrovascular diseases, among others (Moskowitz et al., 2010). Long-term deprivation of oxygen and glucose via hypoperfusion or vasoconstriction of small vessels generates neurovascular unit injury, which is associated with vascular dementia after focal or global cerebral ischemic injury in response to cardiac arrest, coronary artery bypass surgery, cardiorespiratory failure, and other conditions due to drastic reductions in blood flow to the brain (Llinas et al., 2000; Vijayan et al., 2017).

In particular, the incidence of cerebrovascular disease, the third leading cause of death and the first leading cause of physical and mental disability worldwide, is increasing in developing countries (Cardona-Gómez and Lopera, 2016). Particularly, brain ischemia is caused by the occlusion of blood vessels, depriving of oxygen and glucose, resulting in an energy failure that alters mitochondrial ATP synthesis and upregulates the production of oxidative stress, free radicals and lipid peroxidation. Also„ the activation of dopamine and glutamate, as excitatory neurotransmitters, induces intracellular calcium overload, metabolic dysfunction and acidosis (Moskowitz et al., 2010). The increase in intracellular calcium causes activation of enzymes involved in lipid metabolism, such as "sphingomyelinases and phospholipases A2, C, and D, that, in turn, promote the release of second messengers, such as diacylglycerol (DAG), phosphatidic acid (PA), and arachidonic acid (AA), involved in inflammation, excitotoxicity and other cell death pathways" (Phillis and O'Regan, 2004; Tian et al., 2009). However, biomarkers supporting the clinical diagnosis of stroke are in development, and the development of biomarkers used to diagnosis the risk of dementia after stroke and its prevention is a true challenge.

In regard to lipids, these compounds are diverse, complex, and their functions depend on cellular distribution. Lipids are crucial in the homeostasis of cell membrane structure and act as signaling molecules and modulators in the central nervous system (CNS) (Martinez-Gardeazabal et al., 2017). Interestingly membrane lipids can be damaged by lipolysis under ischemia and by peroxidation of polyunsaturated fatty acids (PUFAs) during reperfusion (Schaller and Graf, 2004). Particularly, phospholipids, which are known for their high concentrations in the brain, play an important role both in normal neuronal activity and in pathological processes, even in those associated with memory impairment (Miyawaki et al., 2016). Therefore, we focused on elucidating the changes in lipid profiles of the hippocampus and serum of rats with cognitive impairment induced by global ischemia, as a continue of our previous studies (Marosi et al., 2006).

MATERIALS AND METHODS

Animal Procedures

"All of the animal procedures were performed in accordance with the ARRIVE guidelines, the Guide for the Care and Use of Laboratory Animals, 8th edition published by the National Institutes of Health (NIH) and the Colombian standards (law 84/1989 and resolution 8430/1993). These procedures were approved by the Ethics Committee for Animal Experimentation of the University of Antioquia, Medellin, Colombia.

Male Wistar albino rats from our in-house, pathogen-free colony in the vivarium at SIU (Sede de Investigación Universitaria), University of Antioquia, Medellin, Colombia were kept on a 12:12 h dark/light cycle and received food and water *ad libitum*. Special care was taken to minimize animal suffering and to reduce the number of animals used. Three-month-old rats weighing 400–450 g were used. The rats were randomly divided into two groups, namely, the control and ischemic groups. Nine (9) rats were used per experimental group for behavioral, lipidomic and immunostaining evaluation (Marosi et al., 2006).

Global Cerebral Ischemia (2 VO)

"The animals were anesthetized using ketamine (60 mg/kg) and xylazine (5 mg/kg) and received a 2–4% isofiurane and 96% oxygen mixture via an inhalation anesthesia machine. A variation of the global cerebral ischemic model was implemented, involving a 2-vessel occlusion (2-VO; (Marosi et al., 2006). The right common carotid artery (CCA) was permanently occluded using a 6.0-gauge nylon suture (Corpaul, Bogota, Colombia), and the left CCA was obstructed for 20 min using a vascular clip. After the 20 min, the vascular clip was removed to allow reperfusion. Sham control rats underwent the same procedure without the CCA occlusion. The animals were sacrificed a month postischemia for lipid analyses" (Becerra-calixto and Cardona-gómez, 2017).

Immunochemistry and Immunofluorescence

Twenty four hours after the last behavioral test, animals were perfused intracardially with paraformaldehyde at 4%. Brains were removed and postfixed 48 h. Coronal sections (50 mm) obtained from vibratome were permeabilized, with 0.3% Triton X-100 and blocked with 1% BSA in PBS, using a previously described protocols for immunohistochemistry and immunofluorescence (Marosi et al., 2006), for the following evaluated primary antibodies: anti-NeuN (mouse monoclonal, Millipore, 1:500) anti-GFAP (monoclonal anti-glial fibrillary acidic protein, Sigma, 1:1000), anti-PECAM-1 (rabbit Platelet Endothelial Cell Adhesion Molecule 1, Abcam, 1:500), anti-myelin PLP (rabbit, myelin Proteolipid protein, Abcam, 1:200), COX-2 (rabbit, Cyclooxygenase 2, Abcam, 1:500). For immunofluorescence tissue, we incubated for 90 min at room temperature with mouse Alexa Fluor 488- or Alexa Fluor 594- conjugated anti-rabbit secondary antibodies (1:1000; Molecular Probes, Eugene, OR, United States). The tissues incubated in the absence of primary antibody did not display immunoreactivity.

Morris Water Maze Test

"Nineteen days after ischemia, the animals were evaluated in the Morris water maze (MWM) teste during 10 days (n = 9 per group). The test was performed using a previously described method (Becerra-calixto and Cardona-gómez, 2017). Briefly, a black plastic tank was filled with water (22 ± 2°C), and visual cues around the room remained in a fixed position throughout the experiment. The hidden platform (12 cm in diameter) was submerged 3 cm below the water level during spatial learning and 1.5 cm above the surface of the water during the visible session. Six sessions or trials were performed. Each session consisted of four successive subtrials (30 s intertrial interval), and each subtrial began with the rat being placed pseudorandomly in one of four starting locations. Then, the animals were provided with a 48 h retention period, followed by a probe trial of spatial reference memory, in which the animals were placed in the tank without the platform for 90 s. The latency to reach the exact former location of the platform was recorded during the probe trial. Later, the platform was moved to a new location and the ability of the animals to learn the new location was measured by determining the latency in 4 sessions conducted in the same manner as the learning phase. The latency to reach the platform was evaluated using a visible platform to control for any differences in visual-motor abilities or motivation between the experimental groups; the animals that could not perform the task were excluded. An automated system (Viewpoint, Lyon, France) recorded the behavior of the animals" (Marosi et al., 2006).

Tissue Preparation and Lipid Extraction

A month postischemia, four (4) "animals were sacrificed via decapitation, and the hippocampus of each rat was dissected, immediately frozen in liquid nitrogen and stored at 80°C until analysis. We performed the same procedure to obtain serum samples. The total lipids from the hippocampus and serum were extracted according to the FOLCH technique (Jordi Folch, 1957) using a mixture of 2 mL of chloroform (CHCl3) and 1 mL of methanol (MeOH) in a 2:1 (v/v) ratio. Then, 0.005% butylated hydroxytoluene (BHT) was added, and this mixture was used to homogenize the hippocampus. Subsequently, 1 mL of 0.9% NaCl was added, and the mixture was centrifuged at 3000 rpm for 3 min. The organic layer (lower layer) was removed and transferred to a new glass tube. The solvents were evaporated, and the extract was lyophilized to remove excess humidity. Finally, the lipid composition was analyzed via mass spectrometry" (Villamil-Ortiz et al., 2016).

Mass Spectrometry

"An automated ESI-MS/MS approach was used, and data acquisition and analysis were carried out at the Kansas Lipidomics Research Center using an API 4000 TM and Q-TRAP (4000Qtrap) detection system as described previously (Villamil-Ortiz et al., 2016). This protocol allowed the detection and quantification of low concentrations of the polar lipid compounds. The molecules were determined by the mass/charge ratios, which were compared with the respective internal standard to determine which species of lipids were present in the evaluated extract: 0.30 nmol 14:0 lysoPG, 0.30 nmol 18:0 lysoPG, 0.30 nmol di 14:0 PG, 0.30 nmol 14:0-lysoPE, 0.30 nmol 18:0-lysoPE, 0.60 nmol 13:0-lysoPC, 0.60 nmol 19:0-lysoPC, 0.60 nmol di 12:0-PC, 0.60 nmol di 24:1-PC, 0.30 nmol 14:0 lysoPA, 0.30 nmol 18:0 lysoPA, 0.30 nmol di14:0-PA, 0.30 nmol di20:0 (phytanoyl)-PA, 0.20 nmol di 14:0-PS, 0.20 nmol di Phy PS, 0.28 nmol 16:0-18:0 PI, and 0.10 nmol di 18:0-PI. The system detected a total of 12 different lipid species and their respective subspecies, which were identified by the number of carbons and the degree of unsaturation in the chain. The lipid concentration was normalized according to the molar concentration across all species for each sample, and the final data are presented as the mean mol%" (Villamil-Ortiz et al., 2016).

Profile of Other Lipid Fractions

Lipids were extracted from the hippocampus and serum using the Folch method. The solid-phase extraction (SPE) as described Bermudez-Cardona et al (Bermúdez-cardona and Velásquez-rodríguez, 2016), was used to separate cholesterol esters (CE), triglycerides (TG), and free fatty acids (FFA).

Statistical Analysis

The behavioral test comparisons between two groups were performed using Student's t-tests for parametric data or Mann–Whitney tests for nonparametric data. "The lipid levels of each sample were calculated by summing the total number of moles of all lipid species measured and then normalizing that total to mol%. Comparisons between groups were assessed either by one-way ANOVA, followed by the Tukey *post hoc* test, or the Kruskal–Wallis test, depending on the homoscedasticity and normality of the experimental data. Multivariate statistics were performed using principal component analysis (PCA) and a partial least squares discriminant analysis (PLS-DA)" (Barker and Rayens, 2003). "The PLS-DA was included because this analysis is particularly suitable for the analysis of datasets with a small number of samples and a large number of variables. The PLS-DA was carried out using the protocols described previously by our laboratory" (Villamil-Ortiz et al., 2016). The data are expressed as the mean the standard error of the mean. The statistical significance is indicated in the figures and tables.

RESULTS

Morphological Changes, Cognitive Impairment, and Hippocampal Phospholipid Profile Changes a Month Postischemia

The abilities of spatial learning and memory were examined by using the Morris water maze test. We found that, even a month postischemia, ischemic rats significantly increased their latencies to locate the platform in the MWM from trial 3 to trial 6 (**Figure 1A**). In the memory test, it was found that rats with global ischemia showed significant deficits in locating the submerged escape platform compared with sham rats (**Figure 1A**). In addition, during the relearning test, ischemic rats

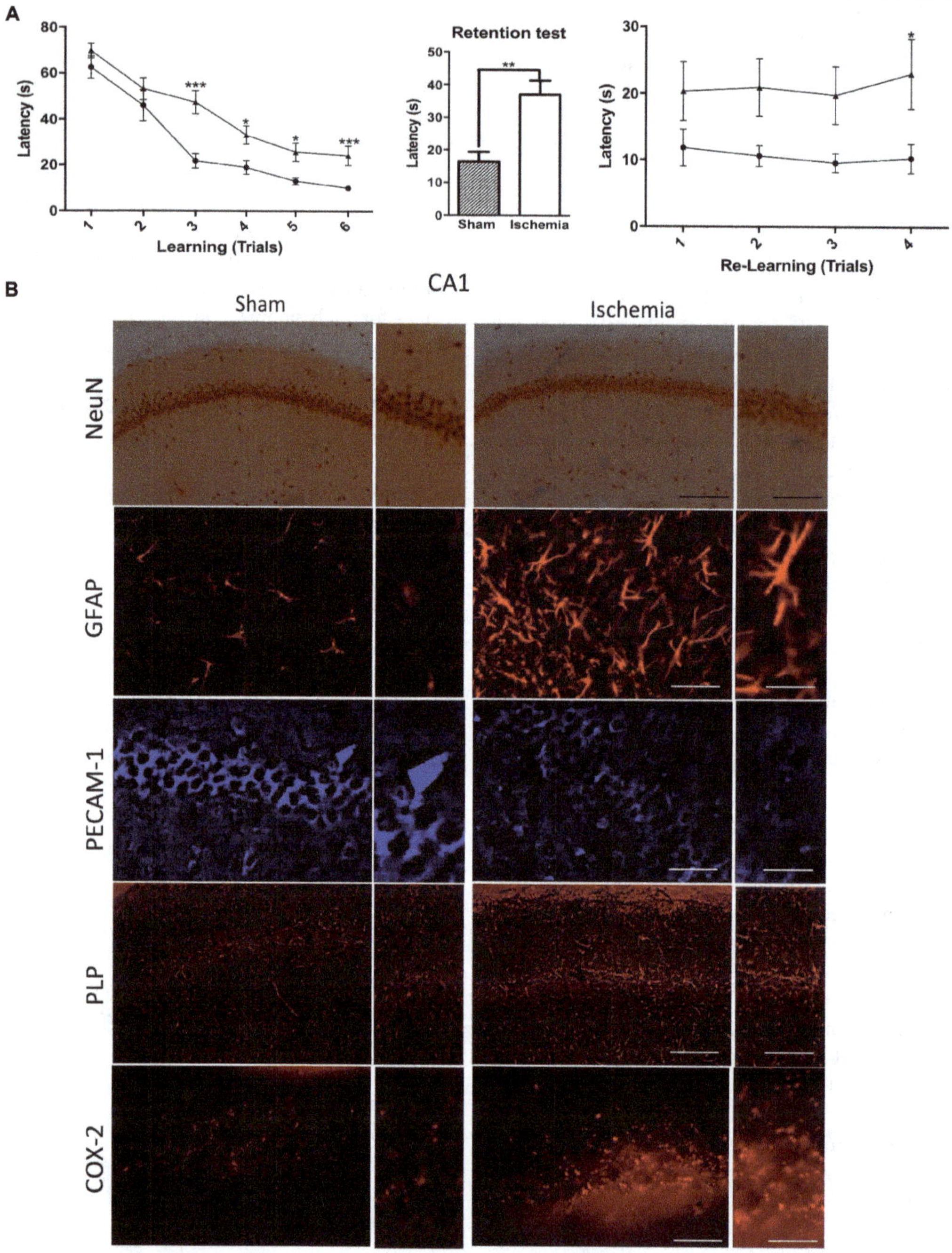

FIGURE 1 | Morphological alterations and cognitive impairment in the rat hippocampus after transient global ischemia. **(A)** The learning and memory task performance was evaluated with the Morris water maze on day 19, starting with the learning test and the first position of the platform. The retention test was conducted after 48 h without the platform. The transference test included the second position of the platform. Data are expressed as group means ± SEM. $^{*}p < 0.05$, $^{**}p < 0.01$, and $^{***}p < 0.001$; $n = 9$ animals/group. **(B)** Immunostaining in pyramidal cell layer in the hippocampus with Neuronal nuclei (NeuN) immunohistochemistry; glial fibrillary acidic protein (GFAP), Platelet Endothelial Cell Adhesion Molecule 1 (PECAM-1), myelin Proteolipid protein (PLP), Cyclooxygenase 2 (COX-2) immunofluorescences. $n = 5$. NeuN and PLP, Magnification: 10×, scale bar: 100 μm; Insert: Magnification 40×; scale bar = 50 μm; GFAP, PECAM, and COX-2. Magnification 20×, scale bar: scale bar = 50 μm; Insert: 60×, scale bar: 15 μm.

exhibited cognitive impairment a month postischemia, and the escape latencies were significantly lower compared with those of the sham group (**Figure 1A**). Which was supported by the morphological alterations of the hippocampus, although there was not a clear neuronal loss, we detected hypertrophic astrocytes with thickened processes and enlarged cell bodies (**Figure 1B**). PECAM-1, a cell adhesion marker, suggested disruption of the parenchima, PLP, a protein involved in the production of myelin, presented aggregation at the CA1, in addition to the increased presence of COX-2, inflammatory marker, suggesting the structural damage in the hippocampus at 1 month post global ischemia respect to healthy rats (**Figure 1B**).

On the other hand, 311 species of phospholipids were evaluated via mass spectrometry in the hippocampus a month postglobal ischemia. At a glance, the analyses indicate that the changes seem to be related to the pathological condition. The lipid profiles of both groups show that they were primarily composed of high-abundance glycerophospholipids, such as PC (48.4 and 47%), PE (23.2 and 23.4%), PS (8.8 and 9.7%), and PI (3.8 and 3.9%); sphingolipids, such as SM-DSM (7.5 and 7.2%); low-abundance ether phospholipids, such as ePC (2.5 and 2.48%), ePE (2.48 and 2.5%), and ePS (0.02 and 0.03%); lysophospholipids, such as LPE (1.68 and 2.35%) and LPC (0.77 and 0.83%); and glycerophospholipids, such as PA (0.74 and 0.76%) and PG (0.11 and 0.12%) (**Figures 2A,B**).

The results of the PCA of the detected lipids indicated that nearly 77% of the total variance might be explained by the first two principal components (PC1 and PC2) (**Figure 2A**). The most relevant variables for these two components were related to reduced PC and increased PS subclasses (**Figure 2B**). The main Rho indices were PC 32:0, 34:1, and 36:1. PC 34:1 was composed of saturated palmitic acid (16:0) and oleic acid (18:1), while PC 32:0 was composed of two palmitic acids. In addition, PS 40:6, conformed by stearic acid (18:0) and docosahexaenoic acid (DHA) (22:6), was represented in the PCA. Complementarily, the PLS-DA showed ellipsoids that were completely different in terms of location; this could explain the reason that the control groups had a more diverse lipid composition compared with the ischemic group. The main changes were shown in LPE 18:1, 20:3, PE 30:0, PC 34:2, and ePC 36:5. Together these findings, based on the abundance by PCA and separability by PLS-DA, suggest decreased PC and increased PS and LPE composed of imbalanced

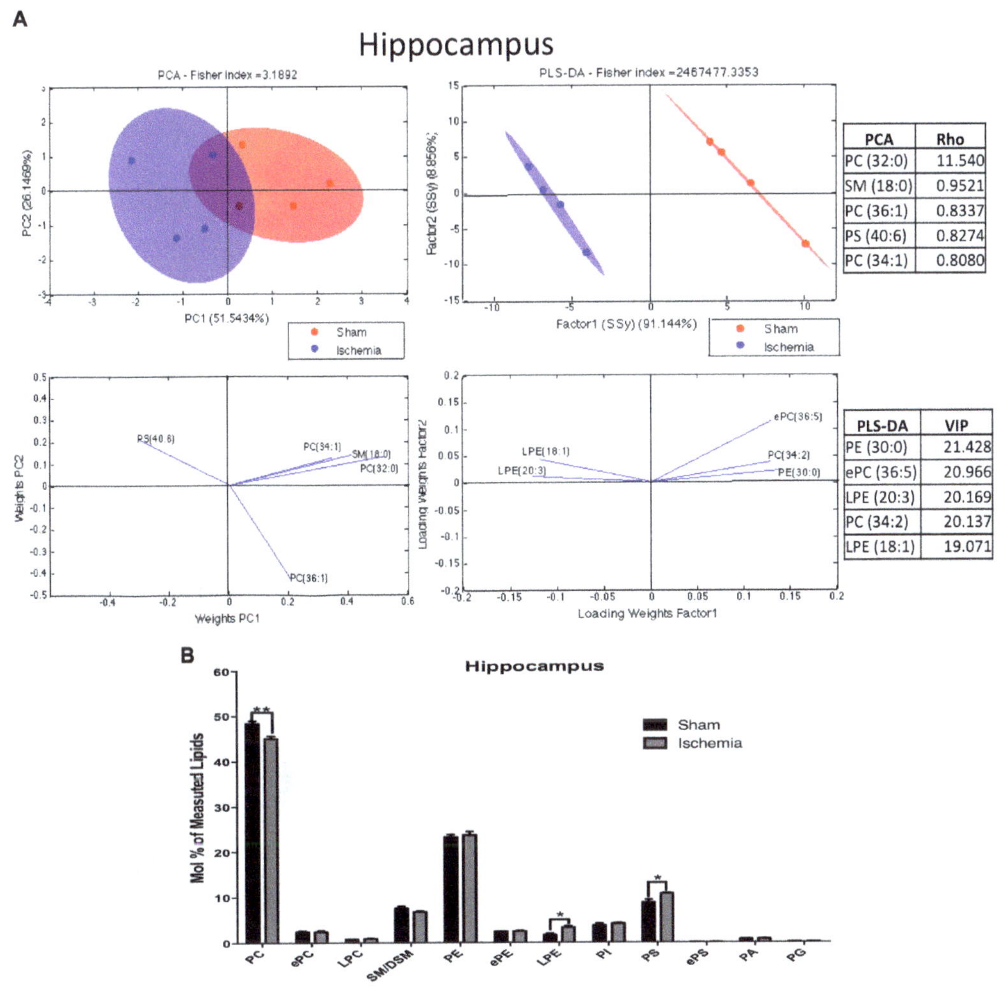

FIGURE 2 | Phospholipid composition in the hippocampus after 1 month postischemia. **(A)** Multivariate analyses of the lipid profiles in the hippocampus. PCA and PLS-DA were performed to discriminate between the lipid classes. The left panel illustrates the factor loadings for PC1 and PC2 with the indices of variance explained for each component. The right panels show the factor score plots for the PLS-DA. **(B)** The lipid class profiles are expressed as % mol composition. All lipid species are represented as the means ± SEM. Data for ischemic group were significantly different from those of the control group (*$p < 0.05$, **$p < 0.01$; Student's *t*-test for parametric data or the Mann–Whitney test for nonparametric data, $n = 4$ per group).

saturated fatty acid (SFA), monounsaturated FA (MFA) and in polyunsaturated FA (PUFA) after ischemia.

Inverse PC and LPE/PS Levels in Postischemic Hippocampus of Rats

PCs are a class of 1,2-diacylglycerophospholipids that are essential components of cell membranes and have structural roles defined primarily by chain length (Billah and Anthes, 1990; Whiley et al., 2014). In previous studies using tMCAO (transient middle cerebral artery occlusion), it has been described that several PC species and sphingomyelin (SM) were significantly decreased after infarction in the cerebral cortex; in the same manner, LPCs were elevated in the tissue (Wang et al., 2010).

We detected that global ischemia had a regulatory effect on the lipid profiles of PC and LPE from the hippocampus. The PLS-DA showed that the ischemic group had ellipsoids in different spaces, explained by the first component in 88% and the second one in 11% approximately (**Figure 3A**). In general, the PC levels decreased (*$p < 0.05$) in the ischemic groups compared with their counterpart in the sham control group (**Figure 2B**). Four PC subspecies showed significant reductions in global ischemia compared with those in the controls: 32:0 (16:0/16:0 - $p < 0.05$), 34:2 (16:1/18:1 ($p < 0.01$), 36:3 (18:1/18:2 - $p < 0.05$), and PC 36:4 (18:2/18:2) (**Figures 3B,C**). In general, considering that PC as the more abundant PL detected in the profile, those results were supported by the tendency and significant reduction of C.16:0 and C 18:0 at the total Free fatty acid (FFA) detected at the hippocampus and inversely C16:0 and C 18:0 were increased in the content of total triglycerides by the global ischemia. However, the CE did not change, lignoceric acid (24:0) FFA increased and a generalized reduction of oleic acid (18:1) was observed in the three analyzed fractions in the ischemic hippocampus (**Supplementary Figures S1A–C**).

On the other hand, LPE, a plasmalogen derived from phosphatidylethanolamine (PE), had significant higher levels ($p < 0.05$) in the ischemia group than in the sham group. The

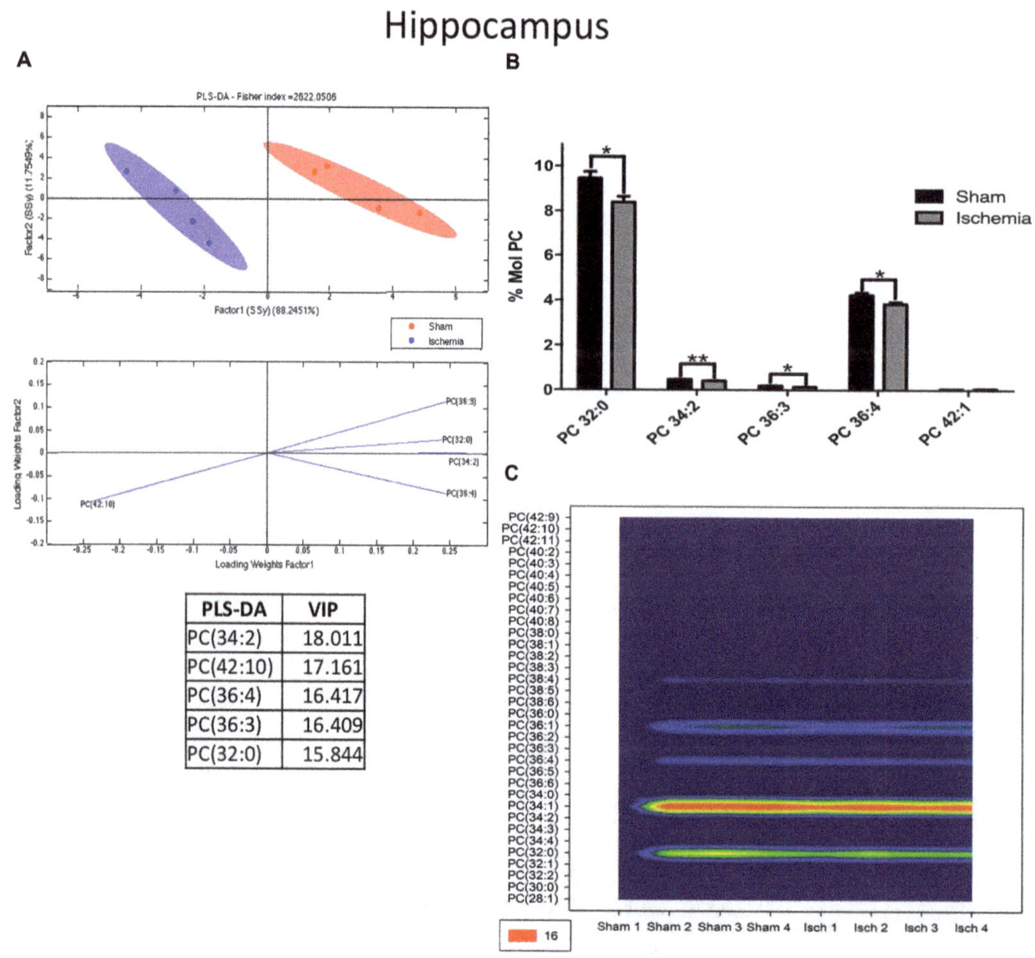

PLS-DA	VIP
PC(34:2)	18.011
PC(42:10)	17.161
PC(36:4)	16.417
PC(36:3)	16.409
PC(32:0)	15.844

FIGURE 3 | Changes in phosphatidylcholine in the hippocampus after global ischemia. **(A)** Multivariate analyses: PLS-DA used to discriminate between the lipid classes in the hippocampus showing the factor score plots. **(B)** The PC profile is expressed as % mol composition. **(C)** Contour plots of the more influential subclasses of PC (variables) in the discriminant analysis for each evaluated variable. Data from the ischemic group were significantly different from those of the control group and are represented as the means ± SEM (*$p < 0.05$, **$p < 0.01$, and ***$p < 0.001$; Student's t-test for parametric data or the Mann–Whitney test for nonparametric data, $n = 4$ per group).

PLS-DA demonstrated that the ischemic group occupied a close area with respect to that of the sham group, having a small overlapping area, however, the separability was explained by the first component at a rate of 75.43% (**Figure 4A**). When the most differential and relevant phospholipidic species was LPE 18:1, 20:3, and 22:6 increased in the ischemic group (**Figures 4A,B**). These results were supported by the contour graphic, which showed increasing levels in these PL subclasses in the global ischemia group, mainly LPE 22:6 and 18:1 (**Figure 4C**).

Complementarily, PS modulates the binding properties of glutamate receptors involved in neurotransmission and long-term potentiation in the brain (Farooqui and Horrocks, 2007). The PLS-DA showed a different distribution of the ischemic group relative to that of the sham group in the PCA graph. These data showed that the main changes occurred in the subspecies of PC 36:4, 38:4, 40:4, 38:5, and 44:11, as was indicated by the VIP index (**Figure 5A**). Most of these subspecies are composed of arachidonic acid (20:4), a proinflammatory molecule. Given that their levels significantly increased in the ischemic group ($^{*}p < 0.05$) (**Figure 5B**), this finding was in agreement with the high abundance shown in the counter plot graphic mainly by PS 40:4, 38:4, and 36:2 (**Figure 5C**).

Phospholipidic Profile Changes in the Serum a Month Postischemia in Rats

Evaluation of the lipid profiles of serum in ischemic rats with cognitive impairment a month postischemia could suggest potential biomarkers. The results of the PCA of the detected lipids indicated that nearly 92% of the total variance might be explained by the first two principal components (PC1 and PC2). The

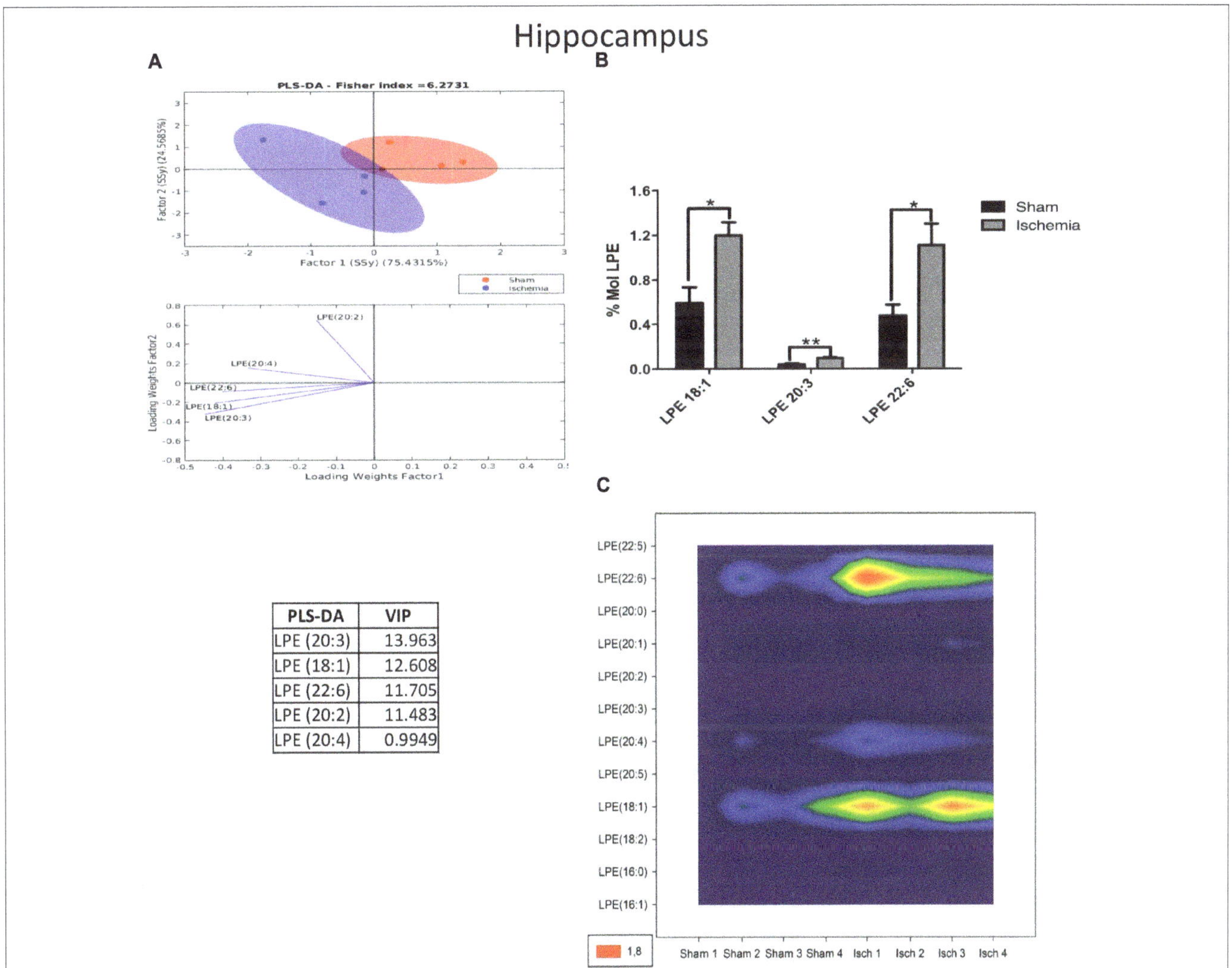

PLS-DA	VIP
LPE (20:3)	13.963
LPE (18:1)	12.608
LPE (22:6)	11.705
LPE (20:2)	11.483
LPE (20:4)	0.9949

FIGURE 4 | Increase in LPE species in the hippocampus after global cerebral ischemia. **(A)** Multivariate analyses: PLS-DA used to discriminate between the lipid classes in the hippocampus showing the factor score plots. **(B)** The LPE profile is expressed as % mol composition. **(C)** Contour plots of the more influential subclasses of LPE (variables) in the discriminant analysis for each evaluated variable. Data from the ischemic group were significantly different than those from the control group and are represented as the means ± SEM ($^{*}p < 0.05$, $^{**}p < 0.01$, and $^{***}p < 0.001$; Student's *t*-test for parametric data or the Mann–Whitney test for nonparametric data, $n = 4$ per group).

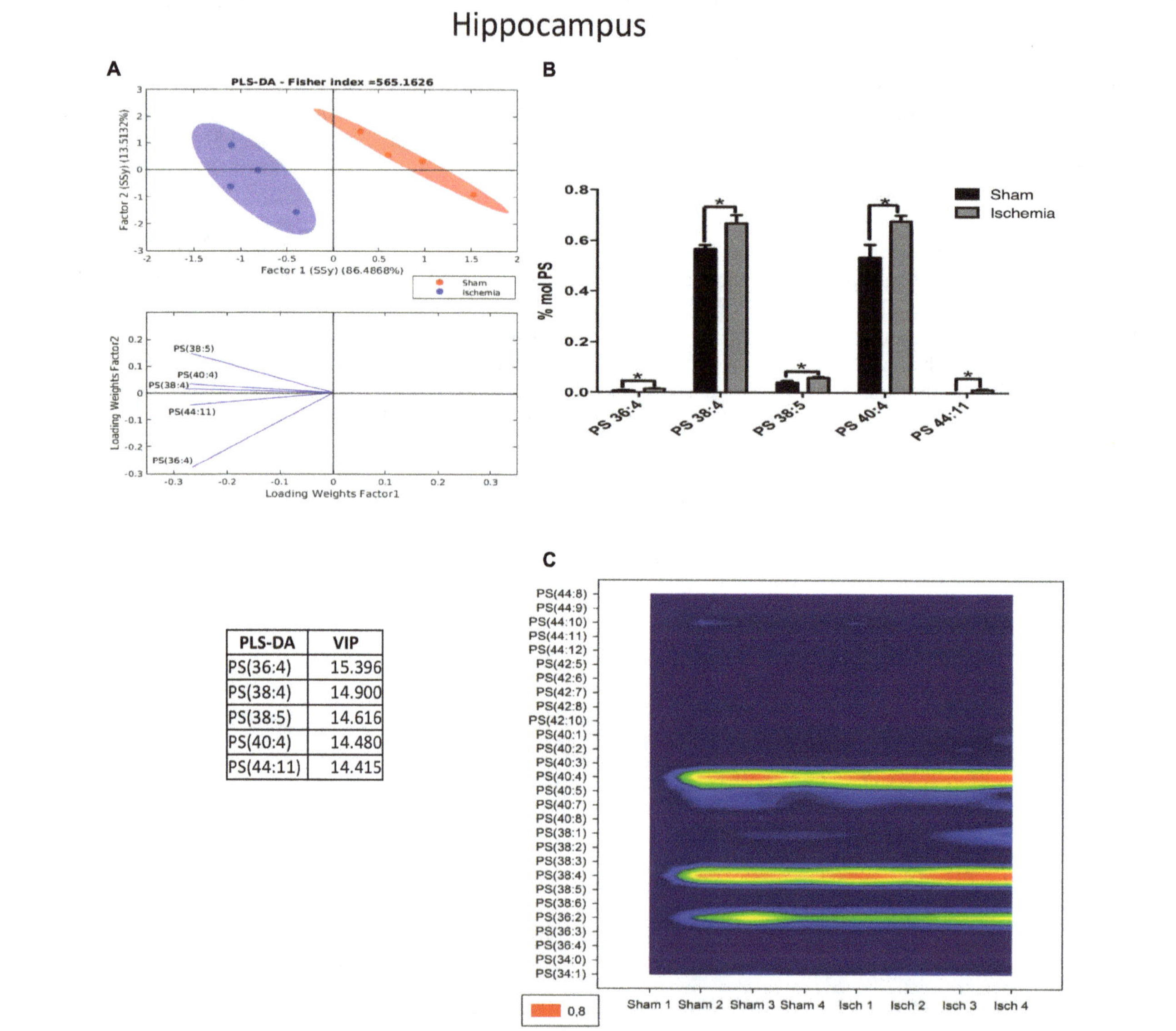

PLS-DA	VIP
PS(36:4)	15.396
PS(38:4)	14.900
PS(38:5)	14.616
PS(40:4)	14.480
PS(44:11)	14.415

FIGURE 5 | PS species increased in the ischemic hippocampus. **(A)** Multivariate analyses: PLS-DA used to discriminate between the lipid classes in the hippocampus showing the factor score plots. **(B)** The PS profile is expressed as % mol composition. **(C)** Contour plots of the more influential subclasses of PS (variables) in the discriminant analysis for each evaluated variable. Data from the ischemic group were significantly different from those from the control group and are represented as the means ± SEM (*$p < 0.05$ Student's *t*-test for parametric data or the Mann–Whitney test for nonparametric data, $n = 4$ per group).

distribution pattern in the plane showed divergent distributions between the ischemic and sham groups in the lipid profiles of the serum (**Figure 6A**). Complementarily, the PLS-DA confirmed a displacement in the left quadrant of the ischemic group, while the sham group occupied a different region on the right side. PCA showed abundant and differential locations of LPC and PC between the control and ischemic groups, with the main divergent phospholipid species being LPC 18:0, 16:0 and PC 34:2 with a Rho of 172.9, 169.25, and 151.74, respectively. While PLS-DA also identified LPC 18:0 and PC 34:2 as the more discriminant species, with a VIP of 18.34 and 18.24, respectively, between others explained by the first component in approximately 80% (**Figure 6A**).

The lipid profiles of both groups showed that they were primarily composed of high-abundance glycerophospholipids, such as PC (53.3 and 47.9%) and LPC (26.43 and 23.55%); sphingolipids, such as SM-DSM (13.7 and 13.2%); low-abundance ether phospholipids, such as ePC (3.07 and 2.85%), ePE (0.05 and 0.03%), and ePS (0.008 and 0.004%); PE (0.48 and 0.32%); PS (0.92 and 0.51%); PI (0.94 and 1.58%); LPE (0.068 and 0.074%); PA (0.05 and 0.04%) and PG (0.03 and 0.02%) (**Figure 6B**). In addition, these analyses showed that the main changes in serum were due to inverse levels of phosphatidylcholine and its plasmalogen, lysophosphatidylcholine, and the intermediate ePC species; together, a significant increase

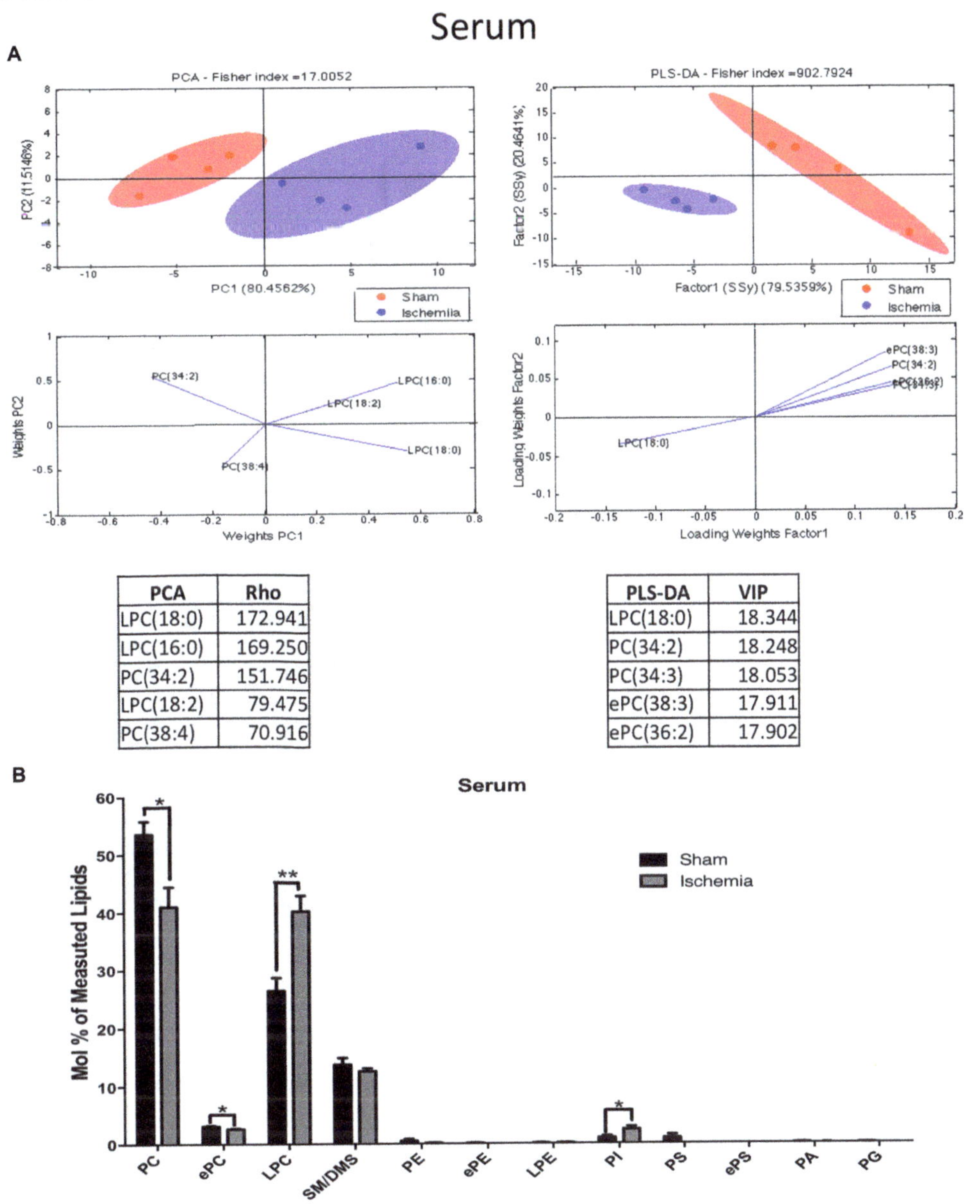

PCA	Rho
LPC(18:0)	172.941
LPC(16:0)	169.250
PC(34:2)	151.746
LPC(18:2)	79.475
PC(38:4)	70.916

PLS-DA	VIP
LPC(18:0)	18.344
PC(34:2)	18.248
PC(34:3)	18.053
ePC(38:3)	17.911
ePC(36:2)	17.902

FIGURE 6 | Altered phospholipid composition in the serum 1 month postischemia. **(A)** Multivariate analyses of the lipid profiles in the serum. PCA and PLS-DA were used to discriminate between the lipid classes. The left panel illustrates the factor loadings for PC1 and PC2 with the indices of variance explained for each component. The right panels show the factor score plots for the PLS-DA. **(B)** The lipid class profiles are expressed as % mol composition. All lipid species are represented as the means ± SEM. Data from the ischemic group were significantly different from those from the control group (*$p < 0.05$, **$p < 0.01$, Student's *t*-test for parametric data or the Mann–Whitney test for nonparametric data, $n = 4$ per group).

in PI subspecies occurred in the serum of the ischemic group.

Inverse PC and LPC-PI Serum Levels in Postischemic and Cognitively Impaired Rats

Our results indicated that lipid phosphatidylcholine molecule subspecies, such as PC 34:2, PC 34:3, PC 36:5, and PC 38:3, significantly decreased in the serum of the ischemic group, showing a notable separability (**Figures 7A,B**) and reduced abundance (**Figure 7C**) relative to those in the sham group (**Figure 7**). Similarly, we observed a reduction in ePC, as shown in **Figure 8A**, and the PLS-DA showed that the sham and ischemic rats had different patterns of distribution, and these changes were reflected by the following subspecies: ePC 36:2, ePC 38:3, ePC 34:2, ePC 34:1, and ePC 38:2 (**Figure 8A**), all of which were significantly reduced with respect to the levels observed in the control group (**Figure 8B**) and supported by the counter graph (**Figure 8C**). Those results could be supported by a general

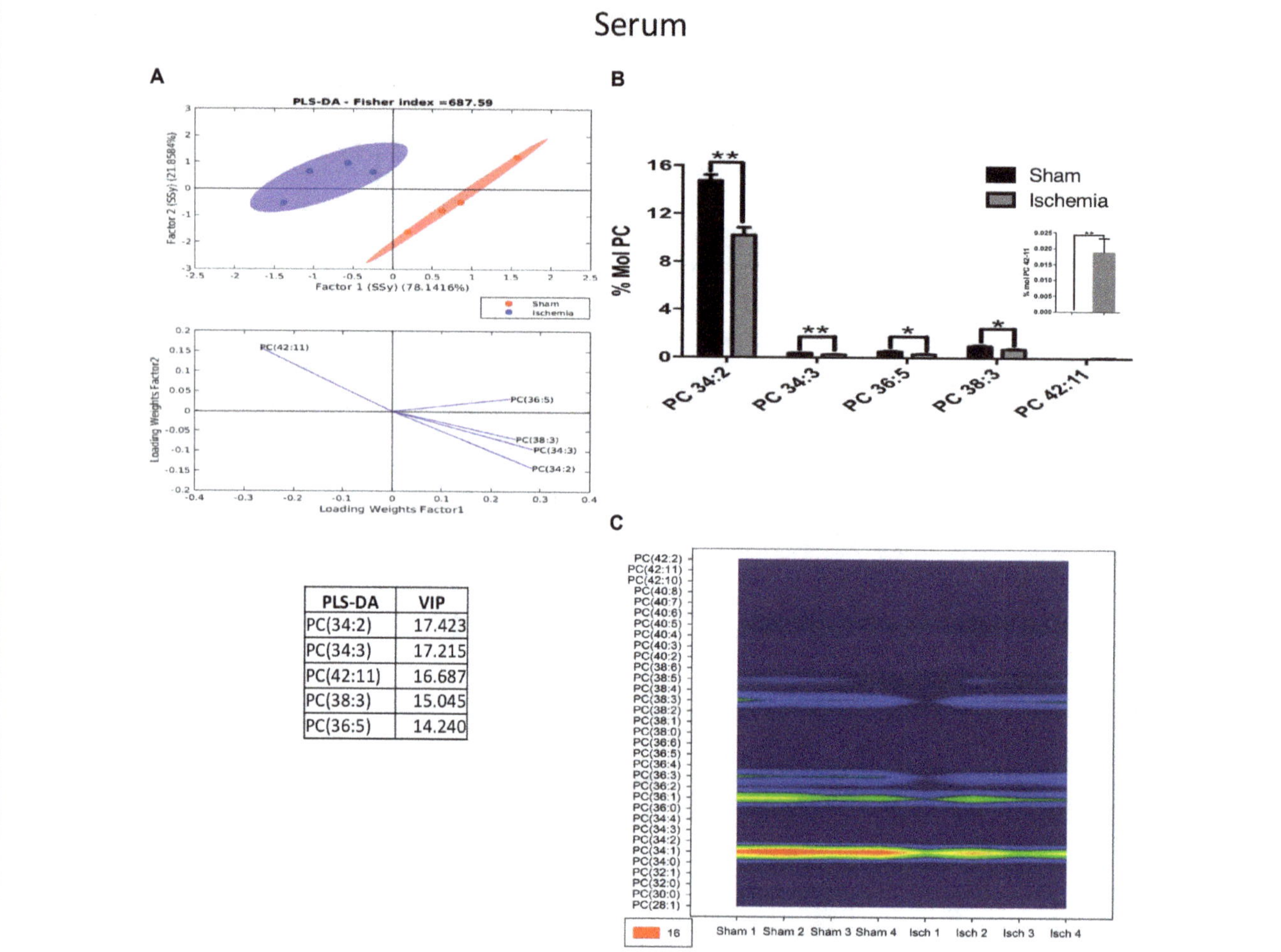

FIGURE 7 | The majority of the species of PC decreased in the serum of postischemic rats. **(A)** Multivariate analyses: PLS-DA analysis used to discriminate between the lipid classes in the serum showing the factor score plots. **(B)** The PC profile is expressed as % mol composition. **(C)** Contour plots of the more influential subclasses of PC (variables) in the discriminant analysis for each evaluated variable. Data from the ischemic group were significantly different from those from the control groups and are represented as the means ± SEM (*$p < 0.05$, **$p < 0.01$, and ***$p < 0.001$; Student's *t*-test for parametric data or the Mann–Whitney test for nonparametric data, $n = 4$ per group).

reduction of C 18 in the total FFA in serum (**Supplementary Figures S1D–F**), and no changes were detected in CE.

Inversely, LPC was shown to have increased in ischemic rats 1 month postischemia. The PLS-DA showed that ischemic and sham ellipsoids occupied different locations, supporting their different profiles (**Figure 9A**). The main subspecies that increased were LPC 18:0, LPC 22:6, LPC 20:5, LPC 18:1, and LPC 20:4 (**Figures 9A,B**) in cases when LPC 18:0, which is a fatty acid involved in inflammatory processes in cerebrovascular disease, detected at a high level also by the counter graph (**Figure 9C**).

For its part, the following PI subspecies demonstrated increased levels in the ischemic group: PI 36: 2 (18: 1/18: 1); PI 38: 4 (18: 0/20: 4), and PI 38: 5 (18: 1 and 20: 4), with PI 38:4 being the most abundant according to the histogram and counter plot analyses (**Figures 10A–C**). Interestingly, PLs composed of fatty acids with long carbon chains, such as 18: 0 (stearic acid) 18: 1 (oleic acid) and 20: 4 (AA), are involved in proinflammatory processes and were detected in the serum of ischemic rats a month postinjury; maybe these results could be in relationship with the general increase of detected C 18:2 in TG and FFA fractions (**Supplementary Figures S1E,F**), future analysis should be done.

DISCUSSION

Novelty, this study described hippocampal and peripheral phospholipid profile changes in long-term postischemia associated with cognitive impairment in rats. The main changes on PLs were associated to hippocampal dysfunction, represented by a downregulation of PC, as precursor of acetylcholine and inverse levels of LPE and PS associated with peroxisome damage, a proinflammatory environment and cell death in the hippocampal parenchyma after 1 month of anoxia, glutamate excitotoxicity and Brain Blood Barrier (BBB) disruption generated by global ischemia in rats (Becerra-calixto and

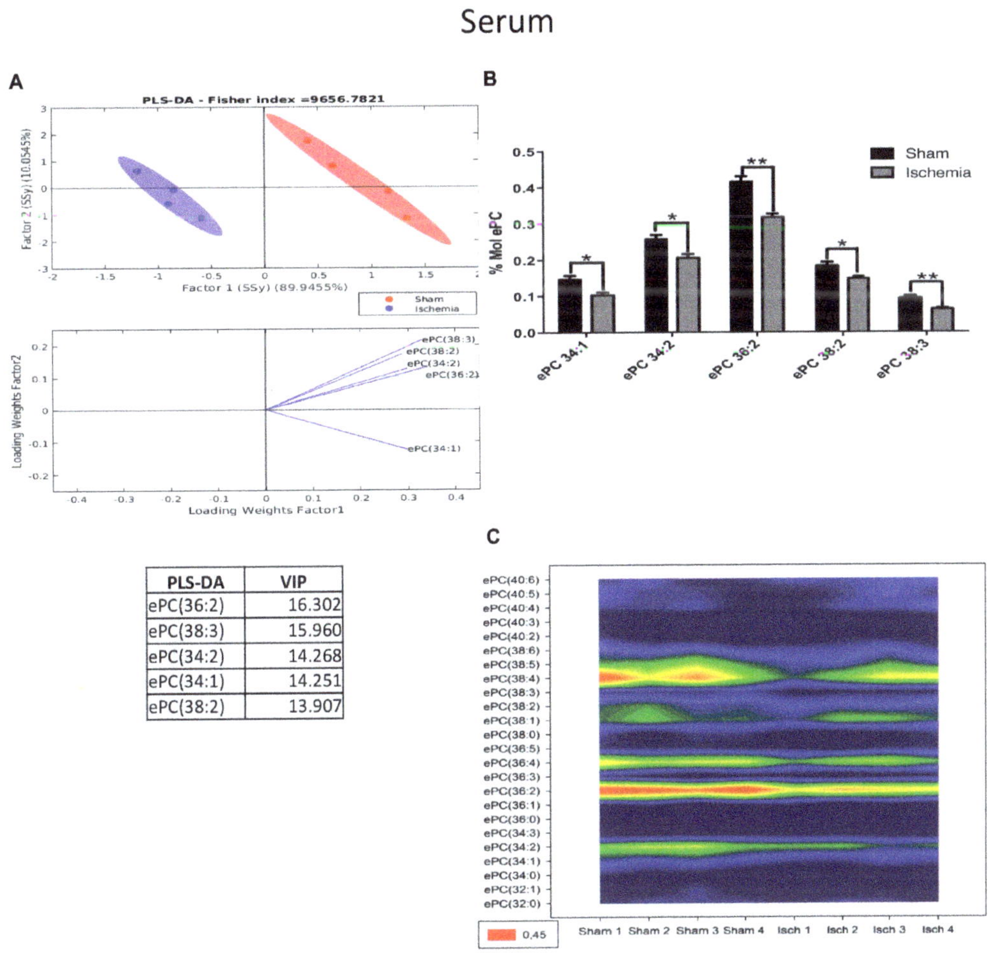

PLS-DA	VIP
ePC(36:2)	16.302
ePC(38:3)	15.960
ePC(34:2)	14.268
ePC(34:1)	14.251
ePC(38:2)	13.907

FIGURE 8 | Changes in ePC in the serum of postischemic rats. **(A)** Multivariate analyses: PLS-DA analysis used to discriminate between the lipid classes in the serum showing the factor score plots. **(B)** The ePC profile is expressed as % mol composition. **(C)** Contour plots of the more influential subclasses of ePC (variables) in the discriminant analysis for each evaluated variable. Data from the ischemic group were significantly different from those from the control group and are represented as the means ± SEM (*$p < 0.05$, **$p < 0.01$, and ***$p < 0.001$; Student's *t*-test for parametric data or the Mann-Whitney test for nonparametric data, $n = 4$ per group).

Cardona-gómez, 2017). Also, these findings are supported by our recent study were proinflammatory phospholipid profile was associated to neurodegeneration and neurological dysfunction (Marosi et al., 2006).

Our data suggested that spatial learning and reference memory were significantly impaired in global ischemic rats, a finding that was in line with those of previous studies (Deng et al., 2017). These results demonstrated that the damage in ischemic rats is large, and the functional outcome can become worse over time. Recently, the high incidence of cognitive impairment after an ischemic stroke event has been described (Sun et al., 2014) and the comorbidity factors, such as atherosclerosis (Knopman et al., 2016). Additionally, plasma phospholipid changes have been suggested in cognitive impairment associated with brain stroke patients but have not been clearly identified by the variability in humans (Li et al., 2016). However, in subcortical ischemic vascular dementia and mixed dementia, an adaptative increase in polyunsaturated fatty acids and elevated membrane degradation (Lam et al., 2014) have been observed. With respect to mild cognitive impairment and its progression to dementia, this condition has been addressed in Alzheimer-type dementia, with lipidomic brain changes in serum PLs being observed, mainly via reductions in PC (Wood et al., 2016). The findings of these studies are in accordance with our current data from an experimental model of global ischemia, however, we showed a specific fatty acid composition imbalance constituted of 18:0, 18:1, 20:4, and 22:6 in the parenchyma and peripheral PLs profile changes in long-term postischemia associated with cognitive impairment. The fatty acid composition of imbalanced PLs in familiar and sporadic Alzheimer's disease in human brains has been commonly found, and in old triple transgenic AD mice with cognitive impairment, the imbalance has mainly been observed in PC and/or LPC, PE, and LPE (Villamil-Ortiz et al., 2016; Villamil-Ortiz et al., 2017).

Until now, few studies have focused on the impact of global ischemia on lipid signaling. Though some of these studies have investigated the first hours to 1 week of the acute phase of

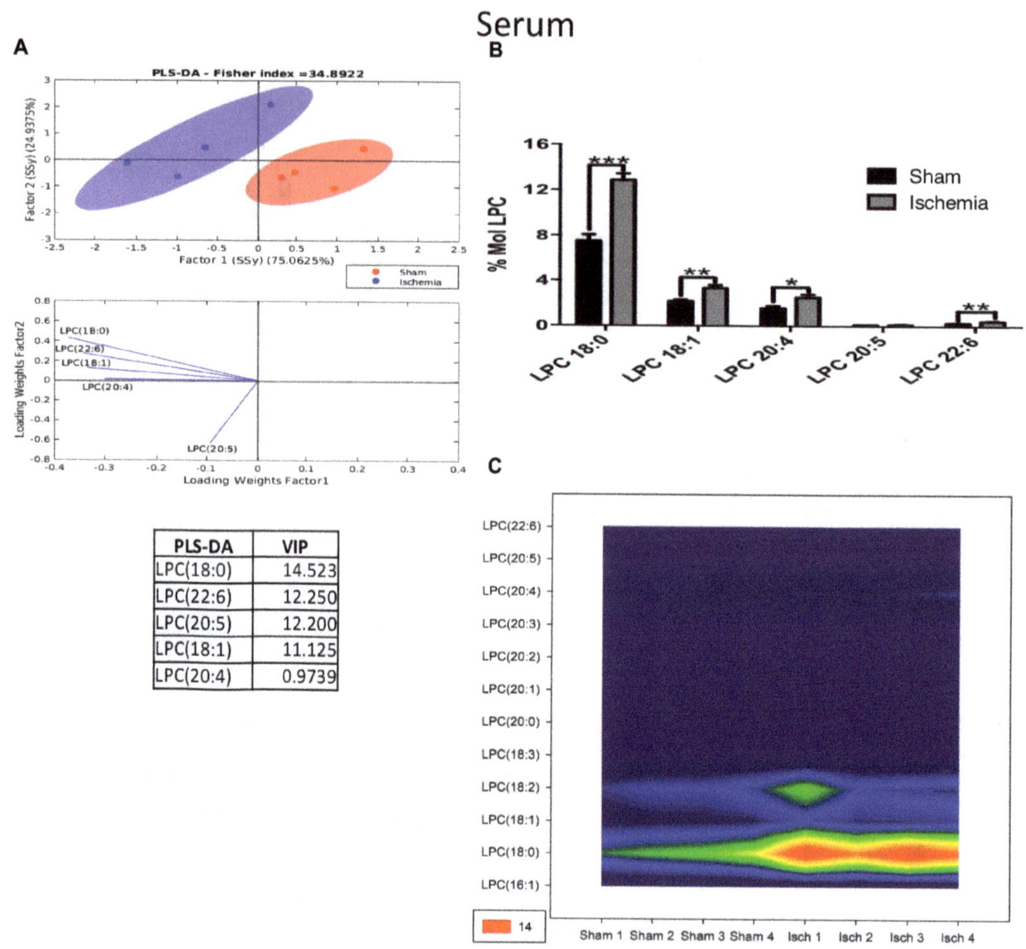

PLS-DA	VIP
LPC(18:0)	14.523
LPC(22:6)	12.250
LPC(20:5)	12.200
LPC(18:1)	11.125
LPC(20:4)	0.9739

FIGURE 9 | Altered LPC in the serum after global ischemia. **(A)** Multivariate analyses: PLS-DA analysis used to discriminate between the lipid classes in the serum showing the factor score plots. **(B)** The LPC profile is expressed as % mol composition. **(C)** Contour plots of the more influential subclasses of LPC (variables) in the discriminant analysis for each evaluated variable. Data from the ischemic group were significantly different from those from the control group and are represented as the means ± SEM (*$p < 0.05$, **$p < 0.01$, and ***$p < 0.001$; Student's *t*-test for parametric data or the Mann–Whitney test for nonparametric data, $n = 4$ per group).

postischemia (Adibhatla and Hatcher, 2007), few have evaluated lipid profiles in the brain or serum, and none have focused on the potential relationship of these profiles with cognitive impairment. Therefore, our data are valuable for the detection of 12 lipid species, six of which had significant concentration changes in the hippocampus and serum, specifically PC, LPE, and PS in the hippocampus and PC, LPC, ePC and PI in the serum of ischemic and cognitively impaired rats during long-term postischemia, possibly suggesting differential lipid signatures under pathological conditions due to ischemia, which has been suggested by some related neurological studies (Lin and Perez-Pinzon, 2013; Shen et al., 2014; Hamazaki et al., 2016).

Glycerophospholipids are multifunctional molecules, are the major constituents of membranes and are responsible for the membrane bilayer, "mainly via choline or ethanolamine and to a lesser extent, inositol, serine or rarely, threonine. Further diversity is introduced by the components at the sn-1 and sn-2 positions, composing subclasses of diacyl and ether GP. Although plasmalogens represent up to 20% of the total phospholipid mass in humans, their physiological roles have been challenging to identify and are likely to vary in different tissues, metabolic processes and developmental stages" (Braverman and Moser, 2012). As plasmalogens serve as storage depots for second messengers and their precursors, membrane activity and ion channels, the study of plasmalogens may also provide insight into neural membrane pathology (Farooqui and Horrocks, 2007).

In particular, PC are composed of fatty acids with polyunsaturated chains, such as 34:2, 34:3, 36:4, 36:5, and 38:3, which are composed of linoleic acid (18:2), a precursor of the biosynthesis of AA (20:4) or AA composition *per se* (Choque et al., 2014), and may be supported by the increased LPC (18:0) catabolism to PC after ischemia. Additionally, elevated LPCs have been related to pathological lipid breakdown and the state of parenchymal inflammation after ischemia as an important source of reactive oxygen species (ROS) (Adibhatla and Hatcher, 2007; Wang et al., 2010), as well as being correlated with macrophage/microglia responses and neuronal death (Nielsen et al., 2016), spatial memory dysfunction (Köfeler et al., 2010)

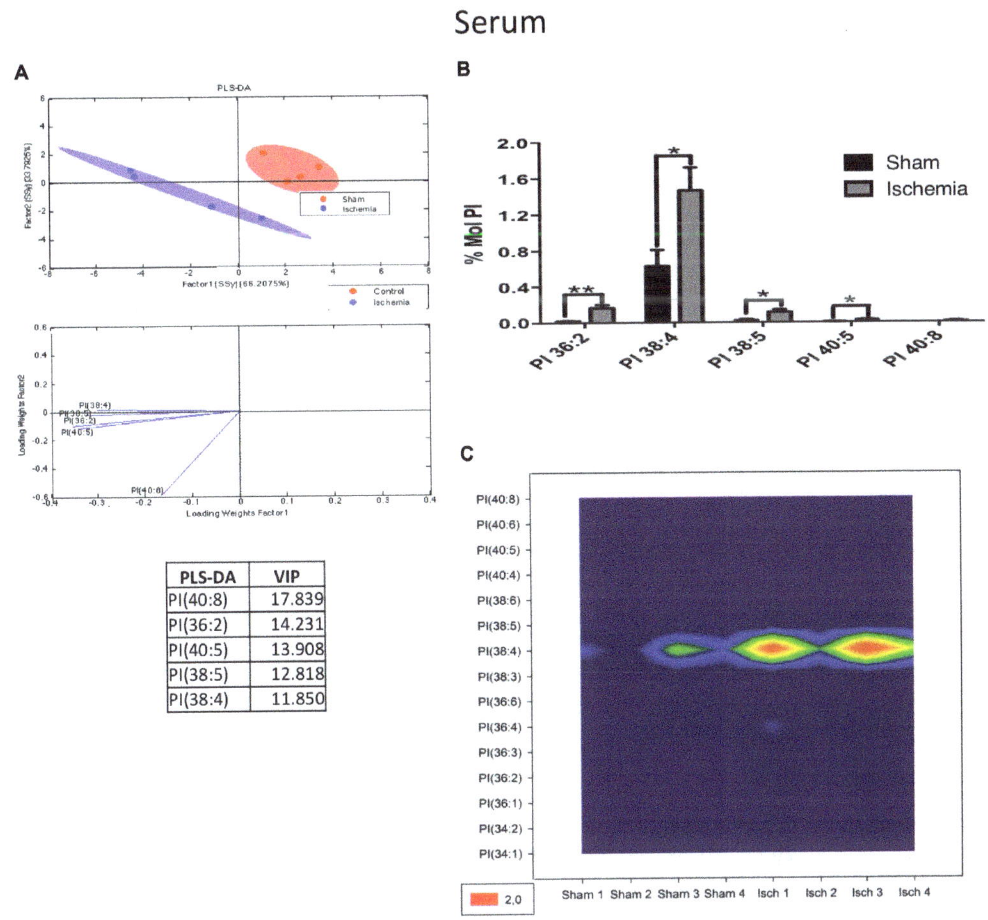

PLS-DA	VIP
PI(40:8)	17.839
PI(36:2)	14.231
PI(40:5)	13.908
PI(38:5)	12.818
PI(38:4)	11.850

FIGURE 10 | PI subspecies increased in the serum in postischemic rats. **(A)** Multivariate analyses: PLS-DA analysis used to discriminate between the lipid classes in the serum showing the factor score plots. **(B)** The PI profile is expressed as % mol composition. **(C)** Contour plots of the more influential subclasses of PI (variables) in the discriminant analysis for each evaluated variable. Data from the ischemic group were significantly different from those from the control group and are represented as the means ± SEM (* $p < 0.05$ Student's *t*-test for parametric data or the Mann–Whitney test for nonparametric data, $n = 4$ per group).

and its efflux and transport by ABCA7 in dementia by AD (Tomioka et al., 2017), also serving as a strategy in the forecast of ischemic stroke (Jickling and Montaner, 2015).

Furthermore, the lipid alterations found in our study suggested that phospholipid- modulating enzymes could be dysregulated in the brain, either due to increased or decreased phospholipase activity catalyzing the hydrolysis of LPC into PC. "The enzymes that catalyze the breakdown of PC to phosphatide (the phospholipase D or PLD enzymes) or to glycerophosphocholine and FFA (phospholipase A2 or PLA2 enzymes) have been directly associated with cerebral ischemia. In addition, alterations in the reaction cascades of PLD enzymes, leading to aberrant phosphatidic acid (PA) signaling, have been linked to neurodegenerative processes, with the activation of PLA2-family enzymes by β-amyloid peptide in neurons, in turn releasing secondary lipid messengers, such as AA. PLA2s also play a role in the modification of physical properties, such as the fluidity of the cellular membrane" (Whiley et al., 2014). It is accepted that, during ischemia and reperfusion, free fatty acid concentrations increase, particularly those of polyunsaturated fatty acids released from membrane PLs through activation of PLA2 (Hamazaki and Kim, 2013).

Another phospholipid that is highly involved is PS is the major acidic phospholipid in human membranes and one that constitutes 2–20% of the total phospholipid mass of adult human plasma and intracellular membranes (Van Meer et al., 2008). Hence, the presence of PS is essential for maintaining cell homeostasis, however, the fatty acid composition of PS is important, with studies of healthy human brains reporting that approximately 20–30% of the PS in human gray matter is composed of DHA (22:6), which is widely reported to be a pro-cell-survival fatty acid in the brain (Tanaka et al., 2012). Therefore, a reduction in the DHA content of PS is associated with the progression of mild cognitive impairment to dementia (Cunnane et al., 2012), possibly because the DHA in the PS conformation is essential for neuroprotection (Zhang et al., 2015). Additionally, PS synthesis may be inhibited by metabotropic glutamate receptor agonists, indicating that metabotropic glutamate receptor stimulation decreases not only the incorporation of serine in PS but also modulates the generation of excitatory postsynaptic currents in rat cerebellar slices. In addition, in neural membrane, PS modulates long-lasting changes in learning and memory according to the membrane composition (Farooqui and Horrocks, 2007). Interestingly, in our study, the increased PS 1 month postischemia was mainly composed of polyunsaturated fatty acids, such as AA 20: 4 (36:4, 38:4, 40:4), possibly suggesting an imbalance between the DHA and AA concentrations in PS. In the context of cerebral ischemia, excess intracellular calcium (Ca_i^{2+}) activates various lipases, including (PLA2) and PLC, which breakdown both intracellular and membrane phospholipids and release AA, thereby enhancing the proinflammatory response (Wang et al., 2007).

Interestingly, we also observed an increase in different species of LPE in the hippocampus of ischemic rats. LPE can be generated from PE via a phospholipase A-type reaction (Farooqui et al., 2000). Currently, the physiological significance of LPE in the brain after global ischemia is unknown. However, increased LPE has been demonstrated in major depressive disorder (MDD) and chronic stress (Liu et al., 2016; Oliveira et al., 2016). It has been reported that LPE has a direct relationship with calcium influx, which is closely related to cell death in neurodegenerative diseases and contributes to the cognitive impairment in transgenic mice with AD (Villamil-Ortiz et al., 2017).

For its part, phosphatidylinositol (PI) is characterized by the phosphorylation of the inositol head group of phosphoinositide, with a rapid and reversible phosphorylation rate, which critically participates in signal cascades and intracellular membrane trafficking (Hammond and Balla, 2015). PI is produced in the ER where its synthesizing enzymes, namely PI synthase (PIS) and CDP-DG synthase (CDS), are located (Kim et al., 2011). Based on the fact that PI is converted to PI3P in early endosomes and PI4P in the Golgi, plasma membrane (PM), and early and late endosomes, it is assumed that PI must be present in all of these membranes, as it has an important role in signaling pathways (Hammond and Balla, 2015). However, one past article mentioned that the four-vessel occlusion model-stimulated [3H]Inositol monophosphate formation via excitatory amino acids was greatly enhanced in hippocampal slices 24 h or 7 days after reperfusion (Seren et al., 1989). Additionally, PI has been recently reported to be a predictive marker of ischemic stroke (Tu et al., 2014).

In summary, our data showed that cognitive impairment in long-term postischemia is associated with a hippocampal phospholipid signature that indicates imbalance, proinflammatory environment, excitotoxicity and cell death, as evidenced in the peripheral PL profile related to cerebrovascular disruption and proinflammatory signaling and concomitantly supporting biomarkers of neurogenerative and cognitive impairment state and progression to long-term postischemia. Finally, this study provided a frame of reference for phospholipids that could be targeted for therapeutic exploration either through pharmacological intervention or enzymatic control, as phospholipases, for example, require further evaluation. Additionally, our findings are potentially useful for improving prediction and intervention after cerebral ischemia and form the basis for a future understanding of phospholipid dysfunction in neurological pathologies and targeting for prevention.

AUTHOR CONTRIBUTIONS

AS-G designed and realized the experiments, analyzed the data, wrote the paper. JV-O analyzed the data and wrote the paper. JA-L analyzed the data and reviewed the manuscript preparation. GC-G designed, analyzed and interpreted the data, prepared the manuscript, and critical revision. All authors read and approved the final manuscript.

FUNDING

This research was funded by grants from COLCIENCIAS # 11565740581 (GC-G), Schorlaship Colciencias # 647 (AS-G).

ACKNOWLEDGMENTS

We thank the Cellular and Molecular Neurobiology Area of the Neuroscience Group of Antioquia for their scientific and technical support during the experiments.

SUPPLEMENTARY MATERIAL

FIGURE S1 | Total changes in lipid fractions from hippocampus and serum after global ischemia. Cholesterol esters **(A,D)** triglycerides **(B,E),** free fatty, acid **(C,F)** from hippocampus and serum, respectively, from ischemic and control rats are shown. Individual concentrations of lipids are expressed as molar percentage. Myristic acid (14:0), palmitic acid (16:0), margaric acid (17:0), stearic acid (18:0), oleic acid (18:1), linoleic acid (18:2), arachidic acid (20:0), arachidonic acid (20:4), Erucic acid (22:1), Lignoceric acid (24:0), nervonic acid (24:1), docosahexaenoic, acid (22:6). Data represent means SEM of 4 mice per group. $^*p < 0.05$, $^{**}p < 0.01$, and $^{***}p < 0.001$; for differences between sham and control groups.

REFERENCES

1. Adibhatla, R. M., and Hatcher, J. F. (2007). Role of lipids in brain injury and diseases. *Future Lipidol.* 2, 403–422. doi: 10.2217/17460875.2.4.403
2. Barker, M., and Rayens, W. (2003). Partial least squares for discrimination. *J. Chemom.* 17, 166–173. doi: 10.1002/cem.785
3. Becerra-calixto, A., and Cardona-gómez, G. P. (2017). Neuroprotection induced by transplanted CDK5 knockdown astrocytes in global cerebral ischemic rats. *Mol. Neurobiol.* 54, 6681–6696. doi: 10.1007/s12035-016-0162-2
4. Bermúdez-cardona, J., and Velásquez-rodríguez, C. (2016). Phospholipids, cholesterol esters and triglycerides metabolic syndrome. *Nutrients* 8, 1–13. doi: 10.3390/nu8020054

5. Billah, M. M., and Anthes, J. C. (1990). The regulation and cellular functions of phosphatidylcholine hydrolysis. *Biochem. J.* 269, 281–291. doi: 10.1042/bj2690281
6. Braverman, N. E., and Moser, A. B. (2012). Functions of plasmalogen lipids in health and disease. *Biochim. Biophys. Acta – Mol. Basis Dis.* 1822, 1442–1452. doi: 10.1016/j.bbadis.2012.05.008
7. Cardona-Gómez, G. P., and Lopera, F. (2016). Dementia, preclinical studies in neurodegeneration and its potential for translational medicine in South America. *Front. Aging Neurosci.* 8:304. doi: 10.3389/fnagi.2016.00304
8. Choque, B., Catheline, D., Rioux, V., and Legrand, P. (2014). Linoleic acid: between doubts and certainties. *Biochimie* 96, 14–21. doi: 10.1016/j.biochi.2013.07.012 Cunnane, S. C., Schneider, J. A., Tangney, C., Tremblay-Mercier, J., Fortier, M.,
9. Bennett, D. A., et al. (2012). Plasma and brain fatty acid profiles in mild cognitive impairment and Alzheimer's disease. *J. Alzheimers Dis.* 29, 691–697. doi: 10.3233/JAD-2012-110629.Plasma
10. Deng, M., Xiao, H., Zhang, H., Peng, H., Yuan, H., Xu, Y., et al. (2017). Mesenchymal stem cell-derived extracellular vesicles ameliorates hippocampal synaptic impairment after transient global ischemia. *Front. Cell. Neurosci.* 11:205. doi: 10.3389/fncel.2017.00205
11. Farooqui, A. A., and Horrocks, L. A. (eds). (2007). "Phospholipases A2 in neurological disorders," in *Glycerophospholipids in Brain* (New York, NY: Springer), 394. doi: 10.1007/978-0-387-49931-4
12. Farooqui, A. A., Horrocks, L. A., and Farooqui, T. (2000). Glycerophospholipids in brain: their metabolism, incorporation into membranes, functions, and involvement in neurological disorders. *Chem. Phys. Lipids* 106, 1–29. doi: 10. 1016/S0009-3084(00)00128-6
13. Hamazaki, K., and Kim, H. Y. (2013). Differential modification of the phospholipid profile by transient ischemia in rat hippocampal CA1 and CA3 regions. *Prostaglandins Leukot. Essent. Fat. Acids* 88, 299–306. doi: 10.1016/j.plefa.2013. 01.003
14. Hamazaki, K., Maekawa, M., Toyota, T., Iwayama, Y., Dean, B., Hamazaki, T., et al. (2016). Fatty acid composition and fatty acid binding protein expression in the postmortem frontal cortex of patients with schizophrenia: a case-control study. *Schizophr. Res.* 171, 225–232. doi: 10.1016/j.schres.2016.01.014
15. Hammond, G. R., and Balla, T. (2015). Biochimica et biophysica acta polyphosphoinositide binding domains?: key to inositol lipid biology ?. *Biochim. Biophys. Acta* 1851, 746–758. doi: 10.1016/j.bbalip.2015.02.013
16. Jickling, G. C., and Montaner, J. (2015). Lysophosphatidylcholine to stratify risk of ischemic stroke in TIA. *Neurology* 84, 17–18. doi: 10.1212/WNL. 0000000000001100
17. Jordi Folch, S. S. (1957). A simple method for isolation and purification of total lipides from animal tissues. *J. Biol. Chem.* 226, 497–509. doi: 10.1016/j.ultrasmedbio.2011.03.005
18. Kim, Y. J., Guzman, M. L., and Balla, T. (2011). A highly dynamic ER- derived phosphatidylinositol synthesizing organelle suplies phosphoinositides to cellular membranes. *Dev. Cell* 21, 813–824. doi: 10.1016/j.devcel.2011.09.005.A
19. Knopman, D. S., Gottesman, R. F., Sharrett, A. R., Wruck, L. M., Windham, B. G., Coker, L., et al. (2016). Mild cognitive impairment and dementia prevalence: the atherosclerosis risk in communities neurocognitive study, *Alzheimer's Dement.* 2, 1–11. doi: 10.1016/j.dadm.2015.12.002
20. Köfeler, H. C., Tiboldi, A., Hoeger, H., and Lubec, G. (2010). Hippocampal lipids linked to spatial memory in the C57bl/6j mouse. *Neurochem. Int.* 57, 935–939. doi: 10.1016/j.neuint.2010.09.013
21. Lam, S. M., Wang, Y., Duan, X., Wenk, M. R., Kalaria, R. N., Chen, C. P., et al. (2014). The brain lipidomes of subcortical ischemic vascular dementia and mixed dementia. *Neurobiol. Aging.* 35, 2369–2381. doi: 10.1016/j. neurobiolaging.2014.02.025
22. Li, D., Misialek, J. R., Boerwinkle, E., Gottesman, R. F., Sharrett, A. R., Mosley, T. H., et al. (2016). Plasma phospholipids and prevalence of mild cognitive impairment and/or dementia in the ARIC neurocognitive study (ARIC-NCS). *Alzheimer's Dement.* 3, 73–82. doi: 10.1016/j.dadm.2016.02.008
23. Lin, H. W., and Perez-Pinzon, M. (2013). The role of fatty acids in the regulation of cerebral vascular function and neuroprotection in Ischemia. *CNS Neurol. Disord.* 12, 316–324. doi: 10.2174/1871527311312030005
24. Liu, X., Li, J., Zheng, P., Zhao, X., Zhou, C., Hu, C., et al. (2016). Plasma lipidomics reveals potential lipid markers of major depressive disorder. *Anal. Bioanal. Chem.* 408, 6497–6507. doi: 10.1007/s00216-016-9768-5
25. Llinas, R., Barbut, D., and Caplan, L. R. (2000). Neurologic complications of cardiac surgery. *Prog. Cardiovasc. Dis.* 43, 101–112. doi: 10.1053/pcad.2000.9030
26. Marosi, M., Rákos, G., Robotka, H., Németh, H., Sas, K., Kis, Z., et al. (2006). Hippocampal (CA1) activities in Wistar rats from different vendors. Fundamental differences in acute ischemia. *J. Neurosci. Methods* 156, 231–235. doi: 10.1016/j.jneumeth.2006.03.010
27. Martinez-Gardeazabal, J., González de San Román, E., Moreno-Rodríguez, M., LLorente-Ovejero, A., Manuel, I., Rodríguez-Puertas, R., et al. (2017). Lipid mapping of the rat brain for models of disease. *Biochim. Biophys. Acta* 1859, 1548–1557. doi: 10.1016/j.bbamem.2017.02.011
28. Miyawaki, S., Imai, H., Hayasaka, T., Masaki, N., Ono, H., Ochi, T., et al. (2016). Imaging mass spectrometry detects dynamic changes of phosphatidylcholine in rat hippocampal CA1 after transient global ischemia. *Neuroscience* 322, 66–77. doi: 10.1016/j.neuroscience.2016.02.013
29. Moskowitz, M. A., Lo, E. H., and Iadecola, C. (2010). The science of stroke: mechanisms in search of treatments. *Neuron* 67, 181–198. doi: 10.1016/j.neuron.2010.07.002
30. Nielsen, M. M. B., Lambertsen, K. L., Clausen, B. H., Meyer, M., Bhandari, D. R., Larsen, S. T., et al. (2016). Mass spectrometry imaging of biomarker lipids for phagocytosis and signalling during focal cerebral ischaemia. *Sci. Rep.* 6:39571. doi: 10.1038/srep39571
31. Nucera, A., and Hachinski, V. (2018). Cerebrovascular and Alzheimer disease: fellow travelers or partners in crime? *J. Neurochem.* 144, 513–516. doi: 10.1111/ jnc.14283
32. Oliveira, T. G., Chan, R. B., Bravo, F. V., Miranda, A., Silva, R., Zhou, B., et al. (2016). The impact of chronic stress on the rat brain lipidome, *Mol. Psychiatry* 21, 80–88. doi: 10.1038/mp.2015.14
33. Phillis, J. W., and O'Regan, M. H. (2004). A potentially critical role of phospholipases in central nervous system ischemic, traumatic, and neurodegenerative disorders. *Brain Res. Rev.* 44, 13–47. doi: 10.1016/j.brainresrev.2003.10.002
34. Schaller, B., and Graf, R. (2004). Cerebral ischemia and reperfusion: the pathophysiologic concept as a basis for clinical therapy. *J. Cereb. Blood Flow Metab.* 24, 351–371. doi: 10.1097/00004647-200404000-00001
35. Seren, M. S., Aldinio, C., Zanoni, R., Leon, A. F. (1989). Stimulation of inositol phospholipid hydrolysis by excitatory amino acids is enhanced in brain slices from vulnerable regions after transient global Ischemia. *J. Neurochem.* 53, 1700–1705. doi: 10.1111/j.1471-4159.1989.tb09233.x
36. Shen, H., Zhou, J., Shen, G., Yang, H., Lu, Z., and Wang, H. (2014). Correlation between serum levels of small, dense low-density lipoprotein cholesterol and carotid stenosis in cerebral infarction patients (65 years of age). *Ann. Vasc. Surg.* 28, 375–380. doi: 10.1016/j.avsg.2013.01.029
37. Sun, J. H., Tan, L., and Yu, J. T. (2014). Post-stroke cognitive impairment: epidemiology, mechanisms and management. *Ann. Transl. Med.* 2:80. doi: 10. 3978/j.issn.2305-5839.2014.08.05
38. Tanaka, K., Farooqui, A. A., Siddiqi, N. J., Alhomida, A. S., and Ong, W. Y. (2012). Effects of docosahexaenoic acid on neurotransmission. *Biomol. Ther.* 20, 152–157. doi: 10.4062/biomolther.2012.20.2.152
39. Tian, H., Qiu, T., Zhao, J., Li, L., and Guo, J. (2009). Sphingomyelinase-induced ceramide production stimulate calcium-independent JNK and PP2A activation following cerebral ischemia. *Brain Inj.* 23, 1073–1080. doi: 10.3109/ 02699050903379388
40. Tomioka, M., Toda, Y., Mañucat, N. B., Akatsu, H., Fukumoto, M., Kono, N., et al. (2017). Lysophosphatidylcholine export by human ABCA7. *Biochim. Biophys. Acta* 1862, 658–665. doi: 10.1016/j.bbalip.2017.03.012
41. Tu, W. J., Liu, X. Y., Dong, H., Yu, Y., Wang, Y., and Chen, H. (2014). Phosphatidylinositol-3,4,5-trisphosphate 5-phosphatase 1: a meaningful and independent marker to predict stroke in the Chinese population. *J. Mol. Neurosci.* 52, 507 511. doi: 10.1007/s12031-013-0206-2
42. Van Meer, G., Voelker, D. R., and Feigenson, G. W. (2008). Membrane lipids: where they are and how they behave. *Nat. Rev. Mol. Cell Biol.* 9, 112–124. doi: 10.1038/nrm2330
43. Vijayan, M., Kumar, S., Bhatti, J. S., and Reddy, P. H., (2017). *Molecular Links and Biomarkers of Stroke, Vascular Dementia, and Alzheimer's Disease.* 1st Edn. Amsterdam: Elsevier Inc.,. doi: 10.1016/bs.pmbts.2016.12.014
44. Villamil-Ortiz, J. G., Barrera-Ocampo, A., Arias-Londoño, J. D., Villegas, A., Lopera, F., and Cardona-Gómez, G. P. (2017). Differential pattern of phospholipid profile in the temporal cortex from E280A-familiar and sporadic Alzheimer's disease brains. *J. Alzheimer's Dis.* 61, 209–219. doi: 10.3233/JAD- 170554

45. Villamil-Ortiz, J. G., Barrera-Ocampo, A., Piedrahita, D., Velásquez-Rodríguez, C. M., Arias-Londoño, J. D., and Cardona-Gómez, G. P. (2016). BACE1 RNAi restores the composition of phosphatidylethanolamine-derivates related to memory improvement in aged 3xTg-AD mice. *Front. Cell. Neurosci.* 10:260. doi: 10.3389/fncel.2016.00260
46. Wang, H. Y., Liu, C. B., Wu, H. W., and Kuo, J. S. (2010). Direct profiling of phospholipids and lysophospholipids in rat brain sections after ischemic stroke. *Rapid Commun. Mass Spectrom.* 24, 2057–2064. doi: 10.1002/rcm
47. Wang, Q., Tang, X. N., and Yenari, M. A. (2007). The inflammatory response in stroke. *J. Neuroimmunol.* 184, 53–68. doi: 10.1016/j.jneuroim.2006.11.014
48. Whiley, L., Sen, A., Heaton, J., Proitsi, P., García-Gómez, D., Leung, R., et al. (2014). Evidence of altered phosphatidylcholine metabolism in Alzheimer's disease. *Neurobiol. Aging.* 35, 271–278. doi: 10.1016/j.neurobiolaging.2013.08.001
49. Wood, P. L., Locke, V. A., Herling, P., Passaro, A., Vigna, G. B., Volpato, S., et al. (2016). Targeted lipidomics distinguishes patient subgroups in mild cognitive impairment (MCI) and late onset Alzheimer's disease (LOAD). *BBA Clin.* 5, 25–28. doi: 10.1016/j.bbacli.2015.11.004
50. Zhang, W., Liu, J., Hu, X., Li, P., Leak, R. K., Gao, Y., et al. (2015). n-3 polyunsaturated fatty acids reduce neonatal hypoxic/ischemic brain injury by promoting phosphatidylserine formation and Akt signaling. *Stroke* 46, 2943–2950. doi: 10.1161/STROKEAHA.115

17

Parkinson's Disease: Biomarkers, Treatment and Risk Factors

Fatemeh N. Emamzadeh[1] *and Andrei Surguchov*[2*]

[1] *Division of Biomedical and Life Sciences, Faculty of Health and Medicine, University of Lancaster, Lancaster, United Kingdom,* [2] *Department of Neurology, Kansas University Medical Center, Kansas City, KS, United States*

Correspondence:
Andrei Surguchov
asurguchov@kumc.edu

Parkinson's disease (PD) is a progressive neurodegenerative disorder caused mainly by lack of dopamine in the brain. Dopamine is a neurotransmitter involved in movement, motivation, memory, and other functions; its level is decreased in PD brain as a result of dopaminergic cell death. Dopamine loss in PD brain is a cause of motor deficiency and, possibly, a reason of the cognitive deficit observed in some PD patients. PD is mostly not recognized in its early stage because of a long latency between the first damage to dopaminergic cells and the onset of clinical symptoms. Therefore, it is very important to find reliable molecular biomarkers that can distinguish PD from other conditions, monitor its progression, or give an indication of a positive response to a therapeutic intervention. PD biomarkers can be subdivided into four main types: clinical, imaging, biochemical, and genetic. For a long time protein biomarkers, dopamine metabolites, amino acids, etc. in blood, serum, cerebrospinal liquid (CSF) were considered the most promising. Among the candidate biomarkers that have been tested, various forms of α-synuclein (α-syn), i.e., soluble, aggregated, post-translationally modified, etc. were considered potentially the most efficient. However, the encouraging recent results suggest that microRNA-based analysis may bring considerable progress, especially if it is combined with α-syn data. Another promising analysis is the advanced metabolite profiling of body fluids, called "metabolomics" which may uncover metabolic fingerprints specific for various stages of PD. Conventional pharmacological treatment of PD is based on the replacement of dopamine using dopamine precursors (levodopa, L-DOPA, L-3,4 dihydroxyphenylalanine), dopamine agonists (amantadine, apomorphine) and MAO-B inhibitors (selegiline, rasagiline), which can be used alone or in combination with each other. Potential risk factors include environmental toxins, drugs, pesticides, brain microtrauma, focal cerebrovascular damage, and genomic defects. This review covers molecules that might act as the biomarkers of PD. Then, PD risk factors (including genetics and non-genetic factors) and PD treatment options are discussed.

Keywords: Parkinson's disease, biomarkers, α-synuclein, microRNAs, orexin

---

Abbreviations: 8-OHdG, 8-hydroxy-2′-deoxyguanosine; BBB, blood–brain barrier; CSF, cerebrospinal fluid; DBS, deep brain stimulation; DLBs, dementia with Lewy bodies; GBA, acid β-glucocerebrosidase; HDLs, high density lipoproteins; LBs, Lewy bodies; LDLs, low density lipoproteins; L-dopa, levodopa; LRRK2, leucine-rich repeat kinase 2; MAOA, monoamine oxidase A; MAOB, monoamine oxidase B; MAPKs, mitogen-activated protein kinases; MAPT, microtubule-associated protein tau; MPTP, 1-methyl-4-phenyl-1,2,3,6 tetrahydropyridine; PD, Parkinson's disease; PDD, Parkinson's disease dementia; PEA, β-phenylethylamine; PINK1, PTEN-induced putative kinase 1; SN, substantia nigra; TBP, TATA box-binding protein; TH, tyrosine hydroxylase; VLDLs, very low density lipoproteins.

INTRODUCTION

Parkinson's disease is the second most common neurodegenerative disease characterized by a progressive loss of dopaminergic neurons in the SN pars compacta. In PD, there is a long latency between the first damage to cells in at-risk nuclei of the nervous system, and the onset of clinical symptoms. The symptoms and signs of PD usually do not develop until 70–80% of dopaminergic neurons have already been lost (El-Agnaf et al., 2006). Thus, identifying patients in the period between the presumed onset of dopaminergic cell loss and the appearance of clinical parkinsonism may be of major importance for the development of effective neuroprotective treatment strategies (Berendse et al., 2001). Staining of LBs, the pathological hallmark of PD, to identify affected neurons throughout the nervous system, revealed six neuropathological stages of this disease based on the localization of the involved brain regions (Braak et al., 2003). Examination of brain samples from hundreds of PD patients revealed that the pathological process was relatively uniform. The pathology in the first stage begins in the lower medulla oblongata, specifically the dorsal motor nucleus of the vagal nerve, and the anterior olfactory structures. In stage 2, lesions in the dorsal motor nucleus worsen, inclusions develop in the lower raphe nuclei, and Lewy neurites can be observed in the locus ceruleus. In stage three the SN is affected. In stage four, lesions appear in the cortex, specifically in the temporal mesocortex. In stage five, the pathology appears in the adjoining temporal neocortical fields, while in stage six cortical involvement is clearly seen. Importantly, cognitive status correlates with the neuropathological stage (Braak et al., 2003). It is also essential to find reliable molecular biomarkers that can distinguish PD from other conditions, monitor its progression, or give an indication of a positive response to therapeutic intervention (Siderowf et al., 2018). α-Synuclein (α-Syn) aggregates are assumed to be harmful to dopaminergic neurons in the SN, and their formation may trigger the transmission of toxic α-syn from affected cells to other adjacent cells, resulting in a cascade of LBs formation and, subsequently, cell death (Angot and Brundin, 2009; Steiner et al., 2018). This promotes further dopaminergic cell loss caused by the spread of pathogenic forms of α-syn to neighboring cells (Luk et al., 2012). The transmission of α-syn between cells can be a normal pathway. However, in a stress condition, the aggregation of α-syn may be initiated within the receiver cells, where pre-aggregated α-syn acts as a 'seed' inducing more aggregation of soluble α-syn in a 'prion-like' fashion (Bernis et al., 2015). Furthermore, because α-syn aggregates are normally cleared by the proteasome system or by the lysosomes, any defect in clearance mechanisms could cause the spread of PD pathology as undigested toxic α-syn transmits to other cells. In accordance with this concept lysosomal inhibition enhances the amount of insoluble α-syn, leading to the elevated release of exosomes containing toxic α-syn (Luk et al., 2012). In healthy neurons unwanted proteins are cleared via an exosome mediated pathway, thus explaining why α-syn can be released from neurons in normal conditions, while any cellular or environmental problem that leads to higher α-syn secretion can be harmful to neurons and can be transmitted to other adjacent cells. There is a hypothesis that the accumulation of α-syn in PD patients begins in the enteric nervous system that is in nerves in the upper gastrointestinal tract (GI). α-Syn produced in GI is spread through vagus to the brain, suggesting a significant role of gut-brain axis in PD development (Liddle, 2018). Therefore, monitoring PD occurrence, diagnosis of early stage of this disease, ability to distinguish it from other parkinsonian syndromes, monitoring of its response to treatment and progression all require the identification of reliable biomarkers. After many years of disease PD can eventually evolve into PDD. The methods of diagnostics and distinctions between PD, PDD, and DLB are described in a recent comprehensive review (McKeith et al., 2017)

NEUROCHEMICAL BIOMARKERS

Orexin

Orexin, also known as hypocretin, is a neuropeptide hormone expressed by a small number of neurons of the dorsolateral hypothalamus. Orexin is secreted by the lateral and posterior neurons of the hypothalamus. The hormone regulates many physiological functions, such as the sleep-wake cycle (Hagan et al., 1999), cardiovascular responses, heart rate, and hypertension (Imperatore et al., 2017). PD patients usually suffer from narcolepsy due to the loss of hypocretin neurons in the hypothalamus. The concentration of orexin A is lower in PD patients than in healthy individuals, and the level of orexin is related to the severity of the disease. The more severe is the disease, the higher loss of hypocretin neurons and the lower orexin levels in the CSF are observed (Fronczek et al., 2007). In the late stages of PD, decreased orexin levels may be responsible for daytime sleepiness (Wienecke et al., 2012). In narcolepsy of PD patients elevated levels of glial fibrillary acidic protein (GFAP) in the CSF seem to be causative for the reduction of orexin levels (Takahashi et al., 2015) pointing to GFAP as another potential biomarker. GFAP is an intermediate filament protein of the cytoskeleton that is expressed mostly in astrocytes. Hypophosphorylation and overexpression of GFAP often occur in PD patients, suggesting that these alterations in astrocytes are associated with the pathogenesis of PD (Clairembault et al., 2014). Astrocytes may be involved in the progression of PD by the production of pro-inflammatory cytokines that damage dopaminergic neurons (Rappold and Tieu, 2010). Therefore, PD can be identified by elevated levels of GFAP as an astroglial marker.

8-Hydroxy-2′-Deoxyguanosine

Reactive oxygen species (ROS) species (such as O_2-, H_2O_2, and·OH) can damage biological molecules basically through irreversible reactions causing degenerative processes associated with aging. One of the DNA lesions caused by ROS is an oxidized form of 8-hydroxyguanine (8-OHG) known as 8-OHdG which can be used as a biomarker of DNA damage (Shigenaga et al., 1989). Likewise, an increase in 8-OHdG serum levels has been measured in PD patients compared to the normal individuals. CSF 8-OHdG levels are also higher in PD patients than in normal cases, but the difference is not as significant as serum levels. Therefore, 8-OHdG could be developed as a potential biomarker for PD (Kikuchi et al., 2002). It has been shown in the rat model that PD stage is directly related to urinary 8-OHdG level, suggesting that it can be used as a severity biomarker for PD (Kikuchi et al., 2011). However, it should be remembered that 8-OHdG is a marker of oxidative DNA damage, but not of progression of PD, so its specificity is limited (Simon et al., 2015).

Peripheral Proteasomes and Caspase Activity

Proteasomes are large protein complexes responsible for degrading and elimination of unwanted and misfolded proteins and therefore are important for cell survival. Damaged proteins that are tagged with ubiquitin molecules by ubiquitin ligase, trigger the ATP-dependent proteolytic activity of the proteasome (Lodish et al., 2004). In PD, the accumulation of proteins within the neurons leads to the formation of pathological intracellular inclusions called LBs. Proteasome dysfunction may be involved in the formation of protein aggregates and associated with LBs (Bentea et al., 2017). In PD mutations disturbing proteasome activity may lead to the accumulation of aggregated α-syn (Shadrina et al., 2010; Ciechanover and Kwon, 2015). In some PD cases, mitochondrial deficiency causes the production of more ROS and higher α-syn oxidation leading to increased ATP-independent proteasomal activity and higher α-syn oligomerization. Depletion of ATP levels in this case inhibits 26S proteasome, but 20S complex still remains active and degrades oxidized α-syn (Martins-Branco et al., 2012). In advanced PD, the severity and duration of PD correlate with reduced proteasome 20S activity and increased caspase 3 activity. The activation of caspase and thus initiation of apoptosis is the main reason of proteasome 20S activity reduction. Therefore, these proteasome and caspase components may be also considered as potential PD biomarkers (Blandini et al., 2006).

Dopamine, Dopamine Receptor, and Dopamine Transporter Activity

A catecholamine neurotransmitter dopamine is secreted by the SN, hypothalamus and some other regions of the brain. TH synthesizes the dopamine precursor (L-DOPA) that is converted to dopamine by L-aromatic amino acid decarboxylase (AADC). In the brain, dopamine is used as the precursor of noradrenaline (norepinephrine) and adrenaline (epinephrine). Loss of dopaminergic neurons in the midbrain and SN of PD brains leads to the reduction of dopamine levels (Obeso et al., 2008). The dopamine transporter (DAT) controls dopamine levels by facilitating its reuptake back to the cytosol. However, free dopamine is toxic for neurons, since its oxidation creates poisonous reactive quinones. Therefore, the vesicular monoamine transporter 2 (VMAT2) stores excess dopamine in vesicles. Thus, any change in dopamine or DAT levels may be an indicator of PD. Moreover, dopamine activates five types of receptors (D1R–D5R) and the severity of PD is related to the decreased expression of the dopamine type 3 receptor (D3R), leading to more severe symptoms because of reduced dopamine signals (Nagai et al., 1996). Therefore, D3R can be also considered as a potential biomarker for PD (Caronti et al., 2001).

Recent studies have point to 3-methoxy-4-hydroxyphenylglycol (MHPG) as a valuable biomarker to distinguish several forms of neurodegenerative diseases. This biogenic amine and norepinephrine's metabolite passes the BBB, and analysis of its level in serum and CSF may be helpful to determine cognitive staging in PD, distinguish PD from non-PD controls, DLB versus AD, etc. (Vermeiren and De Deyn, 2017; van der Zee et al., 2018). This method is promising, since the locus coeruleus becomes affected in an earlier stage than the SN by α-syn.

In another recent article a preclinical phase of PD is identified by analysis of dopamine metabolites in CSF. Low CSF concentrations of 3,4-dihydroxyphenylacetic acid (DOPAC) and DOPA identify pre-clinical PD in at-risk healthy individuals (Goldstein et al., 2018).

Catecholamine neurons are not abundant in the nervous system, and their vulnerability in PD and related diseases (Goldstein et al., 2018) is not explained. A concept of autotoxicity assumes intrinsic cytotoxicity of catecholamines in cells in which it is produced. According to a recent theory, PD might develop when 3,4-dihydroxyphenylacetaldehyde (DOPAL) oligomerizes and aggregates α-syn, providing a link between synucleinopathy and catecholamine neuron loss in LBD (Goldstein et al., 2018).

According to the "catecholaldehyde hypothesis" for the pathogenesis of PD, long-term increased build-up of DOPAL, the catecholaldehyde metabolite of dopamine, causes or contributes to the eventual death of dopaminergic neurons. LBs, a neuropathological hallmark of PD, contain precipitated α-syn. Bases for the tendency of α-syn to precipitate in the cytoplasm of catecholaminergic neurons have also been mysterious. Since DOPAL potently oligomerizes and aggregates α-syn, the catecholaldehyde hypothesis provides a link between synucleinopathy and catecholamine neuron loss in Lewy body diseases. The concept developed here is that DOPAL and α-syn are nodes in a complex nexus of interacting homeostatic systems.

α-Synuclein

α-Synuclein, which is found in an aggregated and fibrillar form, has attracted considerable attention as a potential molecular biomarker of PD. (Emamzadeh, 2016). Human α-syn is predominantly expressed in the brain in the neocortex, hippocampus, SN, thalamus and cerebellum, and is found in LBs (Surguchov, 2015). It is encoded by the SNCA gene that consists of six exons ranging in size from 42 to 1,110 bp (McLean et al., 2000; Yu et al., 2007). As noted above, the predominant form of α-syn is the full-length protein, but other shorter isoforms have been described. Importantly, C-terminal truncation of α-syn induces aggregation, suggesting that C-terminal modifications might be involved in the pathology of α-syn (Venda et al., 2010). Changes in the levels of α-syn have been reported in CSF and plasma of PD patients compared to control individuals (Hong et al., 2010). Recent evidence suggests that α-syn can be secreted into the extracellular space of the brain and spread the pathology of PD by propagating in a prion-like fashion (Masuda-Suzukake et al., 2013). This extracellular form of the protein can also be found in human body fluids, including blood and CSF (Mollenhauer et al., 2011). The gradual spread of α-syn pathology leads to a high concentration of extracellular α-syn that can potentially damage healthy neurons. Moreover, recent biomarker studies have shown changes in the level of α-syn in blood plasma from patients with PD (Li et al., 2007; Foulds et al., 2011), suggesting that α-syn might cross the BBB. Later, radiolabeled α-syn was traced in the bidirectional path from blood to the CNS and vice versa (Sui et al., 2014). Therefore, α-syn can be considered as a potential biomarker for PD.

Apolipoprotein A1 (ApoA1)

ApoA1 is a 28 AA apolipoprotein with ~28 kDa molecular weight which is the main constituent of HDL particles (Brewer et al., 1983). This apolipoprotein is synthesized mostly by the liver and the small intestine and is responsible for gathering extra cholesterol from cells. ApoA1 in cooperation with apoE participates in lipid transport in the brain (Emamzadeh, 2017). ApoA1 together with another apolipoprotein, apoE are responsible for lipid transportation in the brain. Lower levels of one isoform of apoA1 and tetranectin are reported in the CSF of PD patients, suggesting that apoA1 is a potential biomarker for PD (Wang et al., 2010; Swanson et al., 2015). ApoA1 cannot be secreted from neurons, but as the main component of HDL, it is required for cholesterol transportation to the brain. Therefore, it possibly passes through the BBB and contribute to the protective roles of HDL. In PD, lower level of apoA1 means less efficient HDL and reduced brain cholesterol homeostasis and function (Vitali et al., 2014).

RNA-Based PD Biomarkers

Recent investigation of microRNAs (miRNAs) in PD point to their emerging role as potential PD biomarkers, especially due to their presence in CSF and peripheral circulation both free and in exosomes. miRNAs are small 21–24 nucleotide non-coding RNAs that regulate gene expression post-transcriptionally. Due to their ability to cross the BBB miRNAs have a high potential as convenient PD biomarkers. In a recent study Dos Santos et al. (2018) analyzed miRNA expression profile using next generation sequencing (NGS) in the CSF of early stage PD patients and controls. The authors have identified a miRNA-based biomarker panel for the early diagnosis of PD, including the five best ranking variables (Let-7f-5p, miR-125a-5p, miR-151a-3p, miR-27a-3p and miR-423-5p). The analysis showed high predictive value with 90% diagnostic sensitivity. Inclusion of α-syn in the analysis further improves robustness of a miRNA-based panel. Several other teams confirmed that microRNAs may be used as new PD biomarkers suggesting a breakthrough for novel diagnostic and therapeutic approaches to this disease (Arshad et al., 2017; Vitali et al., 2018). Several other biomarkers are under investigation in a number of Medical Centers, the information about which can be found on the website: https://clinicaltrials.gov/ct2/results?cond=Parkinson$+$Disease&term=biomarker&cntry=&state=&city=&dist=.

METABOLITE PROFILING

Metabolic profiling of human tissues and/or biological fluids mirrors the complex interaction of genes, proteins and the environment of an individual. Proton (1H) and phosphorus (31P) magnetic resonance spectroscopy (MRS) are non-invasive imaging techniques that have been used to the study metabolites involved in energy metabolism, including ATP, lactate, creatine and other low molecular weight metabolite (Havelund et al., 2017). Significant alterations in metabolites have been described in PD patients and in animal models, including rise of lactate in striatum (Henchcliffe et al., 2008) and decrease of *N*-acetylaspartate/creatine ratios in advanced PD (Seraji-Bozorgzad et al., 2015). Alterations in alanine, branched-chain amino acids and fatty acid metabolism point to mitochondrial dysfunction in PD (Havelund et al., 2017).

NEUROIMAGING BIOMARKERS

Today's technology is able to detect brain's abnormalities in PD patients using imaging techniques, such as transcranial B-mode sonography (TCS), susceptibility-weighted imaging (SWI), diffusion weighted imaging (DWI) (Chung et al., 2009), positron emission tomography (PET) scan and, single-photon emission computed tomography (SPECT) scan.

Transcranial B-Mode Sonography (TCS)

Transcranial B-mode sonography monitors the blood flow velocity of brain's vessels by measuring the frequency of ultrasounds waves and their echoes. This inexpensive and reliable method shows the higher echogenicity of the SN in PD brains compared to normal group that possibly occurs due to increased iron and gliosis levels in SN of PD patients (Skoloudík et al., 2014). The increased iron level in PD can be due to either alternation or malfunction of the BBB. In PD the increase in the number of iron-transferring receptors including both transferrin receptors of BBB and iron-binding receptors of neurons can lead to accumulation of iron in SN (Hare et al., 2013).

Magnetic Resonance Imaging (MRI)

Diffusion weighted imaging is a form of MRI that measures the rate of water diffusion through a tissue to determine the structural details of that tissue. The higher measured diffusivity means the greater mobility of water molecules that can be due to the death of cells and the reduction of the region volume. This technique can differentiate PD from multiple system atrophy (MSA) in the early stage, while the clinical symptoms of these disorders are similar. In particular, the higher diffusivity of water in middle cerebellar peduncles in MSA patients in comparison to PD patients has been reported using DWI (Chung et al., 2009). DWI can also differentiate patients with progressive supranuclear palsy (PSP) from PD patients by detecting abnormalities in basal ganglia (Seppi et al., 2003). More traditional MRI methods, such as high-resolution 3-Tesla T1-weighted MRI can also detect the reduced volume of caudate and putamen in PD patients in compared to controls (Saeed et al., 2017).

Single-Photon Emission Computed Tomography (SPECT) Scan

Both PET and SPECT scans can detect the early onset of PD and loss of dopaminergic neurons using radiotracers and computer techniques to generate 3D images. The majority of radiotracers are non-invasive radiopharmaceuticals with a short lifetime that usually decay soon after the imaging is complete. Moreover, the 3D images of PET and SPECT scans reveal function of an organ, whereas MRI can only monitor the anatomy and structure (Histed et al., 2012).

The SPECT scan radiotracers have a longer life-time in comparison to PET radiotracers. They mostly are ^{123}iodine (^{123}I) and ^{99m}technetium (^{99m}Tc) that emit gamma rays. The DAT-SPECT imaging can monitor degeneration of presynaptic terminals in dopaminergic neurons by visualizing DAT quantity. This method is a good way to diagnose reduction of DAT in the brain, and importantly it can't distinguish PD and other Parkinsonian Syndromes. The DAT gamma-emitting ligands, such as ^{123}I-iometopane (^{123}I-β-CIT), ^{123}I-ioflupane (^{123}I-FP-CIT), ^{123}I-altropane (^{123}I-IPT) are the most common DAT-density SPECT tracers. These ligands are derivatives of tropane and dopamine reuptake inhibitors that target DAT (Wang et al., 2012; Brooks, 2016).

Single-photon emission computed tomography also employs dopamine D2 receptor radioligands that are dopamine antagonists. They include ^{123}I-iodobenzamide (^{123}I-IBZM) (Reiche et al., 1995), ^{123}I-IBF (Sasaki et al., 2003), and ^{123}I-epidepride (Pirker et al., 1997). ^{123}I-2′-iodospiperone (2′-ISP) is also used in some studies to monitor D2 dopamine receptors. Although this radiotracer can distinguish between PD and other form of parkinsonism due to the pattern of its uptake in basal ganglia, it produces a high imaging background and needs to be modified to improve its performance (Yonekura et al., 1995).

The number of vesicular acetylcholine transporter (VAChT) can be monitored by SPECT radiotracers as an approach for PD early diagnosis. Acetylcholine (ACh) is a neurotransmitter that is in balance with dopamine in healthy people. The death of dopaminergic neurons and reduction of dopamine levels in PD are associated with increased Ach. ^{123}I-iodobenzovesamicol (^{123}I-IBVM) binds to VAChT and reveals the density of acetylcholine containing vesicles. Reduction of VAChT in parietal and occipital lobes in PD patients without dementia and reduced VAChT in all lobes of the cerebral cortex in PD patients with dementia has been established by this SPECT radiotracer (Niethammer et al., 2012).

^{123}I-metaiodobenzylguanidine (^{123}I-MIBG) is another radiotracer that can distinguish between PD and MSA (Goldstein, 2001). The heart-to-mediastinum ration of ^{123}I-MIBG uptake is impaired in idiopathic PD patients, but not in patients with MSA. PET/CT scanning of these PD patients illustrated also decreased FP-CIT striatal uptake (Oh et al., 2015). MIBG scintigraphy allows to distinguish not only between PD versus MSA, but also between PD and DLB (Goldstein, 2001, 2013).

Positron Emission Tomography (PET) Scan

The PET scan radiotracers emit electron anti-particles (positrons) that are positively charged with the same mass as an electron. The presence of presynaptic DAT in dopaminergic neurons of striatum and SN can be assessed with ^{18}F and/or ^{11}C radiolabeled dopamine analogs. These DAT radioligands include ^{18}F-dopamine (^{18}F-dopa) (Ibrahim et al., 2016), ^{18}F-FE-PE2I (Fazio et al., 2015), ^{18}F-β-CFT (Rinne et al., 1999), ^{18}F-LBT999 (Arlicot et al., 2017), and ^{11}C-methylphenidate. The VMAT2 quantification is also possible by using either ^{11}C or ^{18}F radiolabeled dihydrotetrabenazine (DTBZ) (Tong et al., 2008; Lin et al., 2013). Because of dopaminergic cell loss and subsequent loss of VMAT2, the PET signal of radiolabeled DTBZ is lower in PD patients than in controls. Both DAT and VMAT2 radioligands can detect the early signs of dopaminergic damage, although PD may not be differentiated from atypical Parkinsonism with dopaminergic dysfunction. ^{11}C-MP4A is another PET radiotracer that monitors the level of acetylcholinesterase (AChE) activity. AChE hydrolyses deactivates Ach and terminates the signal. Impairment of cholinergic system and reduction of cortical AChE has been assessed by ^{11}C-MP4A-PET scan. AChE activity reduces more in PDD than in PD, indicating that cholinergic dysfunction is correlated with dementia in PD (Bohnen et al., 2006).

PARKINSON'S DISEASE TREATMENT

The development of neuroprotective drugs for PD is an important unmet medical need, since this disease progressively impair the patients' quality of life and functionality in activities of daily living. The identification of new therapeutic targets is therefore of great importance. Although different medications and therapies for controlling PD symptoms are currently available, no cure for PD exists. The development of treatments for PD, based on patients' symptoms and needs, vary from different medications to rehabilitation or even surgery. PD includes different clinical entities observed in several studies investigating the existence of PD subtypes. A cluster analysis permits to identify distinct PD subtypes according to the relevance of both motor and non-motor symptoms and select therapeutic approach according to cluster symptoms presentation (Lauretani et al., 2014).

MEDICATIONS

The most common therapy for PD includes different commercially available medications that treat the lack of dopamine in the SN. These medications can temporarily alleviate PD symptoms in different ways by enhancing dopamine level, mimicking the role of dopamine or inhibiting dopamine oxidative metabolism, which leads to the generation of reactive oxygen species (ROS) (Goldenberg, 2008). Formation of protein aggregates that lead to neuronal cell death is another important target for PD treatment. Among different PD medications, levodopa (L-dopa, L-3,4-dihydroxyphenylalanine) is an effective drug. Levodopa is the immediate metabolic precursor of dopamine which is produced by TH from L-tyrosine. In the dopaminergic neurons, dopa-decarboxylase converts levodopa into dopamine. The orally taken levodopa can be decarboxylated in peripheral sites before reaching the CNS. Therefore, levodopa is available in combination with carbidopa or benserazide that are peripheral inhibitors of Dopa decarboxylase, but do not pass through the BBB. Unchanged levodopa in the presence of decarboxylase peripheral inhibitors can penetrate into the CNS and is used as a precursor of dopamine (Goldenberg, 2008).

Levodopa, is more efficiently transformed into DA after vesicle storage by the serotonergic neurons, rather than the dopaminergic ones of the nigrostriatal system. Since the serotonergic distribution throughout the brain is very different than the dopaminergic one, this causes the well-known side effects of L-DOPA therapy and reduces its efficiency as a drug (De Deurwaerdère et al., 2017).

Sinemet was the first brand of carbidopa/levodopa combination in the pharmaceutical market (Scriabine, 1999). Rytary and duopa are two newly approved medications for PD by the Food and Drug Administration (FDA). Xadago (safinamide) is recently approved medication for PD patients who do not benefit from levodopa/carbidopa. Rytary is manufactured by Impax Laboratories as an oral capsule containing carbidopa-levodopa together with entacapone to prolong its effects. Doupa produced by AbbVie Company is used for the treatment of motor fluctuations in advanced PD. Doupa is an enteral gel made of levodopa-carbidopa that is pumped to patient intestines (Olanow et al., 2014).

A group of dopamine agonists are agents that bind to the dopaminergic post-synaptic receptors and trigger the same signal as dopamine itself. This group include pergolide, pramipexole dihydrochloride, ropinirole hydrochloride, rotigotine, and apomorphine hydrochloride (Jankovic and Aguilar, 2008).

Inhibitors of MAOB – selegiline and rasagiline are also available as PD medications. Monoamine oxidase isoforms, including MAOA and MAOB, located on the outer membrane of mitochondria are involved in the oxidative deamination of biogenic amines, such as neurotransmitters and xenobiotic amines, e.g., 1-methyl-4-phenyl-1,2,3,6-tetrahydropyridine (MPTP) (Bach et al., 1988). The MAOs have a significant effect on the course of PD, because they are involved in the metabolism of dopamine. Oxidative metabolism of dopamine in the dopaminergic cells of SN by MAOs leads to ROS generation, oxidative damage and cell death (Reiter, 1995). Moreover, MAOB catalyzes the conversion of MPTP into 1-methyl-4-phenylpyridine (MPP+) which is responsible for parkinsonism in intravenous drug users (Langston, 1996). Selegiline and rasagiline can protect neurons against oxidative damage induced by dopamine metabolites diminishing MAOB activity. Moreover, several substances, such as entacapone and tolcapone that inhibit catechol-*o*-methyl transferase (COMT) are available as alternative PD medications. These two medications block the conversion of levodopa into methylated levodopa. Therefore, inhibition of COMT activity by these medications can extend the existence of functional levodopa preventing its degradation (Goldenberg, 2008).

Additionally, some other chemicals can be considered as potential PD medicines. Rapamycin can be a useful treatment for PD as an up-regulator of autophagy. Rapamycin induces autophagy in cells by inhibition of a specific kinase activity called mTOR. Autophagy is a potential target for PD treatment, since it initiates the clearance of protein aggregates and inhibits apoptosis (Hochfeld et al., 2013). Adenosine A2A receptor antagonists, such as caffeine also reduces the risk of PD. Transgenic mice with mutant α-syn and deleted adenosine A2A receptor genes are protected against PD. Thus, A2A receptor antagonists are potential candidates for prevention and treatment of PD (Kachroo and Schwarzschild, 2012).

Formation of protein aggregates that leads to neuronal cell death is a promising target for PD treatment. In January 2015, Neuropore Therapies has announced phase I clinical trial of a new drug, NPT200-11 (UCB-1332) that inhibits oligomerization of α-syn (Oertel, 2017). Another potential drug modulating the aggregation of α-syn blocking or reducing the conversion of monomers to oligomers or later on to fibrils is ANLE138b (Levin et al., 2014). Several promising compounds are under development and/or in preclinical testing that may enhance autophagy of α-syn. Recent screening of compounds protecting cells from α-syn induced neurodegeneration identified a non-selective phosphodiesterase (PDE) inhibitor dipyridamole. Importantly, PDE1 inhibition also protects dopaminergic neurons from α-syn induced degeneration in mouse SN. PDE inhibitors are currently at preclinical testing (Höllerhage et al., 2017). Another antiaggregation compound – a natural product squalamine displaces α-syn from the surfaces of lipid vesicles, thereby blocking the first steps in its aggregation process. Furthermore, squalamine suppresses the toxicity of α-syn oligomers by inhibiting their interactions with lipid membranes (Perni et al., 2017).

SURGERY

Deep brain stimulation therapy is rarely used for certain types of brain-related disorders including PD, dystonia, obsessive-compulsive disorder and treatment resistant depression (Herrington et al., 2016). When PD symptoms are very severe and medications cannot moderate them, surgery and DBS can be considered as the final options for the treatment. It involves sending electrical impulses to certain parts of the brain (usually SN or globus pallidus, which communicate with the SN) by a neurostimulator device that is a brain implant known as a 'brain pacemaker.' The target area of DBS is usually the subthalamic nucleus (STN). The stimulation of the dorsolateral STN border alongside the surgery can improve its efficiency (Herzog et al., 2004). Later it was found that stimulation of caudal zona incerta (cZI) can be more effective with fewer complications after the surgery (Plaha et al., 2006). Stimulation of neurons may also lead to neurogenesis and neuroplasticity and thus can improve for a long time motor problems, such as dyskinesia and tremor, and all other levodopa-responsive symptoms, for a long time. However, there are two problems with DBS, namely a 3- to 6-month waiting period required for optimal results and the possibility of brain infection (Bronstein et al., 2011).

GENE THERAPY

The development of gene therapy of PD has made a major progress in a recent decade. Advanced PD does not give a good response to levodopa therapy. Broaden loss of dopaminergic neurons is accompanied by reduction in aromatic amino acid decarboxylase (AADC) levels that converts L-DOPA to dopamine. After successful preclinical studies, adeno-associated viral vectors carrying human AADC gene are recently delivered into putaminal neurons and subthalamic nucleus of PD patients. In this method, sufficient amount of dopamine production can be controlled by taking adequate levodopa dose. Orally taken levodopa can be converted into dopamine by AADC and sooth PD symptoms (Muramatsu et al., 2010). Safety and efficiency of the method have been proven over 4 years by annually PET imaging from patients who received specific dosages of AAV2-hAADC (Mittermeyer et al., 2012). Another target for gene therapy in PD is glutamic acid decarboxylase (GAD) that facilitate production of GABA in GABA-ergic neurons in the subthalamic nucleus. GABA as an inhibitory neurotransmitter regulates muscle tone and improve motor functions (Watanabe et al., 2002). Lack of dopamine in PD causes activation of the subthalamic nucleus and unnecessary muscular responses that GABA by its inhibitory effect can significantly improve. This method can be compared with DBS that by sending electric shocks to subthalamic nucleus reduces its hyperactivity and improve motor impairment (Coune et al., 2012). The human trial of this method was performed by bilateral injection of AAV2-GAD in the subthalamic nucleus of patients with advanced PD. This approach has shown safety and efficiency, although it needs more investigation to be considered as a treatment (LeWitt et al., 2011). Therapeutic effect of glial cell line-derived neurotrophic factor (GDNF) on neuronal function in non-human models of PD encouraged scientists to inject it directly into putamen of PD patients. This surgery helped patients with improved movement, reduced dyskinesia and increased dopamine storage in the putamen (Gill et al., 2003). Therefore, GDNF is a possible option for gene therapy. Neurturin gene is another candidate for PD gene therapy. Neurturin is a neurotrophic factor important for survival and differentiation of dopaminergic neurons (Lin et al., 1993). The human trial of this factor was conducted by bilateral injection of vector AAV2-neurturin (CERE-120) into the putamen biomarkers patients with advanced PD (Bartus et al., 2013). Injected neurturin cannot spread into SN and play its therapeutic role because of vast axonal transport defects in PD patients. Another consequence of this method may be the accumulation of α-syn that leads to downregulation of neurturin expression (Bartus et al., 2014).

NON-GENETIC RISK FACTORS OF PARKINSON DISEASE

Only 10–15% of PD cases are early onset familial PD, while the remaining cases are idiopathic pointing to an important role of non-genetic and environmental factors in PD pathogenesis. Exposure to environmental toxins can cause dopaminergic cell death. The accumulation of heavy metals in the SN enhances the risk of developing PD. The effect of exposure to heavy metals could increase oxidative stress in dopaminergic cells, leading to PD. MAO in the presence of oxygen can mediate dopamine oxidation *in vitro* into 3,4-dihydroxylphenyl-acetaldehyde (DOPAL). DOPAL initiates oligomerization of α-syn into non-fibrillar, SDS-resistant aggregates (Burke, 2003). However, another study has revealed that inhibition of MAO to stop the production of DOPAL is not sufficient to reduce oligomerization of α-syn (Burke, 2003). The auto-oxidation of dopamine to dourmine quinone (DAQ) can also increase both formation and secretion of non-fibrillar α-syn oligomers, thus promoting pathogenic α-syn transmission to adjacent neurons and glia (Lee et al., 2011). Neuromelanin pigment is highly expressed in dopaminergic neurons, preventing oxidative stress related to the accumulation of cytosolic dopamine. On the other hand, dying neurons in PD brains release neuromelanin that activates neuroglia and triggers neuroinflammation (Zucca et al., 2014). Moreover, lipidated neuromelanin can interact with α-syn and trigger its aggregation into the insoluble complex in PD patients (Double and Halliday, 2006).

Genetic polymorphisms of cytochrome P450 2D6 (CYP2D6) – an enzyme involved in metabolizing environmental toxins, are also related to the development of PD. For example, CYP2D6 deficient metabolizers are two times higher at risk of developing PD if they are also exposed to pesticides. Therefore, sufficient levels of CYP2D6 activity are required for the metabolism of pesticides (e.g., organophosphates, atrazine), which are linked to the pathogenesis of PD (Elbaz and Tranchant, 2007).

Reactive oxygen species and thus oxidative stress is also known as a pathological factor in PD. NADPH oxidase-2 enzyme (NOX2) is a membrane-bound oxidase present primarily in phagocytes generating ROS in phagosomes to kill bacteria. NOX2-derived ROS also damages dopaminergic neurons. Dopaminergic neurons in NOX2-knockout mice start to degenerate faster than similar cells in wild-type controls after administration of MPTP (Brieger et al., 2012).

In 1956 two neurologists, Poskanzer and Schwab hypothesized that PD is related to influenza infection (Estupinan et al., 2013). They studied a group of PD patients and revealed that age of disease onset is shifted in the direction of an age group who were born before or during the influenza pandemic in 1918 and mostly had been infected by the flu virus. However, other studies showed that influenza infection can cause PD-like symptoms, but cannot increase the risk of developing PD (Estupinan et al., 2013). Another hypothesis proposes that Toxoplasma gondii, an intracellular parasite causing toxoplasmosis, may increase the risk of PD. The parasite in the brain infected those areas that are affected in PD, including basal ganglia (Miman et al., 2010), although other studies did not get a similar result (Mahami Oskouei et al., 2016).

GENETIC FORMS AND GENETIC RISK FACTORS OF PD

Although most cases of PD are idiopathic forms of the disease, about 15% of PD patients are recognized as having a first-degree family member with this disease. Recently, the genetic factors and gene loci involving in autosomal dominant and autosomal recessive forms of PD have been discovered due to advanced molecular genetics (Samii et al., 2004; Karimi-Moghadam et al., 2018) (**Tables 1, 2**). The mutations in several genes, including α-syn, LRRK2, PINK1, Parkin, DJ-1, VPS35 and GBA1 are linked to PD (Zeng et al., 2018). In addition to mutations in these genetic loci, polymorphisms, and trinucleotide repeats are recognized as PD genes, or susceptibility factors for PD (**Table 3**).

EPIGENETIC RISK FACTORS OF PD

Epigenetics refer to chromatin alternations, including DNA methylation and histone post translational modifications that can alter gene expression without changes in DNA sequence. These modifications can be inherited, but environmental factors including nutritional, chemical and physical factors can also affect epigenetics (Surguchov et al., 2017). In sporadic form of PD involvement of environmental factors in initiation and progression of disease emerging an idea that epigenetic plays an important role in PD (Feng et al., 2015). One of the examples of epigenetic mechanism in PD is modification of α-syn gene (SNCA). SNCA has two CpG islands with the first one being located in exon 1 (CpG-1) and the second one (CpG-2) within intron 1. Transcription factors (TFs) GATA and ZSCAN21 bind to the intron 1 CpG-2 island and modulate transcription of α-syn. CpG-2 methylation prevents the binding of the TFs to SNCA and subsequently inhibits the overexpression of α-syn. Interestingly, binding of transcription factors to α-syn (Iwata et al., 2001) and another member of the synuclein family, γ-synuclein (Surgucheva and Surguchov, 2008), has been

TABLE 1 | Autosomal recessive and X-linked genes involved in Parkinson's disease.

Inheritance pattern	Locus	Chr. location	Mutation site in	Involved protein
Autosomal recessive	PARK2/PARKN	6q25.2-q27	*Parkin*	Ubiquitin-protein ligase (Kitada et al., 1988)
	PARK6	1p36	*PINK1*	PTEN-induced putative kinase 1 (Valente et al., 2004)
	PARK7	1p36.23	*DJ1*	Oncogene DJ1 (van Duijn et al., 2001)
	PARK9	1p36	*ATP13A2*	Lysosomal type 5 P-type ATPase (Ramirez et al., 2006)
	PARK14	22q13.1	*PLA2G6*	Phospholipase A2 (Paisan-Ruiz et al., 2009; Shi et al., 2011)
	PARK15	22q12-q13	*FBXO7*	F-BOX only protein 7 (Paisan-Ruiz et al., 2009)
	PARK19	1p32	*DNAJC6*	Putative tyrosine-protein phosphatase auxilin (Koroglu et al., 2013)
	PARK20	21q22	*SYNJ1*	Synaptojanin-1 (Krebs et al., 2013)
X-linked	PARK12	Xq21-q25	*TAF1*	TFIID subunit 1 (Graeber and Muller, 1992)

TABLE 2 | Autosomal dominant genes involved in Parkinson's disease.

Inheritance pattern	Locus	Chr. location	Mutation site	Involved protein
Autosomal dominant	PARK1	4q21	*SNCA*	α-Syn (Xu et al., 2017)
	PARK3	2p13.2	*SPR*	Sepiapterin reductase in BH4 pathway (Karamohamed et al., 2003)
	PARK4	4q21	Triplication of *SNCA*	α-Syn (Singleton et al., 2003)
	PARK5	4p14	*UCHL1*	Ubiquitin C-terminal hydrolase (Leroy et al., 1998)
	PARK8	12q12	*LRRK2*	Leucine-reach repeat kinase 2 (Zimprich et al., 2004)
	PARK11	2q37	*GIGYF2*	GRB10-interacting GYF protein 2 (Lautier et al., 2008; Tan et al., 2009)
	PARK13	2p12	*HTRA2*	HTRA serine peptidase (Strauss et al., 2005; Lin et al., 2011)
	PARK16	1q32	Multiple independent sites?	Unknown (Satake et al., 2009; Li et al., 2011)
	PARK17	16p12.1-q12.1	*VPS35*	Vacuolar protein sorting 35 (Vilariño-Güell et al., 2011)
	PARK18	3q27	*EIF4G1*	Eukaryotic translation initiation factor 4 gamma 1 (Chartier-Harlin et al., 2011)
	PARK21	3q22	*DNAJC13*	DNAJ-domain-bearing protein (Appel-Cresswell et al., 2014; Vilariño-Güell et al., 2014)

TABLE 3 | Susceptibility factors of Parkinson's disease.

Susceptibility factors	Involved gene	Chr. location	Putative function	Phenotype
	GBA	1q21	Acid β-glucocerebrosidase	Gaucher disease (Pulkes et al., 2014)
	MAPT	17q21.1	Microtubule-associated protein tau	Supranuclear palsy, Dementia (Das et al., 2009)
	MC1R	16q24.3	Melanocyte-stimulating hormone receptor	Albinism (Tell-Marti et al., 2015)
	ADH1C	4q23	Alcohol dehydrogenase 1C	Alcohol dependence (Buervenich et al., 2005)
	ADH4	4q22	Alcohol dehydrogenase 4	Alcohol dependence (Buervenich et al., 2000)
	HLA	6p21.3	Major histocompatibility complex	Imamura et al., 2003
	ATXN2	12q24.1	Ataxin-2	Spinocerebellar ataxia 2 (Charles et al., 2007)
	ATXN3	14q21	Ataxin-3	Machado-Joseph disease (Gwinn-Hardy et al., 2001)
	TBP	6q27	TATA box-binding protein	Spinocerebellar ataxia 17 (Wu et al., 2004)
	ATXN8OS	13q21.33	Ataxin-8 opposite strand	Spinocerebellar ataxia 8 (Wu et al., 2004)
	NR4A2	2q24.1	Nuclear receptor subfamily 4 group A member 2 (transcription factor)	Le et al., 2003

described, suggesting that synuclein family members are involved in various complex mechanisms of gene expression regulation. Therefore, their role in PD is not limited to the formation of toxic aggregates, but may be complemented by participation in regulatory processes.

Matsumoto et al. (2010) found that CpGs in SNCA were hypermethylated in controls, but not methylated in PD patients, suggesting that methylation was an epigenetic risk factor for PD that is related to the pathogenesis of α-syn. In PD, demethylated SNCA codes for a high amount of α-syn that may initiate aggregation and promote neurodegeneration. Additionally, the levels of nuclear DNA (cytosine-5′) methyltransferase 1 (DNMT1) in post-mortem PD brains is lower than in control brains. This methylase epigenetically suppresses gene expression by DNA methylation, and its reduced level in PD may be associated with SNCA hypomethylation.

Epigenetic modifications in other genes are also implicated in contributing to PD, including tumor necrosis factor α (TNF-α), PARK16, transmembrane glycoprotein NMB (GPNMB), and syntaxin-1B (STX1B) genes. Hypomethylation of the TNF-α promoter, hypermethylation of a CpG dinucleotide in synphilin-1, STX1B and hypermethylation of multiple CpG sites proximal to GPNMB are all described in PD (Yang et al., 2017). Moreover, the epigenetic changes in mitochondrial DNA (mtDNA) can also trigger PD. Several studies show the hypo-methylation and hyper-hydroxymethylation of mtDNA displacement loop (D-loop) in the SN of PD brains (Iacobazzi et al., 2013; Chuang et al., 2017).

CONCLUSION

Pathology of PD is complex and include a combination of genetics, epigenetics and environmental factors. Current medical, pathological, and experimental data support the Braak hypothesis (Braak et al., 2003) of spatiotemporal spread of PD pathology involving α-syn propagation from the gastrointestinal and olfactory system via transsynaptic cell-to-cell transfer through the vegetative nervous systems to the CNS. Many non-motor symptoms, including sleep disorders, olfactory deficiency, hyposmia (reduced ability to smell and to detect odors), constipation and others may play an important role as successful, future diagnostic to target PD pathology and mechanisms during the initial stages of disease (Reichmann et al., 2016). Important contributing factors to PD are dysfunctions of mitochondria and endoplasmic reticulum, impairment of autophagy and endocytosis, and deregulation of immunity. Despite intensive investigation of PD mechanism the disease is still incurable. Future challenges for physicians and researchers working in the field of PD and similar disorders will be directed to the identification of biomarkers for an early diagnosis of these diseases at preclinical stage. New biomarkers should follow the progression of the disease and determine key metabolomic alterations to identify potential targets for intervention. Future tasks should be also directed to the development and application of preventive measures to stop or reduce disease progression at pre-symptomatic stages and the finding of novel antiparkinsonian drugs with specific neuroprotective effects on the dopaminergic system. In addition to conservative approach based on the identification of new protein biomarkers in blood, plasma and CSF, there is a growing hope that analysis of microRNAs may greatly contribute to early diagnosis of this disease. The development of induced pluripotent stem cell (iPSC) and genome editing technique open new hopes for the treatment of several human diseases, especially genetic disorders. For PD which is predominantly sporadic disease and a mix of several relatively rare genetic causes these methods gave the opportunity to develop new models and study phenotypes in both genetic and sporadic cases to piece together pathogenic pathways involving their gene products.

AUTHOR CONTRIBUTIONS

FE designed the article contents and wrote the original manuscript. AS revised and edited the manuscript, searched for additional related literature and discussed the writing with FE.

FUNDING

This work was supported by an EC Framework 7 Marie Curie Fellowship Training Network Grant (NEURASYNC) for FE and by VA Merit Review grants 1I01BX000361 and the Glaucoma Foundation grant QB42308 for AS.

ACKNOWLEDGMENTS

FE acknowledges Professor David Allsop for his help and support.

REFERENCES

1. Angot, E., and Brundin, P. (2009). Dissecting the potential molecular mechanisms underlying alpha-synuclein cell-to-cell transfer in Parkinson's disease. *Parkinsonism Relat. Disord.* 15(Suppl. 3), S143–S147. doi: 10.1016/ S1353-8020(09)70802-8
2. Appel-Cresswell, S., Rajput, A. H., Sossi, V., Thompson, C., Silva, V., McKenzie, J., et al. (2014). Clinical, positron emission tomography, and pathological studies of DNAJC13 p.N855S parkinsonism. *Mov. Disord.* 29, 1684–1687. doi: 10.1002/ mds.26019
3. Arlicot, N., Vercouillie, J., Malherbe, C., Bidault, R., Gissot, V., Maia, S., et al. (2017). PET imaging of dopamine transporter with 18F-LBT999: first human exploration. *J. Nucl. Med.* 58:1276. doi: 10.1111/j.1527-3458.2007.00033.x
4. Arshad, A. R., Sulaiman, S. A., Saperi, A. A., Jamal, R., Mohamed Ibrahim, N., and Abdul Murad, N. A. (2017). MicroRNAs and target genes as biomarkers for the diagnosis of early onset of Parkinson disease. *Front. Mol. Neurosci.* 10:352. doi: 10.3389/fnmol.2017.00352
5. Bach, A. W., Lan, N. C., Johnson, D. L., Abell, C. W., Bembenek, M. E., Kwan, S.-W., et al. (1988). cDNA cloning of human liver monoamine oxidase A and B: molecular basis of differences in enzymatic properties. *Proc. Nat. Acad. Sci. U.S.A.* 85, 4934–4938. doi: 10.1073/pnas.85.13.4934
6. Bartus, R. T., Baumann, T. L., Siffert, J., Herzog, C. D., Alterman, R., Boulis, N., et al. (2013). Safety/feasibility of targeting the substantia nigra with AAV2- neurturin in Parkinson patients. *Neurology* 80, 1698–1701. doi: 10.1212/WNL. 0b013e3182904faa
7. Bartus, R. T., Weinberg, M. S., and Samulski, R. J. (2014). Parkinson's disease gene therapy: success by design meets failure by efficacy. *Mol. Ther.* 22, 487–497. doi: 10.1038/mt.2013.281
8. Bentea, E., Verbruggen, L., and Massie, A. (2017). The proteasome inhibition model of Parkinson's disease. *J. Parkinsons Dis.* 7, 31–63. doi: 10.3233/JPD- 160921
9. Berendse, H. W., Booij, J., Francot, C. M., Bergmans, P. L., Hijman, R., and Stoof, J. C. (2001). Subclinical dopaminergic dysfunction in asymptomatic Parkinson's disease patients' relatives with a decreased sense of smell. *Ann. Neurol.* 50, 34–41. doi: 10.1002/ana.1049
10. Bernis, M. E., Babila, J. T., Breid, S., Wüsten, K. A., Wüllner, U., and Tamgüney, G. (2015). Prion-like propagation of human brain-derived alpha-synuclein in transgenic mice expressing human wild-type alpha-synuclein. *Acta Neuropathol. Commun.* 3:75. doi: 10.1186/s40478-015-0254-7
11. Blandini, F., Sinforiani, E., Pacchetti, C., Samuele, A., Bazzini, E., and Zangaglia, R. (2006). Peripheral proteasome and caspase activity in Parkinson disease and Alzheimer disease. *Neurology* 66, 529–534. doi: 10.1212/01.wnl.0000198511. 09968.b3
12. Bohnen, N. I., Albin, R. L., Koeppe, R. A., Wernette, K. A., Kilbourn, M. R., Minoshima, S., et al. (2006). Positron emission tomography of monoaminergic vesicular binding in aging and Parkinson disease. *J. Cereb. Blood Flow Metab.* 26, 1198–1212. doi: 10.1038/sj.jcbfm.9600276
13. Braak, H., Del Tredici, K., Rüb, U., de Vos, R. A., Jansen Steur, E. N., and Braak, E. (2003). Staging of brain pathology related to sporadic Parkinson's disease. *Neurobiol. Aging* 24, 197–211. doi: 10.1016/s0197-4580(02)00065-9
14. Brewer, H. B. Jr., Fairwell, T., Kay, L., Meng, M., Ronan, R., Law, S., et al. (1983). Human plasma proapoA-I: isolation and amino-terminal sequence. *Biochem. Biophys. Res. Commun.* 113, 626–632. doi: 10.1016/0006-291X(83)91772-2
15. Brieger, K., Schiavone, S., Miller, F. J., and Krause, K. H. (2012). Reactive oxygen species: from health to disease. *Swiss Med. Wkly.* 142:w13659. doi: 10.4414/ smw.2012.13659
16. Bronstein, J. M., Tagliati, M., Alterman, R. L., Lozano, A. M., Volkmann, J., Stefani, A., et al. (2011). Deep brain stimulation for Parkinson disease: an expert consensus and review of key issues. *Arch. Neurol.* 68:165. doi: 10.1001/ archneurol.2010.260
17. Brooks, D. J. (2016). Molecular imaging of dopamine transporters. *Ageing Res. Rev.* 30, 114–121. doi: 10.1016/j.arr.2015.12.009
18. Buervenich, S., Carmine, A., Galter, D., Shahabi, H. N., Johnels, B., Holmberg, B., et al. (2005). A rare truncating mutation in ADH1C (G78Stop) shows significant association with Parkinson disease in a large international sample. *Arch. Neurol.* 62, 74–78. doi: 10.1001/archneur.62.1.74
19. Buervenich, S., Sydow, O., Carmine, A., Zhang, Z., Anvret, M., and Olson, L. (2000). Alcohol dehydrogenase alleles in Parkinson's disease. *Mov. Disord.* 15, 813–818. doi: 10.1002/1531-8257(200009)15:5<813::AID-MDS1008>3.0. CO;2-Y
20. Burke, W. J. (2003). 3,4-dihydroxyphenylacetaldehyde: a potential target for neuroprotective therapy in Parkinson's disease. *Curr. Drug Targets CNS Neurol. Disord.* 2, 143–148. doi: 10.2174/15680070334 82913
21. Caronti, B., Antonini, G., Calderaro, C., Ruggieri, S., Palladini, G., Pontieri, F. E., et al. (2001). Dopamine transporter immunoreactivity in peripheral blood lymphocytes in Parkinson's disease. *Neural. Transm.* 108, 803–807. doi: 10.1007/s007020170030
22. Charles, P., Camuzat, A., Benammar, N., Sellal, F., Destee, A., Bonnet, A.-M., et al. (2007). Are interrupted SCA2 CAG repeat expansions responsible for parkinsonism? *Neurology* 69, 1970–1975.
23. Chartier-Harlin, M.-C., Dachsel, J. C., Vilarino-Guell, C., Lincoln, S. J., Lepretre, F., Hulihan, M., et al. (2011). Translation initiator EIF4G1 mutations in familial Parkinson disease. *Am. J. Hum. Genet.* 89, 398–406. doi: 10.1016/j.ajhg.2011. 08.009
24. Chuang, Y. H., Paul, K. C., Bronstein, J. M., Bordelon, Y., Horvath, S., and Ritz, B. (2017). Parkinson's disease is associated with DNA methylation levels in human blood and saliva. *Genome Med.* 9:76. doi: 10.1186/s13073-017- 0466-5
25. Chung, E. J., Kim, E. G., Bae, J. S., Eun, C. K., Lee, K. S., and Oh, M. (2009).
26. Usefulness of diffusion-weighted MRI for differentiation between Parkinson's disease and Parkinson variant of multiple system atrophy. *J. Mov. Disord.* 2, 64–68. doi: 10.14802/jmd.09017
27. Ciechanover, A., and Kwon, Y. T. (2015). Degradation of misfolded proteins in neurodegenerative diseases: therapeutic targets and strategies. *Exp. Mol. Med.* 47:e147. doi: 10.1038/emm.2014.117
28. Clairembault, T., Kamphuis, W., Leclair-Visonneau, L., Rolli-Derkinderen, M., Coron, E., Neunlist, M., et al. (2014). Enteric GFAP expression and phosphorylation in Parkinson's disease. *J. Neurochem.* 130, 805–815. doi: 10.1111/jnc.12742
29. Coune, P. G., Schneider, B. L., and Aebischer, P. (2012). Parkinson's disease: gene therapies. *Cold Spring Harb. Perspect. Med.* 2:a009431. doi: 10.1101/ cshperspect. a009431
30. Das, G., Misra, A. K., Das, S. K., Ray, K., and Ray, J. (2009). Microtubule-Associated Protein Tau (MAPT) influences the risk of Parkinson's disease among Indians. *Neurosci. Lett.* 460, 16–20. doi: 10.1016/j.neulet.2009.05.031

31. De Deurwaerdère, P., Di Giovanni, G., and Millan, M. J. (2017). Expanding the repertoire of L-DOPA's actions: a comprehensive review of its functional neurochemistry. *Prog. Neurobiol.* 151, 57–100. doi: 10.1016/j.pneurobio.2016.07.002
32. Dos Santos, M. C. T., Barreto-Sanz, M. A., Correia, B. R. S., Bell, R., Widnall, C., Perez, L. T., et al. (2018). miRNA-based signatures in cerebrospinal fluid as potential diagnostic tools for early tage Parkinson's disease. *Oncotarget* 9, 17455–17465. doi: 10.18632/oncotarget.24736
33. Double, K. L., and Halliday, G. M. (2006). New face of neuromelanin. *J. Neural Transm. Suppl.* 70, 119–123. doi: 10.1007/978-3-211-45295-0_19
34. El-Agnaf, O. M. A., Salem, S. A., Paleologou, K. E., Curran, M. D., Gibson, M. J., Court, J. A., et al. (2006). Detection of oligomeric forms of (-synuclein protein in human plasma as a potential biomarker for Parkinson's disease. *FASEB J.* 20, 419–425. doi: 10.1096/fj.03-1449com
35. Elbaz, A., and Tranchant, C. (2007). Epidemiologic studies of environmental exposures in Parkinson's disease. *Neurol. Sci.* 262, 37–44. doi: 10.1016/j.jns.2007.06.024
36. Emamzadeh, F. N. (2016). Alpha-synuclein structure, functions, and interactions. *J. Res. Med. Sci.?* 21:29. doi: 10.4103/1735-1995.181989
37. Emamzadeh, F. N. (2017). Role of Apolipoproteins and α-Synuclein in Parkinson's disease. *J. Mol. Neurosci.* 62, 344–355. doi: 10.1007/s12031-017-0942-9
38. Estupinan, D., Nathoo, S., and Okun, M. S. (2013). The demise of Poskanzer and Schwab's influenza theory on the pathogenesis of Parkinson's disease. *Parkinsons Dis.* 2013:167843. doi: 10.1155/2013/167843
39. Fazio, P., Svenningsson, P., Forsberg, A., Jönsson, E. G., Amini, N., Nakao, R., et al. (2015). Quantitative Analysis of ^{18}F-(E)-N-(3-Iodoprop-2-Enyl)-2β-Carbofluoroethoxy-3β-(4'-Methyl-Phenyl) nortropane binding to the dopamine transporter in Parkinson disease. *J. Nucl. Med.* 56, 714–720. doi: 10.2967/jnumed.114.152421
40. Feng, Y., Jankovic, J., and Wu, Y. C. (2015). Epigenetic mechanisms in Parkinson's disease. *J. Neurol. Sci.* 349, 3–9. doi: 10.1016/j.jns.2014.12.017
41. Foulds, P. G., Mitchell, J. D., Parker, A., Turner, R., Green, G., Diggle, P., et al. (2011). Phosphorylated α-synuclein can be detected in blood plasma and is potentially a useful biomarker for Parkinson's disease. *FASEB J.* 25, 4127–4137. doi: 10.1096/fj.10-179192
42. Fronczek, R., Overeem, S., Lee, S. Y., Hegeman, I. M., van Pelt, J., van Duinen, S. G., et al. (2007). Hypocretin (orexin) loss in Parkinson's disease. *Brain* 130, 1577–1585. doi: 10.1093/brain/awm090
43. Gill, S. S., Patel, N. K., Hotton, G. R., O'Sullivan, K., McCarter, R., Bunnage, M., et al. (2003). Direct brain infusion of glial cell line-derived neurotrophic factor in Parkinson disease. *Nat. Med.* 9, 589–595. doi: 10.1038/nm850
44. Goldenberg, M. M. (2008). Medical management of Parkinson's disease. *P T* 33, 590–606.
45. Goldstein, D. S. (2001). Cardiac sympathetic neuroimaging to distinguish multiple system atrophy from Parkinson disease. *Clin. Auton. Res.* 11, 341–342. doi: 10.1007/BF02292764
46. Goldstein, D. S. (2013). Sympathetic neuroimaging. *Handb. Clin. Neurol.* 117, 365–370. doi: 10.1016/B978-0-444-53491-0.00029-8
47. Goldstein, D. S., Holmes, C., Lopez, G. J., Wu, T., and Sharabi, Y. (2018). Cerebrospinal fluid biomarkers of central dopamine deficiency predict Parkinson's disease. *Parkinsonism Relat. Disord.* 50, 108–112. doi: 10.1016/j.parkreldis.2018.02.023
48. Graeber, M. B., and Muller, U. (1992). The X-linked dystonia-parkinsonism syndrome: clinical and molecular genetic analysis. *Brain Pathol.* 2, 287–295. doi: 10.1111/j.1750-3639.1992.tb00706.x
49. Gwinn-Hardy, K., Singleton, A., O'Suilleabhain, P., Boss, M., Nicholl, D., Adam, A., et al. (2001). Spinocerebellar ataxia type 3 phenotypically resembling parkinson disease in a black family. *Arch. Neurol.* 58, 296–299. doi: 10.1001/archneur.58. 2.296
50. Hagan, J. J., Leslie, R. A., Patel, S., Evans, M. L., Wattam, T. A., Holmes, S., et al. (1999). Orexin a activates locus coeruleus cell firing and increases arousal in the rat. *Proc. Nat. Acad. Sci. U.S.A.* 96, 10911–10916. doi: 10.1073/pnas.96.19.10911
51. Hare, D., Ayton, S., Bush, A., and Lei, P. (2013). A delicate balance: iron metabolism and diseases of the brain. *Front. Aging Neurosci.* 18:34. doi: 10.3389/fnagi.2013. 00034
52. Havelund, J. F., Heegaard, N. H. H., Færgeman, N. J. K., and Gramsbergen, J. B. (2017). Biomarker research in Parkinson's disease using metabolite profiling. *Metabolites* 7:E42. doi: 10.3390/metabo7030042
53. Henchcliffe, C., Shungu, D. C., Mao, X., Huang, C., Nirenberg, M. J., and Jenkins, B. G. (2008). Multinuclear magnetic resonance spectroscopy for in vivo assessment of mitochondrial dysfunction in Parkinson's disease. *Ann. N. Y. Acad. Sci.* 1147, 206–220. doi: 10.1196/annals.1427.037
54. Herrington, T. M., Cheng, J. J., and Eskandar, E. N. (2016). Mechanisms of deep brain stimulation. *J. Neurophysiol.* 115, 19–38. doi: 10.1152/jn.00281.2015
55. Herzog, J., Fietzek, U., Hamel, W., Morsnowski, A., Steigerwald, F., and Schrader, B. (2004). Most effective stimulation site in subthalamic deep brain stimulation for Parkinson's disease. *Mov. Disord.* 19, 1050–1054. doi: 10.1002/ mds.20056
56. Histed, S. N., Lindenberg, M. L., Mena, E., Turkbey, B., Choyke, P. L., and Kurdziel, K. A. (2012). Review of functional/ anatomic imaging in oncology. *Nucl. Med. Commun.* 33, 349–361. doi: 10.1097/MNM.0b013e32834ec8a5
57. Hochfeld, W. E., Lee, S., and Rubinsztein, D. C. (2013). Therapeutic induction of autophagy to modulate neurodegenerative disease progression. *Acta Pharmacol. Sin.* 34, 600–604. doi: 10.1038/aps.2012.189
58. Höllerhage, M., Moebius, C., Melms, J., Chiu, W. H., Goebel, J. N., Chakroun, T., et al. (2017). Protective efficacy of phosphodiesterase-1 inhibition against alpha- synuclein toxicity revealed by compound screening in LUHMES cells. *Sci. Rep.* 7:11469. doi: 10.1038/s41598-017-11664-5
59. Hong, Z., Shi, M., Chung, K. A., Quinn, J. F., Peskind, E. R., Galasko, D., et al. (2010). DJ-1 and alpha-synuclein in human cerebrospinal fluid as biomarkers of Parkinson's disease. *Brain* 133, 713–726. doi: 10.1093/brain/awq008
60. Iacobazzi, V., Castegna, A., Infantino, V., and Andria, G. (2013). Mitochondrial DNA methylation as a next-generation biomarker and diagnostic tool. *Mol. Genet. Metab.* 110, 25–34. doi: 10.1016/j.ymgme.2013.07.012
61. Ibrahim, N., Kusmirek, J., Struck, A. F., Floberg, J. M., Perlman, S. B., Gallagher, C., et al. (2016). The sensitivity and specificity of F-DOPA PET in a movement disorder clinic. *Am. J. Nucl. Med. Mol. Imaging* 6, 102–109.
62. Imamura, K., Hishikawa, N., Sawada, M., Nagatsu, T., Yoshida, M., and Hashizume, Y. (2003). Distribution of major histocompatibility complex class II-positive microglia and cytokine profile of Parkinson's disease brains. *Acta Neuropathol.* 106, 518–526. doi: 10.1007/s00401-003-0766-2
63. Imperatore, R., Palomba, L., and Cristino, L. (2017). Role of Orexin-a in hypertension and obesity. *Curr. Hypertens. Rep.* 19:34. doi: 10.1007/s11906-017-0729-y
64. Iwata, A., Miura, S., Kanazawa, I., Sawada, M., and Nukina, N. (2001). alpha- Synuclein forms a complex with transcription factor Elk-1. *J. Neurochem.* 77, 239–252. doi: 10.1046/j.1471-4159.2001.t01-1-00232.x
65. Jankovic, J., and Aguilar, G. (2008). Current approaches to the treatment of Parkinson's disease. *Neuropsychiatr. Dis. Treat.* 4, 743–757. doi: 10.2147/NDT. S2006
66. Kachroo, A., and Schwarzschild, M. A. (2012). Adenosine A2A receptor gene disruption protects in an α-synuclein model of Parkinson's disease. *Ann. Neurol.* 71, 278–282. doi: 10.1002/ana.22630
67. Karamohamed, S., DeStefano, A. L., Wilk, J. B., Shoemaker, C. M., Golbe, L. I., Mark, M. H., et al. (2003). A haplotype at the PARK3 locus influences onset age for Parkinson's disease: the GenePD study. *Neurology* 61, 1557–1561. doi: 10.1212/01.WNL.0000095966.99430.F4
68. Karimi-Moghadam, A., Charsouei, S., Bell, B., and Jabalameli, M. R. (2018). Parkinson disease from mendelian forms to genetic susceptibility: new molecular insights into the neurodegeneration process. *Cell. Mol. Neurobiol.* 38, 1153–1178. doi: 10.1007/s10571-018-0587-4
69. Kikuchi, A., Takeda, A., Onodera, H., Kimpara, T., Hisanaga, K., Sato, N., et al. (2002). Systemic increase of oxidative nucleic acid damage in Parkinson's disease and multiple system atrophy. *Neurobiol. Dis.* 9, 244–248. doi: 10.1006/ nbdi.2002.0466
70. Kikuchi, Y., Yasuhara, T., Agari, T., Kondo, A., Kuramoto, S., Kameda, M., et al. (2011). Urinary 8-OHdG elevations in a partial lesion rat model of Parkinson's disease correlate with behavioral symptoms and nigrostriatal dopaminergic depletion. *J. Cell. Physiol.* 226, 1390–1398. doi: 10.1002/jcp. 22467
71. Kitada, T., Asakawa, S., Hattori, N., Matsumine, H., Yamamura, Y., Minoshima, S., et al. (1988). Mutations in the parkin gene cause autosomal recessive juvenile parkinsonism. *Nature* 392, 605–608. doi: 10.1038/33416
72. Koroglu, C., Baysal, L., Cetinkaya, M., Karasoy, H., and Tolun, A. (2013). DNAJC6 is responsible for juvenile parkinsonism with phenotypic variability. *Parkinsonism Relat. Disord.* 19, 320–324. doi: 10.1016/j.parkreldis.2012.11.006

73. Krebs, C. E., Karkheiran, S., Powell, J. C., Cao, M., Makarov, V., Darvish, H., et al. (2013). The Sac1 domain of SYNJ1 identified mutated in a family with early-onset progressive parkinsonism with generalized seizures. *Hum. Mutat.* 34, 1200–1207. doi: 10.1002/humu.22372
74. Langston, J. W. (1996). The etiology of Parkinson's disease with emphasis on the MPTP story. *Neurology* 47, 153–160. doi: 10.1212/WNL.47.6_Suppl_3.153S Lautier, C., Goldwurm, S., Durr, A., Giovannone, B., Tsiaras, W. G., and Pezzoli, G.
75. (2008). Mutations in the GIGYF2 (TNRC15) gene at the PARK11 locus in familial Parkinson disease. *Am. J. Hum. Genet.* 82, 822–833. doi: 10.1016/j.ajhg. 2008.01.015
76. Lauretani, F., Saginario, A., Ceda, G. P., Galuppo, L., Ruffini, L., Nardelli, A., et al. (2014). Treatment of the motor and non-motor symptoms in Parkinson's disease according to cluster symptoms presentation. *Curr. Drug Targets* 15, 943–947.
77. Le, W., Xu, P., Jankovic, J., Jiang, H., Appel, S. H., Smith, R. G., et al. (2003). Mutations in NR4A2 associated with familial Parkinson disease. *Nat. Genet.* 33, 85–89. doi: 10.1038/ng1066
78. Lee, H., Baek, S. M., Ho, D., Suk, J., Cho, E., and Lee, S. (2011). Dopamine promotes formation and secretion of non-fibrillar alpha-synuclein oligomers. *Exp. Mol. Med.* 43, 216–222. doi: 10.3858/emm.2011.43.4.026
79. Leroy, E., Boyer, R., Auburger, G., Leube, B., Ulm, G., Mezey, E., et al. (1998). The ubiquitin pathway in Parkinson's disease. *Nature* 395, 451–452. doi: 10.1038/ 26652
80. Levin, J., Schmidt, F., Boehm, C., Prix, C., Bötzel, K., Ryazanov, S., et al. (2014). The oligomer modulator anle138b inhibits disease progression in a Parkinson mouse model even with treatment started after disease onset. *Acta Neuropathol.* 127, 779–780. doi: 10.1007/s00401-014-1265-3
81. LeWitt, P. A., Rezai, A. R., Leehey, M. A., Ojemann, S. G., Flaherty, A. W., Eskandar, E. N., et al. (2011). AAV2-GAD gene therapy for advanced Parkinson's disease: a double-blind, sham-surgery controlled, randomised trial. *Lancet Neurol.* 10, 309–319. doi: 10.1016/S1474-4422(11)70039-4
82. Li, D. H., Wang, J., Mao, C. J., Hu, W. D., Xiao, L., Yang, Y. P., et al. (2011).
83. Association of PARK 16 polymorphisms with Parkinson's disease in Han population of Suzhou. *Zhonghua Yi Xue Za Zhi* 91, 296–300. doi: 10.1016/ S1474-4422(11)70039-4
84. Li, Q. X., Mok, S. S., Laughton, K. M., McLean, C. A., Cappai, R., Masters, C. L., et al. (2007). Plasma alpha-synuclein is decreased in subjects with Parkinson's disease. *Exp. Neurol.* 204, 583–588. doi: 10.1016/j. expneurol.2006. 12.006
85. Liddle, R. A. (2018). Parkinson's disease from the gut. *Brain Res.* 1693(Pt B), 201–206. doi: 10.1016/j.brainres.2018.01.010
86. Lin, C.-H., Chen, M.-L., Chen, G. S., Tai, C.-H., and Wu, R.-M. (2011). Novel variant Pro143Ala in *HTRA2* contributes to Parkinson's disease by inducing hyperphosphorylation of HTRA2 protein in mitochondria. *Hum. Genet.* 130, 817–827. doi: 10.1007/s00439-011-1041-6
87. Lin, K. J., Weng, Y. H., Hsieh, C. J., Lin, W. Y., Wey, S. P., Kung, M. P., et al. (2013). Brain imaging of vesicular monoamine transporter type 2 in healthy aging subjects by 18F-FP-(+)-DTBZ PET. *PLoS One* 8:e75952. doi: 10.1371/ journal.pone.0075952
88. Lin, L. F., Doherty, D. H., Lile, J. D., Bektesh, S., and Collins, F. (1993). GDNF: a glial cell line-derived neurotrophic factor for midbrain dopaminergic neurons. *Science* 260, 1130–1132. doi: 10.1126/science.8493557
89. Lodish, H., Berk, A., Matsudaira, P., Kaiser, C. A., Krieger, M., Scott, M. P., et al. (2004). in *Molecular Cell Biology*, 5th Edn, ed. J. Darnell (New York, NY: W.H. Freeman and CO), 66–72.
90. Luk, K. C., Kehm, V., Carroll, J., Zhang, B., O'Brien, P., Trojanowski, J. Q., et al. (2012). Pathological α-synuclein transmission initiates parkinson-like neurodegeneration in non-transgenic mice. *Science* 16, 949–953. doi: 10.1126/ science.1227157
91. Mahami Oskouei, M., Hamidi, F., Talebi, M., Farhoudi, M., Taheraghdam, A. A., and Kazemi, T. (2016). The correlation between *Toxoplasma gondii* infection and Parkinson's disease: a case-control study. *J. Parasit. Dis.* 40, 872–876. doi: 10.1007/s12639-014-0595-3
92. Martins-Branco, D., Esteves, A. R., Santos, D., Arduino, D. M., Swerdlow, R. H., and Oliveira, C. R. (2012). Ubiquitin proteasome system in Parkinson's disease: a keeper or a witness? *Exp. Neurol.* 238, 89–99. doi: 10.1016/j. expneurol.2012. 08.008
93. Masuda-Suzukake, M., Nonaka, T., Hosokawa, M., Oikawa, T., Arai, T., Akiyama, H., et al. (2013). Prion-like spreading of pathological α-synuclein in brain. *Brain* 136, 1128–1138. doi: 10.1093/brain/awt037
94. Matsumoto, L., Takuma, H., Tamaoka, A., Kurisaki, H., Date, H., Tsuji, S., et al. (2010). CpG demethylation enhances alpha-synuclein expression and affects the pathogenesis of Parkinson's disease. *PLoS One* 5:e15522. doi: 10.1371/journal. pone.0015522
95. McKeith, I. G., Boeve, B. F., Dickson, D. W., Halliday, G., Taylor, J. P., Weintraub, D., et al. (2017). Diagnosis and management of dementia with Lewy bodies: fourth consensus report of the DLB consortium. *Neurology* 89, 88–100. doi: 10.1212/WNL.0000000000004058
96. McLean, P. J., Kawamata, H., Ribich, S., and Hyman, B. T. (2000). Membrane association and protein conformation of α-synuclein in intact neurons. Effect of Parkinson's disease-linked mutations. *J. Biol. Chem.* 275, 8812–8816. doi: 10.1074/jbc.275.12.8812
97. Miman, O., Kusbeci, O. Y., Aktepe, O. C., and Cetinkaya, Z. (2010). The probable relation between *Toxoplasma gondii* and Parkinson's disease. *Neurosci. Lett.* 475, 129–131. doi: 10.1016/j.neulet.2010.03.057
98. Mittermeyer, G., Christine, C. W., Rosenbluth, K. H., Baker, S. L., Starr, P., Larson, P., et al. (2012). Long-term evaluation of a phase 1 study of AADC gene therapy for Parkinson's disease. *Hum. Gene Ther.* 23, 377–381. doi: 10.1089/ hum.2011.220
99. Mollenhauer, B., Locascio, J. J., Schulz-Schaeffer, W., Sixel-Döring, F., Trenkwalder, C., and Schlossmacher, M. G. (2011). α-Synuclein and tau concentrations in cerebrospinal fluid of patients presenting with parkinsonism: a cohort study. *Lancet Neurol.* 10, 230–240. doi: 10.1016/S1474-4422(11)70014-X
100. Muramatsu, S., Fujimoto, K., Kato, S., Mizukami, H., Asari, S., Ikeguchi, K., et al. (2010). A phase I study of aromatic L-amino acid decarboxylase gene therapy for Parkinson's disease. *Mol. Ther.* 18, 1731–1735. doi: 10.1038/ mt.2010.135
101. Nagai, Y., Ueno, S., Saeki, Y., Soga, F., Hirano, M., and Yanagihara, T. (1996). Decrease of the D3 dopamine receptor mRNA expression in lymphocytes from patients with Parkinson's disease. *Neurology* 46, 791–795. doi: 10.1212/WNL.46. 3.791
102. Niethammer, M., Feigin, A., and Eidelberg, D. (2012). Functional neuroimaging in Parkinson's disease. *Cold Spring Harb. Perspect. Med.* 2:a009274. doi: 10.1101/ cshperspect.a009274
103. Obeso, J. A., Rodríguez-Oroz, M. C., Benitez-Temino, B., Blesa, F. J., Guridi, J., Marin, C., et al. (2008). Functional organization of the basal ganglia: therapeutic implications for Parkinson's disease. *Mov. Disord.* 23, 548–559. doi: 10.1002/ mds.22062
104. Oertel, W. H. (2017). Recent advances in treating Parkinson's disease. *F1000Res.* 6:260. doi: 10.12688/f1000research.10100.1
105. Oh, J. K., Choi, E. K., Song, I. U., Kim, J. S., and Chung, Y. A. (2015). Comparison of I-123 MIBG planar imaging and SPECT for the detection of decreased heart uptake in Parkinson disease. *J. Neural Transm. (Vienna)* 122, 1421–1427. doi: 10.1007/s00702-015-1409-1
106. Olanow, C. W., Kieburtz, K., Odin, P., Espay, A. J., Standaert, D. G., Fernandez, H. H., et al. (2014). Continuous intrajejunal infusion of levodopa-carbidopa intestinal gel for patients with advanced Parkinson's disease: a randomised, controlled, double-blind, double-dummy study. *Lancet Neurol.* 13, 141–149. doi: 10.1016/S1474-4422(13)70293-X
107. Paisan-Ruiz, C., Bhatia, K. P., Li, A., Hernandez, D., Davis, M., Wood, N. W., et al. (2009). Characterization of PLA2G6 as a locus for dystonia-parkinsonism. *Ann. Neurol.* 65, 19–23. doi: 10.1002/ana.21415
108. Perni, M., Galvagnion, C., Maltsev, A., Meisl, G., Müller, M. B., Challa, P. K., et al. (2017). A natural product inhibits the initiation of α-synuclein aggregation and suppresses its toxicity. *Proc. Natl. Acad. Sci. U.S.A.* 114, E1009–E1017. doi: 10.1073/pnas.1610586114
109. Pirker, W., Asenbaum, S., Wenger, S., Kornhuber, J., Angelberger, P., Deecke, L., et al. (1997). Iodine-123-epidepride-SPECT: studies in Parkinson's disease, multiple system atrophy and Huntington's disease. *J. Nucl. Med.* 38, 1711–1717. Plaha, P., Ben-Shlomo, Y., Patel, N. K., and Gill, S. S. (2006). Stimulation of the caudal zona incerta is superior to stimulation of the subthalamic nucleus in improving contralateral parkinsonism. *Brain* 129, 1732–1747. doi: 10.1093/brain/awl127
110. Pulkes, T., Choubtum, L., Chitphuk, S., Thakkinstian, A., Pongpakdee, S., Kulkantrakorn, K., et al. (2014). Glucocerebrosidase mutations in Thai patients with Parkinson's disease. *Parkinsonism Relat. Disord.* 20, 986–991. doi: 10.1016/ j.parkreldis.2014.06.007
111. Ramirez, A., Heimbach, A., and Grundemann, J. (2006). Hereditary

parkinsonism with dementia is caused by mutations in ATP13A2, encoding a lysosomal type 5 P-type ATPase. *Nat. Genet.* 38, 1184–1191. doi: 10.1038/ng1884
112. Rappold, P. M., and Tieu, K. (2010). Astrocytes and therapeutics for Parkinson's disease. *Neurotherapeutics* 7, 413–423. doi: 10.1016/j.nurt.2010.07.001
113. Reiche, W., Grundmann, M., and Huber, G. (1995). Dopamine (D2) receptor SPECT with 123I-iodobenzamide (IBZM) in diagnosis of Parkinson syndrome. *Radiologie* 35, 838–843.
114. Reichmann, H., Brandt, M. D., and Klingelhoefer, L. (2016). The nonmotor features of Parkinson's disease: pathophysiology and management advances. *Curr. Opin. Neurol.* 29, 467–473. doi: 10.1097/WCO.0000000000000348
115. Reiter, R. J. (1995). Oxidative processes and antioxidative defense mechanisms in the aging brain. *FASEB J.* 9, 526–533. doi: 10.1096/fasebj.9.7.7737461
116. Rinne, J., Ruottinen, H., Bergman, J., Haaparanta, M., Sonninen, P., and Solin, O. (1999). Usefulness of a dopamine transporter PET ligand [18F] β-CFT in assessing disability in Parkinson's disease. *J. Neurol. Neurosurg. Psychiatry* 67, 737–741. doi: 10.1136/jnnp.67.6.737
117. Saeed, U., Compagnone, J., Aviv, R. I., Strafella, A. P., Black, S. E., Lang, A. E., et al. (2017). Imaging biomarkers in Parkinson's disease and Parkinsonian syndromes: current and emerging concepts. *Transl. Neurodegener.* 6:8. doi: 10.1186/s40035-017-0076-6
118. Samii, A., Nutt, J. G., and Ransom, B. R. (2004). Parkinson's disease. *Lancet* 363, 1783–1793. doi: 10.1016/S0140-6736(04)16305-8
119. Sasaki, T., Amano, T., Hashimoto, J., Itoh, Y., Muramatsu, K., Kubo, A., et al. (2003). [SPECT imaging using [123I]beta-CIT and [123I]IBF in extrapyramidal diseases]. *No To Shinkei* 55, 57–64.
120. Satake, W., Nakabayashi, Y., Mizuta, I., Hirota, Y., Ito, C., and Kubo, M. (2009). Genome-wide association study identifies common variants at four loci as genetic risk factors for Parkinson's disease. *Nat. Genet.* 41, 1303–1307. doi: 10.1038/ng.485
121. Scriabine, A. (1999). "Discovery and development of major drugs currently in use," in *The Pharmaceutical Innovation: Revolutionizing Human Health*, ed. A. Scriabine (Philadelphia: Chemical Heritage Press), 222–223.
122. Seppi, K., Schocke, M. F., Esterhammer, R., Kremser, C., Brenneis, C., Mueller, J., et al. (2003). Diffusion-weighted imaging discriminates progressive supranuclear palsy from PD, but not from the parkinson variant of multiple system atrophy. *Neurology* 60, 922–927. doi: 10.1212/01.WNL.0000049911. 91657.9D
123. Seraji-Bozorgzad, N., Bao, F., George, E., Krstevska, S., Gorden, V., Chorostecki, J., et al. (2015). Longitudinal study of the substantia nigra in Parkinson disease: a high-field 1 H-MR spectroscopy imaging study. *Mov. Disord.* 30, 1400–1404. doi: 10.1002/mds.26323
124. Shadrina, M. I., Slominsky, P. A., and Limborska, S. A. (2010). Chapter 6. Molecular Mechanisms of Pathogenesis of Parkinson's disease. *Int. Rev. Cell Mol. Biol.* 281, 229–266. doi: 10.1016/S1937-6448(10)81006-8
125. Shi, C.-h., Tang, B.-s., Wang, L., Lv, Z.-y., Wang, J., Luo, L.-z., et al. (2011). *PLA2G6*
126. gene mutation in autosomal recessive early-onset parkinsonism in a Chinese cohort. *Neurology* 77, 75–81. doi: 10.1212/WNL.0b013e318221acd3
127. Shigenaga, M., Gimeno, C. J., and Ames, B. N. (1989). Urinary 8-hydroxy-2'-deoxyguanosine as a biomarker of in vivo oxidative DNA damage. *Proc. Natl. Acad. Sci. U.S.A.* 86, 9697–9701. doi: 10.1073/pnas.86.24.9697
128. Siderowf, A., Aarsland, D., Mollenhauer, B., Goldman, J. G., and Ravina, B. (2018). Biomarkers for cognitive impairment in Lewy body disorders: status and relevance for clinical trials. *Mov. Disord.* 33, 528–536. doi: 10.1002/mds.27355
129. Simon, D. K., Simuni, T., Elm, J., Clark-Matott, J., Graebner, A. K., and Baker, L. (2015). Peripheral biomarkers of Parkinson's disease progression and Pioglitazone effects. *J. Parkinsons Dis.* 4, 731–736. doi: 10.3233/JPD-150666
130. Singleton, A. B., Farrer, M., Johnson, J., Singleton, A., Hague, S., Kachergus, J., et al. (2003). A-synuclein locus triplication causes Parkinson's disease. *Science* 302:841. doi: 10.1126/science.1090278
131. Skoloudík, D., Jelínková, M., Blahuta, J., Cermák, P., Soukup, T., Bártová, P., et al. (2014). Transcranial sonography of the substantia nigra: digital image analysis. *AJNR Am. J. Neuroradiol.* 35, 2273–2278. doi: 10.3174/ajnr.A4049
132. Steiner, J. A., Quansah, E., and Brundin, P. (2018). The concept of alpha-synuclein as a prion-like protein: ten years after. *Cell Tissue Res.* 373, 161–173. doi: 10.1007/s00441-018-2814-1
133. Strauss, K. M., Martins, L. M., Plun-Favreau, H., Marx, F. P., Kautzmann, S., Berg, D., et al. (2005). Loss of function mutations in the gene encoding Omi/HtrA2 in Parkinson's disease. *Hum. Mol. Genet.* 14, 2099–2111. doi: 10.1093/hmg/ddi215
134. Sui, Y. T., Bullock, K. M., Erickson, M. A., Zhang, J., and Banks, W. A. (2014). Alpha synuclein is transported into and out of the brain by the blood-brain barrier. *Peptides* 62, 197–202. doi: 10.1016/j.peptides.2014.09.018
135. Surgucheva, I., and Surguchov, A. (2008). Gamma-synuclein: cell-type-specific promoter activity and binding to transcription factors. *J. Mol. Neurosci.* 35, 267–271. doi: 10.1007/s12031-008-9074-6
136. Surguchov, A. (2015). Intracellular dynamics of synucleins: here, there and everywhere. *Int. Rev. Cell Mol. Biol.* 320, 103–169. doi: 10.1016/bs.ircmb.2015. 07.007
137. Surguchov, A., Surgucheva, I., Sharma, M., Sharma, R., and Singh V. (2017). Pore- forming proteins as mediators of novel epigenetic mechanism of epilepsy. *Front. Neurol.* 8:3. doi: 10.3389/fneur.2017.00003
138. Swanson, C. R., Berlyand, Y., Xie, S. X., Alcalay, R. N., Chahine, L. M., and Chen-Plotkin, A. S. (2015). Plasma apolipoprotein A1 associates with age at onset and motor severity in early Parkinson's disease patients. *Mov. Disord.* 30, 1648–1656. doi: 10.1002/mds.26290
139. Takahashi, Y., Kanbayashi, T., Hoshikawa, M., Imanishi, A., Sagawa, Y., Tsutsui, K., et al. (2015). Relationship of orexin (hypocretin) system and astrocyte activation in Parkinson's disease with hypersomnolence. *Sleep Biol. Rhythms* 13, 252–260. doi: 10.1111/sbr.12112
140. Tan, E.-K., Lin, C.-H., Tai, C.-H., Tan, L. C., Chen, M.-L., and Li, R. (2009). Non-synonymous GIGYF2 variants in Parkinson's disease from two Asian populations. *Hum. Genet.* 126, 425–430. doi: 10.1007/s00439-009- 0678-x
141. Tell-Marti, G., Puig-Butille, J. A., Potrony, M., Badenas, C., Milà, M., and Malvehy, J. (2015). The MC1R melanoma risk variant p.R160W is associated with Parkinson disease. *Ann. Neurol.* 77, 889–894. doi: 10.1002/ana. 24373
142. Tong, J., Wilson, A. A., Boileau, I., Houle, S., and Kish, S. J. (2008). Dopamine modulating drugs influence striatal (+)-[11C]DTBZ binding in rats: VMAT2 binding is sensitive to changes in vesicular dopamine concentration. *Synapse* 62, 873–876. doi: 10.1002/syn.20573
143. Valente, E. M., Abou-Sleiman, P. M., Caputo, V., Muqit, M. M., Harvey, K., Gispert, S., et al. (2004). Hereditary early-onset Parkinson's disease caused by mutations in PINK1. *Science* 304, 1158–1160. doi: 10.1126/science.1096284
144. van der Zee, S., Vermeiren, Y., Fransen, E., Van Dam, D., Aerts, T., Gerritsen, M. J., et al. (2018). Monoaminergic markers across the cognitive spectrum of Lewy body disease. *J. Parkinsons Dis.* 8, 71–84. doi: 10.3233/JPD-171228
145. van Duijn, C. M., Dekker, M. C., Bonifati, V., Galjaard, R. J., Houwing-Duistermaat, J. J., Snijders, P. J., et al. (2001). Park7, a novel locus for autosomal recessive early-onset parkinsonism, on chromosome 1p36. *Am. J. Hum. Genet.* 69, 629–634. doi: 10.1086/322996
146. Venda, L. L., Cragg, S. J., Buchman, V. L., and Wade-Martins, R. (2010). α-Synuclein and dopamine at the crossroads of Parkinson's disease. *Trends Neurosci.* 33, 559–568. doi: 10.1016/j.tins.2010.09.004
147. Vermeiren, Y., and De Deyn, P. P. (2017). Targeting the norepinephrinergic system in Parkinson's disease and related disorders: the locus coeruleus story. *Neurochem. Int.* 102, 22–32. doi: 10.1016/j.neuint.2016.11.009
148. Vilariño-Güell, C., Rajput, A., Milnerwood, A. J., Shah, B., Szu-Tu, C., Trinh, J., et al. (2014). DNAJC13 mutations in Parkinson disease. *Hum. Mol. Genet.* 23, 1794–1801. doi: 10.1093/hmg/ddt570
149. Vilariño-Güell, C., Wider, C., Ross, O. A., Dachsel, J. C., Kachergus, J. M., and Lincoln, S. J. (2011). VPS35 mutations in Parkinson disease. *Am. J. Hum. Genet.* 89, 162–167. doi: 10.1016/j.ajhg.2011.06.001
150. Vitali, C., Wellington, C. L., and Calabresi, L. (2014). HDL and cholesterol handling in the brain. *Cardiovasc. Res.* 103, 405–413. doi: 10.1093/cvr/cvu148
151. Vitali, M. C. T., Barreto-Sanz, M. A., Correia, B. R. S., Bell, R., Widnall, C., Perez, L. T., et al. (2018). miRNA-based signatures in cerebrospinal fluid as potential diagnostic tools for early stage Parkinson's disease. *Oncotarget* 9, 17455–17465. doi: 10.18632/oncotarget.24736
152. Wang, E. S., Sun, Y., Guo, J. G., Gao, X., Hu, J. W., Zhou, L., et al. (2010). Tetranectin and apolipoprotein A-I in cerebrospinal fluid as potential biomarkers for Parkinson's disease. *Acta Neurol. Scand.* 122, 350–359. doi: 10.1111/j.1600-0404.2009.01318.x
153. Wang, L., Zhang, Q., Li, H., and Zhang, H. (2012). SPECT molecular

imaging in Parkinson's disease. *J. Biomed. Biotechnol.* 2012;412486. doi: 10.1155/2012/ 412486

154. Watanabe, M., Maemura, K., Kanbara, K., Tamayama, T., and Hayasaki, H. (2002). GABA and GABA receptors in the central nervous system and other organs. *Int. Rev. Cytol.* 213, 1–47. doi: 10.1016/S0074-7696(02) 13011-7

155. Wienecke, M., Werth, E., Poryazova, R., Baumann-Vogel, H., Bassetti, C. L., Weller, M., et al. (2012). Progressive dopamine and hypocretin deficiencies in Parkinson's disease: is there an impact on sleep and wakefulness? *J. Sleep Res.* 21, 710–717. doi: 10.1111/j.1365-2869.2012.01027.x

156. Wu, Y. R., Lin, H. Y., Chen, C. M., Gwinn-Hardy, K., Ro, L. S., Wang, Y. C., et al. (2004). Genetic testing in spinocerebellar ataxia in Taiwan: expansions of trinucleotide repeats in SCA8 and SCA17 are associated with typical Parkinson's disease. *Clin. Genet.* 65, 209–214. doi: 10.1111/j.0009-9163.2004. 00213.x

157. Xu, L., Ma, B., Nussinov, R., and Thompson, D. (2017). Familial Mutations May Switch Conformational Preferences in α-Synuclein Fibrils. *ACS Chem. Neurosci.* 8, 837–849. doi: 10.1021/acschemneuro.6b00406

158. Yang, Z., Wang, X., Yang, J., Sun, M., Wang, Y., and Wang, X. (2017). Aberrant CpG methylation mediates abnormal transcription of MAO-A. *Neurotox. Res.* 31, 334–347. doi: 10.1007/s12640-016-9686-5

159. Yonekura, Y., Saji, H., Iwasaki, Y., Tsuchida, T., Fukuyama, H., Shimatsu, A., et al. (1995). Initial clinical experiences with dopamine D2 receptor imaging by means of 2'-iodospiperone and single-photon emission computed tomography. *Ann. Nucl. Med.* 9, 131–136. doi: 10.1007/BF03165039

160. Yu, S., Li, X., Liu, G., Han, J., Zhang, C., Li, Y., et al. (2007). Extensive nuclear localization of α-synuclein in normal rat brain neurons revealed by a novel monoclonal antibody. *Neuroscience* 145, 539–555. doi: 10.1016/j. neuroscience. 2006.12.028

161. Zeng, X. S., Geng, W. S., Jia, J. J., Chen, L., and Zhang, P. P. (2018). Cellular and molecular basis of neurodegeneration in Parkinson disease. *Front. Aging Neurosci.* 10:109. doi: 10.3389/fnagi.2018.00109

162. Zimprich, A., Biskup, S., Leitner, P., Lichtner, P., Farrer, M., Lincoln, S., et al. (2004). Mutations in LRRK2 cause autosomal-dominant parkinsonism with pleomorphic pathology. *Neuron* 44, 601–607. doi: 10.1016/j. neuron.2004.11. 005

163. Zucca, F. A., Basso, E., Cupaioli, F. A., Ferrari, E., Sulzer, D., Casella, L., et al. (2014). Neuromelanin of the human substantia nigra: an update. *Neurotox. Res.* 25, 13–23. doi: 10.1007/s12640-013-9435-y

18

Biomarkers in Vasculitides of the Nervous System

*Daniel Strunk, Antje Schmidt-Pogoda, Carolin Beuker, Lennart S. Milles, Catharina Korsukewitz, Sven G. Meuth and Jens Minnerup**

Department of Neurology, Institute for Translational Neurology, University of Münster, Münster, Germany

***Correspondence:**
Jens Minnerup
jens.minnerup@ukmuenster.de

Besides being affected by the rare and severe primary angiitis of the central nervous system (PACNS) the nervous system is also affected by primary systemic vasculitides (PSV). In contrast to PACNS, PSV affect not only the central but also the peripheral nervous system, resulting in a large array of potential symptoms. Given the high burden of disease, difficulties in distinguishing between differential diagnoses, and incomplete pathophysiological insights, there is an urgent need for additional precise diagnostic tools to enable an earlier diagnosis and initiation of effective treatments. Methods available to date, such as inflammatory markers, antibodies, cerebrospinal fluid (CSF) analysis, imaging, and biopsy, turn out to be insufficient to meet all current challenges. We highlight the use of biomarkers as an approach to extend current knowledge and, ultimately, improve patient management. Biomarkers are considered to be useful for disease diagnosis and monitoring, for predicting response to treatment, and for prognosis in clinical practice, as well as for establishing outcome parameters in clinical trials. In this article, we review the recent literature on biomarkers which have been applied in the context of different types of nervous system vasculitides including PACNS, giant-cell arteritis, Takayasu's arteritis, polyarteritis nodosa, ANCA (anti-neutrophil cytoplasm antibody)-associated vasculitides, cryoglobulinemic vasculitis, IgA vasculitis, and Behçet's disease. Overall, the majority of biomarkers is not specific for vasculitides of the nervous system.

Keywords: PACNS, Primary systemic vasculitides, biomarkers, inflammation, differential diagnoses

INTRODUCTION

Primary angiitis of the central nervous system (PACNS) is a rare and often devastating disease with high morbidity and mortality. Major clinical manifestations include ischemic and hemorrhagic stroke, headache and encephalopathy (1). In addition to PACNS, the nervous system may be also affected by primary systemic vasculitides (PSV), which manifest primarily in the context of vasculitides of small and medium sized vessels, e.g., in ANCA-associated vasculitides and polyarteritis nodosa. Due to the severity of nervous system involvement, aggressive immunosuppressive treatments, e.g., high-dose glucocorticoids and cyclophosphamide, are frequently required for remission induction in both, PACNS and PSV. Nonetheless, chronic neuronal damage and persisting symptoms are frequent, even after early immunosuppressive treatment initiation (1).

With respect to the high disease burden there is an urgent need for additional precise diagnostic tools enabling an early diagnosis and treatment initiation. The use of biomarkers may emerge as a valuable approach to overcome these problems. The term "biomarker" is based on the two words "biological" and "marker." Biomarkers can be extracted from different kinds of body fluids and tissues, and are applied as surrogate parameters for various medical conditions (2, 3).

This review aims to give a concise overview of current areas of application for biomarkers with regard to pathogenesis, clinical manifestation, and management of PACNS and those PSV with nervous system involvement. Although biomarkers derived from biopsy specimens are of unquestionable value, this review puts special emphasis on biomarkers derived from body fluids, because biomarkers that can be isolated from body fluids are more likely to be integrated in daily clinical practice (3).

BIOMARKERS IN PRIMARY ANGIITIS OF THE CENTRAL NERVOUS SYSTEM (PACNS)

PACNS is an important cause of stroke and is difficult to differentiate from other conditions that also result in stroke (4). Men are affected twice as often as women. The mean age at disease onset is 50 years (5). Symptoms of PACNS are diverse and not specific. Among them are, in particular, headache, altered cognition, and focal neurologic deficits such as hemiparesis, hemihypesthesia, ataxia, aphasia, dysarthria, and visual disturbances (6). Further typical clinical manifestations are seizures and encephalopathy. The gold standard for the diagnosis of PACNS is a biopsy of brain parenchyma and leptomeninges. Due to possible sampling errors, a negative result does not necessarily mean that PACNS can be ruled out, though (7). Further examinations, including magnetic resonance imaging (MRI), magnetic resonance angiography (MRA), digital subtraction angiography (DSA), or cerebrospinal fluid (CSF) analysis exhibit a rather high degree of sensitivity whereas specificity assumes low values (8). Well-known markers of inflammation and autoimmunity, such as C-reactive protein (CRP), erythrocyte sedimentation rate (ESR), rheumatic antibodies (ANA, dsDNA, ENA, ANCA), and oligoclonal bands do not play a decisive role in PACNS (9).

Our own group retrospectively analyzed the composition of CSF immune cells in patients with PACNS in comparison with sex- and age-matched patients with ischemic stroke, multiple sclerosis, and somatoform disorders by means of multi-parameter flow cytometry (10). PACNS patients were shown to have higher CSF leukocyte counts than controls (10). Some individuals exhibited a shift toward NK (natural killer) or B cells while proportions of T cell subsets remained unmodified. In other patients, we detected higher numbers of plasma cells and an immunoglobulin synthesis within the central nervous system (10). Altogether, characteristics of the intrathecal immune-cell profile were heterogenous in PACNS patients in this study (10).

Ruland et al. employed ion mobility mass spectrometry for unbiased proteomic profiling to further elucidate the pathophysiologic principles and potential biomarkers of PACNS, and identified fourteen proteins from neuronal structures that might be of importance, among others amyloid—beta A4 protein (APP) (11). Amyloid-beta proteins are metal chelators which reduce metal. They are said to activate mononuclear cells in the central nervous systems and evoke inflammatory processes. Both, APP or its fission product beta-amyloid, respectively, are known to be involved in other diseases of the vasculature of the central nervous system, e.g., Amyloid Beta-Related Angiitis (ABRA) (9, 11). This is why the authors highlight the possibility of inflammatory and degenerative processes being intertwined in PACNS (11).

Thom et al. evaluated the potential role of the proinflammatory cytokine interleukin-17 (IL-17), measured in the CSF by flow cytometry, as a biomarker for cerebral vasculitis in patients with stroke. As a major finding, Thom et al. found a marked and persisting increase in IL-17 production in individuals with PACNS compared to patients with non-inflammatory neurological diseases (12). Another study supports the concept of $CD4^+$ T cells being of major importance in vasculitic conditions by detecting an elevated percentage of this cell type in the CSF of individuals with amyloid-ß related cerebral angiitis (13), thus suggesting intrathecal $CD4^+$ T cells as a possible biomarker in PACNS.

The amount of circulating von Willebrand factor antigen (vWF) seems to correlate with a clinical global assessment of disease activity in childhood PACNS (14). vWF is a glycoprotein important for platelet aggregation and the protection of coagulation factor VIII from proteolysis (15). vWF is released by endothelial cells after vascular injury. Consequently an increase in vFW levels may indicate inflammatory processes of the vasculature (14). vWF seems to be an informative indicator of active inflammation in infants but not in adults due to increasing vWF levels with age (14). In Cellucci's study, increased vWF antigen levels were detected at the timepoint of diagnosis in 65% of children with PACNS and showed a significant decrease after treatment initiation (14). The authors found that elevated values of vWF antigen at the timepoint of diagnosis might be indicative of a less active cPACNS after 12 months of course of disease (14). Therefore, vWF antigen represents a promising biomarker of disease activity in children. One of the study's limitations is that results have been derived from experiences at a single medical center in Canada. Consequently its findings cannot be generalized, the more so as adult patients were not examined (14). To overcome these limitations, further investigations in children and adults should be carried out.

In contrast to vWF, the acute phase reactants C-reactive protein (CRP) and erythrocyte sedimentation rate (ESR) did not show a correlation with disease activity, which is not surprising, given that their levels are known to increase in response to many kinds of inflammatory states not necessarily linked to the vasculature (14).

Taking the above mentioned limitations into consideration, none of these potential biomarkers is sufficiently tested and validated in adult patients with PACNS. For a summary of biomarkers, see **Tables 1, 2**.

BIOMARKERS IN PRIMARY SYSTEMIC VASCULITIDES

The biomarkers currently used for PSV are well-known and were established before the use of the term "biomarker." The majority of such markers are highly useful for diagnosing systemic vasculitis. Among others, antibodies to proteinase-3 (PR3) and myeloperoxidase (MPO) are highly specific for ANCA (anti-neutrophil cytoplasm antibody)-associated vasculitides. ANCA is an autoantibody against endogenous neutrophilic leukocytes. According to their target antigen they can be divided into c- (anti-PR3, elevated in tuberculosis, HIV infection, uveitis, amoebiasis, and cystic fibrosis with superinfection), p- (anti-MPO, of importance to microscopic polyangiitis, eosinophilic granulomatosis with polyangiitis, and pauci-immunen glomerulonephritis), and a-ANCA (Crohn's disease, autoimmune hepatitis) (16). The identification of ANCA is not essential for the diagnosis: About 10–20% of patients with granulomatosis with polyangiitis or microscopic polyangiitis and about 60% of patients with eosinophilic granulomatosis with polyangiitis (EPGA), previously known as Churg-Strauss syndrome, are ANCA negative (17). Erythrocyte sedimentation rate (ESR) and C-reactive protein (CRP), the most common laboratory signs of inflammation in general, are usually considered being helpful in identifying active vasculitis, especially in untreated patients, or ruling out this kind of disease. Nonetheless, all of these markers are much less useful for assessing disease activity in patients with established diagnoses. In the following, this and other aspects will be addressed in the context of the most relevant vasculitides, introducing each section with a brief engram of the respective disease.

TABLE 1 | Summary of traditional and already sufficiently tested biomarkers and their meaning in vasculitides with neurological manifestations.

Type of vasculitis	Biomarker	Meaning
Primary angiitis of the central nervous system	–	–
Giant-cell arteritis	CRP, ESR	Inflammatory markers, diagnosis, monitoring disease activity
	IL-6	Disease activity
Takayasu's arteritis	IL-6	Disease state and activity
Polyarteritis nodosa	–	–
ANCA (anti-neutrophil cytoplasm antibody)-associated vasculitides	CRP to serum albumin ratio	All-cause mortality
	Delta neutrophil index	Correlation with Birmingham vasculitis activity score; Predicting course of disease/relapses
	PR3-ANCA, MPO-ANCA	Diagnosis, Monitoring and predicting course of disease
Granulomatosis with polyangiitis	CRP, ESR, anti-PR3, and anti-MPO titers	Disease activity; Predicting flares
	B cell reconstitution and ANCA-PR3 level	Predicting relapse in patients treated with rituximab
Microscopic polyangiitis	–	–
Eosinophilic granulomatosis with polyangiitis	–	–
Cryoglobulinemic vasculitis	–	–
Henoch-Schönlein purpura	Serum biomarker index	Diagnosis
Behçet's disease	HLA B51	Diagnosis

vWF, Von Willebrand factor; CSF, Cerebrospinal fluid; IL, Interleukin; CD, Cluster of differentiation; NK cells, Natural killer cells; CRP, C-reactive protein; ESR, Erythrocyte sedimentation rate; SGTB, Small Glutamine Rich Tetratricopeptide Repeat Containing Beta; FCGR3A, Fc Fragment Of IgG Receptor IIIa; CCL, chemokine (C-C motif) ligand; sIL-6R, soluble IL-6 receptor; MMP, Matrix-metalloprotease; FCGR2A/FCGR3A and RPS9/LILRB3 and PSMG1, Gene loci; HLA, Human leukocyte antigen; MPO, myeloperoxidase; PR3, Proteinase-3; CXCL, C-X-C motif chemokine; Ig, Immunoglobulin; TARC, Chemokine (C-C motif) ligand 17 (CCL17); TNF, tumor necrosis factor; HCV, Hepatitis C virus; RNA, Ribonucleic acid.

LARGE VESSEL VASCULITIS

Giant-Cell Arteritis (GCA)

Giant-cell arteritis (GCA) most commonly involves vessels of large and medium size and is characterized by a granulomatous inflammatory process affecting the aorta and its main branches, predominantly the extracranial branches of the carotid artery, first of all the temporal artery (18). It is the most frequent type of vasculitis in the Western world, with women being affected more often than men. The annual incidence of GCA amounts to 20–40 per million. The disease rather affects older people, which is also reflected by the classification criteria defined by the American College of Rheumatology (19). The disorder may coexist with polymyalgia rheumatica, whose hallmarks are pain and stiffness in muscles of the pelvis and/or shoulder. Clinical manifestation of GCA comprises visual disturbances that can be temporary (Amaurosis fugax) or permanent in form of a persisting loss of vision, usually in one eye first (20, 21). Further symptoms may consist of headache, pain over the temples, jaw claudication, and a high degree of sensitivity of the temporal artery, which is prominent in many cases. Not only because of increased stroke risk, especially in the vertebrobasilar circulatory system, GCA is considered a serious disease.

Pentraxin proteins (PTX), which are involved in acute immunological responses, are under investigation as potential biomarkers of GCA. Pentraxin-3 (PTX-3), for instance, which originates from endothelial cells, smooth muscle cells and leukocytes, was found to be markedly increased in GCA patients with acute ischemia of the optic nerve compared to both, GCA cases without ischemic signs and healthy controls (22). Most interestingly, PTX-3 showed poor correlation with ESR and CRP, hinting at the potential benefit of using a combination of markers for a laboratory assessment of GCA. Generally speaking, the production of PTX3 is said to be a characteristic

TABLE 2 | Summary of biomarkers of potential clinical value in the future and their area of application in vasculitides with neurological manifestations.

Type of vasculitis	Biomarker	Meaning
Primary angiitis of the central nervous system	Circulating vWF antigen	Disease activity in children
	CSF IL-17; Increased CD 4 T cells in the CSF	Diagnosis
	CSF pleocytosis; Shift toward NK or B cells; Intrathecal immunoglobulin synthesis; Plasma cells	Diagnosis; Differentiating subtypes of PACNS
Giant-cell arteritis	Pentraxin 3	Acute ischemia of the optic nerve; Disease duration <6 months
	Anti-ferritin antibodies	Diagnosis in untreated patients
	Expression of SGTB and FCGR3A	Confirmation of diagnosis; Predicting course of disease
	Serum Osteopontin	Disease activity and relapse; Disease activity in tocilizumab-treated patients
Takayasu's arteritis	Anti-ferritin antibodies	Diagnosis
	IL-8, IL-18, CCL 2, CCL 5	Diagnosis; Disease activity
	sIL-6R, MMP-1,−3, and−9, soluble receptor for advanced glycation and products, Pentraxin 3	Disease activity; Surrogate parameter of arterial inflammation and progression of vascular involvement, i.e., marker of actual arteritis (PTX-3)
	Metabolites N-acetyl glycoprotein and glutamate	Disease activity; Guide to therapy
	Plasma ghrelin level; Leptin/Ghrelin ratio	Monitoring disease activity and creating treatment strategies
	Neutrophil gelatinase-associated lipocalin	Response to treatment with glucocorticoids and tumor necrosis factor-alpha inhibitors
	Anti-endothelial cell antibodies; Antibodies against Annexin V	Disease activity; Management of TA
	Circulating endothelial progenitor cells; Vascular endothelial growth factor	Disease activity
	Serum myeloid-related protein 8/14	Diagnosis; Disease activity; Prognostic biomarker
	FCGR2A/FCGR3A, IL12B, IL6, RPS9/LILRB3, and a locus on chromosome 21 near PSMG1	Non-HLA susceptibility loci
	Serum amyloid A	Disease activity; Treatment response
Polyarteritis nodosa	Vascular endothelial growth factor	Vasculitic neuropathy
ANCA (anti-neutrophil cytoplasm antibody)-associated vasculitides	Level of activated (CD19+/CD38+) B cells; CD 25+ regulatory B cells	Disease activity
	CD8+ T cell expression	Prognosis
	Tissue inhibitor of metalloproteinase 1	Distinguishing between mildly active AAV and remission; Distinguishing active AAV and infectious disease
	Epigenetic modifications of gene loci Proteinase 3 and MPO	Correlation with disease activity, PR 3 and MPO expression
Granulomatosis with polyangiitis	MMP-3, Tissue inhibitor of metalloproteinase 1, CXCL 13	Inflammation, angiogenesis, tissue damage and repair
	Soluble receptor for advanced glycation end products	Cumulative burden of granulomatous inflammation/Disease activity
Microscopic polyangiitis	Carbonic anhydrase III antibodies	Diagnosis in patients without ANCA; Disease activity
Eosinophilic granulomatosis with polyangiitis	Eotaxin-3, IgG4, CCL17/TARC	Diagnosis; Disease activity; Differentiating from other diseases characterized by vasculitis or eosinophilia
Cryoglobulinemic vasculitis	WA B cells	Marker for the development of CV in asymptomatic patients with HCV infection
	IL-6, CXCL10, TNF-alpha serum levels	Distinguishing HCV hepatitis with or without cryoglobulinemia; Active vasculitis (Increase of CXCL10 levels)
Henoch-Schönlein purpura	White blood cells, CRP, IL-6, serum amyloid A, serum biomarker index	Diagnosis
	Fecal secondary colonic bile acids, deoxycholic acid and lithocholic acid	Diagnosis
Behçet's disease	Tyrosine-protein phosphatase non-receptor type 4, threonine synthase-like 2, and ß-actin	Diagnosis
	Serum Amyloid A	Predicting major organ involvement/ ocular disease relapse; Disease activity
	Anti-Tubulin-α-1c antibodies	Diagnosis; Degree of inflammation; Disease activity; Predicting the course/certain manifestations of BD
	Urine and serum derived metabolites	Diagnosis
	Platelet to lymphocyte ratio, Lymphocytes to monocytes ratio	Disease activity; Differentiating BD from differential diagnoses
	Tissue factor-expressing microparticles	Diagnosis; Estimating the risk of thrombosis

vWF, Von Willebrand factor; CSF, Cerebrospinal fluid; IL, Interleukin; CD, Cluster of differentiation; NK cells, Natural killer cells; CRP, C-reactive protein; ESR, Erythrocyte sedimentation rate; SGTB, Small Glutamine Rich Tetratricopeptide Repeat Containing Beta; FCGR3A, Fc Fragment Of IgG Receptor IIIa; CCL, chemokine (C-C motif) ligand; sIL-6R, soluble IL-6 receptor; MMP, Matrix-metalloprotease; FCGR2A/FCGR3A and RPS9/LILRB3 and PSMG1, Gene loci; HLA, Human leukocyte antigen; MPO, myeloperoxidase; PR3, Proteinase-3; CXCL, C-X-C motif chemokine; Ig, Immunoglobulin; TARC, Chemokine (C-C motif) ligand 17 (CCL17); TNF, tumor necrosis factor; HCV, Hepatitis C virus; RNA, Ribonucleic acid.

of damages of the vasculature (23, 24). Being synthesized at the site of vascular injury, its physiological role consists in averting further damage of the affected vessels (23, 25–27). Additional investigations are required to elucidate in how far structural modifications of affected vessels are due to the locally synthesized PTX-3 (23, 28). In the past, diagnosing GCA was sometimes hampered by low values of ESR, especially when glucocorticoids had already been administered. The informative value of biopsies is known to be significantly reduced in this constellation as well. Given that no dependency of PTX-3 levels on the respective glucocorticoid dosage was found, elevated PTX-3 values might facilitate diagnosing GCA in this context (29). A prospective study would be helpful to proof the assumption that PTX-3 levels might be of use in evaluating different types of optic nerve ischemia, i.e., distinguishing (non-) vasculitic forms (23, 30).

In addition to PTX-3, levels of IL-6 and soluble IL-6 receptor (sIL-6R) were shown to be elevated in patients with GCA (31). Il-6 is a pro-inflammatory cytokine of importance in innate immunity serving as a link between innate and specific immune response. IL-6 binds to IL-6-receptors on hepatocytes and leukocytes and soluble IL-6-receptors resulting in the initiation of immunological pathways. Finally acute-phase-reactants are activated. In particular, IL-6 levels were significantly elevated in patients with active disease, whereas sIL-6R levels turned out to be significantly higher irrespective of disease activity. Therefore, IL-6 is considered as potential biomarker for monitoring disease activity. Most importantly, the IL-6 pathway has also emerged as a promising therapeutic target in GCA patients (32). The therapeutic efficacy of IL-6 receptor alpha inhibitor Tocilizumab in the treatment of GCA patients highlights the importance of IL-6 in GCA pathophysiology.

Baerlecken et al. analyzed anti-ferritin antibodies in GCA patients in various stages of the disease. The highest levels of anti-ferritin antibodies were found in untreated individuals with a concomittant polymyalgia rheumatica, whereas treated patients and patients with inactive stages of the disease had lower levels of anti-ferritin antibodies (33, 34). Therefore, these antibodies could be useful as a diagnostic marker.

De Smit et al. suggest new ways to confirm the diagnosis of GCA and to predict the course of disease (35). By means of transcriptional profiling of T-lymphocytes, 4,031 genes in $CD4^{+}$ and $CD8^{+}$ cells were identified that show distinct expression patterns in GCA patients with an active disease (35). Four transcripts in $CD8^{+}$ cells and 179 in $CD4^{+}$ cells were identified which were characterized by alternating expression characteristics over 12 months (35). In $CD8^{+}$ cells transcripts of SGTB [Small glutamine-rich tetratricopeptide repeat (TPR)-containing, β], playing a role in neuronal apoptosis, and FCGR (Fc gamma receptor) 3A, linked to Takayasu's arteritis maintained their altered expression pattern (35). The authors report a connection between genes and clinical aspects in the acute phase, offering the potential to predict prospective disease activity and tailor further therapies (35). The underlying mechanisms linking gene expression to actual symptoms and course of disease and the definite informative values of the aforementioned aspects in terms of a potential biomarker is to be further elucidated (35).

Prieto-González et al. reported that serum osteopontin (sOPN) might be useful in assessing and predicting disease activity in GCA (36). The glycoprotein osteopontin is of importance in the development and specialization of immune cells, inflammatory processes and remodeling in different kinds of tissues (36). Serum osteopontin concentration was significantly elevated in individuals with active disease compared to controls, whereas a significant decline was found as soon as patients entered disease remission (37). Serum osteopontin turned out to correlate with serum IL-6. Additionally, baseline serum osteopontin concentrations were significantly higher in relapsing patients than in non-relapsing patients (37).

Burja et al. investigated existing evidence on the usefulness of already known (potential) biomarkers in GCA by means of a meta-analysis. The results of this meta-analysis highlight the fact that the majority of potential biomarkers in GCA might add valuable information in understanding, diagnosing or treating the disease, but are still not suitable to be integrated in routine clinical use (38). IL-6, CRP, and ESR should, not only because of the meta-analysis by Burja et al., be considered as the best available biomarkers in GCA (for a summary of biomarkers, see **Tables 1, 2**).

Takayasu's Arteritis (TA)

The prevalence of Takayasu's arteritis (TA) is lower than the prevalence of GCA. Pathophysiologically, the aorta and its main branches are affected by a granulomatous inflammatory process with massive intimal fibrosis and vascular narrowing. Takayasu's arteriitis most commonly affects young or middle-aged women of Asian descent (39). Clinical signs may be rather unspecific for several years, comprising fever, fatigue, and joint pains. Circulatory disturbances may lead to complaints in different regions of the body, e.g., in form of Raynaud's phenomenon or angina pectoris. Frequent symptoms of TA include intermittent claudication of the arms or legs, as well as a difference in pulse or blood pressure between the right and left arms or right and left legs (40). Possible neurological symptoms are transitory ischemic attacks (TIA), stroke, syncope, and posterior reversible encephalopathy syndrome (PRES) (41). Stenosis of the renal arteries is capable of causing arterial hypertension with subsequent blood pressure crises and diverse neurological consequences. Furthermore, seizures as a result of stroke or blood pressure crisis, headache, vertigo, and visual disturbances represent additional symptoms of TA. A well-known genetic susceptibility locus for TA is the human leukocyte antigen (HLA) allele HLA-B 52 (4).

Patients with TA usually exhibit an elevation of ESR and CRP. The presence of anti-ferritin antibodies has been described by Große et al. in 62% of patients with TA, compared to 0% in healthy controls and up to 92% in GCA (42). In so far there is a similarity to patients with GCA/PMR (42). Alibaz-Oner et al. found a stronger increase of IL-6, IL-8, and IL-18 in TA patients in comparison with controls, and an association of IL-18 levels with disease activity (43–46). Interleukin-8 (IL-8) is an inflammatory mediator which attracts neutrophils to the site of inflammation. Interleukin-18 (IL-18), a proinflammatory cytokine, induces the release of Interferon (IFN) γ that, in turn, plays a role in the stimulation of macrophages. It is assumed that these cytokines contribute to the emergence of vasculitic lesions in TA (45). The role of IL-6 and also sIL-6R was confirmed by Pulsatelli et al., who reported that the levels of these markers were significantly altered in TA patients compared to healthy controls (47). IL-6 levels were markedly elevated in patients with TA irrespective of disease phase, whereas a significant increase in sIL-6R levels was only detected in individuals with active disease. Longitudinal analysis demonstrated that a significant increase in sIL-6R levels was only apparent at baseline (47). Consequently, sIL-6R is suggested to mirror disease activity in TA (48). Additional research on cytokines and chemokines in TA showed that serum/plasma levels of IL-8, and chemokine (C-C motif) ligands (CCL) 2 and (CCL) 5, cytokines which guide immune cells to the site of inflammation by means of chemotaxis, were increased in TA patients in comparison with healthy controls, and were also elevated when comparing individuals with active TA to those in remission. Consequently, elevated values of pro-inflammatory cytokines, among others CCL2 and 5, in this context may serve as a surrogate parameter for the persisting migration of immune cells to the site of inflammation in affected arteries (37).

Serum IL-6 is considered to be particularly important for assessing disease state and disease activity in TA (37). A presumable significance of IL-6 in the development of TA could be shown by analyzing peripheral blood mononuclear cells (PBMC) from TA patients which produced more IL-6 upon stimulation than their counterparts from individuals with Behçet's disease (37). Apart from that IL-6 was found to be upregulated in inflammatory infiltrates of affected vessels from patients with active TA (37). Monitoring IL-6, which is broadly available and can be performed at relatively low cost, could thus help tailoring therapies to individual patients.

Matrix-metalloproteases might be further suitable markers for distinguishing active and inactive TA (49). Matrix-metalloproteases (MMPs) are enzymes capable of tissue remodeling by modifying the extracellular matrix. Matrix-metalloproteases (MMPs) are found on the surface of immune cells. Consequently, higher MMP levels are required in active inflammatory diseases, since the internal elastic lamina of affected vessels needs to be surmounted in order to allow leukocytes to proceed toward the lamina intima (38).

In addition, low values of the soluble receptor for advanced glycation end products (sRAGE) were suggested as an indicator of active TA (50). sRAGE are membrane spanning receptors and belong to the entity of immunoglobulins (51). Activated cells, e.g., macrophages, release ligands which bind to RAGE, which results in low levels of sRAGE. There are limitations of the mentioned studies: All examinations were performed with specimens from the aorta, limiting potential findings to this part of the vasculature (46). Therefore, a broader range of vessels and cell types should be investigated in future studies.

Similar to GCA, PTX-3 was also found to be involved in TA and might help to distinguish active patients with TA from those in remission (52). One noteworthy point is that an elevation of PTX-3 is not necessarily accompanied by increased CRP levels (53). The concentration of PTX-3 but not that of CRP was, according to Tombetti et al., significantly increased in TA patients who suffered from worsening arterial lesions detected by conventional and computed tomography (CT) angiography. Consequently, plasma PTX-3 levels could serve as a surrogate parameter of disease activity in arteries (48, 52, 54, 55). The reasons for an increase in PTX-3 in TA are similar to those mentioned in the context of GCA. Some authors suggest a local production of PTX-3 in affected vessels by those cells contributing to forming an inflammatory infiltrate (49, 52, 53)).

If these findings can be confirmed in larger cohorts, plasma levels of PTX-3 may in future help to differentiate between active and inactive disease (52).

Nuclear Magnetic Resonance Spectroscopy (NMR) based serum metabolomics has identified distinct profiles in individuals suffering from TA in comparison to age- and sex-matched controls (56). The best discriminatory potential was found for N-acetyl glycoprotein (NAG), an anti-inflammatory metabolite, and glutamate, a neurotransmitter often associated with inflammation (56–58). Upon follow up, changes in metabolic spectra evolved with a change in disease activity. Thus, certain metabolic profiles allow the distinction between clinically active and inactive TA patients, representing potential biomarkers for disease activity and delivering additional information which can serve as a guide to therapy (56). Future studies should further investigate these findings in larger cohorts with a longer follow up duration.

Yilmaz et al. found that plasma levels of unacylated and acylated ghrelin (growth hormone release inducing), a peptide hormone which regulates appetite and energy use, could be of use for intermittently evaluating the activity of TA and identifying the best possible way to treat TA patients. Furthermore, serum leptin levels, with leptin diminishing the feeling of hunger, and the leptin/ghrelin ratio might help to assess disease activity (59). Other studies confirm a bidirectional relationship between Ghrelin, Leptin, and inflammation. (60).

A potential biomarker which is supposed to be informative with regard to the effects of therapy on patients with TA treated with glucocorticoids and tumor necrosis factor-alpha inhibitors was identified by Serra et al. in the form of neutrophil gelatinase-associated lipocalin (NGAL) that modulates the activity of MMP-9 (61). NGAL plasma concentration has been shown to be associated with diseases of the vasculature (62). Furthermore, as mentioned above, MMP levels are known to be increased in inflammation so that changes in NGAL levels can be expected. Apart from the low number of patients an important limitation of the studies is the lack of prospective data.

Further possible biomarkers for TA comprise certain autoantibodies, e.g., anti-ferritin antibodies and anti-endothelial cell antibodies (AECA) (63). Antibodies against Annexin V (AA5A), a factor which contributes to the regulation of (endothelial) cell apoptosis, were identified in a certain percentage of individuals with TA and were associated with AECA, so that AA5A represents another potential biomarker for the management of TA (48, 64). Further data suggest that AECA, which are capable of initiating apoptosis of endothelial cells, are crucially involved in vascular damage observed in TA patients (65–67). The majority of AA5A associated disorders, e.g., systemic lupus erythematosus, and rheumatoid arthritis exhibit AECA as well (64, 68–73). Therefore, AA5A has been proposed as one of the antigen targets of AECA (64). Nonetheless, the actual antigens of AECA have not yet been identified. The differences between isotypes of AECA need to be elucidated in the future. Furthermore, studies on the factors triggering the formation of AA5A and their role under physiological and pathological conditions are required (64).

Dogan et al. focused on markers of destructive and reconstructive processes of the endothelium, such as circulating endothelial cells (CEC), circulating endothelial progenitor cells (CEPC) and vascular endothelial growth factor (VEGF) (49). According to the corresponding study, elevated levels of CEC were detected in patients with TA. Besides, CEC levels showed a slightly positive correlation with CRP levels. Only CEPC and VEGF levels turned out to assume higher values in active compared to inactive patients. Thus, these two markers may correlate with disease activity (74). These findings are based on the following considerations: Systemic vasculitis is, among others, due to endothelial injury (75, 76). This injury causes the detachment of mature endothelial cells, called CEC (74). CEPCs are required for tissue repair in response to various cytokines and growth factors, e.g., VEGF (74).

A limitation of the presented study is that treatment effects on these parameters have not been evaluated. Further larger and prospective studies are required to verify the generated data.

Further promising findings were reported by Goel et al. (77). At the baseline assessment of a longitudinal single center study, median serum myeloid-related protein 8/14 (MRP 8/14) levels, also known as calprotectin, was found to be increased in subjects suffering from TA compared to healthy subjects. In addition, active disease states were characterized by higher MRP 8/14 levels when compared to stable disease states or healthy controls. MRP 8/14 is part of a group of cytosolic calcium-binding protein family called S100 (78). During the course of disease, changes in serial MRP 8/14 levels were linked to disease activity, no matter what the administered glucocorticoid dose has been (77), so that MRP 8/14 has been proposed as another prognostic biomarker in TA (77).

Finally, Nair et al. identified serum amyloid A (SAA), an apolipoprotein which belongs to the group of acute phase proteins, as a biomarker to evaluate disease activity and treatment response in TA (79). At baseline, there were higher SAA levels in individuals with TA than in healthy controls, and also higher values in patients with active disease compared to those with stable disease. SAA exhibited a decreasing trend during follow-up in treatment responders, whereas these changes were not observed in non-responders (79). The study was limited by small sample size and a short duration of follow up (79).

Taking all the above considerations into account, we conclude that IL-6 is particularly valuable for assessing disease state and disease activity in TA. For a summary of biomarkers see **Tables 1, 2**.

MEDIUM VESSEL VASCULITIS

Polyarteritis Nodosa (PAN)

Polyarteritis nodosa exclusively affects medium-sized vessels and is potentially associated with Hepatitis B and C virus (4). In contrast to the aforementioned vasculitides of large vessels PAN is the scarcest type of vasculitis in central Europe. General symptoms include fever, stomach, muscle, and joint pains, and myocardial infarction even in young patients. With regard to neurological complaints, peripheral neuropathy belongs to the most frequent organ manifestations, mostly in the form of mononeuritis multiplex. Also, symmetrical sensorimotor polyneuropathies or an affection of nerve plexi may occur (80). A combination of polyneuropathy in conjunction with Livedo reticularis is highly suspicious of PAN. CNS manifestations in PAN include ischemic stroke, intracerebral and subarachnoid hemorrhage and seizures (4). It has been demonstrated that recessive loss-of-function mutations affecting the gene which encodes adenosine deaminase 2 (ADA2) might lead to polyarteritis nodosa vasculopathy (81).

As far as the pathogenesis of the disease is concerned Shimojima et al. showed an expansion of T-helper cells and an impaired function of regulatory T cells (82). These findings suggest that PAN results, among others, from defects in T-cell-mediated immunity (82). The changes might be due to insufficient suppressive abilities of regulatory T cells with regard to $CD4^+$ T cells and an impaired cytotoxic T-lymphocyte-associated Protein 4- (CTLA-4-) expression of regulatory T cells. CTLA-4 is essential for the inhibition of the proliferation of $CD4^+$ T cells, i.e., T-helper cells. In order to better understand the underlying pathomechanisms, larger cohorts need to be examined.

Manolov et al. found higher levels of plasma VEGF (see remarks on TA) in subjects with vasculitic neuropathy compared to healthy controls (65). This is why plasma VEGF levels could be of use in predicting vasculitic neuropathy (65). However, this finding does not only apply to PAN and the number of included patients was extremely low so that the current practical benefit of this biomarker is very limited.

In PAN patients with cutaneous manifestations, Okano et al. suggested that anti-phosphatidylserine-prothrombin complex (anti-PSPT) antibodies could be regarded as a biomarker for the existence of PAN and therefore support making an early diagnosis (83). These antibodies turned out to decrease to lower levels after treatment with cyclophosphamide and glucocorticoids in comparison with the pre-treatment levels (83). Mechanistically, it is assumed that prothrombin binds to apoptotic endothelial cells and phosphatidylserine (83). The resulting complexes are thought to trigger the production of anti-PSPT antibodies resulting in the development of PAN (83). Apart from that, deteriorations of the clinical disease course might be associated with higher levels of anti-moesin-antibodies. Moesin is an intracellular protein connecting cell membrane and cytoskeleton (83). Anti-moesin antibodies have been suspected to exacerbate PAN via antiphospholipid antibodies, such as anti-PSPT antibodies (83). However, these findings need to be validated in a prospective study.

There have been few studies on biomarkers in polyarteritis nodosa. Autoantibodies against lysosomal-associated membrane protein-2 (LAMP-2) showed an association with dermatological signs of the disease, but in the end there was no significant difference when compared to values measured in healthy controls (66). LAMP-2 is a component of the lysosomal membrane. It has been assumed that LAMP-2 plays a role in the pathogenesis of vasculitis (66). Mechanistically, Takeuchi et al. hypothesize that anti-LAMP-2-antibodies bind to neutrophils, which then infiltrate small vessels of the skin (66). The main limitation of the study consists in the fact that the association with LAMP-2-antibodies seems to exclusively refer to cutaneous manifestation.

To sum up, the tested biomarkers either refer to cutaneous manifestations or bear the potential to predict vasculitic neuropathy, not only in PAN. With regard to the latter aspect, the corresponding study design does not allow to call VEGF an established biomarker. For a summary of biomarkers see **Tables 1, 2**.

SMALL VESSEL VASCULITIS

Granulomatosis with polyangiitis (GPA), Microscopic polyangiitis (MPA), and eosinophilic granulomatosis with polyangiitis (EGPA), previously known as Churg-Strauss syndrome, form the group of ANCA (anti-neutrophil cytoplasm antibody)-associated vasculitides (AAV). The AAV, as well as cryoglobulinemic vasculitis, Ig A vasculitis, and Behçet's disease, potentially affecting all types of blood vessels, will be considered in this chapter.

Before focusing on certain subtypes, biomarkers relevant for AAV in general are reviewed: GPA and MPA patients in remission were shown to have higher levels of $CD25^+$ regulatory B cells in proportion to individuals with active vasculitis (67). CD25 is the α-subunit of the Interleukin-2-receptor, which influences the binding process between receptor and ligand. $CD25^+$ B cells are therefore supposed to have regulatory functions in the mentioned vasculitides (67). To confirm or disprove the role of regulatory B cells as a marker of AAV these shortcomings should be overcome in future investigations.

Effective ways to predict relapse rates have been discovered in both GPA and microscopic polyangiitis. First, anti-MPO positive patients showed lower relapse rates than anti-PR3 positive subjects (84–86). Second, a specific gene expression signature in $CD8^+$ cells was identified, which seems to predict relapses (87): Transcriptional profiling analysis has revealed that $CD8^+$ T cell expression may represent a tool to divide patients into two distinct subgroups (relapse/active disease vs. remission/stable disease) (87, 88). The group of patients with a poor prognosis was characterized by a subset of genes playing a role in the IL-7 receptor pathway and T cell receptor signaling. The $CD8^+$ T cell memory cell population, which has been suspected to promote disease relapses, was also expanded in this group. A possible explanation of these observations could be that altered gene expression in naïve CD 8^+ T cells might be the result of genetic modifications in the phase of T cell maturation in the thymus (87, 89–91). As a reaction to antigen exposure, this could lead to T cell proliferation, at least in part via signaling cascades involving IL-7 receptor and T cell receptor, resulting in an increasing number of memory cells (92, 93). In order to use this information to individualize the therapy in AAV depending on a patient's classification as "active" or "stable," a prospective clinical study is required.

Moon et al. identified the CRP to serum albumin ratio (CAR) as an independent predictor of all-cause mortality in patients suffering from AAV with a similar potency as diabetes mellitus (94). Notably, the combined occurrence of CAR $\geq$ 10.35 and diabetes mellitus had a higher mortality, regardless of the actual reason, than the lack of these characteristics (94). These observations might have the following reasons: Chronic inflammation leads to increased IL-6 release, which increases the levels of CRP in the peripheral circulation" (94, 95). Given that IL-6 also diminishes the hepatic albumin production, the CAR is altered in a specific manner (94). The limitations of this study consist in the small sample size derived from a single center, its retrospective character, and the lack of a clear cut-off value of CAR to predict all-cause mortality in patients with AAV (94).

In AAV patients, myeloperoxidase-(MPO-)ANCA levels returned to values within normal limits during a period of 6 months after the initiation of remission induction therapy. A reappearance of MPO-ANCA could be detected in 40% of these individuals and occurred more often in relapsing subjects than in age- and sex-matched non-relapsing controls (96). Therefore, the reappearance of MPO-ANCA might be a biomarker which bears the potential to predict a relapse in individuals "with MPO-ANCA-positive AAV in" remission (96). Becoming ANCA-negative before maintenance therapy has been initiated was connected to a reduced risk of relapse (96). The frequency of relapses in general is much higher in PR3-ANCA- than in MPO-ANCA-positive disease, whereas there is a reverse relation with regard to mortality.

The so called delta neutrophil index (DNI), a simultaneous view at the number of immature granulocytes and the consumption of neutrophil granulocytes, correlates with the Birmingham vasculitis activity score at diagnosis—an instrument which helps assessing disease activity in patients with PSV (97). DNI values $\geq$0.65% were shown to be a surrogate parameter for a difficult progression of AAV and relapse in GPA and MPA during the observation period (97). This connection may be the result of the following considerations: T cells and macrophages release inflammatory cytokines that prime neutrophils and cause an increase in adhesion molecules on neutrophils and endothelial cells. ANCA promote the interaction of neutrophils and endothelial cells, which results in the diapedesis of neutrophils through the vascular cell layers. Finally, activated neutrophils induce vasculitis by reactive oxygen radicals and degranulation (97–104).

Another potential biomarker for disease activity is the tissue inhibitor of metalloproteinase 1 (TIMP1). TIMP1 is responsible for the regulation of MMPs (105–107). In accordance with MMPs, TIMP1-levels increase in inflammatory states. Additionally, unlike CRP, TIMP1-levels were significantly higher in individuals suffering from active AAV than in infected subjects without disease activity (108). Therefore, TIMP1 can be used to distinguish between AAV with mild activity and remission.

Autoantigen gene loci in ANCA-associated vasculitis Proteinase 3 (PRTN3) and MPO were found to undergo epigenetic modifications, which correlated with disease activity and with PR3 and MPO expression. Epigenetic changes in general may comprise DNA methylation, histone modifications, and non-coding RNA (109–111). Thus, it appears that not only mutations, i.e., changes in the DNA sequence, may have far-reaching consequences for the manifestation of certain diseases. It still has to be elucidated which factors cause certain epigenetic modifications resulting in AAV and, maybe, how they can be avoided or prevented.

Further biomarkers for different types of AAV are, among others, distinct cytokine profiles of PR3-AAV, i.e., IL-6, granulocyte-macrophage colony-stimulating factor (GM-CSF), IL-15, IL-18, CXCL (C-X-C motif chemokine) 8/IL-8, CCL-17/thymus and activation-regulated chemokine, IL-18 binding protein, soluble IL-2 receptor α (sIL-2Rα), and nerve growth factor ß" (NGF-ß). Cytokine profiles of MPO-AAV comprise soluble IL-6 receptor, soluble tumor necrosis factor receptor type II (sTNFRII), neutrophil gelatinase-associated lipocalin (NGAL), and soluble intercellular adhesion molecule 1. Osteopontin, sTNFRII, and NGAL can be attributed to MPA, whereas IL-6, GM-CSF, IL-15, IL-18, sIL-2Rα, and NGF-ß can be attributed to GPA (112). Although these biomarkers bear the potential to improve the handling of ANCA-associated vasculitides, not all of them are suitable for everyday use.

Data derived from the RAVE (Rituximab in ANCA-Associated Vasculitis) trial allow the following conclusions: Patients treated with rituximab, who were anti-PR3 positive and exhibited an increase of calprotectin serum levels between the start of data collection and month 2 or month 6, exhibited a higher risk of relapse at 18 months. Hence, serum calprotectin might guide more intensive or prolonged treatment (113).

Furthermore, anti-PTX3 antibodies were frequently detected in AAV patients and antibody levels were increased in comparison to healthy controls. Comparing the states of remission and active disease, anti-PTX3 antibody values turned out to be higher in the latter case (114). In summary, anti-PTX3 antibody levels allow to distinguish between differential diagnoses and to evaluate disease activity.

Simon et al. hypothesize that Anti-PTX3 autoantibodies attract PTX3-expressing apoptotic neutrophils and enhance their phagocytosis (114). The interaction of PR3- and MPO-expressing neutrophils and ANCA induces phagocytosis and the synthesis of pro-inflammatory cytokines (114–116). Additionally, PTX3 can also be found on the surface of endothelial cells, which, in case of endothelial cell injury, may attract immune cells (114). It still remains to be examined whether the immunogenic capacity of apoptotic cells depends on anti-PTX3 and in how far there is an effect on disease duration (114).

Among others, DNI and CAR seem to be promising, but further studies are required to validate existing findings. For a summary of biomarkers see **Tables 1, 2**.

Granulomatosis With Polyangiitis (GPA)

GPA is a rare form of small vessel vasculitis with an incidence rate of 0.9/100,000/year that affects both sexes equally (4). In the early stage, local inflammatory processes accompanied by granuloma formation take place in the respiratory tract and later on the disease spreads in terms of a generalization into small vessel vasculitis (117, 118). Leading symptoms in the early stadium of GPA is a bloody and barky nasal discharge. As soon as GPA generalizes, the spectrum of potential manifestations includes general symptoms and an affection of the lungs (therapy-resistant pneumonia with coughing, dyspnea, and hemoptysis), the kidneys in terms of glomerulonephritis, the skin in the form of various efflorescences, the eyes (conjunctivitis, episcleritis), the heart (pericarditis, vasculitis of the coronary arteries, cardiomyopathy), and the nervous system. Furthermore, a saddle nose is a symptom of advanced GPA. The latter can be affected by peripheral neuropathies, polyneuropathies, as well as mononeuritis multiplex. These peripheral neuropathies can be the initial disease manifestation of GPA and of other AAV (119). Therefore, neuropathies of unknown etiology should be inspected for signs of AAV, especially when typical stigmata of AAV are present. In AAV patients, peripheral neuropathy manifestation is associated with a higher number of affected organs, an increased ANCA-titer and a more severe disease course compared to individuals without peripheral neuropathy (120, 121). Cerebral small vessel vasculitis is a rather scarce phenomenon in these patients. Additionally, GPA patients might suffer from pachymeningitis and granulomas of the pituitary gland. GPA is associated with ANCA, above all PR3-ANCA, in 50% of cases in the early, local stadium, and in at least 90% of cases in a later, more generalized stage (122–124).

Biomarkers already in use for assessing disease activity and predicting flares are ESR, CRP, anti-PR3, and anti-MPO titers but, as already mentioned, their informative value is limited, since they are much less useful in evaluating the activity of GPA in individuals, in whom a diagnosis has already been made (3). So far, useful markers of inflammation, angiogenesis, tissue damage, and repair have been identified. Observing MMP-3, TIMP-1, and CXCL13 indicated significant differences between groups of patients. Nonetheless, due to the poor correlation of the markers among each other it has been suggested that a combination of these biomarkers might be the most promising approach (125–127). CXCL13 is a chemokine that attracts immune cells to the site of inflammation. The reasons for increased CXCL13 levels are not fully understood, but high CXCL13 levels have been linked to B cell malfunction (127). Furthermore, sRAGE are considered to mirror the cumulative burden of granulomatous inflammation in GPA, so that sRAGE may in future be established as a mean of assessing disease activity (128).

Further studies are required to detect the changes of sRAGE over time with treatment and exacerbations of the disease.

In patients who receive rituximab, the simultaneous consideration of B cell reconstitution after depletion due to the therapy and ANCA-PR3 levels could fulfill the function of a biomarker for a GPA relapse, given that Cartin-Ceba et al. observed that all occurring relapses in the cohort under investigation were accompanied by an increase in B cells, preceded by an increase in ANCA-PR3 levels (129) (for a summary of biomarkers, see **Tables 1, 2**).

Hitherto there are no directly applicable biomarkers in GPA.

Microscopic Polyangiitis (MPA)

Microscopic polyangiitis (MPA) shares some characteristics with GPA regarding the clinical manifestations. Being a necrotizing inflammatory process of small vessels it mostly affects the kidneys and, less often, the lungs, the skin, and the nervous system (4). The latter is mainly affected by peripheral neuropathy, mostly mononeuritis multiplex, by intracranial hemorrhage, seizures, headache and cerebral vasculitis. MPA is strongly associated with ANCA, especially (myeloperoxidase) MPO-ANCA, in 75% of all cases.

Saito et al. demonstrated that carbonic anhydrase III (CAIII) antibodies had a significantly higher prevalence in MPA patients in comparison to healthy controls. Additionally, the authors report, especially in proportion to antibody-negative subjects, elevated values of activity scores for vasculitic disorders in those cases of MPA which came along with anti-CAIII antibodies (130). Therefore, these antibodies might facilitate diagnosing MPA in ANCA-negative patients (70% of MPA patients are pANCA positive) and for assessing disease activity (130). Carbonic anhydrases are zink metalloenzymes that catalyze the hydration of carbondioxide and are present in red skeletal muscle. It is suggested that CA III plays a role in intracellular signaling, particularly in response to oxidative stress (131, 132). Possibly, anti-CAIII-antibodies protect cells from oxidative damage during inflammation (130). The informative value of the results is limited to the low number of patients, highlighting the necessity of future studies involving a higher number of patients.

Hitherto there are no directly applicable biomarkers in MPA.

Eosinophilic Granulomatosis With Polyangiitis (EGPA)

Eosinophilic granulomatosis with polyangiitis (EGPA), previously known as Churg-Strauss syndrome, can be briefly characterized as a granulomatous, necrotizing vasculitis with eosinophilia that is accompanied by pulmonary manifestation with severe asthma attacks as the leading symptom. An ANCA-association, usually MPO-ANCA, is given in 40% of all cases (133). Nervous system manifestations comprise vasculitis of the central nervous system with impaired consciousness as well as sensorimotor deficits. Moreover, EGPA may result in allergic rhinitis/sinusitis, myocarditis, and purpura.

After the initiation of treatment, eosinophilia, the hallmark of EGPA, is not an appropriate biomarker for disease activity, since the eosinophilic cell count tends to drop rapidly as soon as glucocorticoids are administered (134). It has been demonstrated that proteins related to eosinophilia, first of all eoxtaxin-3, and to Th2 immune response in general, particularly IgG4 and CCL17/TARC, were elevated in active EGPA. This elevation was also found when EGPA was compared to inactive disease, other diseases characterized by vasculitis or hypereosinophilia, and healthy controls (135–138). Eotaxins are chemokines which contribute to the accumulation and maturation of eosinophils (136). CCL17/TARC is a chemokine that is released by dendritic and endothelial cells. It is involved in the targeted attraction of activated Th2 lymphocytes to affected foci (135). Further investigations are necessary to increase knowledge on additional characteristics of eotaxin-producing cells in EGPA (136). Higher IgG4 levels might be caused by activated Th2 lymphocytes but the actual pathological role of IgG4 in EGPA is still unclear.

In a cohort of refractory and relapsing EGPA patients treated with rituximab, individuals exhibiting ANCA had a better chance to reach the state of remission (139).

Eotaxin-3, IgG4, and CCL17/TARC are promising future biomarkers, but they are not completely understood yet. For a summary of biomarkers, see **Tables 1, 2**.

Cryoglobulinemic Vasculitis (CV)

Cryoglobulinemic vasculitis (CV) is a rare disease affecting primarily small vessels due to the formation of immune-complexes, and is accompanied by Hepatitis C virus infection in the large majority of all cases. The main symptoms are purpura, ulcerations, arthritis, and, as a late symptom or in severe courses, glomerulonephritis. With regard to neurological affliction, patients have polyneuropathy and less frequently focal neurological signs resulting from cerebral manifestations (140). Cryoglobulinemic vasculitis is mainly characterized by the combination of arthritis, purpura, and polyneuropathy, in conjunction with complement consumption (low C4 levels) and the evidence of rheumatoid factor (141).

Monoclonal rheumatoid factors (mRF) carrying the WA cross-idiotype (Xid) are of major importance in the pathogenesis of cryoglobulinemic vasculitis in individuals with hepatitis C virus (HCV) infection (142). When the WA Xid is found, individuals without symptoms but with HCV infection can be shown to exhibit WA B cells (142). Consequently, WA B cells in asymptomatic individuals with HCV infection might represent a marker for the development of CV (142). Furthermore, B-cells expressing VH1-69 were considered to be the target of treatment of infectious CV. Therefore, using this cell population as a biomarker might provide information on the activity of CV and response to treatment. A possible future perspective consists in the development of an anti-WA Xid antibody as a method for everyday medical use (142). Maybe novel treatment strategies can be derived from such antibodies.

A further study showed that patients with HCV-related mixed cryoglobulinemia (HCV-MC) exhibited significantly higher mean IL-6 values compared to healthy controls and individuals suffering from HCV chronic hepatitis without concomitant cryoglobulinemia (HCV^{+}). IL-6 was also elevated in cryoglobulinemic subjects with active vasculitis, thus representing potential indicator for this state (143). A hallmark of HCV-MC is the synthesis of immune-complexes, primarily cryoglobulins incorporating HCV, evoking vasculitis (143). As a consequence, IL-6 levels rise and enhance inflammation (143). However, the prognostic significance of IL-6 in HCV-MC needs to be examined in larger prospective studies (143).

Moreover, increased values of CXCL10 and TNF-alpha were measured in individuals with HCV-associated cryoglobulinemia (144). In HCV-MC patients, active vasculitis was associated with increased CXCL10 values (144). C-X-C motif chemokine 10 (CXCL10), also known as Interferon gamma-induced protein 10 (IP-10) or small inducible cytokine B10, is a chemokine relevant for chemoattraction of immune cells (144). It is hypothesized that HCV induces the production of CXCL10, which in turn contributes to the development of chronic hepatitis C (144, 145). Further investigations comprising higher numbers of patients will have to test the potential of CXCL10 to predict the disease course of HCV-MC patients and guide the treatment (144).

Hitherto there are no clinically proven biomarkers. For a summary of biomarkers see **Tables 1**, **2**.

Ig A vasculitis

Ig A vasculitis, a vasculitis of small vessels driven by immune complexes, represents the most common vasculitis in childhood (4). Immunoglobulin A (IgA) plays a pivotal role in the disease. Typical clinical manifestations are IgA-nephritis, gastrointestinal symptoms such as stomach pain and hematochezia, purpura, and nephritis. The disease can be associated with cerebral ischemia, intracranial hemorrhage, diffuse cerebral edema, peripheral neuropathies, facial nerve paresis, and Guillain-Barré syndrome (146). Neurological complaints, however, are a rather scarce manifestation of Ig A vasculitis (147).

In pediatric patients with Ig A vasculitis, white blood cells (WBC), serum levels of CRP, IL-6, and SAA (amyloid A) showed a significant increase compared to healthy individuals (148). In addition, a complex serum biomarker index (SAA+IgA/4000+IgM/4000x0.4CRPmeanvalueCRPi) is significantly higher in HSP patients compared to healthy controls (148). The discrimination of these states is enabled by the integration of biomarkers specific and sensitive for Ig A vasculitis, such as SAA, and other biomarkers also connected to inflammatory processes in general, i.e., CRP. The biomarker index can be easily calculated and the number of patients exceeded 100 individuals so that it seems ready for use in discriminating patients with Ig A vasculitis and septicemia or the absence of one of these disorders.

High performance liquid mass spectrometry (HPLC-MS) revealed that levels of fecal secondary colonic bile acids, deoxycholic acid, and lithocholic acid are significantly lower in children with Ig A vasculitis in the acute stage and in remission than in healthy controls (149) (for a summary of biomarkers, see **Table 1**).

The biomarker index is an already available tool that can be used in the treatment of patients with IgA vasculitis.

Behçet's Disease (BD)

Behçet's disease (BD) differs from the aforementioned vasculitides, since both arterial and venous blood vessels of any diameter can be affected. There is a strong association with human leukocyte antigen (HLA) B51 and the leading symptom consists of oral and genital aphthae (4). The peripheral nervous system is rarely affected by polyneuropathies. Manifestations in the central nervous system are divided into a parenchymatic and a non-parenchymatic neurovascular type. The parenchymatic type is characterized by bihemispheric lesions which can cause hemiparesis, hemihypesthesia, vision field losses, seizures, movement disorders, speech disorder, and Parkinson-like symptoms. Furthermore, aseptic meningitis and affections of the brain stem with cranial nerve paralysis, sensorimotor disturbances, and cerebellar symptoms may occur (150–153). The neurovascular type of BD comprises sinus vein thrombosis and increased cerebral pressure, resulting in headache, focal neurological signs, seizures, papilledema, impaired consciousness, and paralysis of the sixth cranial nerve. The affection of arteries may lead to aneurysms, dissections, and consecutive intracranial hemorrhage or cerebral infarction. Peripheral neurological manifestation may consist of Guillain-Barré syndrome, polyneuropathy, autonomous neuropathy, and mononeuritis multiplex (150–153).

In a genome wide association study, the central role of HLA-B51 in regard to BD susceptibility has been confirmed (154). Apart from the connection to HLA-A and HLA-C, BD susceptibility was also associated with cytokines and danger signals IL-10, IL-23R, CCR1, STAT4, KLRC4, GIMAP2/GIMAP4, and UBAC2 genes. These findings hint at an impaired response to danger signals of the human organism and impaired immunological processes in BD patients (154). The presence of HLA-B51 is known to be accompanied by a marked increase in the risk of developing Behcet's disease, but the underlying pathophysiologic mechanisms have not been fully elaborated (154). Case-control studies with higher number of participants could help to elucidate connections between genetic attributes and certain phenotypes of BD (154).

The fact that not only blood but also other body fluids can contribute to the development of new biomarkers was underlined by Ahn et al, who distinguished BD patients from healthy individuals by employing a group of 10 urine derived metabolites, i.e., guanine, pyrrole-2-carboxylate, 3-hydroxypyridine, mannose, l-citrulline, galactonate, isothreonate, sedoheptulose, hypoxanthine, and gluconic acid lactone (155). Similarly, a panel of five metabolic markers derived from serum, i.e., decanoic acid, fructose, tagatose, linoleic acid, and oleic acid, were found to be potential biomarkers of BD with a sensitivity of 100% and a specificity of 97.1% (156). Future studies should include larger sample sizes in order to confirm the results. Apart from that, future studies should take the circadian rhythm of certain metabolites and their dependence on other factors, such as physical activity, into consideration (156).

The expression of Tissue Factor (TF) by microparticles was experimentally shown to contribute to the development of thrombosis (157). Using flow cytometry, it has been demonstrated that the total number of plasma microparticles was elevated in BD patients compared to healthy controls, as were microparticles characterized by TF and Tissue Factor Pathway Inhibitor (TFPI) (157). BD patients who had already presented with thrombosis in the past exhibited elevated counts of total and TF positive microparticles in comparison to individuals without thrombosis, but showed a lower percentage of TFPI positive microparticles. In conclusion, microparticles characterized by TF are elevated in BD and a discrepancy or impaired balance between TF and TFPI could represent a risk factor for thrombosis (157). In order to improve the knowledge about the usefulness of these markers, larger and prospective studies, e.g., in endemic regions, are required.

Yoshioka et al. analyzed protein profiles of peripheral blood mononuclear cells (PBMCs) and compared them to profiles from patients with rheumatoid arthritis (RA) and Crohn's disease (CD), and to healthy controls (HC) (158). Tyrosine-protein phosphatase non-receptor type 4, threonine synthase-like 2, and ß-actin were identified as possible biomarker candidates for BD, since they can be applied to discriminate inflammatory bowel disease from BD and other diseases (158). Tyrosine-protein phosphatase non-receptor type 4 binds to cytoskeletal proteins and is involved in cellular responses to cytokines. Threonine synthase-like 2 exacerbates inflammation, can act as a cytokine and can promote the production of IL-6 in osteoblasts (158, 159). ß-actin is a structural protein which represents a part of the sarcomere of muscle fibers. The changes in ß-actin levels may be due to structural changes in the actin cytoskeleton as soon as T cells are activated in BD (158). In order to learn more about the significance of the identified proteins, the analysis of the protein expression of different kinds of immune cells may be of interest with regard to the pathophysiological mechanisms underlying BD. By doing so, novel biomarkers for everyday use could be developed.

Sota et al. reported that serum amyloid-A (SAA) levels can be useful to predict the affection of organs and repetitive affections of the eyes, but they also found that SAA cannot serve as a surrogate parameter for disease activity (160). SAA plays a role in the acute phase reaction and is frequently elevated in autoimmune disorders. Some authors suggest that SAA interacts with certain cytokines promoting inflammation, e.g., IL-1ß, which might be involved in the development of BD (161, 162). Future studies should be designed as prospective investigations, including a control group because these features are lacking in Sota's study.

A further study identified potential antigens in circulating immune complexes of BD patients but not in those of healthy subjects. Tubulin-α-1c is such an antigen and antibodies directed against it were increased in individuals with BD in comparison to healthy controls and disease controls (systemic lupus erythematosus, recurrent aphthous ulcers, AAV, and TA). In diagnosing BD, the tubulin-α-1c antibody had a sensitivity of 61.4% and a specificity of 88.4% (163). Additionally, an association of anti-tubulin-α-1c with deep venous thrombosis and erythema nodosum, and a significant correlation with the extent of inflammatory processes in BD and indicators of disease activity, such as ESR, CRP and BVAS (Birmingham Vasculitis Activity Score) were found (163). As part of the cytoskeleton, tubulins maintain the shape and structure of cells, GTPase activity and intracellular movement (163). Tubulin-α-1c was moreover shown to increase VEGF levels and cause endothelial damage under vasculitic conditions and in cases of thrombosis (163). However, precise mechanisms have not been elaborated.

As far as the assessment of disease activity in BD is concerned, a substantial gain in information resulted from the analysis of the platelet to lymphocyte ratio (PLR) and the lymphocyte to monocyte ratio (LMR). The PLR was remarkably higher in BD patients, whereas the LMR assumed lower values in subjects with BD compared to controls (164). When comparing active and inactive BD, active BD was characterized by significantly higher PLR, ESR and highly sensitive CRP. Furthermore, PLR and LMR were demonstrated to be independent factors for BD (164). To sum up, PLR may be useful as a novel biomarker to evaluate disease activity in BD which is not expensive but can be easily used. Current data derives from a cross-sectional analysis in a single center. Future studies should be performed in multiple centers over a longer period of time. Beyond, treatment effects should also be evaluated (164).

In summary, there are not no sufficiently tested and established biomarkers for BD apart from HLA B51. For a summary of biomarkers see **Tables 1, 2**.

CONCLUSION

Biomarkers are of importance in improving the diagnostic process, the treatment, and the prognosis for patients suffering from various forms of vasculitis. Nonetheless, the majority of the findings reviewed in this article do not exclusively apply to neurological manifestations of vasculitides. Further studies that employ appropriate control groups, use precise definitions for disease states such as "active" and "remission," and clearly outline the type of neurological manifestation involved are needed to guide our use of biomarkers in vasculitides of the nervous system.

AUTHOR CONTRIBUTIONS

DS conceptualized and wrote the manuscript. AS-P contributed to writing the manuscript. CB, LM, CK, and SM gave valuable suggestions for improving the manuscript. JM conceptualized the manuscript and contributed to writing the manuscript.

REFERENCES

1. Beuker C, Schmidt A, Strunk D, Sporns PB, Wiendl H, Meuth SG, et al. Primary angiitis of the central nervous system: diagnosis and treatment. *Ther Adv Neurol Disord.* (2018) 11:1–16. doi: 10.1177/17562864187 85071
2. Strimbu K, Tavel JA. What are biomarkers? *Curr Opin HIV AIDS.* (2010) 5:463–6. doi: 10.1097/COH.0b013e32833ed177
3. Monach PA. Biomarkers in vasculitis. *Curr Opin Rheumatol.* (2014) 26:24–30. doi: 10.1097/BOR.0000000000000009
4. Magnus T, Melms A, Kötter I, Holle JU. Neurological manifestations of vasculitis and primary central nervous system vasculitis. *Zeitschr Rheumatol.* (2012) 71:551–63. doi: 10.1007/s00393-012-0957-0
5. Birnbaum J, Hellmann DB. Primary angiitis of the central nervous system. *Arch Neurol.* (2009) 66:704–9. doi: 10.1001/archneurol.2009.76
6. Berlit P, Kraemer M. Cerebral vasculitis in adults: what are the steps in order to establish the diagnosis? Red flags and pitfalls. *Clin Exp Immunol.* (2014) 175:419–24. doi: 10.1111/cei.12221
7. Mandal J, Chung SA. Primary angiitis of the central nervous system. *Rheum Dis Clin North Am.* (2017) 43:503–18. doi: 10.1016/j.rdc.2017.06.001

8. Hajj-Ali RA, Calabrese LH. Diagnosis and classification of central nervous system vasculitis. *J Autoimmun.* (2014) 48:149–52. doi: 10.1016/j.jaut.2014.01.007
9. Smith EE, Greenberg SM. β-Amyloid, blood vessels, and brain function. *Stroke.* (2009) 40:2601–6. doi: 10.1161/STROKEAHA.108.536839
10. Strunk D, Schulte-Mecklenbeck A, Golombeck KS, zu Hörste GM, Melzer N, Beuker C, et al. Immune cell profiling in the cerebrospinal fluid of patients with primary angiitis of the central nervous system reflects the heterogeneity of the disease. *J Neuroimmunol.* (2018) 321:109–16. doi: 10.1016/j.jneuroim.2018.06.004
11. Ruland T, Wolbert J, Gottschalk MG, König S, Schulte-Mecklenbeck A, Minnerup J, et al. Cerebrospinal fluid concentrations of neuronal proteins are reduced in primary angiitis of the central nervous system. *Front Neurol.* (2018) 9:407. doi: 10.3389/fneur.2018.00407
12. Thom V, Schmid S, Gelderblom M, Hackbusch R, Kolster M, Schuster S, et al. IL-17 production by CSF lymphocytes as a biomarker for cerebral vasculitis. *Neurol Neuroimmunol Neuroinflamm.* (2016) 3:e214. doi: 10.1212/NXI.0000000000000214
13. Melzer N, Harder A, Gross CC, Wölfer J, Stummer W, Niederstadt T, et al. CD4+ T cells predominate in cerebrospinal fluid and leptomeningeal and parenchymal infiltrates in cerebral amyloid β-related angiitis. *Arch Neurol.* (2012) 69:773–7. doi: 10.1001/archneurol.2011.2441
14. Cellucci T, Tyrrell PN, Pullenayegum E, Benseler SM. von Willebrand factor antigen-a possible biomarker of disease activity in childhood central nervous system vasculitis? *Rheumatology.* (2012) 51:1838–45. doi: 10.1093/rheumatology/kes156
15. Sadler JE. Biochemistry and genetics of Von Willebrand factor. *Ann Rev Biochem.* (1998) 67:395–424. doi: 10.1146/annurev.biochem.67.1.395
16. de Lind van Wijngaarden RA, van Rijn L, Hagen EC, Watts RA, Gregorini G, Tervaert JWC, et al. Hypotheses on the etiology of antineutrophil cytoplasmic autoantibody-associated vasculitis: the cause is hidden, but the result is known. *Clin J Am Soc Nephrol.* (2008) 3:237–52. doi: 10.2215/CJN.03550807
17. Falk RJ, Hoffman GS. Controversies in small vessel vasculitis-comparing the rheumatology and nephrology views. *Curr Opin Rheumatol.* (2007) 19:1–9. doi: 10.1097/BOR.0b013e328011cb80
18. Hunder GG, Bloch DA, Michel BA, Stevens MB, Arend WP, Calabrese LH, et al. The American College of Rheumatology 1990 criteria for the classification of giant cell arteritis. *Arthritis Rheumat.* (1990) 33:1122–8. doi: 10.1002/art.1780330810
19. Reinhold-Keller E, Herlyn K, Wagner-Bastmeyer R, Gross WL. Stable incidence of primary systemic vasculitides over five years: results from the German vasculitis register. *Arthritis Care Res.* (2005) 53:93–9. doi: 10.1002/art.20928
20. González-Gay MA, Blanco R, Rodríguez-Valverde V, Martínez-Taboada VM, Delgado-Rodriguez M, Figueroa M, Uriarte E. Permanent visual loss and cerebrovascular accidents in giant cell arteritis: predictors and response to treatment. *Arthritis Rheumat.* (1998) 41:1497–504.
21. González-Gay MA, García-Porrúa C, Llorca J, Hajeer AH, Brañas F, Dababneh A, et al. Visual manifestations of giant cell arteritis. Trends and clinical spectrum in 161 patients. *Medicine.* (2000) 79:283–92. doi: 10.1097/00005792-200009000-00001
22. Bottazzi B, Garlanda C, Cotena A, Moalli F, Jaillon S, Deban L, et al. The long pentraxin PTX3 as a prototypic humoral pattern recognition receptor: interplay with cellular innate immunity. *Immunol Rev.* (2009) 227:9–18. doi: 10.1111/j.1600-065X.2008.00719.x
23. Baldini M, Maugeri N, Ramírez GA, Giacomassi C, Castiglioni A, Prieto-González S, et al. Selective up-regulation of the soluble pattern-recognition receptor pentraxin 3 and of vascular endothelial growth factor in giant cell arteritis: relevance for recent optic nerve ischemia. *Arthritis Rheumat.* (2012) 64:854–65. doi: 10.1002/art.33411
24. Maugeri N, Rovere-Querini P, Baldini M, Sabbadini MG, Manfredi AA. Translational mini-review series on immunology of vascular disease: mechanisms of vascular inflammation and remodelling in systemic vasculitis. *Clin Exp Immunol.* (2009) 156:395–404. doi: 10.1111/j.1365-2249.2009.03921.x
25. Manfredi AA, Rovere-Querini P, Bottazzi B, Garlanda C, Mantovani A. Pentraxins, humoral innate immunity and tissue injury. *Curr Opin Immunol.* (2008) 20:538–44. doi: 10.1016/j.coi.2008.05.004
26. Norata GD, Marchesi P, Venu VKP, Pasqualini F, Anselmo A, Moalli F, et al. Deficiency of the long pentraxin PTX3 promotes vascular inflammation and atherosclerosis. *Circulation.* (2009) 120:699–708. doi: 10.1161/CIRCULATIONAHA.108.806547
27. Salio M, Chimenti S, De Angelis N, Molla F, Maina V, Nebuloni M, et al. Cardioprotective function of the long pentraxin PTX3 in acute myocardial infarction. *Circulation.* (2008) 117:1055–64. doi: 10.1161/CIRCULATIONAHA.107.749234
28. Lozano E, Segarra M, Corbera-Bellalta M, García-Martínez A, Espígol-Frigolé G, Plà-Campo A, et al. Increased expression of the endothelin system in arterial lesions from patients with giant-cell arteritis: association between elevated plasma endothelin levels and the development of ischaemic events. *Ann Rheum Dis.* (2010) 69:434–42. doi: 10.1136/ard.2008.105692
29. Doni A, Mantovani G, Porta C, Tuckermann J, Reichardt HM, Kleiman A, et al. Cell-specific regulation of PTX3 by glucocorticoid hormones in hematopoietic and nonhematopoietic cells. *J Biol Chem.* (2008) 283:29983–92. doi: 10.1074/jbc.M805631200
30. Hayreh SS. Ischemic optic neuropathy. *Prog Retin Eye Res.* (2009) 28:34–62. doi: 10.1016/j.preteyeres.2008.11.002
31. Roche NE, Fulbright JW, Wagner AD, Hunder GG, Goronzy JJ, Weyand CM. Correlation of interleukin-6 production and disease activity in polymyalgia rheumatica and giant cell arteritis. *Arthritis Rheumat.* (1993) 36:1286–94. doi: 10.1002/art.1780360913
32. Stone JH, Tuckwell K, Dimonaco S, Klearman M, Aringer M, Blockmans D, et al. Trial of tocilizumab in giant-cell arteritis. *N Engl J Med.* (2017) 377:317–28. doi: 10.1056/NEJMoa1613849
33. Perez-Alamino R, Maldonado-Ficco H. New insights on biomarkers in systemic vasculitis. *Curr Rheumatol Rep.* (2015) 17:12. doi: 10.1007/s11926-015-0497-0
34. Baerlecken NT, Linnemann A, Gross WL, Moosig F, Vazquez-Rodriguez TR, Gonzalez-Gay MA, et al. Association of ferritin autoantibodies with giant cell arteritis/polymyalgia rheumatica. *Ann Rheum Dis.* (2012) 71:943–7. doi: 10.1136/annrheumdis-2011-200413
35. De Smit E, Lukowski SW, Anderson L, Senabouth A, Dauyey K, Song S, et al. Longitudinal expression profiling of CD4+ and CD8+ cells in patients with active to quiescent giant cell arteritis. *BMC Med Genomics.* (2018) 11:61. doi: 10.1186/s12920-018-0376-4
36. Prieto-González S, Terrades-García N, Corbera-Bellalta M, Planas-Rigol E, Miyabe C, Alba MA, et al. Serum osteopontin: a biomarker of disease activity and predictor of relapsing course in patients with giant cell arteritis. Potential clinical usefulness in tocilizumab-treated patients. *RMD Open.* (2017) 3:e000570. doi: 10.1136/rmdopen-2017-000570
37. Savioli B, Abdulahad WH, Brouwer E, Kallenberg CG, de Souza AWS. Are cytokines and chemokines suitable biomarkers for Takayasu arteritis? *Autoimmun Rev.* (2017) 16:1071–8. doi: 10.1016/j.autrev.2017.07.023
38. Burja B, Kuret T, Sodin-Semrl S, Lakota K, Rotar Ž, Ješe R, et al. A concise review of significantly modified serological biomarkers in giant cell arteritis, as detected by different methods. *Autoimmun Rev.* (2018) 17:188–94. doi: 10.1016/j.autrev.2017.11.022
39. Arend WP, Michel BA, Bloch DA, Hunder GG, Calabrese LH, Edworthy SM, et al. The American College of Rheumatology 1990 criteria for the classification of Takayasu arteritis. *Arthritis Rheumat.* (1990) 33:1129–34. doi: 10.1002/art.1780330811
40. de Souza AWS, de Carvalho JF. Diagnostic and classification criteria of Takayasu arteritis. *J Autoimmun.* (2014) 48:79–83. doi: 10.1016/j.jaut.2014.01.012
41. Ringleb PA, Strittmatter EI, Loewer M, Hartmann M, Fiebach JB, Lichy C, et al. Cerebrovascular manifestations of Takayasu arteritis in Europe. *Rheumatology.* (2005) 44:1012–15. doi: 10.1093/rheumatology/keh664
42. Große K, Witte T, Moosig F, Hoyer BF, Lansche C, Schmidt RE, et al. Association of ferritin antibodies with Takayasu arteritis. *Clin Rheumatol.* (2014) 33:1523–6. doi: 10.1007/s10067-014-2764-2
43. Alibaz-Oner F, Yentür SP, Saruhan-Direskeneli G, Direskeneli H. Serum cytokine profiles in Takayasu's arteritis: search for biomarkers. *Clin Exp Rheumatol.* (2015) 33:32–5.

44. Noguchi S, Numano F, Gravanis MB, Wilcox JN. Increased levels of soluble forms of adhesion molecules in Takayasu arteritisl. *Int J Cardiol.* (1998) 66:S23–33. doi: 10.1016/S0167-5273(98)00145-4
45. Noris M, Daina E, Gamba S, Bonazzola S, Remuzzi G. Interleukin-6 and RANTES in Takayasu arteritis: a guide for therapeutic decisions? *Circulation.* (1999) 100:55–60. doi: 10.1161/01.CIR.100.1.55
46. Sun Y, Ma L, Yan F, Liu H, Ding Y, Hou J, et al. MMP-9 and IL-6 are potential biomarkers for disease activity in Takayasu's arteritis. *Int J Cardiol.* (2012) 156:236–8. doi: 10.1016/j.ijcard.2012.01.035
47. Pulsatelli L, Boiardi L, Assirelli E, Pazzola G, Muratore F, Addimanda O, et al. Interleukin-6 and soluble interleukin-6 receptor are elevated in large-vessel vasculitis: a cross-sectional and longitudinal study. *Clin Exp Rheumatol.* (2017) 35:102–10.
48. Sun Y, Huang Q, Jiang L. Radiology and biomarkers in assessing disease activity in Takayasu arteritis. *Int J Rheum Dis.* (2019) 22:53–9. doi: 10.1111/1756-185X.13286
49. Ishihara T, Haraguchi G, Tezuka D, Kamiishi T, Inagaki H, Isobe M. Diagnosis and assessment of Takayasu arteritis by multiple biomarkers. *Circul J.* (2013) 77:477–83. doi: 10.1253/circj.CJ-12-0131
50. Mahajan N, Dhawan V, Malik S, Jain S. Serum levels of soluble receptor for advanced glycation end products (sRAGE) in Takayasu's arteritis. *Int J Cardiol.* (2010) 145:589–91. doi: 10.1016/j.ijcard.2010.05.075
51. Neeper M, Schmidt AM, Brett J, Yan SD, Wang F, Pan YC, et al. Cloning and expression of a cell surface receptor for advanced glycosylation end products of proteins. *J Biol Chem.* (1992) 267:14998–5004.
52. Dagna L, Salvo F, Tiraboschi M, Bozzolo EP, Franchini S, Doglioni C, et al. Pentraxin-3 as a marker of disease activity in Takayasu arteritis. *Ann Intern Med.* (2011) 155:425–33. doi: 10.7326/0003-4819-155-7-201110040-00005
53. Ishihara T, Haraguchi G, Kamiishi T, Tezuka D, Inagaki H, Isobe M. Sensitive assessment of activity of Takayasu's arteritis by pentraxin3, a new biomarker. *J Am Coll Cardiol.* (2011) 57:1712–13. doi: 10.1016/j.jacc.2010.10.058
54. Park JH. Conventional and CT angiographic diagnosis of Takayasu arteritis. *Int J Cardiol.* (1996) 54:S16571. doi: 10.1016/S0167-5273(96)88785-7
55. Tombetti E, Di Chio MC, Sartorelli S, Papa M, Salerno A, Bottazzi B, et al. Systemic pentraxin-3 levels reflect vascular enhancement and progression in Takayasu arteritis. *Arthritis Res Ther.* (2014) 16:479. doi: 10.1186/s13075-014-0479-z
56. Jain A, Kumar D, Guleria A, Misra DP, Zanwar A, Chaurasia S, et al. NMR-based serum metabolomics of patients with Takayasu arteritis: relationship with disease activity. *J Proteome Res.* (2018) 17:3317–24. doi: 10.1021/acs.jproteome.8b00456
57. Haroon E, Felger JC, Jung JM, Wommack EC, Woolwine BJ, Chen X, Hu XP, et al. Increased inflammation is associated with increased glutamate in the basal ganglia of depressed patients. *Brain Behav Immun.* (2015) 49:e24. doi: 10.1016/j.bbi.2015.06.100
58. Haroon E, Miller AH, Sanacora G. Inflammation, glutamate, and glia: a trio of trouble in mood disorders. *Neuropsychopharmacology.* (2017) 42:193–215. doi: 10.1038/npp.2016.199
59. Yilmaz H, Gerdan V, Kozaci D, Solmaz D, Akar S, Can G, et al. Ghrelin and adipokines as circulating markers of disease activity in patients with Takayasu arteritis. *Arthritis Res Ther.* (2012) 14:R272. doi: 10.1186/ar4120
60. Dixit VD, Schaffer EM, Pyle RS, Collins GD, Sakthivel SK, Palaniappan R, et al. Ghrelin inhibits leptin- and activation-induced proinflammatory cytokine expression by human monocytes and T cells. *J Clin Invest.* (2004) 114:57–66. doi: 10.1172/JCI21134
61. Serra R, Grande R, Buffone G, Scarcello E, Tripodi F, Rende P, et al. Effects of glucocorticoids and tumor necrosis factor-alpha inhibitors on both clinical and molecular parameters in patients with Takayasu arteritis. *J Pharmacol Pharmacother.* (2014) 5:193. doi: 10.4103/0976-500X.136101
62. Ramos-Mozo P, Madrigal-Matute J, Vega de Ceniga M, Blanco-Colio LM, Meilhac O, Feldman L, et al. Increased plasma levels of NGAL, a marker of neutrophil activation, in patients with abdominal aortic aneurysm. *Atherosclerosis.* (2012) 220:552–6. doi: 10.1016/j.atherosclerosis.2011.11.023
63. Park M, Park Y, Jung SY, Lee KH, Lee S. Anti-endothelial cell antibodies and antiphospholipid antibodies in Takayasu's arteritis: correlations of their titers and isotype distributions with disease activity. *Clin Exp Rheumatol.* (2006) 24:S10–16.
64. Tripathy NK, Sinha N, Nityanand S. Anti-annexin V antibodies in Takayasu's arteritis: prevalence and relationship with disease activity. *Clin Exp Immunol.* (2003) 134:360–4. doi: 10.1046/j.1365-2249.2003.02282.x
65. Manolov V, Petrova I, Vasilev V. VEGF levels in diagnosis of vasculitic neuropathy. *Clin Lab.* (2014) 60:1573–7. doi: 10.7754/Clin.Lab.2013.130622
66. Takeuchi S, Kimura S, Soma Y, Waki M, Yamaguchi M, Nakazawa D,et al. Lysosomal-associated membrane protein-2 plays an important role in the pathogenesis of primary cutaneous vasculitis. *Rheumatology.* (2013) 52:1592–8. doi: 10.1093/rheumatology/ket159
67. Eriksson P, Sandell C, Backteman K, Ernerudh J. B cell abnormalities in Wegener's granulomatosis and microscopic polyangiitis: role of CD25+-expressing B cells. *J Rheumatol.* (2010) 37:2086–95. doi: 10.3899/jrheum.100074
68. Matsuda J, Saitoh N, Gohchi K, Gotoh M, Tsukamoto AM. Anti-annexin V antibody in systemic lupus erythematosus patients with lupus anticoagulant and/or anticardiolipin antibody. *Am J Hematol.* (1994) 47:56–8. doi: 10.1002/ajh.2830470112
69. Kaburaki J, Kuwana M, Yamamoto M, Kawai S, Ikeda Y. Clinical significance of anti-annexin V antibodies in patients with systemic lupus erythematosus. *Am J Hematol.* (1997) 54:209–13.
70. Nojima J, Kuratsune H, Suehisa E, Futsukaichi Y, Yamanishi H, Machii T, et al. Association between the prevalence of antibodies to β2-glycoprotein I, prothrombin, protein C, protein S, and annexin V in patients with systemic lupus erythematosus and thrombotic and thrombocytopenic complications. *Clin Chem.* (2001) 47:1008–15.
71. Satoh A, Suzuki K, Takayama E, Kojima K, Hidaka T, Kawakami M, et al. Detection of anti-annexin IV and V antibodies in patients with antiphospholipid syndrome and systemic lupus erythematosus. *J Rheumatol.* (1999) 26:1715–20.
72. Rodríguez-García MI, Fernández JA, Rodríguez A, Fernández MP, Gutierrez C, Torre-Alonso JC. Annexin V autoantibodies in rheumatoid arthritis. *Ann Rheum Dis.* (1996) 55:895–900. doi: 10.1136/ard.55.12.895
73. Sugiura K, Muro Y. Anti-annexin V antibodies and digital ischemia in patients with scleroderma. *J Rheumatol.* (1999) 26:2168–72.
74. Dogan S, Piskin O, Solmaz D, Akar S, Gulcu A, Yuksel F, et al. Markers of endothelial damage and repair in Takayasu arteritis: are they associated with disease activity? *Rheumatol Int.* (2014) 34:1129–38. doi: 10.1007/s00296-013-2937-3
75. Blake DR, Winyard P, Scott DG, Brailsford S, Blann A, Lunec J. Endothelial cell cytotoxicity in inflammatory vascular diseases–the possible role of oxidised lipoproteins. *Ann Rheum Dis.* (1985) 44:176–82. doi: 10.1136/ard.44.3.176
76. Brogan PA, Shah V, Brachet C, Harnden A, Mant D, Klein N, et al. Endothelial and platelet microparticles in vasculitis of the young. *Arthritis Rheumat.* (2004) 50:927–36. doi: 10.1002/art.20199
77. Goel R, Nair A, Kabeerdoss J, Mohan H, Jeyaseelan V, Joseph G, et al. Study of serial serum myeloid-related protein 8/14 as a sensitive biomarker in Takayasu arteritis: a single centre study. *Rheumatol Int.* (2018) 38:623–30. doi: 10.1007/s00296-017-3881-4
78. Renauer P, Sawalha AH. The genetics of Takayasu arteritis. *La Presse Méd.* (2017) 46:e179–87. doi: 10.1016/j.lpm.2016.11.031
79. Nair AM, Goel R, Hindhumati M, Jayakanthan K, Visalakshi J, Joseph G, et al. Serum amyloid A as a marker of disease activity and treatment response in Takayasu arteritis. *Rheumatol Int.* (2017) 37:1643–9. doi: 10.1007/s00296-017-3786-2
80. Jennette JC, Falk RJ, Andrassy K, Bacon PA, Churg J, Gross WL, et al. Nomenclature of systemic vasculitides. *Arthritis Rheumat.* (1994) 37:187–92. doi: 10.1002/art.1780370206
81. Navon Elkan P, Pierce SB, Segel R, Walsh T, Barash J, Padeh S, et al. Mutant adenosine deaminase 2 in a polyarteritis nodosa vasculopathy. *N Engl J Med.* (2014) 370:921–31. doi: 10.1056/NEJMoa1307362
82. Shimojima Y, Ishii W, Kishida D, Fukushima K, Ikeda S. Imbalanced expression of dysfunctional regulatory T cells and T-helper cells relates to immunopathogenesis in polyarteritis nodosa. *Modern Rheumatol.* (2017) 27:102–9. doi: 10.3109/14397595.2016.1172999
83. Okano T, Takeuchi S, Soma Y, Suzuki K, Tsukita S, Ishizu A, et al. Presence of anti-phosphatidylserine-prothrombin complex antibodies and anti-moesin

antibodies in patients with polyarteritis nodosa. *J Dermatol.* (2017) 44:18–22. doi: 10.1111/1346-8138.13491
84. Harper L, Morgan MD, Walsh M, Hoglund P, Westman K, Flossmann O, et al. Pulse versus daily oral cyclophosphamide for induction of remission in ANCA-associated vasculitis: long-term follow-up. *Ann Rheum Dis.* (2012) 71:955–60. doi: 10.1136/annrheumdis-2011-200477
85. Pagnoux C, Hogan SL, Chin H, Jennette JC, Falk RJ, Guillevin L, et al. Predictors of treatment resistance and relapse in antineutrophil cytoplasmic antibody-associated small-vessel vasculitis: comparison of two independent cohorts. *Arthritis Rheumat.* (2008) 58:2908–18. doi: 10.1002/art.23800
86. Pierrot-Deseilligny Despujol C, Pouchot J, Pagnoux C, Coste J, Guillevin L. Predictors at diagnosis of a first Wegener's granulomatosis relapse after obtaining complete remission. *Rheumatology.* (2010) 49:2181–90. doi: 10.1093/rheumatology/keq244
87. McKinney EF, Lyons PA, Carr EJ, Hollis JL, Jayne DR, Willcocks LC, et al. A CD8+ T cell transcription signature predicts prognosis in autoimmune disease. *Nat Med.* (2010) 16:586. doi: 10.1038/nm.2130
88. Lally L, Spiera R. Current therapies for ANCA-associated vasculitis. *Ann Rev Med.* (2015) 66:227–40. doi: 10.1146/annurev-med-011514-023051
89. Morley M, Molony CM, Weber TM, Devlin JL, Ewens KG, Spielman RS, et al. Genetic analysis of genome-wide variation in human gene expression. *Nature.* (2004) 430:743–7. doi: 10.1038/nature02797
90. Vezys V, Yates A, Casey KA, Lanier G, Ahmed R, Antia R, et al. Memory CD8 T-cell compartment grows in size with immunological experience. *Nature.* (2009) 457:196–9. doi: 10.1038/nature07486
91. Bevan MJ. Helping the CD8+ T-cell response. *Nat Rev Immunol.* (2004) 4:595–602. doi: 10.1038/nri1413
92. Williams MA, Bevan MJ. Effector and memory CTL differentiation. *Ann Rev Immunol.* (2007) 25:171–92. doi: 10.1146/annurev.immunol.25.022106.141548
93. Hou S, Hyland L, Ryan KW, Portner A, Doherty PC. Virus-specific CD8 + T-cell memory determined by clonal burst size. *Nature.* (1994) 369:652–4. doi: 10.1038/369652a0
94. Moon J-S, Ahn SS, Park Y-B, Lee S-K, Lee S-W. C-Reactive protein to serum albumin ratio is an independent predictor of all-cause mortality in patients with ANCA-associated vasculitis. *Yonsei Med J.* (2018) 59:865–71. doi: 10.3349/ymj.2018.59.7.865
95. Rhodes B, Fürnrohr BG, Vyse TJ. C-reactive protein in rheumatology: biology and genetics. *Nat Rev Rheumatol.* (2011) 7:282–9. doi: 10.1038/nrrheum.2011.37
96. Watanabe H, Sada K-E, Matsumoto Y, Harigai M, Amano K, Dobashi H, et al. Association between reappearance of myeloperoxidase-antineutrophil cytoplasmic antibody and relapse in antineutrophil cytoplasmic antibody-associated vasculitis: subgroup analysis of nationwide prospective cohort studies. Arthritis Rheumatol. (2018) 70:1626–33. doi: 10.1002/art.40538
97. Yoo J, Ahn SS, Jung SM, Song JJ, Park Y-B, Lee S-W. Delta neutrophil index is associated with vasculitis activity and risk of relapse in ANCA-associated vasculitis. *Yonsei Med J.* (2018) 59:397–405. doi: 10.3349/ymj.2018.59.3.397
98. Nakazawa D, Tomaru U, Suzuki A, Masuda S, Hasegawa R, Kobayashi T, et al. Abnormal conformation and impaired degradation of propylthiouracil-induced neutrophil extracellular traps: implications of disordered neutrophil extracellular traps in a rat model of myeloperoxidase antineutrophil cytoplasmic antibody-associated vasculitis. *Arthritis Rheumat.* (2012) 64:3779–87. doi: 10.1002/art.34619
99. Schreiber A, Kettritz R. The neutrophil in antineutrophil cytoplasmic autoantibody-associated vasculitis. *J Leukoc Biol.* (2013) 94:623–31. doi: 10.1189/jlb.1012525
100. Kettritz R. How anti-neutrophil cytoplasmic autoantibodies activate neutrophils. *Clin Exp Immunol.* (2012) 169:220–8. doi: 10.1111/j.1365-2249.2012.04615.x
101. Ooi JD, Chang J, Hickey MJ, Borza D-B, Fugger L, Holdsworth SR, et al. The immunodominant myeloperoxidase T-cell epitope induces local cell-mediated injury in antimyeloperoxidase glomerulonephritis. *PNAS.* (2012) 109:E2615–24. doi: 10.1073/pnas.1210147109
102. Furuta S, Jayne DRW. Antineutrophil cytoplasm antibody-associated vasculitis: recent developments. *Kidney Int.* (2013) 84:244–9. doi: 10.1038/ki.2013.24
103. Xiao H, Dairaghi DJ, Powers JP, Ertl LS, Baumgart T, Wang Y, Seitz LC, et al. C5a receptor (CD88) blockade protects against MPO-ANCA GN. *JASN.* (2014) 25:225–31. doi: 10.1681/ASN.2013020143
104. Charles Jennette J, Xiao H, Hu P. Complement in ANCA-associated vasculitis. *Semin Nephrol.* (2013) 33:557–64. doi: 10.1016/j.semnephrol.2013.08.006
105. Brew K, Nagase H. The tissue inhibitors of metalloproteinases (TIMPs): an ancient family with structural and functional diversity. *Biochim Biophys Acta.* (2010) 1803:55–71. doi: 10.1016/j.bbamcr.2010.01.003
106. Graham CH, Lala PK. Mechanism of control of trophoblast invasion *in situ*. *J Cell Physiol.* (1991) 148:228–34. doi: 10.1002/jcp.1041480207
107. Nothnick WB, Soloway P, Curry TE. Assessment of the Role of tissue inhibitor of metalloproteinase-1 (TIMP-1) during the periovulatory period in female mice lacking a functional TIMP-1 gene. *Biol Reprod.* (1997) 56:1181–8. doi: 10.1095/biolreprod56.5.1181
108. Ishizaki J, Takemori A, Suemori K, Matsumoto T, Akita Y, Sada K, et al. Targeted proteomics reveals promising biomarkers of disease activity and organ involvement in antineutrophil cytoplasmic antibody-associated vasculitis. *Arthritis Res Ther.* (2017) 19:218. doi: 10.1186/s13075-017-1429-3
109. Ciavatta DJ, Yang J, Preston GA, Badhwar AK, Xiao H, Hewins P, et al. Epigenetic basis for aberrant upregulation of autoantigen genes in humans with ANCA vasculitis. *J Clin Investig.* (2010) 120:3209–19. doi: 10.1172/JCI40034
110. Jones BE, Yang J, Muthigi A, Hogan SL, Hu Y, Starmer J, et al. Gene-specific DNA methylation changes predict remission in patients with ANCA-associated vasculitis. *J Am Soc Nephrol.* (2017) 28:1175–87. doi: 10.1681/ASN.2016050548
111. Yang J, Ge H, Poulton CJ, Hogan SL, Hu Y, Jones BE, et al. Histone modification signature at myeloperoxidase and proteinase 3 in patients with anti-neutrophil cytoplasmic autoantibody-associated vasculitis. *Clin Epigenet.* (2016) 8:85. doi: 10.1186/s13148-016-0251-0
112. Berti A, Warner R, Johnson K, Cornec D, Schroeder D, Kabat B, et al. Circulating cytokine profiles and antineutrophil cytoplasmic antibody specificity in patients with antineutrophil cytoplasmic antibody-associated vasculitis. *Arthritis Rheumatol.* (2018) 70:1114–21. doi: 10.1002/art.40471
113. Pepper RJ, Draibe JB, Caplin B, Fervenza FC, Hoffman GS, Kallenberg CGM, et al. Association of serum calprotectin (S100A8/A9) level with disease relapse in proteinase 3-antineutrophil cytoplasmic antibody-associated vasculitis. *Arthritis Rheumatol.* (2017) 69:185–93. doi: 10.1002/art.39814
114. Simon A, Subra J-F, Guilpain P, Jeannin P, Pignon P, Blanchard S, et al. Detection of anti-pentraxin-3 autoantibodies in ANCA-associated vasculitis. *PLoS ONE.* (2016) 11:e0147091. doi: 10.1371/journal.pone.0147091
115. Gilligan HM, Bredy B, Brady HR, Hébert M-J, Slayter HS, Xu Y, et al. Antineutrophil cytoplasmic autoantibodies interact with primary granule constituents on the surface of apoptotic neutrophils in the absence of neutrophil priming. *J Exp Med.* (1996) 184:2231–42. doi: 10.1084/jem.184.6.2231
116. Harper L, Cockwell P, Adu D, Savage COS. Neutrophil priming and apoptosis in anti-neutrophil cytoplasmic autoantibody-associated vasculitis1. *Kidney Int.* (2001) 59:1729–38. doi: 10.1046/j.1523-1755.2001.0590051729.x
117. Mueller A, Holl-Ulrich K, Lamprecht P, Gross WL. Germinal centre-like structures in Wegener's granuloma: the morphological basis for autoimmunity? *Rheumatology.* (2008) 47:1111–3. doi: 10.1093/rheumatology/ken202
118. Soukiasian SH, Foster CS, Niles JL, Raizman MB. Diagnostic value of anti-neutrophil cytoplasmic antibodies in scleritis associated with Wegener's granulomatosis. *Ophthalmology.* (1992) 99:125–32. doi: 10.1016/S0161-6420(92)32027-5
119. Cattaneo L, Chierici E, Pavone L, Grasselli C, Manganelli P, Buzio C, et al. Peripheral neuropathy in Wegener's granulomatosis, Churg-Strauss syndrome and microscopic polyangiitis. *J Neurol Neurosurg Psychiatry.* (2007) 78:1119–23. doi: 10.1136/jnnp.2006.111013
120. de Groot K, Schmidt DK, Arlt AC, Gross WL, Reinhold-Keller E. Standardized neurologic evaluations of 128 patients

with Wegener granulomatosis. *Arch Neurol.* (2001) 58:1215–21. doi: 10.1001/archneur.58.8.1215

121. Suppiah R, Hadden RD, Batra R, Arden NK, Collins MP, Guillevin L, et al. Peripheral neuropathy in ANCA-associated vasculitis: outcomes from the European Vasculitis Study Group trials. *Rheumatology.* (2011) 50:2214–22. doi: 10.1093/rheumatology/ker266
122. Falk RJ, Jennette JC. ANCA small-vessel vasculitis. *J Am Soc Nephrol.* (1997) 8:314–22.
123. Hagen EC, Daha MR, Hermans J, Andrassy K, Csernok E, Gaskin G, et al. Diagnostic value of standardized assays for anti-neutrophil cytoplasmic antibodies in idiopathic systemic vasculitis. EC/BCR Project for ANCA Assay Standardization. *Kidney Int.* (1998) 53:743–53. doi: 10.1046/j.1523-1755.1998.00807.x
124. Savige J, Pollock W, Trevisin M. What do antineutrophil cytoplasmic antibodies (ANCA) tell us? *Best Pract Res Clin Rheumatol.* (2005) 19:263–76. doi: 10.1016/j.berh.2004.10.003
125. Monach PA, Kümpers P, Lukasz A, Tomasson G, Specks U, Stone JH, et al. Circulating angiopoietin-2 as a biomarker in ANCA-associated vasculitis. *PLoS ONE.* (2012) 7:e30197. doi: 10.1371/journal.pone.0030197
126. Monach PA, Tomasson G, Specks U, Stone JH, Cuthbertson D, Krischer J, et al. Circulating markers of vascular injury and angiogenesis in antineutrophil cytoplasmic antibody-associated vasculitis. *Arthritis Rheumat.* (2011) 63:3988–97. doi: 10.1002/art.30615
127. Monach PA, Warner RL, Tomasson G, Specks U, Stone JH, Ding L, et al. Serum proteins reflecting inflammation, injury and repair as biomarkers of disease activity in ANCA-associated vasculitis. *Ann Rheum Dis.* (2013) 72:1342–50. doi: 10.1136/annrheumdis-2012-201981
128. Henes FO, Chen Y, Bley TA, Fabel M, Both M, Herrmann K, et al. Correlation of serum level of high mobility group box 1 with the burden of granulomatous inflammation in granulomatosis with polyangiitis (Wegener's). *Ann Rheum Dis.* (2011) 70:1926–9. doi: 10.1136/ard.2010.146456
129. Cartin-Ceba R, Golbin JM, Keogh KA, Peikert T, Sánchez-Menéndez M, Ytterberg SR, et al. Rituximab for remission induction and maintenance in refractory granulomatosis with polyangiitis (Wegener's): ten-year experience at a single center. *Arthritis Rheumat.* (2012) 64:3770–8. doi: 10.1002/art.34584
130. Saito R, Watanabe H, Asano T, Suzuki E, Iwadate H, Kobayashi H, et al. Anti-carbonic anhydrase III autoantibodies in vasculitis syndrome. *Int J Rheumat Dis.* (2013) 16:339–46. doi: 10.1111/1756-185X.12089
131. Cabiscol E, Levine RL. The phosphatase activity of carbonic anhydrase III is reversibly regulated by glutathiolation. *PNAS.* (1996) 93:4170–4. doi: 10.1073/pnas.93.9.4170
132. Räisänen SR, Lehenkari P, Tasanen M, Rahkila P, Härkönen PL, Väänänen HK. Carbonic anhydrase III protects cells from hydrogen peroxide-induced apoptosis. *The FASEB J.* (1999) 13:513–22. doi: 10.1096/fasebj.13.3.513
133. Moosig F, Bremer JP, Hellmich B, Holle JU, Holl-Ulrich K, Laudien M, et al. A vasculitis centre based management strategy leads to improved outcome in eosinophilic granulomatosis and polyangiitis (Churg-Strauss, EGPA): monocentric experiences in 150 patients. *Ann Rheumat Dis.* (2013) 72:1011–17. doi: 10.1136/annrheumdis-2012-201531
134. Schleimer RP, Bochner BS. The effects of glucocorticoids on human eosinophils. *J Allergy Clin Immunol.* (1994) 94:1202–13. doi: 10.1016/0091-6749(94)90333-6
135. Dallos T, Heiland GR, Strehl J, Karonitsch T, Gross WL, Moosig F, et al. CCL17/thymus and activation-related chemokine in Churg-Strauss syndrome. *Arthritis Rheumat.* (2010) 62:3496–503. doi: 10.1002/art.27678
136. Polzer K, Karonitsch T, Neumann T, Eger G, Haberler C, Soleiman A, et al. Eotaxin-3 is involved in Churg-Strauss syndrome-a serum marker closely correlating with disease activity. *Rheumatology.* (2008) 47:804–8. doi: 10.1093/rheumatology/ken033
137. Vaglio A, Strehl JD, Manger B, Maritati F, Alberici F, Beyer C, et al. IgG4 immune response in Churg-Strauss syndrome. *Ann Rheumat Dis.* (2012) 71:390–3. doi: 10.1136/ard.2011.155382
138. Zwerina J, Bach C, Martorana D, Jatzwauk M, Hegasy G, Moosig F, et al. Eotaxin-3 in Churg-Strauss syndrome: a clinical and immunogenetic study. *Rheumatology.* (2011) 50:1823–7. doi: 10.1093/rheumatology/keq445
139. Cornec D, Cornec-Le Gall E, Fervenza FC, Specks U. ANCA-associated vasculitis-clinical utility of using ANCA specificity to classify patients. *Nat Rev Rheumatol.* (2016) 12:570. doi: 10.1038/nrrheum.2016.123
140. Ferri C, Mascia MT. Cryoglobulinemic vasculitis. *Curr Opin Rheumatol.* (2006) 18:54–63.
141. Ferri C. Mixed cryoglobulinemia. *Orphanet J Rare Dis.* (2008) 3:25. doi: 10.1186/1750-1172-3-25
142. Knight GB, Gao L, Gragnani L, Elfahal MM, De Rosa FG, Gordon FD, et al. Detection of WA B cells in hepatitis C virus infection: a potential prognostic marker for cryoglobulinemic vasculitis and B cell malignancies. *Arthritis Rheumat.* (2010) 62:2152–9. doi: 10.1002/art.27490
143. Antonelli A, Ferri C, Ferrari SM, Ghiri E, Marchi S, Colaci M, et al. High interleukin-6 and tumor necrosis factor-alpha serum levels in hepatitis C infection associated or not with mixed cryoglobulinemia. *Clin Rheumatol.* (2009) 28:1179–85. doi: 10.1007/s10067-009-1218-8
144. Antonelli A, Ferri C, Fallahi P, Ferrari SM, Sebastiani M, Ferrari D, et al. High values of CXCL10 serum levels in mixed cryoglobulinemia associated with hepatitis C infection. *Am J Gastroenterol.* (2008) 103:2488. doi: 10.1111/j.1572-0241.2008.02040.x
145. Apolinario A, Majano PL, Lorente R, Núñez O, Clemente G, García-Monzón C. Gene expression profile of T-cell-specific chemokines in human hepatocyte-derived cells: evidence for a synergistic inducer effect of cytokines and hepatitis C virus proteins. *J Viral Hepatitis.* (2005) 12:27–37. doi: 10.1111/j.1365-2893.2005.00540.x
146. Garzoni L, Vanoni F, Rizzi M, Simonetti GD, Simonetti BG, Ramelli GP, et al. Nervous system dysfunction in Henoch-Schönlein syndrome: systematic review of the literature. *Rheumatology.* (2009) 48:1524–9. doi: 10.1093/rheumatology/kep282
147. Saulsbury FT. Clinical update: Henoch-Schönlein purpura. *Lancet.* (2007) 369:976–8. doi: 10.1016/S0140-6736(07)60474-7
148. Purevdorj N, Mu Y, Gu Y, Zheng F, Wang R, Yu J, et al. Clinical significance of the serum biomarker index detection in children with Henoch-Schonlein purpura. *Clin Biochem.* (2018) 52:167–70. doi: 10.1016/j.clinbiochem.2017.11.006
149. Hu HW, Duan J, Zhao B, Xiong JJ, Liu M, Cui JJ, et al. Significance of detection of biomarker fecal bile acids in the diagnosis and treatment of childhood Henoch-Schönlein purpura. *Zhongguo Dang Dai Er Ke Za Zhi.* (2016) 18:517–21.
150. Akman-Demir G, Serdaroglu P, Taşçi B, Group* N-BS. Clinical patterns of neurological involvement in Behçet's disease: evaluation of 200 patients. *Brain.* (1999) 122:2171–82. doi: 10.1093/brain/122.11.2171
151. Serdaroglu P. Behçet's disease and the nervous system. *J Neurol.* (1998) 245:197–205. doi: 10.1007/s004150050205
152. Siva A, Saip S. The spectrum of nervous system involvement in Behçet's syndrome and its differential diagnosis. *J Neurol.* (2009) 256:513. doi: 10.1007/s00415-009-0145-6
153. Al-Araji A, Kidd DP. Neuro-Behçet's disease: epidemiology, clinical characteristics, and management. *Lancet Neurol.* (2009) 8:192–204. doi: 10.1016/S1474-4422(09)70015-8
154. Gül A. Genetics of Behçet's disease: lessons learned from genomewide association studies. *Curr Opin Rheumatol.* (2014) 26:56–63. doi: 10.1097/BOR.0000000000000003
155. Ahn JK, Kim J, Hwang J, Song J, Kim KH, Cha H-S. Urinary metabolomic profiling to identify potential biomarkers for the diagnosis of Behcet's disease by gas chromatography/time-of-flight- mass spectrometry. *Int J Mol Sci.* (2017) 18:2309. doi: 10.3390/ijms18112309
156. Ahn JK, Kim J, Hwang J, Song J, Kim KH, Cha H-S. Potential metabolomic biomarkers for reliable diagnosis of Behcet's disease using gas chromatography/time-of-flight-mass spectrometry. *Joint Bone Spine.* (2018) 85:337–43. doi: 10.1016/j.jbspin.2017.05.019
157. Khan E, Ambrose NL, Ahnström J, Kiprianos AP, Stanford MR, Eleftheriou D, et al. A low balance between microparticles expressing tissue factor pathway inhibitor and tissue factor is associated with thrombosis in Behçet's Syndrome. *Sci Rep.* (2016) 6:38104. doi: 10.1038/srep38104
158. Yoshioka T, Kurokawa MS, Sato T, Nagai K, Iizuka N, Arito M, et al. Protein profiles of peripheral blood mononuclear cells as a candidate biomarker for Behçet's disease. *Clin Exp Rheumatol.* (2014) 32:S9–19.

159. Rifas L, Weitzmann MN. A novel T cell cytokine, secreted osteoclastogenic factor of activated T cells, induces osteoclast formation in a RANKL-independent manner. *Arthritis Rheumat.* (2009) 60:3324–35. doi: 10.1002/art.24877

160. Sota J, Vitale A, Rigante D, Orlando I, Lucherini OM, Simpatico A, et al. Correlation of serum amyloid-a levels, clinical manifestations, treatment, and disease activity in patients with Behçet's disease. *Israel Med Assoc J.* (2018) 20:517–21.

161. Vitale A, Rigante D, Lopalco G, Selmi C, Galeazzi M, Iannone F, et al. Interleukin-1 inhibition in Behçet's disease. *Isr Med Assoc J.* (2016) 18:171–6.

162. Lopalco G, Lucherini OM, Vitale A, Talarico R, Lopalco A, Galeazzi M, et al. Putative role of serum amyloid-A and proinflammatory cytokines as biomarkers for Behcet's disease. *Medicine.* (2015) 94:e1858. doi: 10.1097/MD.0000000000001858

163. Cheng Y, Zhao X, Chen Y, Li Y, Jia R, Zhu L, et al. Circulating immune complexome analysis identified anti-tubulin-α-1c as an inflammation associated autoantibody with promising diagnostic value for Behcet's disease. *PloS ONE.* (2018) 13:e0199047. doi: 10.1371/journal.pone.0199047

164. Jiang Y, Zang M, Li S. Serum PLR and LMR in Behçet's disease: can they show the disease activity? *Medicine.* (2017) 96:e6981. doi: 10.1097/MD.0000000000006981

19

Non-Motor Symptoms as Predictors of Quality of Life in Egyptian Patients with Parkinson's Disease: A Cross-Sectional Study Using a Culturally Adapted 39-Item Parkinson's Disease Questionnaire

Ali S. Shalash[1], Eman Hamid[1], Hanan Hani Elrassas[2], Ahmed Safwat Bedair[1], Abdelrahman Ibrahim Abushouk[3], Mohamed Khamis[1], Mostafa Hashim[2], Nahed Salah-Eldin Ahmed[1], Samia Ashour[1] and Mahmoud Elbalkimy[1]*

[1] Department of Neurology, Faculty of Medicine, Ain Shams University, Cairo, Egypt, [2] Faculty of Medicine, Okasha Institute of Psychiatry, Ain Shams University, Cairo, Egypt, [3] Faculty of Medicine, Ain Shams University, Cairo, Egypt

***Correspondence:**
Ali S. Shalash
ali_neuro@yahoo.com,
drali_shalash@med.asu.edu.eg

Objective: The prevalence of non-motor symptoms (NMSs) and their impact on health-related quality of life (HRQoL) in Parkinson's disease (PD) has been reported inconsistently among different populations. In this study, we aimed to investigate the NMSs and HRQoL profiles and their correlation in Egyptian PD patients, using a culturally adapted Arabic version of the 39-item Parkinson's disease questionnaire (PDQ-39).

Methods: Ninety-seven PD patients were rated using the unified Parkinson's disease rating scale (UPDRS), the non-motor symptoms scales (NMSS), Beck depression inventory (BDI), and the Arabic version of PDQ-39. We used the Spearman's rank correlation and multiple linear regression analyses to evaluate the relationship between NMSs domains and HRQoL dimensions.

Results: Fatigue/sleep (91.3%) and mood/cognitive disturbances (87%) were the most frequently and severely affected NMSS domains. Other common NMSs included urinary (75.9%), memory/attention (72.4%), gastrointestinal (67.8%), and cardiovascular problems (64.8%). The total NMSS scores were positively correlated with UPDRS I, II, and III scores. Depression was prevalent in 76.7% of PD patients. Moreover, all enrolled PD patients reported impairment in different HRQoL dimensions, especially mobility (98.9%), activities of daily living (97.8%), and emotional well-being (95.5%). The summary index of PDQ-39 was correlated to the total NMSS, UPDRS-I, UPDRS-II Off, UPDRS-III (Off and On states), and BDI scores.

Abbreviations: ADL, activities of daily living; BDI, Beck depression inventory; HRQoL, health-related quality of life; H&Y, Hoehn and Yahr scale; NMSs, non-motor symptoms; NMSS, non-motor symptoms scale; PD, Parkinson's disease; PDQ-SI, Parkinson's disease questionnaire-summary index; S&E, Schwab and England scale; UPDRS, unified Parkinson's disease rating scale.

Conclusion: This study showed the high prevalence of NMSs and the value of NMSS and BDI scores as predictors of HRQoL in Egyptian PD patients. Therefore, characterizing the NMSs profile is essential for tailoring management strategies for PD patients.

Keywords: 39-item Parkinson's disease questionnaire, Arabic, Egypt, non-motor, Parkinson's disease, quality of life

INTRODUCTION

Parkinson's disease (PD) is the second most common neurodegenerative disorder worldwide, caused by degeneration of dopaminergic neurons in the substantia nigra, and affects approximately 1–3% of the elderly population (≥60 years) (1). Health-related quality of life (HRQoL) is a multidimensional, self-reported measure of the disease impact on the patients' lives. Improving the HRQoL is the aim of care in chronic diseases, especially PD in which HRQoL is determined by motor, non-motor symptoms (NMSs), and other social factors (2).

The NMSs consist of autonomic dysfunction, sensory symptoms, neuropsychiatric disturbances, sleep problems, fatigue, and gastrointestinal (GIT) disorders. Their impact on HRQoL was reported to be greater than the motor symptoms of PD (3). However, the prevalence of NMSs and their influence on HRQoL in PD patients had been shown to vary among different countries and cultures (4–8). For example, constipation and cognitive deficit were highly prevalent in Asian (especially Chinese) patients (8), compared with Western countries. Moreover, another study showed that bodily discomfort and stigma were the most impaired HRQoL domains among Chinese PD patients, in contrast to other populations (9). These differences could be attributed to several demographic, genetic, and clinical variations in PD patients (10). Moreover, different NMS profiles were identified, resulting in the proposal of NMS subtypes of PD (11). Therefore, identifying the prevalent NMS subtype in various settings will help to personalize the management of PD patients (12).

Despite the high prevalence and genetic variability of PD in Egyptian and Arab populations (13–15), only few studies investigated the NMSs profile in Egyptian PD patients and none—to the best of our knowledge—explored their value as predictors of HRQoL (16, 17). The prevalence of PD among the Egyptian population is the highest compared with other Arabic countries, which may be due to genetic or environmental factors (14, 18). Providing a culturally adapted Arabic version of the 39-item Parkinson's disease questionnaire (PDQ-39) would facilitate epidemiological studies and improve patients' care.

Therefore, this study aimed to explore the NMS and HRQoL profiles and their correlations in Egyptian PD patients. Furthermore, it provides a culturally adapted Arabic version of the PDQ-39 scale.

MATERIALS AND METHODS

Patients

Ninety-seven patients diagnosed with idiopathic PD were recruited from the movement disorders outpatient clinic at Ain Shams University Hospitals (Cairo, Egypt) between 2013 and 2017. The recruited patients were diagnosed according to the British Parkinson's disease Society Brain Bank criteria (19). Patients with atypical or secondary Parkinsonism and those with other comorbid chronic diseases that could affect PD NMSs and/or HRQoL were excluded. Moreover, PD patients who refused or could not complete questionnaires, e.g., due to severe cognitive impairment or being on antidepressants were excluded. The Ethical Committee at the Faculty of Medicine, Ain Shams University approved the study protocol. All subjects gave written informed consent according to the Declaration of Helsinki (1975, as revised in 2008).

Outcome Measurement

All subjects were evaluated using the unified Parkinson's disease rating scale (UPDRS), Hoehn and Yahr scale (H&Y), and Schwab and England scale (S&E) in medication "off" and "on" states by a movement disorders expert. Different UPDRS subscales were estimated, including cognition (UPDRS-I), activities of daily living (ADL, UPDRS-II), motor (UPDRS-III), and total UPDRS scores. Moreover, depression was assessed using the Beck depression inventory (BDI) (20).

The NMSs were assessed in all patients, using the non-motor symptoms scale (NMSS) (21), which consists of 30 items, grouped in nine domains [cardiovascular (CVS), sleep/fatigue, mood/cognition, perception/hallucinations, memory/attention, GIT, urinary, sexual, and miscellaneous symptoms]. The frequency of each NMS (item) was calculated (item score ≥ 1), and the summary index for each domain was estimated (the sum of included items divided by the maximum possible score then multiplied by 100) to allow crude comparisons between the severity of different domains.

The HRQoL of PD patients was measured using a culturally adapted Arabic version of the Parkinson's disease questionnaire (PDQ-39) (22), which is formed of 39 items (ranged from 0 = never to 4 = always) that are grouped into eight dimensions. These dimensions include mobility (1–10, 10 items), ADL (11–16, 6 items), emotional well-being (17–22, 6 items), stigma (23–26, 4 items), social support (27–29, 3 items), cognition (30–33, 4 items), communication (34–36, 3 items), and bodily discomfort (37–39, 3 items). Following answering the questionnaire, a summary index for each dimension (subscales) was calculated by dividing the sum of included items by the maximum possible score then multiplying by 100. Then, the total score [PDQ-39 summary index (PDQ-39 SI)] was calculated by summation of the eight dimensions' scores divided by 8. Consequently, lower scores reflect better HRQoL (23). The frequency of impairment of each dimension to any degree (score > 0) was also estimated.

PDQ-39 Cultural (Same Language) Adaptation

After a written agreement from the scale provider (Isis outcomes), the Arabic version of PDQ-39 (Tunisia) was culturally adapted and changed to an Egyptian version to avoid some words that were not familiar with the Egyptian culture. According to the standard methodology (24), two Egyptian native speakers reviewed the Tunisian Arabic version and identified terms that were unfamiliar separately. The comments of the two reviewers were revised by a third Egyptian individual to confirm their acceptability and cultural relevance. Finally, back-translation of revised items from the Egyptian Arabic version to English was performed to ensure accuracy, followed by a cognitive debriefing with 10 Egyptian patients to confirm that the new version is well understood.

Statistical Analyses

Statistical analyses were performed using the SPSS (version 23 for windows). Categorical data, such as the frequency of NMSs, were described using frequencies and percentages, while continuous data were expressed as mean and standard deviation (SD) values. The comparison between two independent variables was made using the independent *t*-test, while the Spearman's rank correlation coefficient was used to evaluate the association between PDQ-39 dimensions, NMSS domains, and other variables. Moreover, we used the multiple linear regression analysis to determine the predictors of PDQ-SI. The level of statistical significance (*p*-value) was set at 0.05.

RESULTS

Clinical and Demographic Characteristics of PD Patients

Ninety-seven PD [58 males (59.8%) and 39 females (40.2%)] patients were enrolled in this cross-sectional study (mean age at enrollment: 55.3 ± 10.8 years and mean age of disease onset: 50.1 ± 11.2 years). The mean disease staging in the Off state (H&Y Off scale) was 2.8 ± 1.1 (stage 1: 6.4%; 1.5: 12.8%; 2: 13.8%, 2.5: 11.7; 3: 34%; 4: 12.8%; 5: 8.5%), while the mean motor severity in the Off state (UPDRS III Off) was 38.04 ± 19.37. The prevalence of depression was 76.7% in the enrolled cohort (**Table 1**). Females had younger age at study enrollment ($p = 0.007$) and at disease onset ($p = 0.004$), as well as worse S&E Off scores ($p = 0.01$); however, males and females had comparable disease duration, staging, and UPDRS scores.

TABLE 1 | Demographic and clinical motor characteristics of PD patients.

	Mean (SD)	Range
Number	97	
Gender		
Male, *n* (%)	58 (59.8)	
Female, *n* (%)	39 (40.2)	
Age (years)	55.3 (10.8)	23–77
Duration of illness (years)	5.3 (4.1)	0.3–20
Age of onset (years)	50.1 (11.2)	20–70
H&Y off	2.78 (1.1)	1–5
H&Y On	1.00 (0.8)	0–3
S&E Off	56.0 (22)	10–90
S&E On	86.38 (13.9)	40–100
UPDRS I	3.83 (2.87)	0–12
UPDRS II off	17.88 (10.8)	0–44
UPDRS II on	7.38 (8.1)	0–41
UPDRS III off	38.04 (19.4)	4–86
UPDRS III on	15.93 (14.0)	0–92
BDI	17.5 (8.7)	

Data presented are the mean ± SD and range unless otherwise indicated.
BDI, Beck depression inventory; H&Y, Hoehn and Yahr scale; S&E, Schwab and England scale; UPDRS, unified Parkinson's disease rating scale; PD, Parkinson's disease.

NMSs Prevalence and Correlations

All patients (100%) suffered from one or more NMSs. The most common and severely affected domains were sleep/fatigue (91.3%), mood/cognition (87%), miscellaneous symptoms (78.2%), urinary symptoms (75.9%), and memory/attention impairment (72.4%) (**Table 2**). Fatigue was the most frequent NMS (81.8%), followed by mood symptoms (sadness 75%, nervousness 69.6%, and lack of motivation 68.5%), forgetfulness (65.5%), and urinary symptoms (nocturia and urgency 58.6%) (**Figure 1**). No gender differences were detected except that females had worse miscellaneous domain scores ($p = 0.018$, females experienced more pain and sweating) and higher BDI scores ($p = 0.012$).

The total NMSS score was significantly correlated with S&E Off, UPDRS I, UPDRS II (Off & On), UPDRS III (Off & On), and BDI scores, but not with age, duration of the disease, or H&Y staging ($r = 0.204$, $p = 0.06$). Most of NMSs domains (except sexual and urinary domains) were correlated with UPDRS-I and II Off scores (Table A in Supplementary Material).

TABLE 2 | Non-motor and HRQoL characteristics of enrolled PD patients.

	Mean (SD)	Frequency (%)
Non-motor		
NMSS total	61 (42.9)	100
Cardiovascular	2.7 (3.9)	64.8
Sleep/fatigue	10.98 (8.7)	91.3
Mood	18.2 (16.2)	87
Perceptual problems	1.4 (3)	37
Attention/memory	6.1 (6.8)	72.4
Gastrointestinal	5.4 (6.98)	67.8
Urinary	7.3 (9.5)	75.9
Sexual function	3.4 (5.96)	43.5
Miscellaneous	6.7 (6.7)	78.2
HRQoL		
PDQ-39 SI	37.5 (18.6)	100
Mobility	46.8 (29.92)	98.9
ADL	44.4 (28.1)	97.8
Emotional well-being	45.1 (30.1)	95.5
Stigma	50 (31.7)	86.4
Social support	18.3 (24.6)	56.8
Cognition	27.05 (20.94)	88.6
Communication	26.6 (25.2)	73.9
Bodily discomfort	40.15 (24.9)	94.3

Data presented are mean ± SD.
HRQoL, health-related quality of life; NMSS, non-motor symptoms scale; PDQ-39 SI, Parkinson's disease questionnaire-summary index; ADL, activities of daily living; PD, Parkinson's disease.

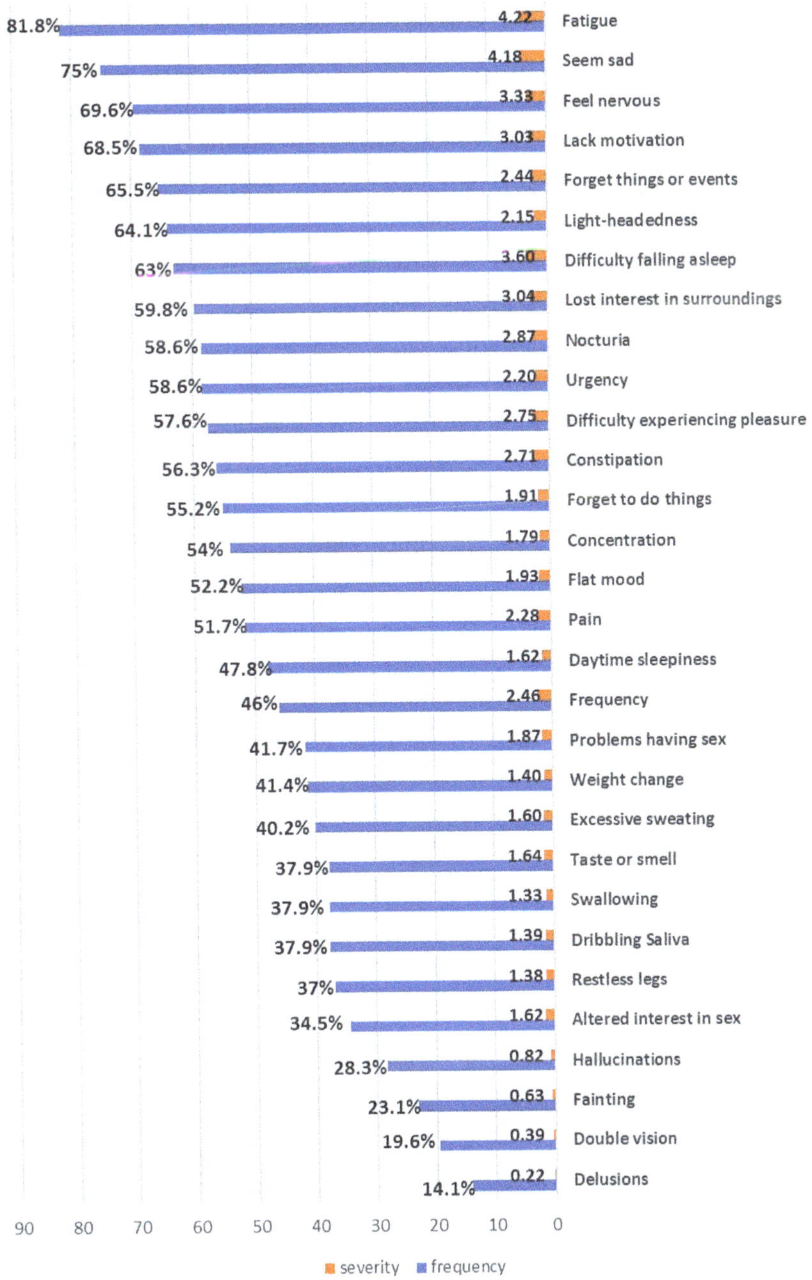

FIGURE 1 | The frequency and severity of individual non-motor symptoms in the enrolled Parkinson's disease patients.

Quality of Life State and Correlations

All enrolled PD patients had impaired HRQoL with comparable values (scores between 40 and 50) and frequency (88.6–98.9%) in most dimensions, except for social support, cognition, and communication (had lower scores, indicating better HRQoL aspects) (**Table 2**). About 86% of PD patients felt stigmatized to some degree, while 56.8% of the cohort reported incomplete social support. Females showed significantly more impaired (higher values) PDQ-SI, mobility, ADL, and bodily discomfort scores ($p = 0.016$, 0.001, 0.003, and 0.047, respectively).

The PDQ-SI score was inversely correlated with the patients' age at enrollment ($r = -0.220$, $p = 0.04$), age of disease onset ($r = -0.272$, $p = 0.01$) and S&E daily activity scores (Off & On scores) ($r = -0.483$ and -0.361, $p < 0.01$, and 0.01, respectively) (Table B in Supplementary Material). This means that younger age at enrollment or disease onset and less independence in daily activity were associated with more impaired HRQoL. In addition, the PDQ-SI was positively correlated with female gender, H&Y (Off and On) disease stage ($r = 0.318$ and 0.298, $p = 0.003$ and 0.006, respectively), UPDRS-I and UPDRS-II Off ($p < 0.001$),

UPDRS-III (Off and On) scores (**Table 3**). Thus, HRQoL impairment was associated with more impaired cognition, daily activity, and "Off and On" motor features. The disease duration did not correlate with PDQ-SI; however, it was correlated with ADL and Stigma dimensions ($r = 0.226, 0.229$; $p = 0.030, 0.036$, respectively).

Moreover, PDQ-SI was strongly correlated to the total and most of NMS subscales' scores (except CVS and sexual domains) and BDI score ($p < 0.001$). The total NMSS score was strongly correlated to PDQ-39 dimensions ($p < 0.001$), except social support. Likewise, most of the PDQ-39 dimensions had a significant correlation with most of NMSS domains, except social support (**Table 4**). In summary, the more severe and frequent NMSs are, the more impaired HRQoL becomes in PD patients.

Multiple linear regression analysis was performed to determine the predictors of the PDQ-SI from different variables including age at enrollment and disease onset, gender, disease duration, UPDDRS I, II, III, BDI, H&Y, S&E, and total NMSS scores. Depression (BDI) and the total NMSS score explained 50.5% of the PDQ-SI. Depression was the primary predictor

TABLE 3 | Correlations between quality of life domains and disease stage, patient disability and UPDRS subscores.

		PDQ-39 SI	Mobility	ADL	Emotional well-being	Stigma	Social support	Cognition	Bodily discomfort	Communication
H&Y off	*r*	0.318	0.281	0.438	0.153	0.168	0.051	0.151	0.118	0.449
	p	0.003	0.008	<0.001	0.160	0.121	0.638	0.165	0.279	<0.001
H&Y On	*r*	0.298	0.291	0.340	0.230	0.096	−0.138	0.249	0.098	0.380
	p	0.006	0.006	0.001	0.034	0.383	0.209	0.022	0.372	<0.001
S&E On	*r*	−0.361	−0.414	−0.402	−0.269	−0.167	−0.001	−0.208	−0.130	−0.305
	p	0.001	<0.001	<0.001	0.013	0.127	0.992	0.057	0.237	0.005
S&E Off	*r*	−0.438	−0.433	−0.463	−0.294	−0.285	−0.099	−0.252	−0.214	−0.375
	p	<0.001	<0.001	<0.001	0.006	0.007	0.364	0.018	0.047	<0.001
UPDRS I	*r*	0.599	0.514	0.495	0.612	0.338	0.234	0.459	0.377	0.452
	p	<0.001	<0.001	<0.001	<0.001	0.002	0.032	<0.001	<0.001	<0.001
UPDRS II off	*r*	0.548	0.539	0.552	0.467	0.335	0.122	0.270	0.410	0.390
	p	<0.001	<0.001	<0.001	<0.001	0.003	0.282	0.016	<0.001	<0.001
UPDRS II on	*r*	0.217	0.209	0.178	0.189	0.085	0.048	0.180	0.108	0.302
	p	0.057	0.061	0.112	0.098	0.457	0.675	0.115	0.348	0.007
UPDRS III off	*r*	0.384	0.415	0.426	0.280	0.208	0.004	0.169	0.217	0.375
	p	<0.001	<0.001	<0.001	0.011	0.061	0.971	0.129	0.051	0.001
UPDRS III on	*r*	0.283	0.276	0.275	0.202	0.076	0.042	0.276	0.079	0.364
	p	0.010	0.010	0.010	0.067	0.492	0.703	0.012	0.478	0.001

Data presented are p values and correlation coefficients (r).
H&Y, Hoehn and Yahr scale; S&E, Schwab and England scale; UPDRS, unified Parkinson's disease rating scale; ADL, activities of daily living.

TABLE 4 | Correlations between NMSs and quality of life domains.

		Mobility	ADL	Emotional well-being	Stigma	Social support	Cognition	Communication	Bodily discomfort	PDQ-39 SI
CVS	*r*	0.221	0.150	0.237	0.079	0.027	0.242	0.197	0.154	0.198
	p	0.039	0.163	0.030	0.475	0.807	0.026	0.072	0.161	0.071
Sleep and fatigue	*r*	0.643	0.548	0.563	0.389	0.148	0.508	0.559	0.415	0.659
	p	<0.001	<0.001	<0.001	<0.001	0.176	<0.001	<0.001	<0.001	<0.001
Mood and cognition	*r*	0.518	0.444	0.742	0.423	0.182	0.501	0.471	0.531	0.681
	p	<0.001	<0.001	<0.001	<0.001	0.096	<0.001	<0.001	<0.001	<0.001
Perception	*r*	0.202	0.164	0.348	0.013	0.007	0.382	0.234	0.412	0.263
	p	0.058	0.125	0.001	0.905	0.953	<0.001	0.031	<0.001	0.015
Memory	*r*	0.289	0.303	0.378	0.137	0.242	0.669	0.404	0.174	0.421
	p	0.008	0.005	0.001	0.223	0.029	<0.001	<0.001	0.120	<0.001
GIT	*r*	0.455	0.343	0.433	0.148	0.049	0.474	0.415	0.466	0.452
	p	<0.001	0.001	<0.001	0.188	0.666	<0.001	<0.001	<0.001	<0.001
Urinary	*r*	0.333	0.359	0.383	0.182	0.099	0.308	0.335	0.340	0.414
	p	0.002	0.001	<0.001	0.104	0.380	0.005	0.002	0.002	<0.001
Sexual	*r*	0.060	0.164	0.217	0.035	0.154	0.261	0.201	0.053	0.151
	p	0.593	0.140	0.054	0.760	0.176	0.020	0.076	0.643	0.184
Total	*r*	0.625	0.573	0.697	0.400	0.160	0.613	0.594	0.526	0.723
	p	<0.001	<0.001	<0.001	<0.001	0.155	<0.001	<0.001	<0.001	<0.001
BDI	*r*	0.671	0.578	0.745	0.524	0.309	0.569	0.574	0.387	0.765
	p	<0.001	<0.001	<0.001	<0.001	0.005	<0.001	<0.001	<0.001	<0.001

Data presented are p values and correlation coefficients (r).
ADL, activities of daily living; BDI, Beck depression inventory; CVS, cardiovascular; GIT, gastrointestinal; PDQ-SI, Parkinson's disease questionnaire-summary index; NMSs, non-motor symptoms.

(adjusted R^2 0.497, $p < 0.0001$). On removing BDI score from the model, the total NMSS score and UPDRS-I (cognition) were the independent predictors of HRQoL and explained 53.7% of patients' HRQoL. The total NMSS score was the primary predictor (adjusted R^2: 0.480, $p < 0.0001$).

DISCUSSION

This study explored the non-motor and HRQoL profiles of PD patients in an African country with a high prevalence of PD. It confirmed the marked impact of NMSs and depression on HRQoL impairment. Moreover, it provides a culturally adapted Arabic version of the PDQ-39 to promote further research and care of Arabic PD patients. To the best of our knowledge, this is the first study to investigate the HRQoL and its association with NMSs in Egyptian PD patients.

Our study showed a high prevalence of NMSs in Egyptian PD patients (100%). Fatigue, mood disturbances (sadness, nervousness, and lack of motivation), and memory impairment were the most frequent NMSs. Likewise, the most severe and frequently affected domains were sleep/fatigue and mood/cognition domains. Gender differences were minimal and restricted to miscellaneous symptoms. A similar high prevalence of NMSs and frequency of NMS domains were reported in Upper Egypt by Khedr and colleagues (16). This NMS profile in the Egyptian patients is more consistent with the depression/anxiety PD subtype (11).

Previous studies have identified differences in NMS profile between different countries and races. Reports from different Asian countries identified GIT symptoms, especially constipation as the most frequent NMS (8). Nocturia was the most frequent NMS, followed by fatigue and dribbling of saliva in a multicenter European study (3). Cognition, sleep followed by urinary symptoms were the most common NMS in an Estonian cohort (25), while fatigue followed by urinary symptoms were more common in the Spanish population (26). These differences could be attributed to several demographic, genetic, and clinical variations in enrolled patients (age, the age of onset, disease duration, and severity), as well as different assessment questionnaires (10, 12).

The different dimensions of HRQoL were impaired in all patients and markedly correlated to NMSS total score and depression severity. Moreover, it was associated with motor severity, disease staging, and impaired daily activity in Off and On states. However, regression analysis confirmed the independent predicting effect of NMSs for HRQoL. This is consistent with the findings of former studies in different populations in which the total NMSS score was the main predictor of QoL. Mood/cognition and sleep/fatigue had the strongest correlation with PDQ-SI in accordance with prior studies (3, 7, 27).

Neuropsychiatric symptoms, especially depression, were reported as independent determinants of HRQoL (28). In consistence with previous studies (25, 26, 29), depression was recognized as the main independent predictor of HRQoL. This could be explained by the high prevalence of depression (76.7%) and the strong correlation between depression and all HRQoL dimensions, several NMS domains and total NMSS scores. Consequently, depression affects HRQoL directly and indirectly through its impact on the NMSs, especially emotional well-being and cognition (28). In agreement with several previous studies, depression was recognized as the main predictor of poor HRQoL in PD patients (29, 30). Antonini et al. reported improvement in mobility and ADL after depression treatment, indicating that mood problems affect how PD patients perceive their motor functions (31).

Intriguingly, 86.4% of PD patients felt stigmatized, while 56.8% of the cohort reported incomplete social support. Stigma was associated with younger age of enrollment, younger age of disease onset, disease severity, impaired daily activities and cognition, as well as depression. This is consistent with prior studies (32, 33). Furthermore, it was correlated with fatigue/memory, mood/cognition domains, and total NMSS scores. Stigma is an important determinant of HRQoL, related to cultural and social factors (32, 34). Consequently, the identification and management of this feature are crucial for the improvement of HRQoL of PD patients.

Although this study provides a comprehensive assessment of the impact of different NMS domains on HRQoL for the first time in Egyptian patients, it has some limitations. The relatively small sample size and the fact that the majority of enrolled patients came from a low socioeconomic class restrict the generalizability of our findings. Moreover, as a clinic-based study [plus the relatively short disease duration (5.3 years)], patients with advanced stages and cognitive impairment were under-represented. Furthermore, some NMSs are prevalent in the elderly population without PD; therefore, a case–control study would elucidate whether the investigated NMSs are PD related.

In conclusion, this study demonstrated the high prevalence of NMSs in Egyptian PD patients and the significant impact of NMSs and depression on HRQoL. Thus, the assessment and management of NMSs are as important as the motor aspects of PD. Future larger studies can use our culturally adapted questionnaire to evaluate the correlation between NMSs domains and HRQoL dimensions in patients with advanced PD.

AUTHOR CONTRIBUTIONS

All authors made substantial contributions, revised the manuscript, and approved the final version. AS, HE, SA, and ME: con ception and design of the study. AS, AB, MH, MK, and EH: data collection and analysis. AS, AB, AA, and HE: first draft writing All authors: revision of the manuscript.

ACKNOWLEDGMENTS

We thank Ms Enas Shalash, MSc in written and simultaneous translation, for her help in the cultural adaptation of the PDQ-39.

REFERENCES

1. Hirsch L, Jette N, Frolkis A, Steeves T, Pringsheim T. The incidence of Parkinson's disease: a systematic review and meta-analysis. *Neuroepidemiology* (2016) 46:292–300. doi:10.1159/000445751
2. Martinez-Martin P. What is quality of life and how do we measure it? Relevance to Parkinson's disease and movement disorders. *Mov Disord* (2017) 32:382–92. doi:10.1002/mds.26885
3. Martinez-Martin P, Rodriguez-Blazquez C, Kurtis MM, Chaudhuri KR. The impact of non-motor symptoms on health-related quality of life of patients with Parkinson's disease. *Mov Disord* (2011) 26:399–406. doi:10.1002/mds.23462
4. Barone P, Antonini A, Colosimo C, Marconi R, Morgante L, Avarello TP, et al. The PRIAMO study: a multicenter assessment of nonmotor symptoms and their impact on quality of life in Parkinson's disease. *Mov Disord* (2009) 24:1641–9. doi:10.1002/mds.22643
5. Dotchin CL, Jusabani A, Walker RW. Non-motor symptoms in a prevalent population with Parkinson's disease in Tanzania. *Parkinsonism Relat Disord* (2009) 15:457–60. doi:10.1016/j.parkreldis.2008.11.013
6. Leonardi M, Raggi A, Pagani M, Carella F, Soliveri P, Albanese A, et al. Relationships between disability, quality of life and prevalence of nonmotor symptoms in Parkinson's disease. *Parkinsonism Relat Disord* (2012) 18:35–9. doi:10.1016/j.parkreldis.2011.08.011
7. Song W, Guo X, Chen K, Chen X, Cao B, Wei Q, et al. The impact of non-motor symptoms on the health-related quality of life of Parkinson's disease patients from Southwest China. *Parkinsonism Relat Disord* (2014) 20:149–52. doi:10.1016/j.parkreldis.2013.10.005
8. Yu RL, Wu RM, Chan AY, Mok V, Wu YR, Tilley BC, et al. Cross-cultural differences of the non-motor symptoms studied by the traditional Chinese version of the International Parkinson and Movement Disorder Society-Unified Parkinson's Disease Rating Scale. *Mov Disord Clin Pract* (2017) 4:68–77. doi:10.1002/mdc3.12349
9. Zhao YJ, Tan LC, Lau PN, Au WL, Li SC, Luo N. Factors affecting health-related quality of life amongst Asian patients with Parkinson's disease. *Eur J Neurol* (2008) 15:737–42. doi:10.1111/j.1468-1331.2008.02178.x
10. Konno T, Al-Shaikh RH, Deutschlander AB, Uitti RJ. Biomarkers of nonmotor symptoms in Parkinson's disease. *Int Rev Neurobiol* (2017) 133:259–89. doi:10.1016/bs.irn.2017.05.020
11. Sauerbier A, Jenner P, Todorova A, Chaudhuri KR. Non motor subtypes and Parkinson's disease. *Parkinsonism Relat Disord* (2016) 22(Suppl 1):S41–6. doi:10.1016/j.parkreldis.2015.09.027
12. Titova N, Chaudhuri KR. Personalized medicine and nonmotor symptoms in Parkinson's disease. *Int Rev Neurobiol* (2017) 134:1257–81. doi:10.1016/bs.irn.2017.05.015
13. Al-Kurdi AA, Mubaidin AM, Bohlega S. Problems of Parkinson's disease in the Arab world. *Neurosciences (Riyadh)* (2001) 6:188–91.
14. Lesage S, Dürr A, Tazir M, Lohmann E, Leutenegger A-L, Janin S, et al. LRRK2 G2019S as a cause of Parkinson's disease in North African Arabs. *N Engl J Med* (2006) 354:422–3. doi:10.1056/NEJMc055540
15. Benamer HT, De Silva R, Siddiqui KA, Grosset DG. Parkinson's disease in Arabs: a systematic review. *Mov Disord* (2008) 23:1205–10. doi:10.1002/mds.22041
16. Khedr EM, El Fetoh NA, Khalifa H, Ahmed MA, El Beh KM. Prevalence of non motor features in a cohort of Parkinson's disease patients. *Clin Neurol Neurosurg* (2013) 115:673–7. doi:10.1016/j.clineuro.2012.07.032
17. Khedr EM, Fawi G, Abbas MA, Mohammed TA, El-Fetoh NA, Attar GA, et al. Prevalence of parkinsonism and Parkinson's disease in Qena governorate/Egypt: a cross-sectional community-based survey. *Neurol Res* (2015) 37:607–18. doi:10.1179/1743132815Y.0000000020
18. Ahmed H, Abushouk AI, Gabr M, Negida A, Abdel-Daim MM. Parkinson's disease and pesticides: a meta-analysis of disease connection and genetic alterations. *Biomed Pharmacother* (2017) 90:638–49. doi:10.1016/j.biopha.2017.03.100
19. Hughes AJ, Daniel SE, Kilford L, Lees AJ. Accuracy of clinical diagnosis of idiopathic Parkinson's disease: a clinico-pathological study of 100 cases. *J Neurol Neurosurg Psychiatry* (1992) 55:181–4. doi:10.1136/jnnp.55.3.181
20. Beck AT, Ward CH, Mendelson M, Mock J, Erbaugh J. An inventory for measuring depression. *Arch Gen Psychiatry* (1961) 4:561–71. doi:10.1001/archpsyc.1961.01710120031004
21. Chaudhuri KR, Martinez-Martin P, Brown RG, Sethi K, Stocchi F, Odin P, et al. The metric properties of a novel non-motor symptoms scale for Parkinson's disease: results from an international pilot study. *Mov Disord* (2007) 22:1901–11. doi:10.1002/mds.21596
22. Peto V, Jenkinson C, Fitzpatrick R. PDQ-39: a review of the development, validation and application of a Parkinson's disease quality of life questionnaire and its associated measures. *J Neurol* (1998) 245(Suppl 1):S10–4. doi:10.1007/PL00007730
23. Martinez-Martin P, Jeukens-Visser M, Lyons KE, Rodriguez-Blazquez C, Selai C, Siderowf A, et al. Health-related quality-of-life scales in Parkinson's disease: critique and recommendations. *Mov Disord* (2011) 26:2371–80. doi:10.1002/mds.23834
24. Wild D, Grove A, Martin M, Eremenco S, Mcelroy S, Verjee-Lorenz A, et al. Principles of Good practice for the translation and cultural adaptation process for patient-reported outcomes (PRO) measures: report of the ISPOR Task Force for Translation and Cultural Adaptation. *Value Health* (2005) 8:94–104. doi:10.1111/j.1524-4733.2005.04054.x
25. Kadastik-Eerme L, Rosenthal M, Paju T, Muldmaa M, Taba P. Health-related quality of life in Parkinson's disease: a cross-sectional study focusing on non-motor symptoms. *Health Qual Life Outcomes* (2015) 13:83. doi:10.1186/s12955-015-0281-x
26. Santos-Garcia D, de la Fuente-Fernandez R. Impact of non-motor symptoms on the quality of life of patients with Parkinson's disease: some questions beyond research findings. *J Neurol Sci* (2013) 335:239. doi:10.1016/j.jns.2013.09.019
27. Scaravilli T, Gasparoli E, Rinaldi F, Polesello G, Bracco F. Health-related quality of life and sleep disorders in Parkinson's disease. *Neurol Sci* (2003) 24:209–10. doi:10.1007/s10072-003-0134-y
28. Balestrino R, Martinez-Martin P. Neuropsychiatric symptoms, behavioural disorders, and quality of life in Parkinson's disease. *J Neurol Sci* (2017) 373:173–8. doi:10.1016/j.jns.2016.12.060
29. Gallagher DA, Lees AJ, Schrag A. What are the most important nonmotor symptoms in patients with Parkinson's disease and are we missing them? *Mov Disord* (2010) 25:2493–500. doi:10.1002/mds.23394
30. Sławek J, Derejko M, Lass P. Factors affecting the quality of life of patients with idiopathic Parkinson's disease – a crosssectional study in an outpatient clinic attendees. *Parkinsonism Relat Disord* (2005) 11:465–8. doi:10.1016/j.parkreldis.2005.04.006
31. Antonini A, Tesei S, Zecchinelli A, Barone P, De Gaspari D, Canesi M, et al. Randomized study of sertraline and low-dose amitriptyline in patients with Parkinson's disease and depression: effect on quality of life. *Mov Disord* (2006) 21:1119–22. doi:10.1002/mds.20895
32. Ma HI, Saint-Hilaire M, Thomas CA, Tickle-Degnen L. Stigma as a key determinant of health-related quality of life in Parkinson's disease. *Qual Life Res* (2016) 25:3037–45. doi:10.1007/s11136-016-1329-z
33. Tu XJ, Hwang WJ, Ma HI, Chang LH, Hsu SP. Determinants of generic and specific health-related quality of life in patients with Parkinson's disease. *PLoS One* (2017) 12:e0178896. doi:10.1371/journal.pone.0178896
34. Maffoni M, Giardini A, Pierobon A, Ferrazzoli D, Frazzitta G. Stigma experienced by Parkinson's disease patients: a descriptive review of qualitative studies. *Parkinsons Dis* (2017) 2017:7203259. doi:10.1155/2017/7203259

Permissions

All chapters in this book were first published by Frontiers; hereby published with permission under the Creative Commons Attribution License or equivalent. Every chapter published in this book has been scrutinized by our experts. Their significance has been extensively debated. The topics covered herein carry significant findings which will fuel the growth of the discipline. They may even be implemented as practical applications or may be referred to as a beginning point for another development.

The contributors of this book come from diverse backgrounds, making this book a truly international effort. This book will bring forth new frontiers with its revolutionizing research information and detailed analysis of the nascent developments around the world.

We would like to thank all the contributing authors for lending their expertise to make the book truly unique. They have played a crucial role in the development of this book. Without their invaluable contributions this book wouldn't have been possible. They have made vital efforts to compile up to date information on the varied aspects of this subject to make this book a valuable addition to the collection of many professionals and students.

This book was conceptualized with the vision of imparting up-to-date information and advanced data in this field. To ensure the same, a matchless editorial board was set up. Every individual on the board went through rigorous rounds of assessment to prove their worth. After which they invested a large part of their time researching and compiling the most relevant data for our readers.

The editorial board has been involved in producing this book since its inception. They have spent rigorous hours researching and exploring the diverse topics which have resulted in the successful publishing of this book. They have passed on their knowledge of decades through this book. To expedite this challenging task, the publisher supported the team at every step. A small team of assistant editors was also appointed to further simplify the editing procedure and attain best results for the readers.

Apart from the editorial board, the designing team has also invested a significant amount of their time in understanding the subject and creating the most relevant covers. They scrutinized every image to scout for the most suitable representation of the subject and create an appropriate cover for the book.

The publishing team has been an ardent support to the editorial, designing and production team. Their endless efforts to recruit the best for this project, has resulted in the accomplishment of this book. They are a veteran in the field of academics and their pool of knowledge is as vast as their experience in printing. Their expertise and guidance has proved useful at every step. Their uncompromising quality standards have made this book an exceptional effort. Their encouragement from time to time has been an inspiration for everyone.

The publisher and the editorial board hope that this book will prove to be a valuable piece of knowledge for researchers, students, practitioners and scholars across the globe.

List of Contributors

Pawel J. Winklewski
Department of Human Physiology, Medical University of Gdańsk, Gdańsk, Poland
Department of Clinical Anatomy and Physiology, Pomeranian University in Słupsk, Słupsk, Poland
2-nd Department of Radiology, Medical University of Gdańsk, Gdańk, Poland

Agnieszka Sabisz, Edyta Szurowska and Arkadiusz Szarmach
2-nd Department of Radiology, Medical University of Gdańsk, Gdańsk, Poland

Patrycja Naumczyk and Krzysztof Jodzio
Institute of Psychology, University of Gdańsk, Gdańsk, Poland

Bruno Stuhlmüller, Udo Schneider and Eugen Feist
Department of Rheumatology and Clinical Immunology, Charité-Universitätsmedizin, Berlin, Germany

José-B. González-González
Department of Rheumatology and Clinical Immunology, Charité-Universitätsmedizin, Berlin, Germany
Labor Berlin-Charité Vivantes GmbH, Berlin, Germany

Andreas Johnen
Section for Neuropsychology, Department of Neurology, University Hospital Münster, Münster, Germany

Maxime Bertoux
Univ Lille, Inserm UMR 1171 Degenerative and Vascular Cognitive Disorders, CHU Lille, Lille, France

Mohamed H. M. Ali and Tariq Ahmed
Neurological Disorders Research Center, Qatar Biomedical Research Institute, Hamad Bin Khalifa University, Qatar Foundation, Doha, Qatar

Fazle Rakib and Khalid Al-Saad
Department of Chemistry and Earth Sciences, Qatar University, Doha, Qatar
Diabetes Research Center, Qatar Biomedical Research Institute, Hamad Bin Khalifa University, Qatar Foundation, Doha, Qatar

Essam M. Abdelalim
Diabetes Research Center, Qatar Biomedical Research Institute, Hamad Bin Khalifa University, Qatar Foundation, Doha, Qatar
Department of Cytology and Histology, Faculty of Veterinary Medicine, Suez Canal University, Ismailia, Egypt

Andreas Limbeck
Institute of Chemical Technologies and Analytics, Vienna University of Technology, Vienna, Austria

Raghvendra Mall and Ehsan Ullah
Qatar Computing Research Institute, Hamad Bin Khalifa University, Qatar Foundation, Doha, Qatar

Nasrin Mesaeli
Weill Cornell Medicine-Qatar, Qatar Foundation, Doha, Qatar

Donald McNaughton
Centre for Biospectroscopy, School of Chemistry, Monash University, Clayton, VIC, Australia

Janik Goltermann, Ronny Redlich, Katharina Dohm, Dario Zaremba, Jonathan Repple, Dominik Grotegerd, Katharina Förster, Susanne Meinert, Verena Enneking, Emily Schlaghecken, Lara Fleischer, Tim Hahn, Udo Dannlowski and Nils Opel
Department of Psychiatry, University of Münster, Münster, Germany

Claas Kaehler
Department of Psychiatry, University of Münster, Münster, Germany
Department of Mathematics and Computer Science, University of Münster, Münster, Germany

Harald Kugel
Institute of Clinical Radiology, University of Münster, Münster, Germany

Andreas Jansen
Department of Psychiatry, University of Marburg, Marburg, Germany
Core-Facility BrainImaging, Faculty of Medicine, University of Marburg, Marburg, Germany
Center for Mind, Brain and Behavior, University of Marburg, Marburg, Germany

Axel Krug, Katharina Brosch, Igor Nenadic, Simon Schmitt, Frederike Stein, Tina Meller, Dilara Yüksel, Elena Fischer and Tilo Kircher
Department of Psychiatry, University of Marburg, Marburg, Germany
Marcella Rietschel and Stephanie H. Witt Department of Genetic Epidemiology, Central Institute of Mental Health, University of Heidelberg, Mannheim, Germany

Andreas J. Forstner
School of Medicine & University Hospital Bonn, Institute of Human Genetics, University of Bonn, Bonn, Germany
Centre for Human Genetics, University of Marburg, Marburg, Germany
Department of Biomedicine, University of Basel, Basel, Switzerland

Markus M. Nöthen
School of Medicine & University Hospital Bonn, Institute of Human Genetics, University of Bonn, Bonn, Germany

Anbupalam Thalamuthu
Centre for Healthy Brain Ageing, School of Psychiatry, University of New South Wales Sydney, Sydney, NSW, Australia

Bernhard T. Baune
Department of Psychiatry, University of Münster, Münster, Germany
Department of Psychiatry, Melbourne Medical School, The University of Melbourne, Melbourne, VIC, Australia
The Florey Institute of Neuroscience and Mental Health, The University of Melbourne, Parkville, VIC, Australia

Stefan J. Teipel
German Center for Neurodegenerative Diseases-Rostock/Greifswald, Rostock, Germany
Department of Psychosomatic Medicine, University of Rostock, Rostock, Germany

Enrica Cavedo
AXA Research Fund and Sorbonne University Chair, Paris, France
Sorbonne University, GRC n° 21, Alzheimer Precision Medicine, AP-HP, Pitié-Salpêtrière Hospital, Boulevard de l'Hôpital, Paris, France
Brain and Spine Institute (ICM), INSERM U 1127, CNRS UMR 7225, Boulevard de l'Hôpital, Paris, France
Department of Neurology, Institute of Memory and Alzheimer's Disease (IM2A), Pitié-Salpêtrière Hospital, AP-HP, Boulevard de l'Hôpital, Paris, France
IRCCS Istituto Centro San Giovanni di Dio-Fatebenefratelli, Brescia, Italy

Harald Hampel
AXA Research Fund and Sorbonne University Chair, Paris, France
Sorbonne University, GRC n° 21, Alzheimer Precision Medicine, AP-HP, Pitié-Salpêtrière Hospital, Boulevard de l'Hôpital, Paris, France
Brain and Spine Institute (ICM), INSERM U 1127, CNRS UMR 7225, Boulevard de l'Hôpital, Paris, France
Department of Neurology, Institute of Memory and Alzheimer's Disease (IM2A), Pitié-Salpêtrière Hospital, AP-HP, Boulevard de l'Hôpital, Paris, France

Michel J. Grothe
German Center for Neurodegenerative Diseases-Rostock/Greifswald, Rostock, Germany

Bendix Labeit, Sigrid Ahring, Rainer Dziewas, Paul Muhle, Sonja Suntrup-Krueger, Jens Burchard Schröder, Thomas Marian, Inga Claus, Matthias Pawlowski, Heinz Wiendl, Rainer Dziewas, Tobias Ruck and Tobias Warnecke
Department of Neurology, University Hospital Münster, Münster, Germany

Jun Chen, Wei Huang, Chao-Hui Cheng and Lan Zhou
Department of Neurology, Taihe Hospital, Hubei University of Medicine, Shiyan, China

Guang-Bin Jiang
Department of Radiology, Suizhou Central Hospital, Suizhou, China

Yuan-Yuan Hu
Department of Stomatology, Taihe Hospital, Hubei University of Medicine, Shiyan, China

Sven G. Meuth
Department of Neurology, University Hospital Münster, Münster, Germany
Department of Neurology, Institute for Translational Neurology, University of Münster, Münster, Germany

Ruth L. O'Gorman Tuura
Center for MR Research, University Children's Hospital Zurich, Zurich, Switzerland

Christian R. Baumann and Heide Baumann-Vogel
Department of Neurology, University Hospital Zurich, Zurich, Switzerland

Christian Gatz, Stephan Buchkremer, Joachim Weis and Thomas Labisch
Institute of Neuropathology, RWTH Aachen University Hospital, Aachen, Germany

Denisa Hathazi
Leibniz-Institut für Analytische Wissenschaften -ISAS-e.V., Dortmund, Germany
Department of Clinical Neuroscience, University of Cambridge, Cambridge, United Kingdom

Ute Münchberg
Leibniz-Institut für Analytische Wissenschaften—ISAS—e.V., Dortmund, Germany

Ben Munro and Rita Horvath
Department of Clinical Neuroscience, University of Cambridge, Cambridge, United Kingdom

Ana Töpf
International Centre for Life, Institute of Genetic Medicine, Newcastle upon Tyne, United Kingdom

Andreas Roos
Department of Neuropediatrics, Developmental Neurology and Social Pediatrics, Centre for Neuromuscular Disorders in Children, University Children's Hospital Essen, University of Duisburg-Essen, Essen, Germany
Leibniz-Institut für Analytische Wissenschaften -ISAS-e.V., Dortmund, Germany
Institute of Neuropathology, RWTH Aachen University Hospital, Aachen, Germany
Pediatric Neurology, Faculty of Medicine, University Childrens Hospital, University of Duisburg-Essen, Essen, Germany

Ju-Wan Kim, Hee-Ju Kang, Kyung-Yeol Bae, Sung-Wan Kim, Il-Seon Shin, Jin-Sang Yoon and Jae-Min Kim
Department of Psychiatry and Depression Clinical Research Centre, Chonnam National University Medical School, Gwangju, South Korea

Robert Stewart
Institute of Psychiatry, King's College London, London, United Kingdom

Corinna Preusse and Hans-Hilmar Goebel
Department of Neuropathology, Charité - Universitätsmedizin Berlin, Corporate Member of Freie Universität Berlin, Humboldt-Universität zu Berlin, and Berlin Institute of Health, Berlin, Germany

Werner Stenzel
Department of Neuropathology, Charité - Universitätsmedizin Berlin, Corporate Member of Freie Universität Berlin, Humboldt-Universität zu Berlin, and Berlin Institute of Health, Berlin, Germany
Leibniz Science Campus Chronic Inflammation, Berlin, Germany

Anna M. Wirth
Department of Neurology, University Hospital of Regensburg, Regensburg, Germany
Department of Experimental Psychology, University of Regensburg, Regensburg, Germany

Andrei Khomenko, Dobri Baldaranov, Ines Kobor, Ohnmar Hsam, Thomas Grimm, Siw Johannesen, Tim-Henrik Bruun, Wilhelm Schulte-Mattler and Ulrich Bogdahn
Department of Neurology, University Hospital of Regensburg, Regensburg, Germany

Mark W. Greenlee
Department of Experimental Psychology, University of Regensburg, Regensburg, Germany

Alessia Manni, Antonio Iaffaldano, Domenico Maria Mezzapesa, Vincenzo Felica, Pietro Iaffaldano, Maria Trojano and Damiano Paolicelli
Department of Basic Medical Sciences, Neurosciences and Sense Organs, University of Bari "Aldo Moro", Bari, Italy

Giuseppe Lucisano
Department of Basic Medical Sciences, Neurosciences and Sense Organs, University of Bari "Aldo Moro", Bari, Italy
Center for Outcomes Research and Clinical Epidemiology, Pescara, Italy

Mariangela D'Onghia
Operative Unit of Neurology, "Dimiccoli" General Hospital, Barletta, Italy

Angelica Maria Sabogal-Guáqueta, Javier Gustavo Villamil-Ortiz and Gloria Patricia Cardona-Gómez
Neuroscience Group of Antioquia, Cellular and Molecular Neurobiology Area - School of Medicine, Sede de Investigación Universitaria (SIU), University of Antioquia, Medellin, Colombia

Julian David Arias-Londoño
Department of Systems Engineering, University of Antioquia, Medellín, Colombia

Fatemeh N. Emamzadeh
Division of Biomedical and Life Sciences, Faculty of Health and Medicine, University of Lancaster, Lancaster, United Kingdom

Andrei Surguchov
Department of Neurology, Kansas University Medical Center, Kansas City, KS, United States

Daniel Strunk, Antje Schmidt-Pogoda, Carolin Beuker, Lennart S. Milles, Catharina Korsukewitz and Jens Minnerup
Department of Neurology, Institute for Translational Neurology, University of Münster, Münster, Germany

Ali S. Shalash, Eman Hamid, Ahmed Safwat Bedair, Mohamed Khamis, Nahed Salah-Eldin Ahmed, Samia Ashour and Mahmoud Elbalkimy
Department of Neurology, Faculty of Medicine, Ain Shams University, Cairo, Egypt

Hanan Hani Elrassas and Mostafa Hashim
Faculty of Medicine, Okasha Institute of Psychiatry, Ain Shams University, Cairo, Egypt

Abdelrahman Ibrahim Abushouk
Faculty of Medicine, Ain Shams University, Cairo, Egypt

William T. Hu
Department of Neurology, Emory University, Atlanta, GA, United States
Center for Neurodegenerative Disease, Emory University, Atlanta, GA, United States

Jennifer Christina Howell
Department of Neurology, Emory University, Atlanta, GA, United States
Alzheimer's Disease Research Center, Emory University, Atlanta, GA, United States

Index

N

O

P

R

S

T

V

Printed in the USA
CPSIA information can be obtained
at www.ICGtesting.com
LVHW080737221023
761596LV00011B/2171